P9-CFM-616

Back to Eden

A Human Interest Story of Health and Restoration
To be Found in Herb, Root, and Bark

JETHRO KLOSS

REVISED AND EXPANDED
SECOND EDITION

KLOSS FAMILY HEIRLOOM® EDITION

BACK TO EDEN BOOKS® PUBLISHING CO.
Loma Linda, California 92354
An Enterprise of The Jethro Kloss Family

COVER
Harry Anderson's painting, "Man's First Home,"
copyright® 1949 by Review and Herald
Publishing Association, is used by permission
given to the Kloss Family 15 October 1971.

PUBLISHING HISTORY
Original copyright 1939 by Jethro Kloss.
Published continuously by the Kloss Family since 1946.
Copyright © 1972, 1973, 1974, 1981, 1982, 1983, 1985, 1988, 1992, 1994, 1995
by Promise Kloss Moffett and Doris Kloss Gardiner.

Library of Congress Catalog Card Number: 88-072032

All rights reserved. No part of this book may be
reproduced or transmitted in any form or by any means,
electronic or mechanical, including photocopying,
recording or by any information storage and retrieval
system without written permission.

BACK TO EDEN® PUBLISHING CO.
P.O. Box 1439
Loma Linda, California 92354

ISBN 0-940985-10-1

Published in the United States of America.

792-100M-H

CONTENTS

A PERSONAL MESSAGE TO THE READER

If my father, Jethro Kloss, were living now, I am sure that he would still be updating, improving, and adding valuable new health information to his beloved lifelong project, *Back To Eden,* which we are now reissuing in this newly updated format.

I know he would continue to incorporate new material from the subjects in his range of interest, including herbs, natural remedies, nutrition, and healthful cooking, home health care, and the latest medical information. He was forward-looking and eager to adopt whatever was valuable, as long as it did not conflict with the basic laws of nature.

Readers and users of the original *Back To Eden* (called by some a "classic") know that Jethro Kloss was continually striving to make available a large amount of practical knowledge that would help others to achieve and maintain healthful and productive lives.

The completion of this revised edition of *Back To Eden,* therefore, would surely please Jethro Kloss. A great deal of time and effort have been expended to enhance its content, organization, factual clarity, and readability. Undoubtedly, readers will be pleased to find the new volume more convenient to use than the earlier version.

All the essential original material has been retained in this revised edition. Sections and paragraphs on the same or similar topics (scattered in various places throughout the first edition) have now been brought together and arranged in a logical order for ease and speed of reference.

Medical terms have slowly but continually changed over the years. For example, few people today know the meaning of such words as "gleet," "tetters," and similar terms used during the 1920s and 1930s when *Back To Eden* was first written. Therefore, the vocabulary has been brought up to date, even though the old names are also retained for their historical interest.

A number of vital topics (such as vitamins, minerals, proteins, etc.), which were mentioned only briefly in the early work, have been substantially expanded, and many other timely topics have been incorporated. In addition, this revised text has new illustrations and photographs, new charts, new appendix and glossaries, and a new comprehensive index.

To all those seeking improved health through natural means, this new edition of *Back To Eden* is dedicated. My sincere hope is that this revised and expanded *Back To Eden* will prove to be of even greater benefit than was the original book written by my father nearly fifty years ago.

Promise Kloss Moffett

PREFACE

It is with godly fear and much humility that I undertake the task of writing this book, as I am in no sense of the word a writer. My purpose in sending forth this book is to help humanity and give courage to those who may have thought their case hopeless. My prayer is that God may make this book a blessing to many.

I wish to present the truth in a practical manner, to help the human family, and to prevent others from becoming slaves to erroneous ideas, so that mothers and fathers may better care for their families.

This book contains inexpensive remedies for the prevention of disease and sickness; treatments that are the result of my own practical experience of nearly forty years.

Many recipes are given herein that are not found elsewhere. They are inexpensive and can be made in any home. They contain all the elements the body requires, and are very palatable when properly prepared. Millions today who have little food would be better able to keep body and soul together if they knew which foods to eat to really sustain life. In addition, I have provided much information on the uses of nonpoisonous herbs, in response to the public's need for such practical knowledge.

Actual facts about the true healing art are given in this book, as handed down by physicians beginning with Hippocrates, who was called "the father of medical literature," until 1541, when Hohenheim started the practice of using chemicals and promoted his idea that the human body could be purified chemically, as were the metals at Tyrol, where he worked after giving up his medical profession.

I wish to bring to the notice of the general public the untold blessings that our Heavenly Father has provided for all the world. It can be truly said, "My people are destroyed for lack of knowledge." Hosea 4:6. A lack of knowledge based on truth is accountable for much of the untold sufferings and miseries of humanity. The advice contained in this book, if heeded, will save money, suffering, and often premature death.

From practical experience, I explain how to be healthy, mentally and physically. No matter how many germs get into the body, if the bloodstream is clean and the blood corpuscles are in a healthy condition, you will be safe. Everyone comes in contact with many kinds of germs; but these organisms will not harm you or cause sickness and death unless they have a place in which to propagate themselves.

Many who violate the laws of health are ignorant of the relation of the laws of living (eating, drinking, and working) to their health. Until they have some kind of sickness or illness, they do not realize that their condition is caused by violating the laws of nature and health. If then they would resort to simple means and follow the basic laws of health that they have been neglecting – nature's remedies, herbs, etc. – nature would restore the body to its original health. Had the body been supplied with these remedies all along, it would always be in good condition. When a course such as is outlined above is followed, patients will generally recover without being weakened.

There is a wonderful science in nature, in trees, herbs, roots, and flowers, which man has never yet fathomed. All the science of ancient Egypt when it was in its glory, and the science of ancient Babylon when it was at its height, and the wisdom of Solomon when he lived in obedience to God, plus the science and knowledge of our present enlightened age, as taught in the colleges and universities, does not equal the science in nature; and yet that science is little understood even by the most intelligent people.

God has provided a remedy for every disease that might afflict us. Satan cannot afflict anyone with any disease for which God has not provided a remedy. Our Creator foresaw the wretched condition of mankind in these days, and made provision in Nature for all the ills of man.

If our scientists and medical colleges would put forth the same effort in finding the virtues in the "true remedies" as found in nature for the use of the human race, then poisonous drugs and chemicals would be eliminated and sickness would be rare indeed. If they would make use of only these remedies that God has given for the "service of man" it would bring an untold blessing to the world.

In these distressing days, the use of a simple natural diet would prevent much suffering and would also save money. The most important subject for people to study should be; "How can we live out our allotted time without suffering?" God has surely made this possible. *Revolutionize the common manner of living, eating, and drinking, and you will have a happier and healthier people.*

Recently a Chicago firm advertised very extensively some little tablets, claiming that they contained all the elements needed by the body, and were prepared by scientifically combining foods. But the most learned scientists who ever lived on this earth cannot separate natural foods and then combine them in a better manner than nature herself has prepared them!

The fundamental principle of true healing consists of a return to natural habits of living.

We must return to God's original plan for maintaining health, by restoring the sick, and rediscovering the miraculous truths that were covered up by commercial graft, ignorance, or neglect. Miraculous things are found in the Bible and Nature.

The Creator of this universe made man in the beginning from "the dust of the ground." The different properties that are found in the earth are found in man, and the fruits, grains, nuts, and vegetables contain the same elements that are in the soil as well as in man. When these fruits, grains, nuts, and vegetables are eaten in their natural state, instead of being perverted and robbed of their life-giving properties during preparation, human health, beauty, and happiness will be the sure reward.

The scripture that says, "My people are destroyed for lack of knowledge," is surely being fulfilled. But our loving Heavenly Father sees the world's untold suffering and wretchedness; He has made provision that if we use these things that He has provided they will surely bring relief. Read in this book about the wonderful properties that are in trees, herbs, flowers and roots, and leaves of the trees, which the Holy Book says are for our medicine. Ezekiel 47:12. There are also wonderful life-giving properties in fruit, if properly eaten and not combined with certain other foods. Improper combination of foods causes fermentation and other disturbances and thus destroys their life-giving properties.

Jethro Kloss

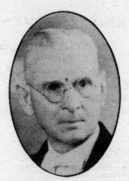

1863-1946

Who is she that goeth forth as the morning — fair
as the moon, clear as the sun, and with banner
floating above her? The true healing art.

Whence art thou? — I come from nature.

What art thou? — Herbs, water, food, pure air,
sunshine, exercise, and rest.

Where art thou going? — On the wings of the
morning to the ends of the earth.

What is thy commission? — To go to every
physician and nurse and whosoever will,
to restore many families, prevent
much suffering and premature death, and wipe
the tears from many eyes.

Speed on thy flight, thou message of health and joy.

The Author

Jethro Kloss

ACKNOWLEDGMENTS

Our warmest thanks and appreciation to Ruth H. Hoover for her collaboration in the editing and indexing of this revised manuscript. Her gentle, kind persistence enabled it to all come together. We also want to extend our thanks to Charlotte and Lee Schamadan, graphic artists, par excellence.

WARNING – DISCLAIMER

This book is intended to be read and used only as a book containing the recommendations and personal opinions and experiences of the author, Jethro Kloss. If the symptoms of any illness are persistent, or become worse, or if there is any reason whatever for believing that the services of a medical practitioner would be helpful to the patient, professional aid should be sought without delay, as recommended by the author. No responsibility is assumed on the part of the author, publishers, or distributors of this book if you choose to use the information contained herein to treat yourself or others.

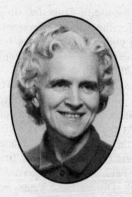

MEMOIRS OF HIS DAUGHTER

By Promise Kloss Moffett

My father was born on a large farm near Manitowoc, Wisconsin, on April 27, 1863. The ninth of eleven children born to his pioneering parents, he lived a healthy and happy life in that primitive Indian country. The stories he told us about his childhood and youth on their farm in Wisconsin, where the foundation of his knowledge and interest in natural living was laid, are well told in this book.

It was here, led by his industrious, hard-working, provident parents that Jethro Kloss first learned the value of wild and cultivated herbs, grains, nuts, fruits, and vegetables. As a child he was taught to gather from the land many kinds of leaves, barks, and berries for his parents, who prepared and used them to help ailing neighbors.

When he was about twenty, he went to Florida and worked in the orange groves, finally owning a large grove at Deland. Later he attended school in Nebraska and then in Battle Creek, Michigan. While in Battle Creek he worked closely with the then revolutionary medical leadership of the world-renowned Battle Creek Sanitarium. He saw clearly the disastrous results of the use of dangerous drugs then commonly used in caring for the sick. He developed further his own philosophy and understanding of the laws of nature; still remembering those things so deeply implanted in his mind from his early childhood.

He was married March 5, 1900 to Miss Carrie Stilson, who had trained as a Bible worker and teacher, had labored in a mission in Madison, Wisconsin, and taught several terms of grade school. At that time he was a licensed minister in Wisconsin and they established their home at Rose Lawn. Two children were born to this union, first Promise Joy and then my brother Paul, who died when only four weeks old of whooping cough. During these years, besides my father's ministerial work, my parents operated a branch of the Battle Creek Sanitarium and also sold Battle Creek Sanitarium health foods. My mother died in July 1905.

In March 1907, my father married Mrs. Amy Ponwith, a widow with a small daughter, Mabel. My father and step-mother owned and operated an attractive sanitarium in pleasant surroundings in St. Peter, Minnesota, which they named The Home Sanitarium. This was conducted much as a small hospital would be today, and included an operating room where local surgeons performed surgery while my father administered the anesthetic. He and Mrs. Kloss operated men's and women's wards as well as private rooms for the care of patients. They were well equipped for electrical treatments and hydrotherapy and were unusually successful in treating cases of nervous breakdown. Their daughter Lucile was born here in St. Peter in 1908 and their son, Eden, in 1910.

Next the Klosses became interested in the self-supporting work being conducted in the south and they visited some of the schools in North Carolina and Tennessee. About 1911 they sold the sanitarium in Minnesota and moved to Fountain Head, Tennessee, where their youngest daughter, Naomi, was born in 1913. Here they bought a 250-acre farm, built a large house and barn, and raised many kinds of fruits and vegetables. They also raised Shetland ponies for a time.

A later development in good health was his creation of a significant health food manufacturing operation in Amqui, Tennessee after receiving a request from the owners to take charge of their food factory. While he was operating this factory he would be up at two, three, or four o'clock in the morning; as early as necessary to build the fires for the steam cooker or the large oven and whatever else needed to be done to have everything in readiness for the workers to begin the day processing, canning, or baking. When that big oven was hot, he would often pop into it some special weekend treat for his family — some delicious health coffee cake or raisin buns like no one else could make, for he was an excellent baker.

Before this factory was sold to the Nashville Agricultural Normal Institute, he was shipping health foods all over the United States and Canada. It was also during this time and at this place that he originated many new health food recipes. This establishment later became a part of what has since become the well-known Madison College near Nashville, Tennessee.

Our next move was to Brooke, Virginia, where Papa established a health food factory and retail market. Each of us children was pressed into service in one way or another with this family enterprise. At times we would be helping with some food experiment, or perhaps we were typing and retyping the material that later became *Back To Eden,* which was many years in preparation. Jethro Kloss's son Eden was for many years his right-hand helper. Whatever my father did in spreading the gospel of health and natural living, he did with all his might, and he trained his children in that same pattern of living.

He was always an early riser. If some urgent work did not call him, he would be studying or writing while others were still sleeping, and many times I have overheard his earnest prayers spoken in his study corner or as he walked out-of-doors.

One of my favorite memories as a family is the daily worship hour when Father would gather his family of six about him and we would sing hymns, read Bible verses around the circle, and pray together. He was a gentle but firm family leader.

Although a strict disciplinarian, my father was warm-hearted and affectionate, devoted to his family. When he was away from home, we invariably received a letter from Papa every day. We knew he loved us and was thinking of us. When he came home, there were always the little gifts, a lovely piece of material for a dress, some choice fruit, or something else he knew we would like and enjoy.

We often read aloud to him from new books and magazines in the field of health; for his interests extended far beyond even his own vast experiments and studies. We read to him to spare his eyesight, which was not the best for reading, and he could cover more ground this way. As we read along, with pencil poised, he would now and then say, "Mark!" Then a little check mark in the margin would be his guide for further study as he checked author with author and compared with his own rich experience.

Eventually this health food factory at Brooke, Virginia was taken over by my stepsister, Mabel, and her husband.

The Klosses then moved to Washington, D.C. and Papa carried on his work of treating the sick, lecturing on health and engaged in a more intensive study of herbs and the preparation of his book, *Back To Eden*. I still have in my possession an attractive menu, with a colored picture of the Washington Monument and cherry blossoms on the cover, for a Demonstration Dinner he gave March 27, 1933, at the Dodge Hotel in Washington, D.C. The menu was completely vegetarian and included "Sweetbreads a la Kloss." The pumpkin pie and strawberry sundae were made with soy milk.

Requests poured in for his services as a lecturer and he traveled widely throughout the country, all the while refining and perfecting the manuscript for *Back To Eden;* and continuing personally to treat the sick, often taking them into his own home where they could have a proper diet and the necessary herbs and treatments.

Back To Eden was at last published in 1939, the fruition of much toil and sacrifice for many years by the entire Kloss family.

After the death of his wife, Amy Kloss, in 1944 at Fredericksburg, Virginia, he visited me in my home in Northern British Columbia. He delighted in the rich harvest of giant fruits and vegetables produced by that land of long summer daylight hours. I remember how he enjoyed picking peas from the tall vines, and how he measured the length of the huge boysenberries with his pocket ruler. How my father rejoiced in the fruits of God's green earth! And how he did relish every new and different food flavor! He loved life, and often talked of the joys and bounties of Heaven, where he was preparing to go.

In 1945 Papa became acquainted with Mr. and Mrs. Deloe Robert Hiatt on a trip to Madison, Tennessee. Together they found a property at Coalmont, Tennessee, where the Hiatts took over the promotion and publication of *Back To Eden*. Here my father continued treating the sick and teaching health principles as advocated in his book. He hoped to establish a sanitarium and health center in this beautiful area. But he had driven himself mercilessly, early and late, and now he found himself in failing health.

When I was finally called across the continent to my father in his last illness, when the candle that for so many years had been burned at both ends was almost spent, I remember how his face would light up and his eyes shine as he spoke of the Sanitarium he was going to build, where he could do a still greater work for "suffering humanity."

He did not know that his greatest work had already been accomplished, nor could he know then how many thousands of lives would be benefitted by his book, *Back To Eden*.

And so he peacefully went to sleep in June 1946, his eighty-fourth year, and today rests in a little cemetery in

Tennessee.

But the legend of Jethro Kloss, the promoter of natural health and healing, continues to grow. And as multiplied thousands continue to refer to this, his handbook of good health, his work goes on today — perhaps even stronger than in his lifetime.

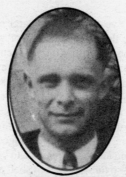

A SON'S RECOLLECTIONS

By Eden Pettis Kloss

I was born in St. Peter, Minnesota, on February 10, 1910, to Jethro and Amy Kloss. My memories of St. Peter, and of the home sanitarium my parents operated there, are few because we moved away when I was very young. But I do remember visiting St. Peter later with my mother and seeing soldiers march to the depot to go off to World War I. The band was playing, flags were flying, and people were saying their goodbyes.

After the move to Tennessee, my parents developed a plant for the manufacture of a line of vegetarian meat substitutes, cereals, crackers, and other items. It was located at Amqui, near Nashville. (Our business was called the Nashville Sanitarium Food Factory.) Many of my early memories center on that large two-story factory, where raw materials were transformed into good-tasting, healthful food products.

Up a long lane from the factory was our home, bordered on one side by a grove of persimmon trees and on the other by Papa's orderly garden. My father was an untiring worker. He would be up hours before the rest of the family — building fires, starting cracker dough, and making everything ready so that the work could go full speed ahead when the workers arrived in the morning.

I recall the massive dough mixer (large enough for several men to stand in), the dough-brakes for kneading, and the stamping machines for marking and cutting the cracker dough. Also I can still see, in my mind's eye, the huge oven with the swinging shelves on which crackers and zwieback were baked. This oven reached from the basement to the second floor. The coke fire would be stoked to just the right heat. The sheets of crackers were first shoved onto a shelf from the front door. Then a pulley arrangement would move that shelf and swing another into place to be loaded, and then another shelf, and so on. When each shelf arrived back at the starting point, the crackers would be baked exactly right and were ready to be transferred to racks for cooling, then packaging, and finally shipping.

Papa would remove many of several different kinds of crackers that happened to get broken in handling — whole wheat, bran, white, and oatmeal. These he would process with malt honey into the most delicious breakfast cereal — called Dixie Kernel. I wish I had some right now!

One way Papa expressed his loving care for his family was to include in the Friday baking a large pan of good old German coffee cake for our weekend pleasure. Also, often a steaming kettle of rice, sprinkled with raisins, would be brought out of the fireless cooker for our breakfast.

Malta syrup or honey made at our plant was one of the products that I remember especially, because of the long process necessary to prepare it. The process began with a huge tank of liquid starch, which looked like milk. This was the residue that had been washed from the flour in the preparing of gluten. This liquid starch was treated with barley malt and left to stand overnight. Then the clear liquid was siphoned into another large tank with many steam pipes on the bottom. Here, for a whole day, with close watching, this liquid was boiled down to the right syrupy consistency — a job often done by one of my sisters. When the syrup was finally ready, it was run into a copper kettle with a faucet at the bottom. From there the cans were filled, sealed, and labeled for the market.

It was here also, on tomato canning day, that I fell across and partly into a tub of hot tomatoes. That could easily have been the end of me. But my father grabbed me, held me under the cold water faucet to stop the burning, and then rushed me to the Madison Sanitarium. In spite of careful treatment, my deep burn took many painful weeks of recovery and left a scar I still carry.

As a boy I was fascinated with all of this manufacturing activity. Papa wanted us all to watch, for he expected us to learn and to take responsibility as soon as we were able. Once when one of the men needed to go to a meeting, he questioned whether or not I could take care of one of the machines that was washing flour to separate the gluten. Papa assured him that indeed I could. Sure enough, when the meeting ended, I had the gluten all properly washed.

Life wasn't all work, though. There were excitement and fun too. I'll never forget the day the big smokestack on the furnace-room blew over — just after Lucile and I had run past. We had many good times with our ponies — Fannie, Maud S., and Blackey. We would saddle and ride them, or we'd hitch one to our small buggy or two to the little wagon. Once Lucile, who was always the daring one, drove into the pasture where our stallion was kept; and when he came running, the pony turned so sharply that the wagon tipped over on Lucile. Fortunately she was not hurt.

Great carloads of coal and coke were switched onto our railroad siding and spilled out for use in the big furnace that kept all the machinery running. This same sidetrack brought carloads of empty tin cans to be sterilized, filled, sealed, packed in cases, labeled, and reloaded into the same cars, along with other packaged foods, for shipping out.

When I was nine or ten years old, the factory was sold to the private school at Madison and transferred to that campus, and our family traveled in our pickup truck, camping en route, from Tennessee to Virginia. Here, at a town named Brooke, we found an ideal location — a plot of ground with a building in which we could make and sell health foods and teach people about healthful living.

Alongside the garden spot below the house ran a little stream where luscious watercress grew in abundance. Here our father planted a fine garden that we all worked in, helping to raise many varieties of vegetables. Also he prepared hotbeds for strawberry, tomato, and other plants. and one of my jobs, when frost threatened, was to keep the fire going in the stove beneath.

I helped my father remove an old sawmill from the lower floor of the house and pour cement for a floor to hold equipment used for the manufacture of health foods. These foods were processed, canned, labeled, and hauled in a light truck to the Brooke depot for shipping to various destinations. We also cleaned out the old well, covered it, and installed pipes and pumps to provide running water for the house and the basement factory. My father, it seemed to me, could do anything!

The mixer, sealer, and other equipment were run by a gasoline engine. Also we had a buzz saw for cutting wood for the furnace and cook-stove. Papa hauled in discarded ties from the railroad near our place, and my sister Naomi and I would saw them into stove and furnace lengths with the crosscut saw.

Not far from the old building, where we lived and had our factory, Papa built a lecture hall where he could give lectures and food demonstrations. We also had a store where we sold both health foods and fresh produce. Papa baked bread for home use and for sale in our store. His whole wheat cinnamon rolls were a special treat for our family.

On a hill across the road from us was a beautiful little Methodist church, where Father was invited to teach a Sunday school class. Mother often played the organ for services there and also at another church not far away.

It was here at Brooke, Virginia, that Papa started to put in uncounted hours working on the beginnings of his book, *Back To Eden*.

After some years, my oldest sister and her husband took over the food factory, and my parents moved to Takoma Park (on the outskirts of Washington, D.C.). Here Papa could spend more time working on his favorite project, *Back To Eden,* giving lectures from time to time, and helping someone on a one-to-one basis to understand the important principles of healthful living.

Papa's travels to give lectures and food demonstrations took him to places like Miami, Florida, and Houston, Texas. My younger sister and I went with him and helped. He took along some of his products (cough syrup and liniment), which I would sell for him, and herb preparations for various ailments.

My father was a very fine Christian man. And of course he wanted his family members to exemplify to other people the benefits of healthful living. Like many fathers, he enjoyed bringing home surprises for his children. Sometimes these were pets of different kinds, which he then taught us to take care of and be responsible for. We knew he loved his family and wanted us to be happy. And we knew he was also dedicated to his work of helping people maintain, or regain, their health through intelligent use of natural means.

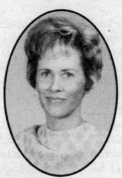

MY REMARKABLE GRANDFATHER

By Doris Kloss Gardiner

My first memories of Grandpa are of his winsome smile, his cheeriness, and his playfulness. His nicknames for me delighted me. One was Bluebird — doubtless because my mother usually dressed me in her favorite color, blue. And the other was Sunbeam. I'm not sure what the second name signified. Of course I'd like to believe it had to do with my personal qualities, but the thought hasn't escaped me that he might have been encouraging me to accentuate the positive.

One thing about which Grandpa was utterly faithful was going outside every morning, summer and winter (weather permitting), to do a certain number of "jumping jack" exercises. Afterward he came to the kitchen for a glass of fresh orange or grapefruit juice, which he drank precisely one-half hour before breakfast. Drinking that juice was a hard-and-fast rule in the Kloss household — one that I follow to this day. Another rule that was equally firm was that never, under any circumstance, did we eat between meals. I never saw Grandpa break this rule.

Today, even this far removed from childhood, one recollection still makes me cringe — my grandparents' insistence on a cold-water rubdown as soon as one tumbled out of bed in the morning. Afterward, Grandma would rub me briskly with a thick, rough cotton towel. This rite of the morning is guaranteed to give a running start to anyone's day.

Wherever he and Grandma lived, Grandpa always built shelves to cover one wall of his room. There he arranged his innumerable boxes, his bags of herbs, and his formulations, in neat array. I can never forget the aromas and pungence that distinguished Grandpa's quarters.

Grandpa would keep on hand large slabs of slippery elm, from which he would carve small pieces for my cousins and me to chew. That was our "chewing gum." Grandpa's herbal liniment was poured generously on every cut and scrape I acquired. And since climbing trees was one of my favorite activities, I usually had an abundance of wounds under treatment. An application of liniment felt like liquid fire, but it did get results. I loved Grandpa's herbal cough syrup, though, and I can remember exaggerating coughing spells sometimes to obtain an extra swig!

One thing Grandpa especially enjoyed was to have his feet rubbed and massaged. This proved to be a boring chore for a small child whose most important goal in life was to "go outside and play." On the other hand, my second most important goal was to earn money to buy "penny candy" — something frowned upon by my grandparents. (And, oh, the difficulty of choosing from the numerous assortments in the stores in those days.) So Grandpa outsmarted his grandchildren's reluctance by appealing to our mercenary side. He offered to pay a nickel for a ten-minute foot rub!

I was the only child of Jethro Kloss's youngest daughter, Naomi. But because Aunt Mabel (my mother's oldest sister) made up for my "only-ness" by having nine children, Grandpa had lots of little foot massagers that he kept busy throughout a good number of years.

Grandpa gave me a whole dollar to memorize the Ten Commandments, and other sums were earned for memorizing the Twenty-Third Psalm and some of his other favorite Bible texts. Of course the money would be forthcoming only after each selected passage was repeated "word perfect" to him.

As I grew and became able to take on responsibility, I filled hundreds (it just seemed like thousands) of gelatine capsules with the powdered herbs that Grandpa prepared for his patients. This was not my favorite pastime. Nor was I happy to stand at the stove stirring and stirring large kettles of soybean milk (so the milk wouldn't stick and be scorched) — a laborious and time-consuming process. But Grandpa's soybean milk was delicious, and so were the twenty or so other soy products that he originated and produced — including meat substitutes and soybean bread, butter, cheese, and ice cream.

Throughout all his life Grandpa used his strength and mind and ingenuity in experimenting to develop food products and other practical products, and to share with others what he read or learned firsthand or invented. Often Grandpa would prepare soybean ice cream to serve at the close of his lectures or cooking demonstrations. One of my favorite treats was to lick the paddle from the ice cream freezer before we left home to go to the lecture. Perhaps this treat was an incentive for me to sit quietly through the lecture without complaining.

Grandpa loved to hear my grandmother play the piano. Often he would stand behind her and sing. "He Leadeth Me" was one of his favorite hymns. In my mind I can still hear him singing that song, even today.

Sometimes my grandfather's early morning prayers were said aloud. I remember his voice, praying for his family, praying for his patients, thanking God for helping him in the work he loved so well.

There seemed to be a continuing stream of humanity seeking Grandpa out for treatment, advice, and reassurance. Many persons were taken directly into my grandparents' home for periods of time and treated successfully with herb therapy, water therapy, nourishing diet, and massage. Grandpa liked to travel, and that was fortunate, for often he would go to see those who were disabled or too sick to come to him. When he came home he would be bearing gifts of food — perhaps a sack of oranges, or avocados, or mangoes.

Grandpa and Grandma Kloss died when I was in my mid-teens. Having had the pleasure of being in their company much and often, for many long and short visits, I count myself fortunate. The memory of them as persons, of their strength of character, and their goodness of heart has been an anchor to my life.

I am proud of Grandfather Kloss for the initiative and ingenuity with which he forged ahead in his times to amass a great deal of knowledge of Nature's many resources and to put what he learned to practical use for the welfare of his "neighbors" everywhere.

Section I
Natural Health

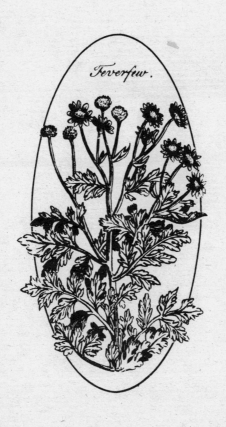

Feverfew.

1

PERSONAL EXPERIENCES

During my long years of experience along medical lines, I have worked out things that are of value to the human family. There is a crying need for an old-fashioned remedy book that people can use themselves. I have been asked many times to write out my experiences so that others may have the benefit of what I have found to be true.

When presenting the subjects on which this book treats, I have many times been asked the reason for my interest in these matters and what my purpose is in endeavoring to interest others also. It is only fitting that now, in putting my experience and knowledge in printed form, I should answer these questions. This I can best do by giving a brief sketch of personal experiences during my youth and early manhood.

I was born and reared on a truck and nursery farm in the northern part of Wisconsin. We raised all kinds of vegetables, as well as growing seeds for large seed houses. My father was a practical farmer and nursery man. We raised nearly everything that we needed, and had very few things to buy. We made our own syrup and sugar from beets and carrots, and had an abundance of all kinds of fruits, such as apples, cherries, plums, blackberries, raspberries, strawberries, grapes, and currants. We lived almost entirely upon the natural products of the earth.

After I left home I lived in boarding houses and hotels, eating little except devitalized foods, until my health began to fail. See Section III, Liquor Habit, pg. 386. This continued until I suffered a complete breakdown. My nerves gave way completely, and I became so weak that at one time I was in bed for three months, suffering with pains no tongue can describe. Death would have been a welcome release.

Finally, when I was able to be up and around again, I went to various sanitariums and consulted with doctors and specialists. Sometimes it seemed as though I was getting a little better and then I would get worse again. Even when I could walk around, if anyone talked to me for only five minutes, holding the most pleasant conversation, I would collapse. Some of the very best doctors said that they did not see how I lived at all, and that I certainly could not live long. My nerves were in such condition that sometimes when I had my eyes open, I would seem to see flashes of lightning in broad daylight. In this condition I lingered for a number of years.

I had tried every remedy known to the medical profession, but none of my doctors gave me one ray of hope. I had no thought of ever getting well again. I had made my will and was not looking for any further help from the medical profession.

It was while in this condition that I came across some books written by Mrs. E. G. White, who, though not a physician, was a great medical missionary. In those books I found statements like these: "Nine out of every ten could get well if they would use simple God-given means." "Do not eat food robbed of its life-giving elements." "Do not eat food that makes you sick." This was an entirely new line of thought to me. Up to that time I had never heard such things mentioned.

Anyone desiring any of Mrs. E. G. White's writings on healthful living can procure them from the Review and Herald Publishing Association, 55 West Oak Ridge Drive, Hagerstown, Maryland 21740.

A.   MY SEARCH FOR GOD'S REMEDIES

These were the first things that began to open my eyes and they gave me encouragement that there might be hope for me. This brought back to my mind that while at home in my youth, we never needed a doctor. For food we depended on the nuts of the forest, the fruits of the orchard, and the grains of the field. For medicine we used the herbs of the fields and gardens, teas made from the inside barks of certain trees and shrubs, and the health-giving, cooling juices of wild and cultivated fruits that grew in abundance all around us. Our herbs we gathered and dried in the summertime, and saved to have on hand in case of sickness, either for ourselves or our neighbors. Well do I remember how I gathered herbs, barks, and blossoms. I recalled many times when my parents were called to a neighbor's home after someone there had been given up to die. They, with their herbs, fruit juices, and vegetable broths, helped the sick one back to health again.

One time smallpox broke out in a community a little distance from us. Our whole family was exposed before we knew it; and though we did not have a doctor, we recovered by means of these simple herbs, water, and plain foods. There were also other nearby families who used only the herbs and not one of them died.

In those pioneer days, doctors were scarce in that northern country. The people depended upon each other and upon simple means of treatment, for they had a practical knowledge of its effectiveness, gained from experience. All these things came vividly to my mind at this time when I was in such hopeless physical and mental condition.

I began to search further in those books written by Mrs. E. G. White and I found many useful things. It was not long until my health began to improve, and by the continued use of these simple God-given remedies, it improved until I was a well man.

The Typhoid Epidemic

One time there was an epidemic of typhoid fever in the locality where I was living. Most of the people were deathly afraid of it, because a great many died. Someone told me of a man and wife who were afflicted with typhoid and had no one to wait on them. The neighbors would come and place food on the porch, but would not go into the house. I went to see this family. As I approached the house, I met the doctor outside the door and asked him if he had any objections to my doing something for these folks. He said "No, no objection," and he added that the woman would recover, but the man would die.

I found this man in very critical condition. He was hemorrhaging from the bowels and was in severe pain, with ulcers in his mouth and doubtless throughout the entire digestive tract. He was very low. From all appearances, there was no hope for him. But I obtained a cot, put it in his room, and began to treat the man with the simple remedies that I had found in the books of Mrs. E. G. White. I stopped all poisonous drugs and gave him plenty of water and fruit juices, and used other simple means, such as hot and cold fomentations, which proved a great means of allaying his pains.

In about six weeks the man was up and around. When he asked me how much he owed me, I told him he owed me nothing, as I myself had been lingering for years with no hope of ever being well again, and I was glad and happy to be able to do something for him. But the man said, "No sir. You will never do this for nothing," and he gave me a check for $75.

This was the beginning of my medical missionary work, as I had never before done anything for the sick. I was so pleased and happy that I had been successful in doing something for someone that I continued nursing, having the same good results. I nursed for several doctors who were surprised that one having had no medical training of any kind could get such results. I have had the same results many times since. The means are so simple that anyone can use them in their own home.

I studied every case that I had because I had to see what I could learn further on the subject of simple methods of treating the sick. I was so aroused by this time that I began to search for and buy books on these subjects, and also to subscribe to medical magazines. I have continued this search for many years, writing many letters in search of things that might be a blessing to man. I studied the Bible on cooking and baking, and also learned the remedies that were used in

Bible times. I have found that the methods of healing that God gave to man to maintain and restore health were to be practiced by ministers and gospel workers. And God has never changed that plan.

I have also studied many bulletins from the government in which I have found valuable information, analysis of various products, etc. I read the *Journal of the American Medical Association* and many of the books that the Medical Association publishes, from which I learned much.

Man's methods of treating disease are truly complicated and mystifying, but God's ways are so simple that anyone can understand them without a medical education. This led me to think of the simple herbs, fruits, fruit juices, and barks that my parents used, and the means which Mrs. White used, which are so simple and harmless and so inexpensive that everyone can use them for themselves. This is God's plan. His remedies can be used at small expense.

Here are the simple means that Mrs. White, with the aid of her helpers and many others, used: pure air, sunshine, properly prepared food, nonpoisonous herbs, water treatments, pure water to drink, abstemiousness (moderation), foods not robbed of their life-giving properties during manufacture, and cleanliness of body and premises. When we heed these things, God will do for us what we cannot do for ourselves. He lets the sun shine on the just and the unjust. If any man or woman would apply these simple, God-given remedies, the results would be the same for both saint and sinner. When physical law is obeyed by any human being, whether good or bad, he will reap the reward God has promised. When a man, who does not believe in God, tills his soil properly and sows and plants properly, God gives him sunshine and rain the same as he does a righteous man, for God is no respecter of persons.

I have heard many health lectures and have read a great deal on health topics, but it was the books of Mrs. White that first opened my eyes. I have been told that she employed as medicine the common red clover blossoms. She used them as a beverage throughout her life and lived to the age of 87 years.

It is now nearly 40 years since I was given up by my doctors without hope of ever being able to do anything again in this world. Part of the time I have done the work of two or three, and many times the circumstances were such that I could not take proper care of myself, and I would work beyond my strength. Now I am getting to be an old man and have more strength and endurance than many young people. I feel grateful to my heavenly Father for all these simple God-given remedies. It was the reading of such statements as the following which led me to believe that there must be a remedy for me. "Do not eat food that makes you sick." "Eat food as much as possible in its natural state." "Foods that require cooking should be prepared in a simple, palatable way without the use of spices." God has a remedy for every ill of man, and I certainly found those remedies.

Remedies For Infections

A short time after I had begun to help people with these simple remedies, as I was driving along the road, a man who had heard about my work called to me and said, "Can't you do something for my boy?" A large, strapping young fellow was sitting in the house suffering with an ingrown toenail. His toe was so sore and inflamed that he could not walk. I washed the foot with soap and water, and trimmed away the toenail down to the quick. Then I took some peroxide and kept putting it on until the pus and foul matter was cleaned away. Finding there was proud flesh, I put on burnt alum powder. This killed the proud flesh. I then asked him to place his foot in water as hot as he could stand it for several minutes, then plunge it into cold water for a few seconds, repeating this several times a day. Then I had them get an old shoe and cut the leather away at the toe, so his sore toe would not touch it. Then I put a little cotton between the toes so they would not touch each other. Three days later I stopped by to see the boy. His father said he was out in the field working.

Along that same road the farmers were threshing. The man who was doing the feeding was cut in the palm of the hand by the bundle cutter. There was a deep cut in the flesh and the gash was nearly an inch wide. I put a little disinfectant in water and some astringent and soaked his hand in hot water for over an hour. Hot water, of course, was added at intervals to keep it hot. This almost entirely closed the wound. Then I cut some narrow strips of adhesive plaster. I pressed the wound together so it was tightly closed, and put these narrow strips across it to hold it in place. Then I put his arm in a sling. In one week, his wound had entirely knit together, and in less than two weeks the man began to work again.

For a disinfectant and astringent, a tea made of white oak bark or bayberry bark is excellent. Use a heaping teaspoonful in powder form to a cup of boiling water and steep it thirty minutes, or it can be made a little stronger. Wild alum root, golden seal, and myrrh are also excellent for such purposes. Use a half teaspoonful of any of these three to a cup of boiling water.

An excellent liniment for strains and bruises is made from a mixture of a small teaspoonful each of myrrh and golden seal and a half teaspoonful of red pepper added to a pint of alcohol, which is allowed to stand for seven days. Shake well every day. This is also an excellent liniment for any sore, fresh wound, or ulcer. Kerosene is also excellent for wounds and bruises.

Following are a number of my experiences with these simple remedies that anyone can use in his own home.

A Swollen Foot

On another occasion I came to a home where a young man was sitting with a swollen foot. The thick part under his foot near the toes was very badly swollen and inflamed so that he was not able to walk. I had them get a large pan of hot water and one of cold. He soaked his foot in the hot water until it was thoroughly heated, then plunged it into the cold for just a second or two, putting it immediately back into the hot water, alternating in this manner for one hour. I then took a pan with some kerosene in it, and put his foot into this cold kerosene while the foot was hot and the pores open. We went through this process several times during the evening and then repeated it the first thing in the morning. The young man went to work that same day. I advised him to continue this treatment every evening for a few evenings, and this entirely cured the soreness in his foot.

Treating a Sore Toe With Peroxide

Many years ago I had occasion to treat a young man who had been wearing a shoe that was too tight, or at least it did not fit his foot well, causing his large toe to become very sore. It was swollen and had become so painful that he could not work. There was nothing available except some of that old household remedy, hydrogen peroxide. I washed his foot in very warm water and then applied peroxide every two or three minutes, until the foot was perfectly clean and the peroxide did not bubble anymore. This treatment alone relieved the inflammation so much that the young man could resume his work. I told him that for several evenings he should soak his foot, first in hot and then cold water, and then apply the peroxide or kerosene until the soreness was entirely gone. The toe got well.

Cases of Rheumatism

One time four men came to see me and told me of a man who was crippled with rheumatism. They insisted that I go with them to see him. We found a man about 35 years of age lying in bed with both legs drawn up so tightly that they could not be moved to a normal position. His arms were the same way. His wife fed him with a spoon, as one would feed a little baby.

This man had been doctored for years by specialists, and

spent hundreds of dollars without receiving any help. What the doctors were doing for him at this time was injecting strychnine and morphine. Without this the man would groan night and day.

I gave him hot blanket packs to sweat in, then later I gave him baths in the washtub. I covered him with blankets and put his feet in a pan of hot water as you would give a sitz-bath, and then rubbed him with oil. (For herbs used, see index under Rheumatism.) For food I gave him zwieback, whole wheat flakes (adding a tablespoonful of lime water to alkalinize every cup of milk), an abundance of fresh fruits and vegetables, and had him drink a great deal of pure water. In one week there was decided improvement, and in a comparatively short time he was well and resumed his work again, with both his arms and legs perfectly limber.

Another time an elderly minister came to me, saying he was full of aches and pains, all stiffened up, and feeling very ill in general, and asked me if I would do something for him. I gave him an enema and some herbs to cleanse his system thoroughly. I put him in a tub of hot water, keeping him there several hours, massaging his body while in the water, and at the last, gave him a vigorous salt glow to open the pores and stimulate the circulation, using half Epsom salts and half common salt. I gave him several glasses of water to drink while in the bath, then gave him some herbs for his rheumatism. In a few days he had recovered and went about his work.

Ulcerated Stomach With Spasm

This case was brought to my attention by the man mentioned in the preceding section who had the case of rheumatism. He suggested that I might be able to do something for his aunt, who had not been able to work for a number of years. She had a bad case of ulcerated stomach and bowel trouble. When I met her I inquired about her troubles. She told me that every few days, aside from the constant pain, she would get a spell in the form of a spasm with terrible pain. I told her that if I could see her in one of those spells I could tell more about what was the matter. She said, "If you can do anything for me to keep me from having another spell, for God's sake do it, for I'd sooner die than have another spell." I ordered a sitz bath and a sweat bath, followed by a salt glow and a high enema. I put her on a liquid diet and also gave her whole wheat flakes dissolved in boiling water with a little cream. She also had some whole wheat zwieback with hot milk. A teaspoonful of lime water was added to each cup of milk. We gave her daily hot and cold applications over the stomach, liver, and spine. I gave her herbs to heal the ulcers in her stomach and to cleanse the system. In three weeks this woman had improved so much that she was able to go home and continue her treatment.

Fifteen years later I received a letter from Mr. Gilson, the woman's nephew who had been healed of rheumatism, saying that he wished he could get a few more treatments as he was again feeling a touch of rheumatism. He added in the same letter, "It might please you to know that my aunt has been well ever since, and has not suffered another spell, but is just now feeling a little touch of that old trouble." I had thoroughly instructed them both that the things which had caused the trouble originally would do so again. I could not go to see them, but instructed them by letter what to do, and they got along all right.

Cured of Tuberculosis

About 35 years ago a man by the name of Stevens, who lived in the northern part of Wisconsin, called me very urgently to come to see his wife. I found her sick in bed with tuberculosis. She was a young woman with one child less than a year old. Upon inquiry, we found that three in this family had already died of tuberculosis; her mother, one brother, and one sister. This lady was the fourth in the family to be afflicted with the disease. The doctors had given her up. She was a frail woman with a small, round chest and very small lungs. A number of my friends advised me not to try to do anything for the woman, as they thought it would be impossible for a cure to be effected.

I told both the woman and her husband just what it would mean to undertake this case. I said that if they would not live up to everything I asked them to do to the last detail, that I would not undertake it, and that just as soon as I might find out that they did not live up to every requirement, I would drop the case at once.

Suffice it to say, that it was not more than two weeks before the woman was so much improved that she could walk around. I asked them to get her some warm felt shoes, woolen stockings, and woolen underwear extending down to her ankles; then I had her exercise outdoors every day. As her strength increased I had her exercise more and more. Nearby was a high hill which I had her walk up every day, rain or shine, unless the weather was too stormy. Walking uphill is very beneficial as it compels one to breathe deeply.

This woman got entirely well, and the last I heard of her she had reared a family of children. There is no need for failure in such cases unless the disease has gone so far that the organs of the body have been destroyed and you have nothing to build on. I could cite many more instances of this kind, but will only give a few more to show the results of the use of simple means that can be used in your own home.

Child Given Up To Die

One time I was called to a home where there was a little four-year-old child. Her fever was over 104° and she had been unconscious for some time. The doctor had pronounced it pneumonia. This child was clothed in a heavy woolen under-suit, and also wore a jacket made of batting to cover her lungs, both in front and back. The house was full of people, as they expected the child to die at any minute. I asked them to remove her clothes. The grandfather, who was standing on one side of the bed, objected very seriously, saying that it would cause the child's death. But her father said to leave me alone. The doctor had said that the child would die, and unless a decided change came they all knew that she would.

They asked me the cause of the fever. I told them I did not know the cause, but that no matter what the cause was, the fever must be reduced. We put the child, without any clothes on, between cotton blankets, gave her an enema, then sponged her with tepid water every five minutes, letting the water evaporate. I raised her head every few minutes and filled her mouth with cold water. She would take only one swallow. We kept this treatment up all night. When she seemed to get a little chilly, I would stop the sponging and put a hot water bottle to her stomach or feet, keeping her well covered. As soon as she got warm we would continue the sponging. At three o'clock in the morning, when I raised her head and gave her a drink of cold water, she opened her eyes for the first time and said, "Thank you." Her father, who was standing on the other side of the bed, burst into tears and said, "Now I know she is going to get better."

By this time the fever had gone down more than 2°. We kept this treatment up until three o'clock in the afternoon, a little more than twenty-four hours from the time we started. By this time the child was quite normal, and began to talk, but she would get a coughing and choking spell every little while. Upon inquiry as to what might have been the cause of this fever, I found that at suppertime three or four days before this, the child had eaten very freely of beefsteak. Shortly after, she became ill. I told them I thought the child was full of worms, and that her choking spells were caused by the worms crawling up in her throat. I sent them to their own physician to get some worm medicine. In three or four days the child was entirely well. The cause of this fever was the beefsteak she had eaten. She was unable to digest it. The worms had a feast on it and caused a large amount of poison to accumulate. The poison in the large bowel was removed by the enema, the pores were opened and the skin was made active by sponging. Then by constantly giving her water to drink, we reduced the fever to normal.

Hemorrhage From the Uterus

Once I assisted in saving the life of a person who had bled so much that she was near death. I use the word assisted because ultimately only God saves lives. She could only whisper faintly, and could not be heard except by listening close to her mouth. I elevated the foot of the bed, and gave her hot malted nut cream, diluted half and half with grape juice. After giving her several very hot cups, she was so strengthened that I could understand what she said while standing at the foot of the bed. I followed this with more treatment for hemorrhage as given in the chapter on the use of herbs for special diseases.

Infantile Paralysis (Poliomyelitis)

A few years ago, a woman brought to me a three-year-old boy who had infantile paralysis. His head was drawn clear over to his shoulder, his arm was drawn up to his chest, and his shoulder blade stuck far out. This child had been permitted all the candy, ice cream, cakes, and cookies he wanted, and nearly all the food he had been eating had been robbed of its life-giving properties. The mother said they had consulted several physicians in the city where they lived, and had also taken him to another city to some of the best specialists they could find. All the physicians gave her no hope for the boy's recovery and said that it would probably take years for him to outgrow it.

I told them to give the child plenty of fresh fruits and vegetables, but no candy, ice cream, cake, or cookies of any description, and no white flour or cane sugar products. I had them give the boy hot and cold applications to the spine, stomach, and liver, and then taught them how to massage his entire body. He was also to have alternate hot and cold baths, finishing with a short cold bath. I had him take lots of exercise in the open air. Anyone could notice improvement after the first few days. In six weeks this boy could throw a ball with the hand that had been drawn up to his chest. His head, which had been drawn down on his shoulder, was perfectly straight and the shoulder blade was almost entirely normal. All that was done for this child was what anyone can do in his own home. This was quite a number of years ago. The child has been well ever since and is a normal high school student today. Following is a letter from the boy's mother.

1817 Downing Street,
New Smyrna Beach, FLA.
September 22, 1938

Dear Mr. Kloss:

I had a letter from my sister, Mrs. Burkhard, several days ago, telling me about the letter she had received from you. I will be glad to give the date of Harry's illness and other particulars.

Harry Peyton Cobb, Jr., became ill of infantile paralysis in April 1925, at the age of three. It paralyzed his right side from his waist up and his lower limbs were very weak, as he could only walk a short distance without falling. He could not hold his head up and it dropped forward badly. When he would lie down, he could not sit up without being helped, nor could he stand up by himself. After three treatments from Mr. Kloss and the proper diet, he was able to sit and stand up unassisted. After taking six weeks of treatments, he could hold his head erect, throw a ball, ride his tricycle and walk without falling. Harry is 17 years old now and is in good health. He enters in all high school sports and no one knows he had infantile paralysis unless we tell them. We certainly owe his strong physical condition to Mr. Kloss and enough cannot be said of his treatments.

When I see other children left so crippled from infantile paralysis, it makes me so thankful for Mr. Kloss's help and for God's help that my boy has grown to be a big, fine young man. I do wish you folks could see him.

All send their best regards to you, Mrs. Kloss, Naomi, and Eden.

Yours truly,
MRS. HARRY P. COBB

Another Case of Paralysis

Not long ago my wife asked me to go and see a neighbor's child who had been stricken with infantile paralysis that day. Upon entering the home I found the mother holding in her arms a plump baby who was not yet a year old. The mother also was fleshy. This child was nursed exclusively by the mother and had never had any other food. Upon inquiring about the mother's diet, I found that she was practically living on white bread, white biscuits made with soda, pork, and peeled potatoes with white flour gravy. For breakfast she would have pancakes and syrup. She also used some milk, but very few vegetables. All these foods are high in calories but have few life-giving properties in them. This is what caused the baby's paralysis, because the mother was not eating food that would properly nourish the nerves. We at once gave the woman oatmeal and bran water to drink, and fresh fruits. My wife cooked her a kettle of vegetable soup, with carrots, onions, potatoes, and natural brown rice. We gave the baby oatmeal water and tomato juice. We then gave the baby some baths, both hot and cold, and rubbed her well, repeating this treatment several times. In a few days every symptom of paralysis was gone, and the child got well. Of course we thoroughly instructed the mother about how to eat in order to have a healthy baby and to avoid sickness.

Complete Paralysis

Many years ago, a man awoke me about one in the morning saying that his wife was paralyzed all over. I went with him to his home and began treatment at once. First, we gave her an enema, followed by hot and cold applications to the spine, stomach, and liver. We then gave her a hot towel rub, just as hot as we could give it, followed by a cold towel rub and a thorough massage from head to foot. We kept this up practically all the rest of the night, giving alternate hot and cold treatments to the spine, then percussion, hacking movements, and spatting. (See chapter on massage.) In the morning there was a marked improvement in the pulse, but there was as yet no sign of life or any feeling. In a short while, we repeated the treatment in full.

The second day we began to see signs of life when we pricked her gently with a needle. We kept this treatment up for hours each day and part of the night. The fourth day she could stand alone, without any assistance, but as yet was not able to walk. We continued this treatment for some time, but not so vigorously or so prolonged. In less than two weeks she was up doing her housework again. I knew this lady for years afterward, and know that she stayed well. This was nearly thirty years ago and the last I heard she was rearing a family.

I have had many experiences with treating spinal meningitis and paralysis. I will mention just one more case, an extremely severe one.

Two Strokes Resulting in Paralysis

This was my own wife. We had been married only a short time. One morning when I got up I noticed that my wife did not act as she usually did. Upon examination I found that half her body was paralyzed from her head down to her feet. I could take a needle and stick it gently into one side of her face, arm, leg, or foot and there was no sign of life. I at once called the best doctor that we knew and in whom we had the most confidence. He gave her a thorough examination and said that nothing could be done aside from giving general good care. He said that she would be likely to die at any time, that this stroke would be followed by another stroke, which would cause her death.

I started the same course of treatments which I had used with my neighbor's wife, related in the preceding incident, "Complete Paralysis." In the course of three weeks my wife was up and around the house in the usual way and we could again listen to the beautiful tones that she is capable of producing on the piano.

Not long after that I arose at an early hour, as my custom was, and went about my work. When I came in for breakfast, I inquired as to where Mrs. Kloss was and the answer was that they had not seen her yet that morning. I went to the bedroom and found her lying in bed. When I talked to her there was no response. When I took hold of her it felt as if I was taking hold of a dead person, only she was not entirely cold. I tried to get her to say something, but she gave not a sound of any kind. Then I took a needle and gently pricked her face and neck. But she did not flinch or blink her eye. I went down her body to her feet on both sides, but there was not a flinch or response of any description. I called into her ear and asked her if she could hear me. Then I put my finger on her eyeballs but she did not blink. Her pulse was so weak that I could not find a pulse at all on her wrist. There was just a very faint pulse in her neck.

After I saw the situation, I again called the doctor. He thoroughly examined Mrs. Kloss and said that she was liable to drop off at any minute. Then I began to work along the same line of treatment already mentioned. After one day's treatment, her pulse had increased materially, and in four weeks she was able to walk around. In five or six weeks she was playing the piano again and going about her work as usual. This happened about 26 years ago, and she has been well ever since. I wish you could see her today. She is active, well, and cheerful.

I am sure that many would be interested in knowing how her health ever came to be in such a bad condition. Before I met her, she would sleep for a week or two and no one could awaken her. The cause of this was that she was a bookkeeper for 12 years and instead of working six or eight hours a day, she would work twelve to fourteen hours. Sometimes she kept two or three sets of books. That was not the worst of it. She would hurry at lunch to get a white bread sandwich and then go back to work. She did not get the proper food to nourish her nervous system. Besides auditing the books and working late into the night, she did not get enough sleep or proper exercise. She kept this up until she had a complete breakdown. There was no one to advise her to do the right things.

Thank God, there is a remedy for every ill of man. The angels in Heaven weep because of the dreadful suffering that is going on because of ignorance. And I have wept until I could not weep any more, when I have seen the untold amount of suffering in the world and knew that most of it might be prevented if people only knew what to do to prevent it. The only thing that I feel conscience stricken about is that I have not done more to bring to the notice of the public and show by practical experience what really can be done for suffering humanity with simple remedies that can be used in every ordinary home. I could write volumes, giving my personal experiences, but will mention only a few more for practical lessons.

Pneumonia

Another time I was called to see a young lady who had been given up to die with a relapse of pneumonia. When I arrived at her house, I found her in bed with a very high temperature. She had been sick for some time and was very low. They had a graduate nurse, but she knew little about water treatments. The patient's lungs were in very bad shape. I could hardly hear the sound of air with the stethoscope in any part of her lungs.

I sent at once for one of my best graduate nurses who understood water treatments. We started in by giving an enema. Then we placed her between cotton blankets and sponged her with tepid water, giving her frequent sips of cold water and also short hot and cold applications to both the front and back of the chest. In the course of two hours with this treatment, her lungs began to open up, and we could hear air in her lungs through the stethoscope. In four hours we had lowered her temperature 2°.

We kept up the treatment, sponging her body with tepid water and letting the water evaporate. Sometimes she would show signs of chilliness and we would stop the treatment, put a hot water bag to her stomach, and cover her up. We continued giving her sips of cold water and also wrapped a cold towel around her head and neck, changing it frequently. Never let a cloth on the head or neck get hot. *Just as soon as it starts to get warm, replace it with a cold one.*

We also gave her a liquid diet and fruit juices. In four days her temperature was normal. This woman, who is my wife's niece, is alive today. Her illness occurred nearly 25 years ago.

Many cases of pneumonia would recover if treated early, and the right treatment given. I mention these cases to show what can be done in the home by using these simple treatments. There will be many times when you cannot get a doctor or nurse, and it is a most blessed thing to know how to relieve suffering.

Pneumonia Resulting From Wrong Habits of Living

Many years ago, before there were any automobiles, I was in the extreme northern part of Wisconsin, at a country club. The manager was a drinking man and a high liver. He had had frequent spells of pneumonia. The last time he had pneumonia, the doctor told him that if he got another spell there would be no means on earth to save him: he told the man not to call him, that he would not come if he were called.

There was, therefore, great excitement when the manager became very sick and came down with a high fever of 104°. They were fifteen miles away from a doctor. They had a fine driving team, which he ordered hitched up at once. He did not know about any of my medical experience, but his wife had heard something about it. She called me in to see him and asked the driver to wait a few minutes.

The man was very much excited and urged them to hurry on for a doctor; but his wife reminded him of what the doctor had said. She said I had had splendid results with such cases, and urged him to give me a trial. When he got over his excitement a little, he consented for me to go ahead. The team was unhitched. I removed all his clothing, had him lie between cotton blankets, gave him an enema, and began sponging him with tepid water all over, giving him cold water to drink. During such treatments the room should be 75°F. and well ventilated; I kept on sponging him every five minutes. Sometimes he would get a little chilly and we would stop for a while and cover him up. I kept up the cold water drinking and tepid sponging. Tepid sponging feels very agreeable to a patient with a high fever.

The next day at three o'clock, just twenty-four hours from the time the fever began, it was almost entirely gone. His temperature was below 100°. The man said he felt as well as he ever had in his life and wanted to get up. I advised him not to get up for a day or two at least. I knew this man for years afterward, and he never had another attack of pneumonia while I knew him.

In this case, and I might say in all cases, I constantly hold before the patients the things that put them in that condition and how to avoid sickness. Never forget that water, which puts out fire, is one of the best known remedies to cure fevers, and is to be used both internally and externally.

B.   POSTMORTEMS REVEAL SECRETS

At one time I connected with an emergency hospital just to get the experience. It was a wonderful help to me in many ways. I witnessed scores of postmortems performed by competent surgeons. It was very interesting to see the organs of people whose lives and eating and drinking habits we had previously known about.

We opened up a middle-aged man, quite fleshy, who had died of heart failure. Here is his story: one evening at about six o'clock as he prepared to take a bath, he reached up to get a drinking glass standing on a shelf about as high as his head. As he reached for it he fell dead. This man had been a great eater of meats, rich pastries, pies, cakes, puddings, white bread, peeled potatoes, etc. We found his liver about three times its normal size. There were tumors all around the liver, and some in the liver, ranging in size from a small marble to a small-sized potato. The heart was also very much enlarged, more than once again its normal size, and the walls of the heart were very thin and flabby and a dark color as if bloodshot. The spleen and pancreas were both enlarged and diseased and he had stones and gravel in the gallbladder. His stomach was also very much prolapsed and diseased.

Another man, past middle age, was cancerous. He had always complained of pain around his navel, but there was no outward sign of cancer. The only indication that could be seen on the outside of his body was a little lump under his jaw. After he died we did a postmortem examination. His bowels were full of cancerous growths where he had complained of his pain. The cancer had eaten right through the bowels, which resulted in his death. He was full of cancerous growth from his head clear down to his feet. You could not cut him anywhere without finding cancer. All his organs were in bad shape.

One person who was very fleshy had layers of pure fat almost three inches thick. The colon in some parts was three or four times its natural size. But in some parts it had shrunk to the diameter of a finger and in other places it was so small that it was almost impossible for anything to pass through. The small intestines had shrunk in some places to the size of a lead pencil, with a heavy hard growth on the outside. Only a very small portion of the intestine was of natural size. The spleen was very much enlarged, and the stomach hung far down in the abdomen. The kidneys were very enlarged and flabby, the lungs were much enlarged and almost black, and the liver was enlarged and hard.

In another case, the lungs and liver were very much enlarged and almost as hard as a rock. The colon and small intestines were also much enlarged, although in some places they had shrunk so that almost nothing could pass through. The stomach was enlarged and flabby and hung far down out of its place. The kidneys were spongy and the whole intestinal tract was out of its regular order.

In another case the liver was very much enlarged. Over and around it were tumors, from the size of a small marble to that of a small potato. The heart was very much enlarged, very flabby, and in each part was a bunch of pure fat the size of a small potato. Both the colon and the small intestines were very much enlarged, with pockets that were filled with fecal matter.

In another case, the intestines had shrunk very much, with pockets in various parts of the colon; and the entire intestines were full of small growths. There were little hard growths under the skin over this person's entire body, from the top of his head to the soles of his feet.

Another case was one that was mere skin and bones. The liver was almost entirely eaten away, with just a little fibrous slush left; and all the intestines were deformed. There was not a drop of blood in the whole system, and the body was full of pus and slime.

But some patients, whose X-rays revealed that the colon was full of deformities and that it and the stomach hung far down in the abdomen, are alive after treatment and are able to be up and working.

One such case had a colon that was shrunken in several places. In other places there were big pockets, and the rectum was full of hard growths. Through an operation the narrowed places were cut out and the colon was sewed back together. The patient recovered enough to be up and working, and to have normal bowel movements.

These cases, and others that I might mention, give unfailing evidence and proof of what effect a wrong diet will have upon the system. All of the preceding examples lived largely on foods that had been robbed of their life-giving properties, and ate mixtures that could not make good blood but only cause suffering and disease. If everyone would follow the health principles as outlined in this book, they would avoid an untold amount of suffering and premature death.

One finds no such irregularity in the bodies of the other animals. They eat their food as God has prepared it for them. Man has spoiled the food by poor preparation and has robbed it of its life-giving properties. If man would eat the food as God has made it, his body would be symmetrical, beautiful, and healthy.

"Lo, this only have I found, that God hath made man upright; but they have sought out many inventions." Ecclesiastes 7:29.

Man has made many inventions that are good and very useful, but also many that destroy both soul and body.

C.   EXPERIENCE IN A SMALL SANITARIUM

Some years ago, much was said about the wonderful cures effected by operations and the use of electricity. Much expensive electrical apparatus was manufactured, and it was advertised extensively.

I, like thousands of others, thought there might be something to it; so I equipped a small sanitarium in the best part of the beautiful little town of St Peter, Minnesota, near a lovely park.

I provided it with bathrooms for both men and women, so that we could give Turkish and Russian baths, electric baths, showers, tub baths, etc. It was also equipped with a very fine operating room and a room with electrical apparatus, containing one of the best X-ray units, static and high frequency current, galvanic and sinusoidal current, German ultraviolet rays, sun-rays, and several other rays.

I took a medical electrical course at Battle Creek, Michigan, at that time one of the best medical electrical schools. I hired by the year one of the finest medical doctors. He had graduated as a nurse and had learned the water cure and had then graduated from the regular medical course. He had also studied in Europe and had taken several postgraduate courses. I hired graduate nurses from recognized institutions. Then I extended invitations to the doctors in that city to bring their cases to this institution, which they did. I gave the anesthetics for about five years, prepared the patients for their operations, and took care of them after the operations, assisted by my corps of workers.

Here, in my own institution, with a well-trained physician and graduate nurses, together with all the necessary equipment, I obtained much valuable experience.

D.   THE TENNESSEE HEALTH FOOD FACTORY

Many years ago I purchased a large food factory near Nashville, Tennessee. Here I gained a most wonderful experience along food lines, as we were making a large variety of foods in larger quantities than I had ever made before. Here we had a large reel oven and an up-to-date cracker machine. We made a very fine line of crackers, five different kinds. Our capacity was from 1200 to 2000 pounds per day. Besides this, we made a very fine cereal coffee, and various breakfast foods, whole wheat flour and quite a line of gluten and nut food preparations to take the place of meat. We also made malt honey and malt extract.

I hired an experienced baker and health food maker. I subscribed to various journals on cracker making, bread making, etc., and bought the best books obtainable on bread making, canning, and cooking. I had a regular experimental outfit, which I have till this day. I am experimenting with foods all the time, for the sole purpose of giving to the public the best.

My purpose in this was not to establish some commercial business, but to get before the public healthful things, which can take the place of the harmful articles of foods that are filling the world with chronic invalids. While I was operating this food factory, I took in people at different times who were interested and wanted to learn the business. I gave them my recipes and helped them to find the proper machinery and materials and much other necessary information needed to make health foods.

Since then I have helped others to start food businesses in different parts of the United States, and they are successful. I will not be satisfied until I have so many of these factories in operation — to make the foods of various sorts in the baking line as well as others — that the people who want to live right and avoid sickness can get these wholesome products everywhere.

I am now spending my time conducting public food demonstrations, cooking schools, and health lectures. My main object is to have everyone learn how to make these things in his own home. I have spent a good deal of money to simplify these things so that everyone can make the foods in an ordinary home.

I tell the people where they can get the various products that are wholesome at a reasonable price, and I condemn the hurtful articles. I help manufacturers everywhere to make wholesome products that will take the place of many injurious articles. Anyone wishing to manufacture any of these health foods in the baking line or in canning, etc., may obtain from me my best information on where to get the machinery and other needed articles.

I am also especially interested in having people everywhere start health restaurants combined with health food stores, so that these products can be sold and served at the same time.

After I had run this large factory at Nashville for a number of years, I sold it to an industrial school, Madison College. The factory was moved to their school campus and is still operating in connection with their school.

In 1921 I opened another factory at Brooke, Virginia, and equipped it with machinery for large capacity production. After operating this factory for a number of years I sold it. During this time I was teaching others how to make health foods, and they are now operating factories in different parts of the United States.

There should be a large number of factories so that these healthful articles could be obtained in every grocery store. I have developed a number of new products that have not yet been put on the market; and I am still experimenting for the sole purpose of giving these products to those who will make good use of them.

E.   THE COUNTRY DOCTOR

The following is an extract from "The Sawdust Trail," by Rev. William (Billy) Sunday, in the *Ladies Home Journal*, September 1932.

The Country Doctor

During the first three years of my life, I was sickly and could scarcely walk. Mother used to carry me on a pillow which she made for that purpose. There were no resident physicians in those pioneer days, and itinerant doctors would drive up to our cabin and ask, "Anybody sick here?"

One day, Doctor Avery, a Frenchman, called at our cabin and mother told him, "I have a little boy three years old who has been sick ever since he was born."

The old doctor said, "Let me see him." He gave me the once over while I yelled and screamed like a Comanche Indian. Then he said to Mother, "I can cure that boy."

She asked him how much he would charge, and he replied, "Oh, if you will feed me and my old mare, that will pay the bill."

Mother said, "All right, but you will have to sleep up in the garret. We have no stairs and you'll have to climb the ladder."

He replied, "That suits me." He then went into the woods and picked leaves from various shrubs, including mulberry leaves and elderberries, dug up roots, and from them made a syrup and gave it to me. In a short time I was going like the wind and have been hitting on all eight ever since. From that day to this, elderberries and mulberries have been my favorite wild fruits, and I like sassafras tea.

I do not believe that there is a disease to which human flesh is heir but that somewhere there is growing a weed or an herb or plant that will cure it. Somewhere there is a remedy for the dread plagues of the human race, consumption and cancer. God has made the cure and is waiting for man to discover it.

The greatest doctor this world ever knew is an old Christian mother, and my mother was the greatest of all. I regret that I did not write down the names of all the herbs and roots she knew, and the diseases they would cure. When she put on the "specks" to look at the sore and spread salve on it, that made it almost well.

You may name this suggestive therapeutics or the power of mind over matter. All these designations are as useless as the name of the horse that Paul Revere rode. The fact remains.

SOIL PREPARATION AND FARMING

A. PLOWING AND SOIL PREPARATION

"Back to the farm" is my message. It is really very interesting to take a piece of poor soil and make it productive in a short time by plowing deep and plowing under soybeans, green crops, etc., for fertilizer.

To make some interesting experiments, plow your soil 8 or 10 inches deep in the fall with a turn-plow. Plant corn on a piece of poor ground the first year. You will have to fertilize it so you will get big cornstalks. When you lay the corn by, plant soybeans between the rows. These beans will get big enough so you can have green shelled beans, an excellent food. Just as soon as the corn is glazed, pull it and haul it from the field, then spread it out to dry. Mow or cut down the cornstalks and soybean vines close to the ground, then plow the ground with a 12- or 14-inch plow with a rolling cutter on it. This will bring soil that has not been worn out to the surface. The green cornstalks and soybean vines put a wonderful mulch of the very best kind of fertilizer into the soil. This will emulsify the soil. If the soil has a clay subsoil, cultivate it at once with a disc harrow to pulverize it and keep it from getting hard on top.

Sow a winter crop to cover and protect the soil. The next spring plow the ground 6 or 7 inches deep, turning under your cover crop, then harrow thoroughly and plant your corn. Shallowly cultivate the corn and when ready to lay by, plant soybeans again and harvest and plow the soil just the same as you did the year before, only plow it crossways from the way you plowed it the year before. This loosens up the soil so the roots can go down deep and the moisture can come up. I have raised a fine crop of corn in this way during what was considered a year of crop failure.

Plant alfalfa or any grain on this ground the following year, and you will see a real crop of grain. If the ground is worked this way for a few years it will make real fertile soil, which will produce wonderful vegetables or any kind of fruit that will contain all the mineral and vitamin elements.

Those who have tractors can do this work easily with great satisfaction and big rewards. Anyone that has any land should work it this way, whether he raises fruits or vegetables. I have set out an orchard in this kind of soil and obtained growth in three years that would ordinarily have taken five or six years. This way of handling the soil holds the moisture and keeps the water from running off. There are many other ways to improve the soil.

If one does not have sufficient horsepower and machinery to cultivate the soil deeply, he should get together with his neighbors and obtain the necessary power and machinery. Bring the deep soil up to the surface and thoroughly pulverize it; then the fine and tender roots will have a nice mellow bed in which to run in every direction and get their nourishment.

All the plants — wheat, corn, oats, flowers, fruit trees — in fact, all plants and trees will have many more roots if they have a nice finely pulverized bed of soil. This kind of soil will also produce stronger plants that will yield better and more abundant grains and fruits, and the planter will be more than doubly paid for all the work he has put in on the land.

Shown following is a regular subsoiling plow, which can be used on ground that has not been plowed to subsoil 18 inches deep. Follow with this subsoiler and another team of horses in the furrow that has been made by the regular turning plow, to stir the ground deeper. If you do not have two teams, unhitch from the turning plow and hitch to the subsoiler.

Also shown is an attachment that can be used on a regular turning plow. It can be set so that it digs the dirt 4 to 6 inches deeper than the turning plow goes. A heavy team is necessary to use this attachment with the turning plow; if your team is not heavy put on more horses. Or if you have a tractor, it will

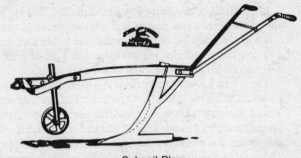

Subsoil Plow

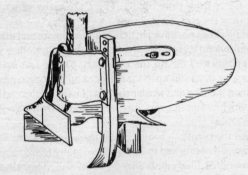

Subsoil Attachments

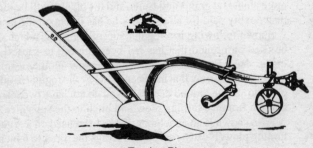

Turning Plow

draw the regular turning plow with the subsoiler without any difficulty, and even two plows could be used.

This is a regular turning plow with a rolling, cutting coulter. If your plowing ground is covered with vines of any kind, or long hay or straw, this plow will cut such material in two so that it will not drag in front of the plow.

The most effective way to work ground is to first plow it 8 or 10 inches deep in the fall, and subsoil it. Then work the soil in thoroughly with a disc harrow, and put in a winter crop, letting it grow until spring as much as it will. Then plow it again crossways, turning under the winter crop, so that the subsoil is crossways. The deep stirring of the ground in this way will give the moisture a chance to come up, and will also hold the moisture from rainfall in the ground, and give the roots of your grain and corn a chance to go down deep.

People who have not already used this method will be surprised at how it will increase the production of their grains or corn. As mentioned earlier, I have raised a fine crop by this method when my neighbors had very little or nothing. This method of farming is intensely interesting and profitable. Thoroughly pulverize your ground, because those fine roots cannot grow when there are hard clods of dirt, nor will they hold moisture.

It is of very great importance to have the soil worked deep enough so that the roots of all the plants can go far into the ground to draw nourishment and moisture. It is wonderful for both wet and dry seasons. When it is wet, the water can go down into the soil, and when it is dry there is a deep mellow mulch of soil for the roots to penetrate deep enough to get the moisture from beneath. Therefore, when the soil is loose deep down, the moisture will come up and it will not dry out so quickly.

When the soil is loose and finely pulverized, the sun, oxygen, and other life-giving elements can penetrate deeply and give life and proper nourishment to the plants.

It is my desire to arouse the people to thoroughly cultivate their soil, plant at the right time, and thoroughly cultivate their crops. In so doing they will be well repaid for their labor.

Fruits grown in the shade or raised on worn-out ground where commercial fertilizer has been used have very few life-giving properties. Many times even wheat is raised year after year on the same ground without properly taking care of the soil; however, you can put all the minerals back into poor depleted soil by handling your soil right. Just as soon as your crop is harvested, plow the ground and sow it with soybeans, cowpeas, rye, or buckwheat. When the crop is full grown, drag it down and plow it under, plowing deep. In the northern states it must be plowed under before it freezes. This will wonderfully help to make fertile soil. In the fall the ground should be plowed deeply in order to expose it to the sun and air. Red clover, which was formerly used so much for improving soil, does not grow as well as it used to. But with soybeans the ground can be improved much more successfully and more rapidly than with other crops.

It is very easy to raise hay in some of the southern states where hay is scarce by sowing oats and cutting them just before they turn yellow, when the oats are full grown and the straw is yet green. These oats, when cut, make an excellent hay that is real medicine for stock, and the grain is splendid. I have kept work stock in good shape on this kind of hay.

In raising vegetables and truck gardening, I have many times raised two and three crops on the same ground during the same year. When one crop begins to ripen you can work the ground between the rows and plant your second crop so when you harvest the first crop, your second crop is well under way. In this way you can keep on raising two or three crops of some things.

It is well to have a good book on farming and gardening, of which there are many on the market that are not expensive. Learn about the things that grow very quickly and will produce a large amount of food in a short time on a small piece of land. Furthermore, in every state there is a government experimental station that has valuable bulletins on all kinds of farming subjects and many of them are free.

B. FARMING AND GARDENING

Farming and gardening are intensely interesting when you learn to do them correctly. Many people have land but do not make the right use of it to have an abundance of food. Here are some of my personal experiences:

To have EARLY TOMATOES in the extreme northern states where it is very cold and the growing season short, plant the tomatoes in February in a box in the house, if you do not have a greenhouse or a hotbed. Then transplant the plants two or three times before it is time to set them out in the field or garden. The transplanting makes them sturdy and produces large roots, so when they are set out they have lots of vitality and soon make large plants that bear fruit much earlier. Later when it gets warm enough, plant the seeds right out in the garden or field, and do not transplant them at all. Plant a number of seeds in the same place, leaving the strongest plant, and transplant the others.

For EARLY LETTUCE: Sow in the fall early enough for it to make two or three leaves, then get some brush and throw over the bed. Put some straw or hay of some sort over this to shield it against the fierce winter. The brush and straw protect it against the snow and keep it from packing solid and smothering the plants. In the spring, after the hard frosts are over, remove the brush and straw.

For EARLY ONIONS: Plant in the fall. There are a number of varieties with which you can do this. The potato onion is an excellent variety for this. If you write to your seedhouse, they will send you directions for fall planting.

There are varieties of spinach that can be planted in the fall. Let the spinach grow three or four leaves, the same as lettuce, before covering. This will give you spinach, onions, and other greens very early in the spring, much earlier than if you do all your planting in the spring after the ground gets warm enough. In the southern states you can have greens the year around.

For EARLY POTATOES: Plant much earlier than they are

usually planted. I have had potatoes frozen off three or four times, but they seem to grow right along. When they are small it does not hurt them to have the tops frozen off. Thus for early potatoes, I have had them three or four weeks sooner than if I had waited until potatoes are generally planted.

For EARLY STRAWBERRIES: Buy the early varieties and plant them on a southern slope or southeastern slope. Protect them with a little light straw; then when they start to bloom early the frost will not hurt them. When the danger of frost is over, rake the straw off, but leave some between the rows for mulching the strawberries. Plant the late varieties of strawberries on a northern or western slope. Cover them lightly with straw and leave it on until quite late. This will produce a later crop. Then for a general crop, raise them wherever they grow best. Working it this way you will have berries for a much longer time. Get early, late, and everbearing varieties. In this way you can have berries for a long season. I have kept a strawberry bed in good bearing condition for five or six years. After all the berries have been picked, harrow the ground with a fine-toothed harrow, crisscrossing the patch as if you were going to harrow the plants out. This will take out the old plants, thus giving the new ones a better chance.

Keep planting various other garden vegetables at different times so as to have green shelled peas and beans nearly all summer long. You can also plant green corn at different times and have roasting ears all summer. I planted some of the evergreen sweet corn so that it would produce roasting ears just before the frost. Then we would cut the corn, shock it up, and gather roasting ears out of the shocks for a long time after there had been many a hard frost. When you get farther south where the winters are not so long and severe, it is much easier. You can have an abundance of garden stuff all the year around as there are a number of greens and vegetables that will stand light frosts.

Everyone who has any ground at all should have a patch of ground cherries. They grow abundantly and make a fine sauce.

In the fall when fruits and vegetables are cheap, can a lot of food so you will have an abundance during the winter. There are small canners and can sealers that can be used in homes where goods may be canned just as well as in the canning factories. Tin cans are very cheap, but it is really better to use glass jars because they can be reused.

Many years ago I helped a man buy a canner. He had eighty acres of land with a heavy mortgage on it, which he paid off with the help of his canning outfit in just a few years. If you could listen to this man tell his experience with this canning outfit it would be extremely interesting. He said that one time he bought a large two-horse load of pumpkins for $3. He canned them and the proceeds from this one load of pumpkins was nearly $35. Aside from being very practical, canning is a very interesting thing for the children. Give them a share in it and a part of the profits. Every farmer's child should have a garden space of his own, and the profits of that space should be his. When I was on the farm I had but very little to buy and always something to sell.

All farmers should produce an abundance of feed for their stock. I used to cut our grain as early as possible and do my best to get it threshed before it rained on the shocks in order to preserve the straw in the best possible condition. Grain also brings a better price when this is done, and the straw makes excellent feed when it is well taken care of. Always save the cornstalks and do not let them weather out in the field. I always had plenty of feed for my stock using such materials, which could not be readily turned into cash on the market. Thus my feed cost me very little.

We kept our stock in good healthy condition by cutting up red clover, pea hay, and well-preserved cornstalks, and feeding a little bran or shorts over it. The animals would eat this with great relish.

The farm is an intensely interesting place when you work it right. Children get interested in it if you give them some part, and let them have some of the proceeds. I was born and raised on a farm, as I have said before, and the farm has always been interesting to me. Many years afterwards I became interested in the manufacture of health foods. While I experimented extensively in raising food from the soil, I also experimented on a large scale in preparing food that could perfectly nourish the body. I have developed many nice foods and made palatable dishes that are really healthful, invigorating, and life-sustaining. I have a regular experimenting outfit and am continually working to develop food to meet the needs of every disease of the young and old.

Although I have worked at different things during my lifetime, no work is more interesting to me than work on the farm and in the garden. How rewarding it is to take some barren land and make it fertile, straightening out and cleaning up the corners, planting seeds, cultivating and seeing the plants grow and develop, continually adding new and better varieties, trying to produce as early a crop as possible, and then having a continual supply all season long of fresh garden products. It is also satisfying to grow new varieties of flowers and enjoy the old-fashioned varieties that we used to have when we were children. When we were youngsters, and later on young men and women in my parent's home, the farm was heaven on earth for us.

All the good things in the city do not equal the good things that my mother and my sisters would prepare, such as the big panfuls of baked apples with fresh cream over them, and a good piece of old-fashioned coffee cake made from whole-wheat flour. Show me a dish in the city nowadays that beats that. And a dish of clabbered milk that comes out of the icebox on a hot day. Leave the cream on the milk, grate some genuine rye bread over the top of it, together with a little cinnamon and sugar, and then a soup spoon to eat it with. What have you that could beat that? So very delicious and healthful you could practically live and work on it. In those days we made it of cow's milk, but now we make it of soybean milk, which is far better. Also in those days we used cane sugar, but now we use malt sugar, which is infinitely better and like the juice in ripe fruits.

Then I often think about the wonderful dish of fruit soup that we relished so much, made of prunes, raisins, apricots, and various other fruits.

Another dish that we appreciated very much was new potatoes and peas served with Mother's dumplings, which she made with whole wheat flour and which we enjoyed more than any spaghetti that was on the market. Now we have soybean spaghetti, which is even better.

Then when I think of those wonderful pieces of baked squash, which we always enjoyed so much, made of those hard squashes that we had to take an axe to split open and served with nice fresh butter, my mouth waters. We also feasted on parsnips, carrots, and vegetable oysters (salsify), cooked until nearly done and then put in the oven and baked with a little cream.

When strawberry season came on, we relished those big dishes of red-ripe strawberries fresh from the vines with a large piece of homemade coffee cake and some of that wonderful cream. Can you beat that in the city? Most of the strawberries sold in the city are picked too green and are almost worthless. They do not have the delicate flavor that they have when they are picked fresh and ripe from the vines. When fruit is picked fresh from the trees or vines, thoroughly ripened, it is without question an antidote for disease and premature death.

Then when the cherries got ripe, oh! how we did enjoy climbing up in the trees and eating that fruit. We had three different varieties; red, white, and black cherries. We liked the black ones best.

We had an abundance of currants also; red, white, and black. When the raspberries, of which we had an abundance in the garden and also in the woods, were ripe, we used to pick them by the water-buckets full and make juice of them. This is infinitely better than any soft drink that you buy in the cities, and it does not contain any harmful ingredients as they do.

Both the red raspberry leaves and the juice are a wonderful

medicine. It will break any kind of a fever. When we were working out in the fields on a hot day, how we used to enjoy seeing Father or Mother coming with a nice cold pitcher of raspberry juice. I do not believe there is anyone who goes to a counter for a soft drink that enjoys it as much as we enjoyed this fresh juice. Sometimes they would come with a big pitcher of lemonade with fruit juice in it.

When we would pick the different berries, cherries, and currants, my mother would pay us so much a quart. Then we would go downtown on the Fourth of July and other special days and Mother would tell us how much she thought we should spend of the money we had. With most children nowadays, when they get hold of a little money, it burns their pockets, and they are just seeking an opportunity to spend it for some knickknack. Our great ambition was to try and see how big we could make our little pile so we could buy something worthwhile with it. I shall never forget when I was a little lad I had never had a jackknife of my own, so I saved quite a little bit of money. I wanted a jackknife so much that my mother told me I could buy one and she told me just about how much I should spend for it. I bought the knife, and my mother said she thought I did very well. Many times during the day I would put my hand in my pocket and take my knife out and look at it.

It was intensely interesting for us youngsters on the farm as the years rolled around. There was always something to look forward to. When the harvest was gathered, we always enjoyed the threshing and harvesting as the neighbors helped one another. We always had a great time with plenty of good things to eat and all kinds of sports. The children had many innocent sports on the farm. Once we saw the circus man keep three or more apples in the air at the same time and not let them fall to the ground; so when we had spare time we practiced it and got so we could keep four apples in the air without letting them fall to the ground.

Both my younger brother and I were pretty good shots with a rifle. We would throw a bottle in the air, just as high as we could throw it, and when it began to come down we would shoot at it and break it in the air. Sometimes we would have other sports. We would run and jump until we got so we could jump over a fence as high as our heads. Then we would jump off something quite high onto a straw pile and make two somersaults before we would strike the straw.

There were no automobiles in those days, but we had nice horses. My father would let us ride them sometimes. We practiced until we could stand on them and gallop. There were so many interesting things that space will not permit me to mention them all, but suffice it to say that seed time was interesting — to watch the various things grow and have an abundance of foods on our own table.

Harvest time was also extremely interesting. Then we would get wood ready for winter. At times when there was not much to do, we would gather beechnuts, hazelnuts, walnuts, and cranberries, and my sisters would make a fine cranberry jelly. We would make a barrel of sauerkraut and a barrel of string beans, which we sliced up and put up just about like sauerkraut. We made a big crock full of tomato jam. Now we make it without cane sugar.

In those days only 7 to 10 percent of the people were in the cities, while now there are some 80 percent of the people in the cities, cooped up in tenements and apartments. The shows, movies, and pleasures people have in the cities are not wholesome. They are physically and mentally destructive. The pleasures that we had on the farm were of a different nature and would make real men and women out of the people. They were elevating and inspiring, instead of degrading and debasing. The pleasures of the city usually do not make noble men and women, good fathers and mothers, good husbands and wives, or good citizens. On the farm you do not have to be afraid to go out into the dark nor do you have to be afraid that you will not have something to eat. It is a very small matter to arrange to have something to eat, even if there should be a drought. It is very easy to can enough to eat for two or three years. Then if there is a crop failure you would not go hungry. You should also have enough wheat, rye, and barley to last two seasons should there be a crop failure.

Our place was often called "The Garden of Eden." Both my mother and father were lovers of flowers, and we had various trees and hedges, and plenty of fruit at all times. We children were always interested, as we had never learned to run the streets in the cities at night. We had our different little sports evenings, then we would go to bed. Mother and Father always knew where we were at night. We never had that craving for money that young folks in the cities have, because they can never get enough to carry out all their plans and schemes, which are so expensive nowadays.

C. WILD HERBS

One of the most interesting things on the farm was herbs, used both for food and as a medicine. When I was just a very small child, I used to gather red clover blossoms and our father would carry them to the postmaster in town, who was afflicted with cancer. This was over sixty years ago, and I cannot remember the particulars, but I do know that my father took the red clover blossoms to him every year. The postmaster lived to be a very old man.

Then our groceryman had a daughter who was afflicted. What the trouble was I do not remember, but I very distinctly remember that we would gather the wintergreen, which grows very abundantly in that country, and my mother would take it to her. The outcome of that also I do not remember, as it was over half a century ago.

I used to gather the mullein flowers and other herbs for an old doctor. We had what we called the draw-shave, a long narrow knife with two handles, one on each end. We used to shave off the rough bark from the white ash trees, slippery elm, birch, wild cherry, willows, pines, poplars, and a number of other trees, and then after we had the outer bark off, we would shave off the inner fresh bark, which contained the medical properties, and dry this bark so as to have it ready for use. I do not know what people used these barks for then, but I know perfectly well what I am using them for now, because I have been using them for many years and have seen wonderful results. I know from actual experience what they can do for mankind.

Many of the things that occurred when I was a child are as vividly before my mind today as if it were only a short time ago.

ANNOTATION: Much of the farming equipment illustrated and described in this chapter is no longer in use. But the type of plowing recommended in this chapter is definitely standard procedure for organic farming.

It is interesting to note the reception that organic principles of growing have had from government and big business alike for a number of years. Both have been strongly against such methods longer than we'd like to see. One reason for this opposition is the vested interest of special power groups in their own methods of farming. As one scientist recently explained, "All the big-time agricultural research in the west is financed either by the chemical industry or by governments and we all know where the interest of the chemical industry lies, and it *isn't* in organic farming." (John Seymour in "Organic Farming," *New Scientist*, September 27, 1979, page 946.)

Recently, however, the tide has been turning more than ever before in favor of organic farming. Several recent studies give certain aspects of organic farming high marks of praise. Bob S. Bergland, Secretary of Agriculture during the Carter Administration, wrote in 1980, "We need to gain a better understanding of these organic farming systems. As we strive to develop relevant and productive programs for all of agriculture, we look forward to increasing communication between organic farmers and the U. S. Department of Agriculture." Here at last are some extremely positive and very open-minded statements from one of the world's largest agricultural bureaucracies, in guarded favor and careful support of a system that has been maligned and slandered for many years. Astonishingly enough, the recent USDA report on organic farming praised its methods of tilling the ground as compared to the moldboard plowing frequently used by conventional farmers. USDA said the organic methods improve water conservation better than conventional ways do. It is interesting to note that the organic plowing methods favorably recommended by USDA are identical to the ones described by Jethro Kloss in this chapter. (*Report and Recommendations on Organic Farming;* USDA, July 1980, Washington, D. C.; p.iii; 58; and Luther J. Carter, "Organic Farming Becomes 'Legitimate'"; *Science* 209; 254, July 11, 1980.)

Jethro Kloss states that his way of preparing the soil holds the moisture and keeps the water from running off. These same principles which he advocated some 50 years ago were recently evaluated by agricultural scientists and soil biologists independent of the knowledge he had left in this book. Their conclusions were to the effect that "Water erosion was about one-third less" for the crop rotation and plowing methods used on organic farms, (these being the same kind previously suggested by Jethro Kloss). (William Lcokeretz et al., "Organic Farming in the Corn Belt"; *Science* 211:545, Feb. 6, 1981.)

Section II
Herbs for
Healthful Living

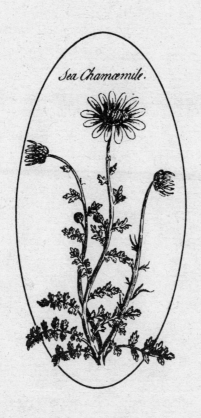

Sea Chamæmile.

1

HISTORY OF HERBAL MEDICINE

A. EARLY PRACTITIONERS

Hippocrates (460-377 B.C.), known as the "father of modern medicine" was, so far as we know, the first man who practiced medicine as an art. The following is the oath Hippocrates took.

I swear by Apollo the physician and Aesculapius, and Health, and All-Heal, and all the gods and goddesses, that, according to my ability and judgment, I will keep this Oath and this stipulation — to reckon him who taught me this Art equally dear to me as my parents, to share my substance with him, and relieve his necessities if required; to look upon his offspring in the same footing as my own brothers, and to teach them this Art, if they shall wish to learn it, without fee or stipulation; and that by precept, lecture, and every other mode of instruction, I will impart a knowledge of the Art to my own sons, and those of my teachers, and to disciples bound by a stipulation and oath according to the law of medicine, but to none others. I will follow that system of regimen which, according to my ability and judgment, I consider for the benefit of my patients, and abstain from whatever is deleterious and mischievous. I will give no deadly medicine to anyone if asked, nor suggest any such counsel; and in like manner I will not give to a woman a pessary to produce abortion. With purity and with holiness I will pass my life and practice my Art. I will not cut persons laboring under the stone, but will leave this to be done by men who are practitioners of this work. Into whatever houses I enter, I will go into them for the benefit of the sick, and will abstain from every voluntary act of mischief and corruption; and further, from the seduction of females or males, of freemen and slaves. Whatever in connection with my professional practice, or not in connection with it, I see or hear, in the life of men, which ought not be spoken of abroad, I will not divulge, as reckoning that all such should be kept secret. While I continue to keep this Oath unviolated, may it be granted to me to enjoy life and the practice of the Art, respected by all men, in all times, but should I trespass and violate this Oath, may the reverse be my lot.

Hippocrates

Hippocrates is also known as the "father of medical literature." His treatises are filled with practical knowledge of the difficulties of the human race and this knowledge may be derived from studying his works at the present time. We find that he believed in natural healing and left many things to the "effort of nature." In his oath, he swore he would give no deadly medicine, which means he would not knowingly give anything of a harmful or destructive nature. He belonged to the "regular school," but he was also an herbal practitioner. He used no minerals, unless salt was considered to be a mineral by some physicians. His methods of treatment were used until the year A.D.1500. History seems to indicate that during this long period of time no "regular" physicians were unwise enough to attempt chemical poisoning of the body.

ADDENDUM: Hippocrates was truly "the father of medical science." Prior to his time, the treatment of disease was in the hands of the priests, but Hippocrates showed that disease had only natural causes and removed the treatment of disease from the temple priests. He insisted that only nature could heal the body and that the physician was only nature's helper. He used this rule in his practice, treating his patients with herbs, proper diet, fresh air, proper exercise, and attention to correct habits and living conditions. Between 300 and 400 plants are mentioned in the Hippocratic writings and nearly a third of these plants are still in use at the present time. The Hippocratic oath is still used by the medical profession, providing a sense of duty to mankind that has not been lost.

The Greek god Apollo was believed to bring on illness and plagues by shooting certain types of "arrows." He was addressed as the "two-horned god" in Orphic hymns. But there was only one original two-horned god, Nimrod, who founded the Chaldean monarchy. Nimrod was the original Apollo. Apollo was the mighty hunter who went before the Lord and was the husband of Semiramis. Aesculapius, also called Asclepios, (Fig.1) the legendary son of Apollo, eventually became the predominant Greek and Roman god of healing. Numerous temples were dedicated to him throughout the kingdoms of Greece and Rome. These temples were extremely popular among all classes of people, and even though Asclepios was the god of healing, the temples seem mostly to have been a mixture of a religious shrine and what today would be known as a health spa. The vast majority of the illnesses treated at these temples were most likely psychologically based, and the most important part of the temple "cures" was faith.

Many members of Asclepios's family were also involved in different aspects of health and healing. His wife Epione was known as a soother of pain. A daughter, Hygeia, eventually came to represent healthful living and the prevention of disease, while another daughter, Panacea, represented the treatment of illness. Two of his sons, Machaon and Podalirios, became patron gods of surgeons and physicians.

The name Aesculapius is not in the Greek, Egyptian, Assyrian, or Hebrew languages, but is found in the Chaldean language. There are three words that make up the word Aesculapius — ashe, skul, aphe. The word ashe means man, skul means instruct, aphe means snake. Aesculapius, therefore, means man-instructing-snake. In the Bible we are told that Satan working through the serpent was the only man instructing snake, a menace to all mankind.

Among other early healers, and as prominent as any, was Scribonius Largus, a Roman, who lived during the reign of Nero. He wrote a book containing a cure-all formula made up of 61 ingredients. This preparation was first used as a

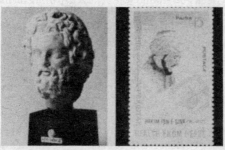

FIG. 1   FIG. 2

treatment for snakebite. Snake flesh was first added to the
formula in the first century A.D. by Andromachus, the physician of Nero. Nero was one of the best known but cruelest
of the Roman emperors. It was at about this time that this
multi-ingredient formula first came to be called theriac, the
name coming from the Greek word that means "wild beast."
As time passed, more and more ingredients were added until
during the Middle Ages the number reached more than one
hundred. Theriac was used by persons in all walks of life, not
only as a means of preventing illness, but also to treat all
manner of plagues, infections, poisonous bites, and pestilences. The fact that it contained opium may well have
accounted for some of its widespread popularity. It was still
being used in a variety of forms in some countries of Europe
as recently as the nineteenth century.

But the physicians who followed Hippocrates's teachings
were convinced that they should not give any deadly medicine. Those kinds of medicines were eagerly sought for by
the ignorant people, who thought that if medicine made the
bowels active it was good and would heal them, as people
think of present-day cathartics. When taking these harmful
medicines, however, they defied the life force of the body.

Avicenna (980-1037), the most influential of the Arabic
contributors to medicine, was commemorated on a postage
stamp during the Pakistani Health Institute in 1966 (Fig.2).

Because he believed that somewhere in the world there

was a specific plant that could be used to cure each illness, Avicenna traveled far from his homeland of Persia into distant countries, collecting hundreds of herbs, roots, and seeds. In recognition of this, the words "health from herbs" can be seen printed across the bottom of the stamp.

While he wrote nearly 100 books during his lifetime of 58 years, by far the best known is his *Canon of Medicine,* containing nearly one million words. This was largely a systematic compilation of the works of Hippocrates and Galen, but it was used as a standard text for medical education throughout Asia and Europe until the mid-seventeenth century.

B.   CHEMISTRY AND ALCHEMY

Near the end of the fifteenth century there was a physician and chemist living in Europe named William Bombast von Hohenheim. A son was born to him in 1493 near Einsiedeln, Switzerland whom he named Theophrastus Bombastus von Hohenheim. The son was carefully taught in the same schools as his father, but he soon became dissatisfied with the instruction of his father and teachers and left school to wander about Europe, learning all he could about alchemy, chemistry, and metallurgy in relation to their application to medicine. He finally went to work in the mines of Tyrol. There he saw minerals purified by the action of other minerals and he conceived the idea of purifying the human body in the same manner. He began using minerals to treat his patients, but kept no record of these experiments. He was the first to point out the relation between goiter in the parent and the condition called cretinism in the child. He wrote an excellent description of hospital gangrene and preceded Lister in declaring that "In wounds, nature is the real healer. All that is necessary is to prevent infection and wound diseases." He called himself Paracelsus, for what reason we do not know, unless to designate that he was above Celsus (53 B.C.-A.D.7) who, although not a physician, was well-known as a great medical encyclopedist.

An alchemist, his ideas about the human body were those of a chemist. He salivated his patients when they had "actions of the bowels," so that it seemed as though he knew what to do for them. Even though he believed that the stars and planets were the main influence that caused human illness, and that all diseases should be treated with minerals, he eventually came to be called the "father of pharmacology."

He was one of the first men, while making a profession of practicing medicine, to give mercury to his patients. He used it in both large and small doses. At least two thousand years earlier, however, history tells us that the Chinese were using mercury to treat ulcers. Even to the present day, the use of minerals has increased until now the majority of doctors in the civilized world use minerals to purify the body.

The herbalists in Great Britain are called botanic practitioners and are the successors of the Greek physicians, Galen and Hippocrates, but the conventional doctors of today are successors of Hohenheim of the fifteenth century.

From 460 B.C. to A.D. 1500, a period of over nineteen hundred years, we have no record of anyone giving large doses of poisonous minerals for the cure of disease until Hohenheim thought of using them after he worked in the mines at Tyrol. During those 1900 years there had been very little deviation from the beliefs and teachings of Hippocrates that "in nature there is strength" to cure disease.

From 1526 to 1528, Hohenheim lectured at the University of Basel, but was dismissed because of his refusal to accept time-honored traditions. It is stated that he publicly burned the books of Galen and Hippocrates, threw aside all of their ideas and instead went in for chemically purifying the body by the use of minerals. Wherever he went, however, he was met by opposition to his theories.

Several stories are told to account for his death in Salzburg, Austria where he was living at the time. It is commonly believed that he was thrown from a window by his rivals in 1541 when he was only 50 or 51 years old. (*World Book Encyclopedia,* volume 13, 1959, page 6090.)

Although he did not live a long life, he transformed the practice of medicine. After his death, hundreds of people took up his practice of treating illnesses with minerals in place of herbs, roots, and barks.

There seems to be no doubt that when Columbus returned to the Old World after discovering America in 1492, either he or some of his men brought with them the germs that cause syphilis. There are people, however, who have doubts that this disease originated in America. The Italians called it a French disease and the French people said it originated in Spain. Syphilis and gonorrhea have been recognized for thousands of years, and may even have existed during the time the pharaohs ruled in Egypt. It is probably safe to say, whether syphilis originated in America or not, that during this time there was apparently one of the periodical increases in the prevalence of this disease. It was called the "new disease" in the early part of the fifteenth century. In fact, Hohenheim tried his mercurial compounds on his patients who had syphilis, and in his works stated that this treatment seemed to "drive out humor." The mercury was sometimes given in such large doses, however, that the end results proved fatal. This is the way that mercury came into general medical use in the treatment of syphilis.

Chemical reactions which take place in the human body do not necessarily follow the same chemical laws that minerals do, and therefore the body cannot be purified by taking another mineral. This practice led the world into the deception of dosing the body with a poison to counteract another poison, but in reality this method merely added another poison to one already in the body. Mercury cures absolutely nothing, but creates a far worse condition in the system than was there before. The giving of quicksilver (mercury or Quack Salber) resulted in the naming of physicians who treated patients with quicksilver "quacks."

In the early part of the eighteenth century, a German physician by the name of Hahneman set forth the idea that it would be better to give smaller doses of medicines. He started giving medicines in powdered form, and in such small doses that it had little effect. He did not discard the old *materia medica*, but in addition to giving mercury, arsenic, and many other minerals, he included some of the most filthy serums, unsanitary preparations from bees, bedbugs, snake poisons, etc. Anyone who would take the time to study and learn about the composition and functions of the human body would realize that minerals and such unsanitary medicines could not prove a remedy for any of the ills of man. Hahneman was wrong when he ignored the fact that it is the strength of nature that restores the body.

C. HERBAL MEDICINE

Herbs have been used from antiquity and were the first medicine used by man, while allopathic medicine (the use of minerals to treat disease) is only about 500 years old.

The use of herbs in the written record actually dates back for several thousands of years B.C. The Chinese, Sumerians, and Egyptians all used plants for medicinal purposes. A Chinese book on herbs, dated around 2700 B.C., lists over 300 plants with their medicinal uses. In Old Testament times, several herbs are mentioned, including aloe.

In 1926 a large stone slab was discovered in the tomb of an Egyptian official, located near the great pyramids. The figures carved into the stone indicate that the man buried here had been named Iry and was the Chief of Court Physicians. Also revealed on the slab is that "doctor" Iry, and probably other physicians during this same period of Egyptian history, was a specialist. Among other things he was called the Eye Doctor of the Palace, and the Doctor of the Abdomen. Herodotus, often called "the father of history," seems to endorse this concept of specialization among Egyptian physicians. He wrote the first account of Egyptian medicine that we have available (c.450 B.C.). In it he notes that each Egyptian "physician treats a single disease and no more."

The painstaking work of deciphering Egyptian papyri has

shown that probably one-third of the medicinal plants and herbs listed in a modern pharmacopoeia were known and used by the Egyptians. Among these are garlic, flaxseed, fennel, juniper, sycamore, pine, senna, thyme, celandine, cinquefoil, black hellebore, tamarisk, celery, mandrake, henbane, willow, mulberry, myrrh, saffron, thyme, and onion, to name but a few.

In the first century A.D., a Greek physician by the name of Dioscorides composed a long treatise on the properties and uses of over 500 medicinal plants. This exhaustive and authoritative reference work remained in use until about the seventeenth century. The preservation of the knowledge of herbal medicine during the Middle Ages can be attributed to the monks, who not only copied the ancient manuscripts, but also cultivated their own herbal gardens in the monasteries and used the herbs for the treatment of many common disorders.

In England during the Elizabethan era, herbalism experienced a golden age, from which most of our present day herbal lore derives. Following the invention of the printing press in the fifteenth century, a large number of books on herbs were printed.

In 1551, William Turner published his *Newe Herball* with detailed illustrations of a variety of medicinal plants, and this initiated a renaissance in herbalism.

By far the best known and best liked of the English herbalists, however, was John Gerard, who published his herbal book, *The Herball or General Historie of Plantes*, in 1597. Gerard was a Tudor surgeon, apothecary to James I and superintendent of the gardens of the court of Queen Elizabeth, where he cultivated over 1,000 herbs. Gerard's herbal lists 2,000 plants. Common and scientific names are given in a variety of languages, descriptions of each plant, and finally the virtues of each herb, in a noble attempt to separate effective folk medicine from fiction.

The next noteworthy English herbalist was John Parkinson, director of the Royal Gardens at Hampton Court, who in 1640 wrote *Theatrum Botanicum,* Man encyclopedic work covering over 3,000 plants and their medicinal uses.

The *English Physician Enlarged* was written in 1653 by Nicholas Culpepper. Culpepper was the most controversial of the English herbalists. During the Dark Ages, it had been noted that certain parts of a plant might resemble in form or color some part of the human body, and it was believed that diseases affecting a particular part or organ in the body could be cured by the application of the corresponding plant. For example, the unusual appearance of the two-pronged root of the mandragora, or mandrake plant, was thought to resemble the two legs of a human, as shown in this old illustration (Fig.3). Thus, the healing properties of the plant were indicated by its "signature"; that is, its shape, texture, or manner of growing, so it was only necessary to develop the "insight" or "sensitivity" to perceive the plant's "signature" in order to discover its medicinal use. The relationship between humans and plants was perceived as vital, dynamic, and entailing mutual communication on the level of vibrations. According to Culpepper, "Modern writers may laugh about it, but I wonder in my heart how the virtues of herbs first came to be known if not by their signatures. The moderns have them from the writings of the ancients — the ancients had no writings to have them from."

Culpepper's complete herbal incurred the wrath of the medical establishment of the seventeenth century, because he included an authorized translation of a portion of the Latin pharmacopoeia of the Royal College of Physicians. He also believed that astrology had a strong influence on the healing powers of plants and that the positions of stars affected human health and behavior. The medical establishment accused Culpepper of being a drunkard and a lecher (which he was, according to other sources) and he denounced the Royal College of Physicians as "proud, insulting, and domineering dunces." (From *Herbal Connection* by Ethan Nebalcouf, May 1981, pages 21 and 22.)

Two large and beautifully illustrated books on English

herbs were published in the eithteenth century. William Salmon's *The English Herbal or History of Plants*, published in London in 1710 (Fig. 4), and *An History of Plants and Trees, Natives of Britain, Cultivated for Use, or Raised for Beauty*, by John Hill, was also published in London a few years later, in 1756.

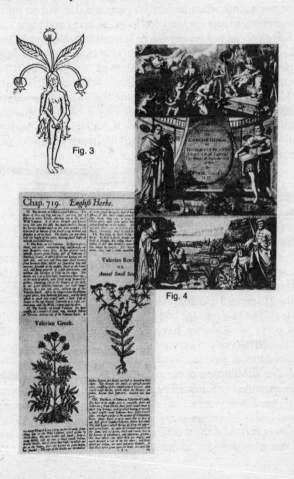

Fig. 3

Fig. 4

In 1769, Samuel Thomson was born in Alstead, New Hampshire. He was one of six children, the son of a poor New Hampshire farmer and learned the use of herbs from local practitioners of folk medicine. He was often taken to the woods to help a botanic practitioner and midwife by the name of Benton gather herbs and plants. He went to school for one month when he was 10 years old. He had no other education, except for the knowledge of herbs and roots and their effect on sick people that he learned from Benton. When Thomson was very young, he experimented with the herb lobelia. He chewed it and swallowed the juice until he vomited, and called it the emetic herb. When about 19 years old, Thomson was laid up for some time when he severely injured his leg. But instead of cutting it off, he applied a poultice of comfrey root and saved his leg. When he was about 24 years old, he remembered the action of lobelia and started to make use of it.

The saying "History repeats itself" was certainly true in the career of Samuel Thomson. Although he was an uneducated farmer without medical training and knew nothing of Roman history, he perfected the same treatment that was practiced by the Romans 2,000 years earlier. Hippocrates, the "father of medicine," also lived in poverty during his youth.

There is no doubt that Thomson demonstrated the emetic qualities of lobelia and that his ideas were correct about the necessity of eliminating waste materials from the body in order to restore it to a natural condition of health. Thomson's idea was to cleanse the body. His idea of steaming the body is what the Russians have been doing for centuries. He steamed the body to get outward (surface) heat and used herb stimulants to produce inward heat.

The introduction of naturopathy in America can probably be attributed to Samuel Thomson. Along with herbs, Thomson used steam baths, diet, and massage. Samuel Thomson's motto was "To make every man his own physician." Many people followed the theories of Thomson after he died. His ideas of relaxation, stimulation, and the use of astringents were used by many doctors because they were satisfied with the correctness of the results.

Dr. Curtis of Cincinnati, Ohio, chartered one of the first colleges that followed Dr. Thomson's teachings from the Ohio legislature and W. H. Cook took charge of another. When Dr. Curtis died, the institution was moved to Chicago under the name of College of Medicine and Surgery.

Along natural medical lines, England and many other countries are far ahead of the United States. Many years ago naturopathic doctors were given permission to practice in England, and herbal doctors are fast growing in popularity and favor with the people. Even English royalty now employs herbal doctors.

For centuries the American Indians, as well as natives of other countries, have used all kinds of herbs, roots, and barks in the healing art, and they are still using them today.

As more and more settlers arrived in the New World from Europe, their knowledge of herbs was combined with the herbal lore of the native Americans and this combination produced a distinctly American folk medicine. But during this same time, the orthodox medical establishments in Europe and America were moving farther away from natural methods of healing and relying more on chemicals, leeches, and bloodletting.

2

HERBS

The great remedial properties of herbs and the juices of fruits and vegetables have been recognized and appreciated from time immemorial. Only since Theophrastus von Hohenheim started using chemicals during the sixteenth century have people been looking for, and depending on, medicines artificially prepared from chemicals. People have been diverted from the true healing remedies by misleading advertising. It seemed as though false science had succeeded. Chemical poisons are now very convenient to obtain and are quick-acting. People were deceived for a time, but at last they are seeing the effects of drugs and their evil aftereffects, and are looking for something better.

When the Saxon invaders entered Great Britain they took with them much knowledge concerning herbal healing. It is well-known that they made frequent use of the dandelion, comfrey, nettle, burdock, and other common wayside herbs in treating the sick. The girls were taken into the fields by their parents and taught the names and healing virtues of the plants. And so a knowledge was planted that grew until it has become customary to have an "herb garden" in England. What a blessing it would be to the homes in this land if our children were taught the value of raspberry leaves, thyme, sage, peppermint, yarrow, and dozens of other wayside herbs. More than half the sickness and deaths in early life would be unknown, and chronic sufferers would be a curiosity. Only those who know the value of herbal remedies can appreciate the wonderful effects that a knowledge of the herbs we tread underfoot daily would produce.

With all our boasted knowledge, we have to admit that the North American Indians and the natives of other countries, though unskilled in letters and without any knowledge of anatomy, physiology, or chemistry, use simple herbs to prevent and cure many diseases that baffle the best efforts of the medical doctors.

Herbal healing was the first system of healing that the world knew. My parents, originally from Germany, brought with them much knowledge of these simple herbs, as told elsewhere in this book. I gathered many of them as a small child, and was taught their use.

Why use herbs? They are Nature's remedies and have been placed here by an all-wise Creator. There is an herb for every disease that the human body may be afflicted with. The use of herbs is the oldest medical science. Herbs were mentioned in the Bible from the beginning of creation. Much has been written about herbs all down through history, to the present day.

A. THE BIBLE ON HERBS

When God created this world and planted a beautiful garden in Eden, He placed the tree of life in the center of the garden (Genesis 2: 8,9). This tree corresponds to the tree of life, found in the Paradise of God, of which the redeemed will some day eat freely. "The angel also showed me the river of the water of life, sparkling like crystal, and coming from the throne of God and of the Lamb and flowing down the middle of the city's street. On each side of the river was the tree of life, which bears fruit twelve times a year, once each month; and its leaves are for the healing of the nations" (Revelation 22:1,2 *Good News Bible*).

On the third day of creation He also made all kinds of plants for food. "Then He commanded, 'Let the earth produce all kinds of plants, those that bear grain and those that bear fruit — and it was done. So the earth produced all kinds of plants, and God was pleased with what he saw." (Genesis 1:11,12, *Good News Bible*). After He had created human beings, God told them what He had made for them to eat. "And God said, Behold, I have given you every herb bearing seed, which is upon the face of all the earth, and every tree, in the which is the fruit of a tree yielding seed; to you it shall be for meat (food)" (Genesis 1:29).

After man was driven from the Garden of Eden and no longer had access to the tree of life, God added herbs to man's diet. He also advises us to partake of them to keep from getting sick. "Thorns also and thistles shall it bring forth to thee; and thou shalt eat the herb of the field" (Genesis 3:18). Herbs are one of God's remedial agents for afflicted humanity. His plan was that everyone should raise herbs in his garden, and also gather those that grow wild everywhere and use them when needed.

This is what my parents and many others did. We were never sick, and we never had to call a doctor. If we would only return to God's original design for the human family, sickness would be rare instead of common.

Some of the first things Moses taught the Israelites after they left Egypt was to keep their premises clean, wash their clothes and their bodies, and discard all the harmful articles, including the lustful diet of flesh that they had been eating while they were slaves in Egypt. They were taught to live on simple nourishing food and to use herbs for their medicine. David, in the Psalms, wrote that the grass was caused to grow for the cattle, and herbs for the service of man (Psalms 104:14).

The Prophet Ezekiel said that the fruit of the tree was for man's meat (food), and the leaves for man's healing (Ezekiel 47:12).

The great Apostle Paul said, when referring to the human body, "Don't you realize that you yourselves are the temple of God, and that God's Spirit lives in you? God will destroy anyone who defiles his temple, for his temple is holy — that is exactly what you are!" (1 Corinthians 3:17, *Phillips.*)

After he was taken as a captive to Babylon as a young man, and while studying in the royal court of King Nebuchadnezzar, Daniel decided not to defile himself with the king's rich food, nor with the wine. After partaking of nothing but vegetables and water for a period of only ten days, he was found to be healthier and stronger than all the young men who had been eating the royal food. You can read this interesting story for yourself in the Bible. It is found in Daniel 1:1-16.

Solomon, the wisest man that ever lived, said: "Better is a dinner of herbs where love is than a fatted ox and hatred with it" (proverbs 15:17, *R.S.V.*).

When Samuel, one of God's foremost prophets, was training young men for the ministry or the priesthood, he taught them the use of herbs.

Following are some other texts in the Bible that refer to the use of herbs.

"And Ahab (King of Israel) spake unto Naboth, saying, Give me thy vineyard that I may have it for a garden of herbs, because it is near unto my house" (I Kings 21:2).

"They were as the grass of the field, and as the green herb" (2 Kings 19:26).

"For they shall soon be cut down like the grass, and wither as the green herb" (Psalms 37:2).

"How long shall the land mourn, and the herbs of every field wither?" (Jeremiah 12:4).

"For the land, whither thou goest in to possess it, is not as the land of Egypt, from whence ye came out, where thou sowedst thy seed, and wateredst it with thy foot, as a garden of herbs" (Deuteronomy 11:10).

The priests in Christ's time were well acquainted with herbs. They used to take herbs to counteract their gluttonous living, as well as using them for food. Rue, which they used quite freely, is a wonderful medicine to quiet and soothe the nerves and give clearness to the head. "You tithe mint and rue and every herb, and neglect justice and the love of God" (Luke 11:42, *Revised Standard Version*).

"Then one went into the field to gather herbs and gathered from a wild vine his lap full of wild gourds, and returned and cut them up into the pot of pottage; for they were unknown to them. So they poured out for the men to eat. But as they ate of the pottage, they cried out, 'Oh man of God, there is death in the pot!' and they could not eat it" (2 Kings 4:39,40, *Amplified Bible*). This Scripture teaches everyone that when using herbs they should learn to know the plants thoroughly, so that they will gather the nonpoisonous instead of the poisonous herbs.

ADDENDUM: We quote from the *FDA Consumer,* October 1983, as follows. "If you gather your own herbs to brew a cup of tea, be *absolutely 100 percent certain* that the herb you pick is the herb you seek.... There are half a million known plant species. Less than 1 percent are poisonous. But it takes only one error." This is good advice.

B.   GATHERING AND PRESERVING HERBS

It must be understood that both wide experience and knowledge of herbs are needed to successfully gather and preserve them. It is a study of a lifetime. Lack of knowledge in the gathering and preserving of herbs may render them of little or no medicinal value. Knowledge of the soil is also necessary. Plants grown in virgin soil will contain far greater medicinal value than those grown on poor, nutritionally depleted soil. The same plants grown in different localities will show a great difference in the amount of curative properties they contain. There is a difference between cultivated plants and those growing in their natural wild state. For instance, the dandelion growing wild has rare medicinal properties that are almost entirely lost when the plant is cultivated. Wild herbs are more effective for use in medicines than those grown in the garden.

Gather herbs only in dry weather, preferably when the plant is in full bloom or the seeds are getting ripe.

Barks: The barks should be taken when the sap is rising in the spring. Shave off the rough outer part; then peel the inner part from the trunk of the tree. To dry, put in the sun for a short time (if desired), then complete the drying in the shade. Be sure the pieces of bark are thoroughly dry. If there is any moisture left in them when they are put away, they will mold.

Roots: Dig up the roots either in the spring when the sap is rising or in the late autumn, after the sap has gone down. Slice and dry the roots in the shade, tie them up in small bundles, and put them in the attic or some place where they are sure to keep dry.

Flowers, Seeds, and Leaves: Flowers, seeds, and leaves should be gathered when they are in their prime, gathering only the perfect ones. These should also be dried in the shade. When thoroughly dry, put them in heavy brown paper bags.

Do not preserve herbs in glass, because sometimes the glass sweats. If any moisture comes in contact with the herbs they will become moldy.

When barks, roots, or other herbs are thoroughly dried and kept dry, they will retain their medicinal value for years.

Bark, roots, flowers, seeds, or leaves may all be dried for a short time in the sun, but always complete the drying process in the shade. Too much exposure to the sun tends to lessen the medicinal value. They may be dried entirely in the shade in an airy place. The only thing gained by putting them in the sun for a short time is to hasten the drying process.

GENERAL DIRECTIONS FOR THE PREPARATION AND USE OF HERBS

Herbal preparations should be made fresh every day: the only exceptions are the herbal salves, liniments, and ointments and also those preparations that are made with alcohol, such as tinctures.

Eating a good, diversified diet, getting regular rest and outdoor exercise, and following the other rules for good health given in this book will all be a great help in assisting the herbs to do their work of restoring the normal healthy balance in the system. Don't forget that herbs do not usually give rapid results as drugs do. *Because of their milder action, herbs must be taken over a period of weeks or even months, depending on the condition being treated, in order to produce a lasting, beneficial effect.* In general, the longer the disease has been present in the body, the longer it will take the herbs to have a noticeable effect.

It is also important to remember that when herbal preparations are used for children, weak or debilitated persons, or the elderly, the doses given in this book must be adjusted downward to one-third to two-thirds of the average adult dose.

While the proper use of herbs can be of very great importance in the maintenance or recovery of one's health, the careless or excessive use of certain herbs can result in a real health hazard. There is a common saying that if a little is good, more is even better. This must be interpreted with great care when it is applied to taking medicine, even natural products such as herbs. A more accurate paraphrase of this saying might be: if taking 3 capsules of a certain herb makes you feel better, taking 6 capsules will not necessarily make you feel twice as good, nor will it help you to recover your health twice as fast. In fact, taking more than the recommended dose may result in serious health consequences, for plants may contain chemicals, as well as other substances, that can prove dangerous if they are not recognized and treated with proper respect.

A. TYPES OF HERBAL PREPARATIONS

Infusion: An infusion is usually made just like a tea. Boiling water is poured onto a certain amount of the herb, usually the leaves or flowers, in a cup or other suitable container. This is covered with a saucer or other cover and allowed to steep, in order to give the ingredients in the herb time to pass into the water. The aromatic and volatile ingredients, vitamins, and essences are removed by the infusion. The average amount of herb used is 1/2 to 1 ounce in a pint of water or 1 teaspoon of the herb in 1 cup of water. After the boiling water has been poured on the plants, let them set, covered, for about 10 to 20 minutes. Never allow an infusion to boil. After the water has cooled sufficiently, strain carefully into a cup or other container and drink when it is cool or lukewarm. Some honey may be added if desired, to improve the taste. Take the infusion while it is still hot for colds, influenza, coughs, or to produce sweating. Most infusions are taken in small doses, regularly spaced during the day, using a total of about 1 to 3 cups, depending on the condition and the herb used.

When the twigs, stems, or other larger parts of the plant are used, they should be cut into small pieces and let steep for a longer period of time.

Always use glass, porcelain, or enamel cooking utensils.

Decoction: A decoction is made by simmering the plant part in water, in a nonmetal container, for 3 to 5 minutes or even up to 30 minutes if the material is very hard. Keep the container covered. Use 1 teaspoon of the powdered herb or 1 tablespoon of the cut herb to a cup of water. If you are planning to simmer the decoction for 30 minutes, always start with about 30 percent more liquid to allow for evaporation. For example, if you would usually use 1 ounce of the herb to a pint of water, start with one and a half pints instead, so that there will be about one pint left after 30 minutes. Strain carefully before using. Directions for taking are the same as for infusions. This method is used for extracting the active ingredients from the tougher parts of the plant, such as roots, bark, and seeds. Roots must be simmered one-half hour or more in order to extract their medicinal value. Simmer only; DO NOT BOIL HARD.

When you gather the roots and bark yourself, cut or crush them fine. If you raise or gather herbs and barks, use good judgment in making teas; if you find them too strong, add more water.

Tincture: A tincture is a very concentrated extract of an herb in liquid form. Tinctures are useful when it is unpleasant to take the herb in another form because of its bad taste or if it must be taken over a long period of time. Tinctures are also used to rub on the skin as a liniment. Tinctures are usually made from potent herbs that are not commonly used as teas.

Extract: An extract is a highly concentrated liquid form of an herb, about 10 times as potent as a tincture. It is made by a variety of means such as high pressure, evaporation by heat, or cold percolation. Each herb is treated in a manner that is best suited to extract its medicinal properties.

Extracts are a popular and convenient way of taking and storing herbs and they are faster acting than teas, capsules, or powdered herbs.

Herbal extracts are readily obtained at most herb shops. The usual dose is from 6 to 8 drops. This amount is about equal to 1 teaspoon of the tincture.

Teas: There are some general rules that should be followed when making herb teas. The usual amount of herb used is 1 teaspoon of the dried herb or 3 teaspoons of the freshly crushed herb to one cup of boiling water. Pour the cup of boiling water over the herb and let set (steep) for 5 to 10 minutes. To make the tea stronger, use more of the herb; do not steep for a longer time as this will tend to make the tea bitter. Milk or cream added to the tea will cover up the natural flavor of the herb.

In warm weather, herb tea must be made fresh every day to prevent souring. It can be kept longer in a refrigerator, but not for more than one week.

How much to take? Good judgment must be exercised in the amount of herbs taken, usually four cups a day – one cup an hour before each meal, and one cup upon retiring. Each person has a different constitution; therefore, if good results are not obtained by taking as directed, increase or decrease as may be best. For instance, if the herbs are not laxative enough, increase the dose; if too laxative, decrease the dose. The bowels should move one or two times a day if three meals are eaten.

Most herb teas now come already prepared in tea bags, either as a single herb or in various combinations. Some feel that the bag filters out the delicate flavor of the herb. You may wish to try both methods to see which one you prefer. When using a tea bag, it should be placed in a cup and boiling water added. Cover and let steep for 3 to 5 minutes. Never use aluminum pans.

For example, golden seal may be taken in three ways, as follows:

1. Take one-fourth to one-half teaspoonful golden seal dissolved in one-fourth glass of water. Follow by drinking one glass of water. Take one to four doses a day. One No.00 capsule equals one-fourth to one-half teaspoonful of powder. This varies somewhat according to the size of the powder grains, with the finer powders being less potent.

2. Steep a heaping teaspoonful of golden seal in a pint of boiling water for 20 minutes, stir thoroughly, let settle, and pour off the clear liquid. Take eight table-spoonfuls a day, taking two tablespoonfuls 15 minutes before each meal and the remainder upon retiring. You

may double the above amount and take even more with benefit. For some, taking this amount of golden seal only every other week or two weeks out of three, is more beneficial than using it constantly.

3. Take in gelatin capsules and drink one or more glasses of water with the capsules. Gelatin capsules may be purchased at most retail or wholesale drug stores. I make most use of No. 1, No. 0, and No. 00 sizes, but there are smaller sizes. As a rule, take two of the No. 00 size for a dose, more or less according to need.

Granulated or finely cut herbs: Steep a heaping teaspoonful of herbs in a cup of boiling water for 20 minutes, strain, and take one cup one hour before each meal and one cup on retiring. You may take more or less as the case requires. If too strong, use less herbs per cup.

Powdered herbs: The powdered herbs may be mixed in hot or cold water. The herbs take effect quicker if taken in hot water. Use 1/2 teaspoonful of the herb to 1/4 glass of water. Follow by drinking one glass of water, either hot or cold. This is about the same as taking one No.00 capsule.

Capsules: Most herbs may be purchased in either powdered or capsule form. The average dose is two capsules two or three times a day. Whichever form you decide to use, capsules or powder, follow the directions as given on the container. A No.0 capsule contains about 10 grains of the herb, while a No.00 capsule holds approximately 15 grains. Notice that a No.00 capsule does not contain twice as much material as a No.0 capsule, but holds roughly half again as much.

Herbs for sensitive patients and children: Persons who have very sensitive stomachs, stomach ulcers, etc., may at times become nauseated and sick after taking some of the best old-fashioned herbs. If this happens, do not become alarmed. It is not the herbs that are at fault, but the sensitive condition of the stomach. In cases where the stomach is very sensitive, start by taking teaspoonful doses of tea often – say, every 15 minutes – and increase the amount until it becomes possible to take the required amount.

Powdered herbs may be mixed with foods such as mashed potatoes, mashed vegetables of any kind, or ground-up sweet fruits such as figs or dates.

To the herb tea you can add a little honey or malt sugar, especially for children, to make it more palatable. Do not use refined sugar or sugar substitutes.

NEVER TAKE DRUGS WHEN TAKING NONPOISONOUS HERBS. THE TWO DO NOT WORK TOGETHER.

DO NOT PREPARE HERBS OR FOOD IN ALUMINUM COOKING UTENSILS.

B.   HOW TO MAKE SYRUPS

A Simple Syrup: Dissolve three pounds of brown sugar in a pint of boiling water and boil until thick. To this you may add any medicinal substance.

Malt honey, bee's honey, or Karo syrup may also be used in making syrups. To make an herb syrup, you simply add the cut herbs (or if using granulated herbs, sift them first so there will not be any dust or sediment). Boil to a syrupy consistency and stir thoroughly; then strain through a double cheesecloth, and bottle.

Lemon Syrup: Boil one pint of lemon juice ten minutes, strain, add three pounds of brown sugar, and boil a few minutes longer.

Wild Cherry Syrup:
    2 ounces wild cherry bark
    2 ounces cubeb berries
    2 ounces mullein
    2 ounces skunk cabbage
    2 ounces lobelia herb
    4 pounds brown sugar
    Juice of 4 lemons

Place the first five ingredients in a large kettle. Add four quarts of boiling water, simmer ten minutes, let stand until nearly cold, then strain through a double cheesecloth. Put in a large porcelain cooking pan and add four pounds of brown sugar. Boil this down to a medium thick syrup – it must be thick enough so it will not sour. Add the juice of four lemons and let boil two or three minutes longer. Strain again. When cool, it is ready for use or for bottling.

C. HERBAL SALVES

Use fresh leaves, flowers, roots, barks, or the dried granulated or powdered herbs. If you gather the herbs yourself and use them fresh, be sure to cut them up fine.

Use one pound of herbs to one and a half pounds of cocoa fat, or any pure vegetable oil, and four ounces of beeswax. It is necessary to use a little more beeswax in the warmer climates, as this is the ingredient that keeps the salve firm.

Mix the above together, cover, and place in the hot sun or in an oven with the fire turned low for three or four hours. Strain through a fine sieve or cloth. When it is cold, it will be firm and ready for use. It can be used, however, before it is cold.

D. POULTICES

The following herbs are especially useful for making poultices: balm, flaxseed, gum arabic, hyssop, marshmallow, mustard, slippery elm, virgin's bower, wintergreen, chickweed, poke root, cayenne pepper, flaxseed meal, smartweed and charcoal, red sage, burdock, lobelia, and comfrey.

To make herb poultices it is best to have the herbs in a ground or granulated form. When using the herbs in powdered form, mix with just enough water to make a thick paste. When using them granulated, mix with water, cornmeal, and flaxseed meal to make a thick paste. Apply the paste in a layer about one-quarter inch thick onto a piece of muslin or linen cloth large enough to cover the area completely. Cover this with a piece of plastic. This can readily be found in today's kitchen, such as in a plastic trash bag. The plastic should be several inches larger than the poultice and held in place with pins or some kind of cloth binder. Leave it on for one to eight hours. Wash the skin thoroughly after removing. If fresh green leaves are used, beat them well, steep, and apply to the affected parts. Once a poultice has been used, do not warm it over. Do not allow a poultice to become cold. Have a second poultice ready immediately upon removing the first one.

Poultices are excellent for enlarged glands of any kind, such as neck, breast, groin, prostate, etc. They are also excellent for eruptions, boils, carbuncles, and abscesses. Occasionally the use of a poultice will increase the amount of pus in a sore. If this should occur, stop the use of the poultice. Be careful when using a mustard poultice as it may cause blistering of the skin. They are also good to relieve pain and congestion, to reduce inflammation and swelling, and to relax tense muscles.

An excellent thing to do first in any case where poultices are to be used, is to bathe the affected part thoroughly with mugwort tea. If this is not available, cleanse the area with hydrogen peroxide before applying the poultice. It must be remembered that many herbs are used for poultices, so study these herbs and use those best suited or those recommended for that condition.

Slippery elm poultice: This has no superior in the line of poultices, used either alone or combined with other herbs. Stir ground slippery elm bark in water or any strong herb tea, to the consistency of a thick paste. It is excellent for inflamed sores.

Lobelia and slippery elm poultice: Mix one-third part lobelia with two-thirds part slippery elm. Is excellent for blood poisoning, boils, and abscesses. Also use it for rheumatism.

Charcoal and hops poultice: This poultice will relieve gallstone pain quickly.

Charcoal and smartweed poultice: Excellent for inflammation of the bowels or inflammation in other parts of the body. When using for old and inflamed ulcers and sores, add powdered echinacea, golden seal, myrrh, or a small amount of all three. They all have powerful healing properties and are also disinfectant. See also Section IX, Chapter 4, The Value of Charcoal.

Poke root and cornmeal poultice: Very excellent for caked and inflamed breasts. Also good for blood poisoning.

Burdock leaf poultice: A burdock leaf poultice is very cooling and drying. It is good to use on old skin ulcers and sores. A poultice made of the root, adding a teaspoonful of salt, eases the pain of a wound caused by the bite of a dog.

Plantain poultice: This is excellent in rabid dog bites and to prevent blood poisoning.

A poultice made of any of the following herbs is very good for dissolving tumors: origanum, nettle, wintergreen, fenugreek, and mullein.

To bring a boil to a head quickly, apply poultices at a temperature of 100°F and repeat as often as necessary to keep the temperature above body heat. When a soothing effect is desired, as in painful wounds or bee stings, apply a poultice agreeably warm, and renew sufficiently often to prevent souring or becoming dry.

When applying poultices, the aim is to have the warmth and moisture retained as long as possible.

Yeast poultice: In making a yeast poultice, dilute ordinary cake or powdered yeast with enough liquid to make a stiff batter. It can be diluted with strong infusions of the desired herb tea and cornmeal to make a stiff batter. In sluggish conditions, such as gangrene, old sores, etc., mix either myrrh, charcoal, ginger, or golden seal with the batter before applying.

To decrease or stop discharges from ulcers, add witch hazel or wild cherry bark tea. When there is much inflammation and tenseness, sprinkle lobelia over the poultice, either the herb or crushed seeds.

Potato poultice: Scrape or grate a raw Irish potato and apply to any feverish part, such as a carbuncle or boil. It has a very soothing and cooling effect and will draw the infection to ahead.

Bayberry poultice: This poultice is used in the treatment of foul ulcers, old sores, and cancerous sores.

White pond lily poultice: This poultice, either used alone or combined with slippery elm or linseed, is one of the best for old sores, inflamed tumors, and similar ailments.

Sage poultice: Excellent for sore breasts or for any local inflammation.

Charcoal and slippery elm poultice: Use equal parts of each to make the poultice and use for gangrenous sores.

Slippery elm and yeast poultice: Make a regular slippery elm poultice. Mix a yeast cake with warm water and add to the slippery elm. The poultice will bring boils and abscesses to a head and keep gangrene from setting in.

Hyssop poultice: A small handful of this herb (used fresh), boiled in water for a few minutes, then drained and applied, will remove discoloration from bruises, or from a black eye. If you use the dried herbs, steep in boiling water.

Comfrey, ragwort, and wood sage poultice: Use equal parts of these three herbs and steep in boiling water. Apply poultice to external cancers and tumors. It is most beneficial and will give excellent results.

Bread and milk poultice: A poultice of bread and milk, with a little lobelia added, is very soothing and will bring boils to ahead.

Bran poultice: Use enough hot water to make a paste of the bran and apply as hot as can be borne. Use for inflammations of any kind, sprains, or bruises. When there is great pain, mix equal parts of lady's slipper and lobelia with the bran. Cover the poultice with several thicknesses of flannel or oiled silk to retain the heat. This is an unusually excellent poultice.

Carrot poultice: Boil carrots until soft, or they can be used raw. Mash to a pulp, add some vegetable oil to keep them from hardening, spread on a cloth, and apply. Excellent for offensive sores.

Garden carrots, grated raw, and applied as a poultice, will cleanse old sores and ulcers. Follow with an application of healing lotion or a wash of golden seal and myrrh solution.

Onion poultice: Make in the same way as carrot poultice. Very stimulating to indolent sores, and for boils that are slow to heal.

Lobelia poultice: Mix 1 ounce of powdered lobelia and 1 ounce of powdered slippery elm; excellent for wounds, fistulas, boils, felons, erysipelas, insect bites and stings.

Elderberry poultice: Use elderberry leaves, bruised or steamed just enough to wilt them; add a little pure olive oil. This makes an excellent poultice for inflammation and for piles and hemorrhoids. Apply as warm as can be borne for an hour or more to relieve pain.

E.   HERBAL LINIMENT

Good for all pains, painful swellings, bruises, boils, skin eruptions of any kind, and pimples. Apply herbal liniment every few minutes for an hour or two. It will stop a sty from developing on the eye in a short time if used freely. BE CAREFUL NOT TO GET IT INTO THE EYE.

Herbal liniment is also very useful for headaches. Apply to the temples, the back of the neck, and the forehead. It is very effective for rheumatism. For toothache, apply in the cavity and all around on the gums and on the outside of the jaw if necessary. It will take the swelling and soreness away. It is excellent for pyorrhea and sores in the mouth. Saturate a piece of cotton and thoroughly wash the mouth with liniment; or take a mouthful, rinse the mouth with it and spit it out. It is very good for pain located in any part of the body. It is also useful for the control of athlete's foot. Apply frequently, saturating the affected parts thoroughly.

To make herbal liniment, combine two ounces powdered myrrh, one ounce powdered golden seal, one-half ounce cayenne pepper and one quart rubbing alcohol (70 percent). Mix together and let stand seven days; shake well every day, decant off, and bottle in corked bottles. If you do not have golden seal, make the liniment without it.

F. HERBAL LAXATIVE

To make herbal laxative, combine equal parts of buckthorn bark, rhubarb root, cascara sagrada bark, calamus root, and fennel seed. Mix thoroughly. These herbs are nonpoisonous, are soothing to the stomach and will help to prevent gas and fermentation.

Dose: One-fourth teaspoonful in one-fourth glass of water. Follow with a glass of hot water. Take after each meal if the digestion is slow, or you can take a half-teaspoonful in the same manner upon retiring. Increase or decrease the amount taken to suit your personal need, but take enough so that you have a good elimination every day or at least so the bowels stay open. Children should be given proportionately less according to age.

This laxative should be made of the powdered herbs as it can then be used in the gelatin capsules. Two No.00 capsules are the usual dose for an adult. If making a tea of granulated herbs, steep a teaspoonful to a cup of boiling water for thirty minutes and drink.

If you do not have on hand or cannot obtain all the herbs used in the above laxative, any one of the following three will bring good results when used singly in the same dose as given in the preceding paragraph: buckthorn bark, rhubarb root, or cascara bark.

Other herbs that act as a laxative are: horehound, hyssop, mandrake, mullein, peach leaves, psylla, sage, senna, wahoo, blue flag, wild Oregon grape, fringe, and aloes.

G. A NERVINE AND TONIC

Combine equal parts of gentian root, skullcap, burnet root,

wood betony, and spearmint. This will prove a blessing to anyone who takes it. It is soothing and relaxing, quiets the nerves, has many good qualities, and is perfectly harmless.

Dose: One-half teaspoonful of the powdered herbs, combined and mixed in one-half glass of cold water, followed by a glass of hot water, one hour before each meal, and upon retiring. This tonic can be put in gelatin capsules. Two No.00 capsules would contain the required amount for one dose. More can be taken with benefit.

H. COMPOSITION POWDER

Composition powder is a fine remedy for colds, flu, hoarseness, colic, cramps, sluggish circulation, and the beginning of fevers. It should be kept in every home, and used when the need arises. It is safe and effective.

In fevers and colds, give a cup of composition tea every hour until the patient perspires freely. This will clear the body of the cold, and bring the fever down.

To make composition powder, combine the following herbs.

4 ounces bayberry
2 ounces ginger
1 ounce white pine
1 dram cloves
1 dram cayenne

Use all herbs in powdered form. Mix and put through a fine sieve twice. Steep one teaspoonful in a covered cup of boiling water for fifteen minutes. Drink the clear liquid poured off from the sediment.

I. ANTISPASMODIC TINCTURE

Antispasmodic tincture may be used either internally or externally. It is very effective for cramps in the bowels when taken internally. Take eight to fifteen drops, according to age, in one-half glass of hot water in cases of snake bites, mad dog bites, or any dangerous illness. Increase the dose to one teaspoonful every two or three hours; children less according to age. It is a mild stimulant without any harmful reaction as it is nonpoisonous. It is very effective for pyorrhea and sores in the mouth, and is an excellent remedy for tonsillitis, diphtheria, or any other throat trouble. As a gargle, use one-half teaspoonful to a glass of water. Gargle with this solution until the throat is perfectly clear. Repeat as often as necessary. It will cut all the mucus and kill the germs. It is also a very good voice tonic.

Apply externally to any kind of swelling or muscle cramps: it is very beneficial in rheumatism and lumbago. It is an excellent remedy for lockjaw. Put it into the mouth, getting it behind the teeth so that it will get on the tongue. It will invariably unlock the jaw in a few minutes. For small children, when it is hard to get it behind the teeth, bathe the neck and jaws frequently with it until relief is obtained.

To make antispasmodic tincture, combine the following herbs.

> 1 ounce lobelia seed, granulated
>
> 1 ounce skullcap, granulated
>
> 1 ounce skunk cabbage, granulated
>
> 1 ounce gum myrrh, granulated
>
> 1 ounce black cohosh, granulated
>
> 1/2 ounce cayenne, powdered
>
> 1 pint boiling water
>
> 1 pint apple (cider) vinegar

Steep the herbs in the pint of water just below the boiling point for one-half hour, strain, add the apple vinegar, and bottle for use.

J.   EMETICS

Emetics have been used from time immemorial. Hippocrates called them "upward purges." When Rome was the chief city of the earth, the fashionable had their palaces built with a special room in which to take "upward purges."

Such rooms were called "vomitories." In these vomitories there was a marble rail, where, after they had eaten a feast, the Romans would go and lean over and have a slave tickle their throats, after drinking some warm water or decoction. Then they would go back and finish their feast.

An emetic is given when it is necessary to empty the stomach or cleanse it. In nausea, when there is a lot of undigested food, it must be cleaned out. When a person has been bitten by a rabid dog, or poisonous snake, or poisons of any kind have been taken internally, an emetic is one of the remedies. It is also good to take a high enema, and rid the body of as much poison as possible in that way. Poisonous materials in the stomach are much more easily thrown out by emetics than any other means, but anyone who is weak or subject to hemorrhages of the stomach should not take emetics. The stomach, in those cases, should be cleaned out by fasting, mild herb laxatives, and enemas used to cleanse the rest of the system.

How to take an emetic: Drink five or six cups of lukewarm water. If vomiting does not occur freely, touch the back of the throat far down. This will bring up the contents of the stomach. In some cases it may be necessary to drink more. This should be repeated until the stomach is entirely cleansed and the water comes back clear. The addition of a teaspoonful of salt is very helpful.

Herb emetics are very beneficial. Use a tea made of boneset, pennyroyal, or Canada snakeroot. Other herbs that are good for emetics and antiemetics are: bayberry bark, buckbean, lobelia (large doses: small doses will stop spasmodic vomiting), mint (antiemetic), mustard, myrica, peach leaves (antiemetic), peppermint (antiemetic), giant Solomon seal (antiemetic), spearmint (antiemetic), white willow, colombo (antiemetic), ragwort (emetic).

A cup of peppermint, spearmint, or catnip tea taken after an emetic has a soothing and settling effect on the stomach. Golden seal taken afterwards is very healing and destroys mucus and fermentation in the stomach.

After taking the emetic, followed by an herb tea to settle and soothe the stomach, take a tonic herb, such as wild cherry bark, skullcap, valerian, or calamus root. Make the tea according to directions given earlier in this chapter. Take one-half cupful every two hours.

Some herbs that act as stimulants are: cayenne, elder, prickly ash, peppermint, ginger, cloves, red sage, raspberry, nettle, pennyroyal, rue, shepherd's purse, valerian.

The following herbs can be used in place of quinine: fit root, golden seal, magnolia, white poplar (bark), yarrow, willow (excellent), Peruvian bark, skullcap, gentian root, dogwood blossoms, peach, sage, vervain, wahoo, wood betony, willow bark, and red pepper (these act quickly; they are tonic and stimulating without any harmful reaction), boneset, turnips (grated, skin and all). Any of these can be given in tablespoonful doses whenever a dose of quinine is indicated. Use instead, because they are better than quinine.

4

TONIC HERBS

A tonic is an agent that is used to give strength to the system. The remedies that are given in this book all work toward the strengthening of the body and are not like any of the patent medicines or drugs generally given for that purpose.

One of the best things to do to tone up the body is to accustom it to a cold shower or a cold towel rub in the morning, followed by a vigorous dry towel rub. A fruit diet to begin with is advisable, as this makes it easier to rid the system of poisons.

These tonics may be taken with great benefit by anyone who is not overflowing with health and vitality. It is always good, of course, to take tonic herbs when convalescing from any disease or ailment. If the millions working in offices and those having taxing brain work knew what these things would do for them with no harmful aftereffects, the herb business would increase a hundredfold. To overtaxed mothers and overtaxed nurses with too many household duties and peevish sick children, they would prove an untold blessing that no pen could fully describe. No one can overestimate the benefits to be derived from using the simple treatments given in this book.

Be sure to study the following list of herbs. In Chapters 5 and 6 there are descriptions of herbs and medicinal trees, arranged alphabetically. You will be surprised to discover all the valuable properties these herbs have.

The following are all tonic herbs:

agrimony	gentian root	quassia
angelica	ginger root	red clover
apple tree bark	ginseng	blossoms

balmony
bayberry
bitterroot
boneset
broom
camomile
capsicum
celery
centaury
colombo
comfrey
coriander
cudweed
dandelion
elder
elecampane
fireweed
fringe tree

golden seal
ground ivy
heal-all
hops
horehound
hyssop
lavender
magnolia
marjoram
meadow sweet
mistletoe
mugwort
myrrh
Oregon grape
root
poke root
poplar bark
prickley ash

red raspberry
 leaves
sage
sanicle
sassafras
self-heal
skullcap
sweet flag
turkey corn
valerian
vervain
white oak bark
white pond lily
white willow
wild cherry bark
wood betony
yarrow
yellow dock

Specific nerve tonics: Golden seal is a pure tonic to the nervous system. It acts as a tonic and powerful cleanser to all of the mucous membranes in the body. In my estimation, there is no herb that can take the place of golden seal.

White willow, called Nature's aspirin, is a very effective tonic.

Skullcap is one of the finest nerve tonics; used alone, it gives excellent results.

Valerian, taken cold several times during the day, acts powerfully on the nerves.

Mistletoe is good for nerves.

Equal parts of wood betony, agrimony, and self-heal are good for nervous tremors.

Tonic for lungs: One teaspoonful of each of the following: comfrey, black horehound, cudweed, ground ivy, elecampane, ginger root, and one-half teaspoonful of cayenne: take as directed for use of herbs in Section II, Chapter 3, General Directions for the Use of Herbs.

Tonics for general debility and loss of appetite: Centaury, dandelion, ground ivy, meadow sweet, mugwort, wood betony, self-heal, agrimony, capsicum, balmony, poplar bark, black horehound, broom sanicle, yarrow, and sage. Boneset by itself is a specific tonic whenever one is needed. Take as directed in Section II, Chapter 3, General Directions for the Use of Herbs.

5

HERBS USED TO TREAT DISEASE

In reading the following descriptions of herbs, it may seem that many of them have the same qualities. This is true. I give the descriptions so that if you are unable to obtain a certain herb, you can get a different one having the desired qualities. Moreover, different herbs grow in different parts of the earth, and knowing their qualities enables you to obtain one having the elements that are needed. So no matter where you live, a remedy can be found locally. See also Section III, Treating Disease with Herbs, as well as the Glossary of Medical Properties of Herbs. For definition of the medical terms used in the Medicinal Properties lines of the descriptions, see the Glossary of Medical Terms in the Appendix.

In the **Part Used** line of the description, some of the terms used are readily understood, such as "leaves" and "roots," but a few require explanation. **Herb** means all of the plant above ground, except for large, tough stems and branches. **Plant** refers to all the plant, including the roots. **Rootstock or rhizome** is the part of a plant's stem that grows horizontally, just below the surface of the ground; and sends roots downward and stems or leaves upward. It remains alive from year to year, putting out new growth each season.

ADDENDUM: The following herbs should not be used in foods, beverages, or drugs, according to a list compiled by the FDA in October 1983: Bittersweet, bloodroot, broomtops, calamus, lily of the valley, lobelia, mandrake, mistletoe, St. John's wort, wahoo bark, and wormwood. Please heed the cautions that are included in the information about each of these herbs.

ALOES (Aloe socotrina)
Common Names: Bombay aloes, Turkey aloes, mocha aloes, Zanzibar aloes, Barbados aloes, and Curacao aloes.

Part Used: Leaves.

Medicinal Properties: Cathartic, stomachic, aromatic, emmenagogue, emollient, vulnerary.

Description and Uses: Promotes menstruation when it is suppressed. Will expel pinworms after several doses.

Aloes is one of the most healing agencies we have among the herbs. It is used in many cathartics since it is one of the best herbs to clean out the colon. The writer is personally acquainted with a lady who could not find anything that would move the bowels. She has used aloes alone for many years with most splendid results. I have used aloes for many years in connection with other herbs in the following mixture: 1 ounce powdered buckthorn bark, 1 ounce powdered rhubarb root, 1 ounce powdered mandrake root, 1/4 ounce powdered socotrina aloes, 1 ounce powdered calamus root.

Dose: Each person should take the amount necessary to move the bowels freely one or two times a day. For instance, start with one-fourth teaspoonful, then increase or decrease the dose as needed. Some need much more than others, so everyone must take the amount needed in his own case. Some who have very slow digestion do well if they take the full amount needed the first thing in the morning, an hour or more before breakfast. Others prefer to take it just before retiring in the evening. Do not take it during pregnancy or while nursing.

This is one of the finest body cleansers and brings most gratifying results. It cleans the morbid matter from the stomach, liver, kidneys, spleen, bladder, and is the finest colon cleanser known. It should be used in any case where a laxative is needed. It does not gripe and is very healing and soothing to the stomach and the rest of the body. Aloes may be used alone for any kind of sore, cut, burn, or wound on the outside of the body, and is a very excellent remedy for piles or hemorrhoids. Take a heaping teaspoonful to a pint of water, strain, and use. Two teaspoonfuls of boric acid may also be added, which, besides being healing, will keep the mixture from souring.

ALUM ROOT (Geranium maculatum)

Common Names: Cranesbill, spotted cranesbill, geranium, wild geranium, tormentil, spotted geranium, wild dovefoot, American tormentil, storksbill, wild cranesbill, alum root, crowfoot, American kino root.

Part Used: Root.

Medicinal Properties: Astringent, styptic, antiseptic.

Description and Uses: A powerful astringent. Very useful as an infusion in cholera, diarrhea, and dysentery. Should be used both internally and externally. Rinse the mouth often with a strong tea for sores in the mouth and bleeding gums. When there is bleeding from extracted teeth, rub some of the powder on. Excellent in hemorrhage, bleeding wounds, nosebleed, and profuse menstruation. The dry powder sprinkled on a wound or cut will stop bleeding immediately. Useful in old chronic ulcers. In womb troubles, use as a douche. A strong solution of the tea rubbed on the breast will dry up milk, or if rubbed just on the nipples will harden them. For internal piles and hemorrhoids, inject as an enema two or three tablespoonfuls of the strong tea several times a day, and after each stool. Excellent for mucus and pus in the bladder and intestines, and for leukorrhea or mucous discharges from any part of the body. Very useful in diabetes and Bright's disease. For mucous discharges, it is excellent when used with an equal part of golden seal. Use a teaspoonful of each to a pint of boiling water.

Let steep thirty minutes. Use this liquid as an injection for piles or any trouble in the rectum, as a douche, or take internally, a tablespoonful four to six times a day. For general use, steep a heaping teaspoonful in a cup of boiling water thirty minutes. Drink one or more cupfuls a day, a large mouthful at a time; children less according to age.

ANGELICA (Angelica atropurpurea)

Common Names: Dead nettle, purple angelica, masterwort, high angelica, archangel, American angelica.

Part Used: Root, seed, herb.

Medicinal Properties: Stimulant, carminative, emmenagogue, tonic, aromatic, diuretic.

Description and Uses: Angelica is a good tonic and a remedy for stomach pain, sour stomach, heartburn, gas, and cramps. It is also good for flu, colds, and fevers. Tea made from this herb when dropped into the eyes helps dimness of sight, and, dropped into the ears, it helps deafness. It should be taken hot to break up a cold quickly. For a general tonic, one to three cupfuls should be taken every day. Angelica is a most effective remedy in epidemics and is used to strengthen the heart. Such wonderful results have been obtained from this plant that it has been given the name "archangel." Christ is an archangel and the results of this agent are compared with the mighty working power of God Himself. Excellent in diseases of the lungs and chest. Eases stoppage of urination, good for suppressed menstruation, and helps expel the afterbirth. Good in sluggish liver and spleen. A tea made of angelica when dropped into old ulcers will cleanse and heal them. An infusion is made by taking one ounce of the dried herb to one pint of boiling water and drinking wineglassful doses frequently. The powder of the root may also be used for this purpose.

But do not take angelica if you are pregnant or have severe diabetes.

ANISE (Pimpinella anisum)

Common Names: Anise seed, common anise.

Part Used: Seed, root.

Medicinal Properties: Aromatic, diaphoretic, relaxant, stimulant, tonic, carminative, stomachic.

Description and Uses: Anise is one of the old-fashioned herbs and has many valuable properties. It will prevent fermentation and production of gas in the stomach and bowels, check griping in the bowels when taken as a hot tea, and relieves flatulence. Anise is a very good stomach remedy to overcome nausea and colic. It is useful when mixed with or taken with other herbs to give them a palatable flavor and is frequently used in cough medicines.

BALM (Melissa officinalis)
Common Names: Garden balm, sweet balm, lemon balm, honey plant, cure-all, balm mint, bee balm.
Part Used: Herbs, flowers.
Medicinal Properties: Diaphoretic, carminative, febrifuge, tonic.
Description and Uses: A warm tea of balm will produce perspiration. To make the tea, pour one pint of boiling water on one ounce of the herb, let stand for 15 minutes, cool, strain, and then drink freely. Liquid extract can be used; one-fourth to one teaspoonful. It is very helpful in painful or suppressed menstruation. Aids digestion and is valuable in nausea and vomiting. Useful in low-grade fever, liver, spleen, kidney, and bladder troubles, griping in the bowels, and dysentery. A warm poultice of balm will bring a boil to a head and then it will break. For insect stings and rabid dog bites, take the tea internally and make a poultice to apply to the bite or sting. It is good also as a toothache and headache remedy.

BALMONY (Chelone glabra)
Common Names: Snake head, turtle bloom, turtle head, fishmouth, shell flower, bitter herb.
Part Used: Leaves.
Medicinal Properties: Tonic, antibilious, stimulant, detergent, anthelmintic.
Description and Uses: Specific tonic for enfeebled stomach and indigestion, general debility, biliousness, jaundice, constipation, dyspepsia, and torpid (sluggish) liver. An excellent remedy for worms in children. Increases the gastric and salivary secretions, and stimulates the appetite. Good for sores and eczema. This herb may be difficult to obtain. An

infusion of one ounce of the herb in one pint of water can be used freely, a wineglassful at a time.

BARBERRY (Berberis vulgaris)
Common Names: Berberidis, European barberry, jaundice berry, pepperidge bush, sowberry.

Part Used: Root, root-bark, berries.

Medicinal Properties: Tonic, purgative, hepatic, antiseptic.

Description and Uses: The berries must be ripe when used and can be taken as a drink for fever or diarrhea. The fresh juice is also good as a mouthwash or gargle. The root-bark contains berberine, a bitter alkaloid, that aids in the secretion of bile and is therefore good for all liver problems, acts as a mild purgative, and helps regulate the digestive processes. There may also be a beneficial effect on the blood pressure by causing a dilatation of the blood vessels.

BASIL (Ocimum basilicum)
Common Names: Common basil, sweet basil, St. Josephwort, garden basil.

Part Used: Leaves.

Medicinal Properties: Stimulant, condiment, nervine, aromatic.

Description and Uses: The tea taken hot is good in suppressed menses. It helps to stop vomiting and eases stomach cramps. It is effective when applied to snake bites and insect stings. It is a well-known culinary herb and is used in cooking as a flavoring agent.

Use two teaspoonfuls steeped in a cup of hot water. Take one cup a day.

BAYBERRY (Myrica cerifera)
Common Names: Bayberry bush, American bayberry, American vegetable tallow tree, bayberry wax tree, myrtle,

wax myrtle, candleberry, candleberry myrtle, tallow shrub, American vegetable wax, vegetable tallow.

Part Used: Bark, leaves, flowers.

Medicinal Properties: Astringent, tonic, stimulant. Leaves – aromatic, stimulant.

Description and Uses: One of the most valuable and useful herbs. The tea is a most excellent gargle for sore throat. It will thoroughly cleanse the throat of all putrid matter. Steep a teaspoonful in a pint of boiling water for thirty minutes, gargle thoroughly until the throat is clear, then drink a pint of lukewarm tea to thoroughly cleanse the stomach. If it does not come up easily, tickle the back of the throat. This restores the mucous secretions to normal activity.

For chills make tea as given in the preceding paragraph, adding a pinch of cayenne, and take a half cup warm every hour. This is very effective.

Bayberry is excellent as an emetic after narcotic poisoning of any kind. It is good to follow the bayberry with an emetic, such as lobelia.

Bayberry is also valuable when taken in the usual manner for all kinds of hemorrhages, whether from the stomach, lungs, or excessive menstruation, and when combined with capsicum it is an unfailing remedy for this. Very good in leukorrhea. Has an excellent general effect on the female organs, also has an excellent influence on the uterus during pregnancy, and makes a good douche. Excellent results will be obtained from its use in goitre. In diarrhea and dysentery, use the tea as an enema.

For gangrenous sores, boils, or carbuncles, use as a wash and poultice, or apply the powdered bayberry to the infection. The tea is an excellent wash for spongy and bleeding gums.

The tea taken internally is useful in jaundice, scrofula, and canker sores in the throat and mouth. The tea taken warm promotes perspiration, improves the whole circulation and tones up the tissues. Taken in combination with yarrow, catnip, sage, or peppermint, it is unexcelled for colds.

An excellent formula made with bayberry and used by the famous Dominion Herbal College for colds, fevers, flu, colic, cramps, and pains in the stomach, is as follows:

bayberry	4 ounces
ginger	2 ounces
white pine	1 ounce
cloves	1 dram
capsicum	1 dram

This is prepared by mixing the herbs (in powdered form) and passing them through a fine sieve several times. Use one teaspoonful, more or less as the case may require, in a cup of hot water. Allow the herbs to stand so they will settle, then drink the clear liquid, leaving the settlings. Anyone knowing the benefit of this wonderful composition would not be without it. This formula may now be available in capsule form. Take one to three capsules daily. Bayberry is high in tannin content. Taking some milk with the herb will tend to counteract the effect of the tannin.

BETH ROOT (Trillium pendulum)
Common Names: Birthroot, milk ipecac, three-leaved nightshade, trillium, Indian shamrock, cough root, nodding, wakerobin, lamb's quarters, ground lily, snake bite, rattlesnake's root, Jew's harp plant.
Part Used: Root.
Medicinal Properties: Astringent, tonic, antiseptic, emmenagogue, diaphoretic, alterative, pectoral.
Description and Uses: Useful in coughs, bronchial troubles, pulmonary consumption, hemorrhages from the lungs, excessive menstruation, leukorrhea, lax conditions of the vagina, and fallen womb. Remedy for diarrhea and dysentery. One of the common names for this herb, birthroot, is an indication of its use by the American Indians as an aid during childbirth. Bethroot is available in whole, cut, or powdered form. It may also be obtained as a tincture and used in a solution of one-fourth teaspoonful daily in a cup of water.

BISTORT ROOT (Polygonum bistorta)

Common Names: Patience dock, snake weed, sweet dock, dragonwort, red legs, Easter giant.

Part Used: Root.

Medicinal Properties: Astringent, diuretic, styptic, alterative.

Description and Uses: Bistort is one of the strongest herb astringents. It is excellent for gargles, injections, and is used for cholera, diarrhea, dysentery, and leukorrhea. Excellent wash for sore mouth or gums and running sores. Combined with equal parts of red raspberries, it will cleanse internal ulcers. Makes a good wash for the nose. Useful in smallpox, measles, pimples, jaundice, ruptures, insect stings, snake bites, and expels worms. Combined with plantain, it is useful in gonorrhea. The powdered bistort will stop bleeding of a cut or wound when applied directly to the injury. Used in a douche to decrease or regulate the menstrual flow.

BITTERROOT (Apocynum androsaemifolium)

Common Names: Dogsbane, milkweed, honey bloom, milk ipecac, flytrap, wandering milkweed, catchfly, bitter dogsbane, western wallflower, wild cotton.

Part Used: Root.

Medicinal Properties: Emetic, diuretic, sudorific, cathartic, stimulant, expectorant.

Description and Uses: This is a very good remedy for intermittent fever, typhoid fever, and other fevers. Has an excellent effect on the liver, kidneys, and bowels. Increases the secretion of bile. Excellent for poor digestion. Bitterroot has been known to cure dropsy when everything else has failed. Expels worms. Is very useful in syphilis, and to rid the system of other impurities. Especially valuable in gallstones. Good in rheumatism, neuralgia, diseases of the joints and mucous membranes. Wonderful for diabetes.

BITTERSWEET (Solanum dulcamara)

Common Names: Woody nightshade, wolfe grape, nightshade, violet bloom, scarlet berry, bittersweet herb, bittersweet twigs, nightshade vine, garden nightshade, fever twig, felonwort, staff vine, felonwood.

Part Used: Root, twigs.

Medicinal Properties: Emetic, anodyne, deobstruent, herpatic, resolvent, depurative, aperient, laxative.

Description and Uses: Has a splendid effect on the liver, pancreas, spleen, and other glandular organs of the body. Excellent in all skin troubles, and will purify the blood. It is very soothing and allays general irritability. Good in piles, jaundice, syphilis, gonorrhea, and rheumatism. It makes the skin and kidneys active, increases the menstrual flow, is helpful in leprosy, and is an important part of many salves. The tea is very healing to sores when they are bathed with it, and it is especially good for burns and scalds. A salve made of equal parts of bittersweet and yellow dock makes an excellent ointment for various skin conditions. A poultice made of the bruised berries will help to cure felons. Bittersweet may be combined with camomile as an ointment that is useful for minor injuries such as bruises, sprains and abrasions.

Caution: Bittersweet may have some toxic effects and should be used with caution when taken internally. It is usually used externally.

BLACKBERRY (Rubus villosus)

Common Names: Bramble, cloudberry, thimbleberry, dewberry.

Part Used: Root, leaves.

Medicinal Properties: Astringent, tonic.

Description and Uses: Blackberry is a fine remedy for dysentery and diarrhea. It is also good for bleeding; either internally or from the rectum or mouth. This herb has a high tannin content and should be taken for a limited time only, not more than one week at a time. A little honey or cinnamon makes it a more palatable medication. It is available as a tincture, one half to one teaspoonful twice daily in water.

BLACK COHOSH (Cimicifuga racemosa)

Common Names: Black snakeroot, bugwort, bugbane, squawroot, rattleroot, rattleweed, rattlesnake's root, richweed.

Part Used: Root.

Medicinal Properties: Emmenagogue, nervine, alterative, expectorant, diaphoretic, astringent, antispasmodic.

Description and Uses: A powerful remedy in hysteria, St. Vitus dance (or chorea), epilepsy, convulsions, and all spasmodic afflictions. Good for pelvic disturbances, female complaint (menstrual cramps), all uterine troubles, and relieves pain in childbirth. Dependable herb to bring on menstrual flow that has been retarded by cold or exposure. Splendid for dropsy, rheumatism, spinal meningitis, asthma, delirium tremens, poisonous snake bites, and poisonous insect bites. A wonderful remedy for high blood pressure and for equalizing the circulation. By making it into a syrup, black cohosh is effective in coughs, whooping cough, and in liver and kidney troubles. *This herb should not be used during pregnancy.* Because of its potency it should not be used constantly over a long period of time without a break. One to three capsules a day is the average dose.

BLACK ROOT (Leptandra virginica)

Common Names: Culver's physic, tall speedwell, tall veronica, Culver's root, beaumont root, bowman's root, leptandra, hini, oxadoddy, physic root, whorlywort.

Part Used: Root.

Medicinal Properties: Cathartic, cholagogue, tonic, emetic, hepatic.

Description and Uses: The fresh root is too toxic to use safely. The dried root is an excellent laxative and tonic and is useful in cases of sluggish liver to stimulate the normal flow of bile.

Even the dried root must be used with caution as it contains leptandrin, a very strong purgative and emetic. It is best to use only with medical supervision. Steep a teaspoonful of the dried root, cut into small pieces, in a cup of boiling water for half an hour. Drink cold, one mouthful before each meal. Start with a small dose and gradually increase the amount taken, as tolerated, to no more than one cup a day.

BLADDERWRACK – See Seawrack.

BLOODROOT (Sanguinaria canadensis)
Common Names: Red puccoon, Indian plant, pauson, red paint root, red root, Indian paint, tetterwort.

Part Used: Root.

Medicinal Properties: Emmenagogue, tonic, diuretic, stimulant, febrifuge, emetic, sedative, and rubefacient.

Description and Uses: It is an excellent agent in adenoids, nasal polyps, sore throat, and syphilitic troubles. When the condition is not easily overcome, combine with equal parts of golden seal. Bloodroot is also excellent for piles by using the strong tea as an enema. Effective remedy in coughs, colds, laryngitis, bronchitis, typhoid fever, pneumonia, catarrh, scarlatina, jaundice, dyspepsia, ringworm, whooping cough, running sores, eczema, and skin diseases. Small doses stimulate the digestive organs and heart. Large doses act as a sedative and narcotic. Bloodroot was used as a body paint by the American Indians.

Caution: Bloodroot is a powerful herb and should be used only under competent supervision.

BLUE COHOSH (Caulophyllum thalictroides)
Common Names: Blueberry, squaw root, papoose root, blue ginseng, yellow ginseng.

Part Used: Root.

Medicinal Properties: Stimulant, sudorific, parturient, emmenagogue.

Description and Uses: Used to regulate menstrual flow and for suppressed menstruation. It is a common remedy among the Indians to make childbirth easier and to bring on labor pains when the proper time arrives. Good for chronic uterine trouble, leukorrhea, rheumatism, neuralgia, vaginitis (inflammation of the vagina), dropsy, cramps, colic, hysteria, palpitation of the heart, high blood pressure, and diabetes. Good for hiccough, whooping cough, spasms, and epilepsy. Blue cohosh contains the following vital minerals: potassium, magnesium, calcium, iron, silicon, and phosphorus. These minerals help to alkalinize the blood and urine. This herb can be quite irritating to mucous surfaces and therefore should be used with some caution.

It should not be used during pregnancy and should be taken for only one week at a time, one to three capsules daily.

BLUE FLAG (Iris versicolor)

Common Names: Poison flag, water flag, water lily, flag lily, fleur-de-lis, liver lily, snake lily, flower-de-luce, iris.

Part Used: Rhizome.

Medicinal Properties: Alterative, resolvent, sialagogue, laxative, diuretic, vermifuge.

Description and Uses: Useful in cancer, rheumatism, dropsy, impurity of blood, constipation, syphilis, skin diseases, liver troubles, and as a laxative. It is very relaxing and stimulating.

BLUE VIOLET — See Violet.

BORAGE (Borago officinalis)

Common Names: Burrage, bugloss, common bugloss.

Part Used: Leaves, flowers.

Medicinal Properties: Pectoral, tonic, febrifuge, aperient, demulcent.

Description and Uses: It is excellent to bathe sore inflamed eyes with the tea. Taken internally, the tea cleanses the blood and is effective for fevers, yellow jaundice, to expel poisons of all kinds due to snake bites, insect stings, etc. Strengthens the heart and is good for cough, itch, ringworms, tetters, scabs, sores, and ulcers. Use as a gargle for ulcers in the mouth and throat, and to loosen phlegm. Steep three teaspoonfuls of the herb in one cup of hot water and take three tablespoonfuls two times a day for one week at a time.

BROOM (Cytisus scoparius)

Common Names: Broom tops, common broom, broom flowers, Irish broom.

Part Used: Tops, seed.

Medicinal Properties: Tops – cathartic, diuretic. Seed – cathartic, emetic.

Description and Uses: Excellent for dropsy, toothache, ague, gout, sciatica, swelling of the spleen, jaundice, kidney and bladder troubles, especially in cases of gravel in the bladder. Makes an excellent remedy when used with uva-ursi, cleavers, and dandelion for cleansing the kidneys and bladder, and to increase the flow of urine. Broom is of great service in dropsy caused by a weak heart. Makes a good ointment for lice or vermin. Contains forty-two parts potash. The stomach readily receives the nutritive salts found in the plant, since they are natural.

Caution: Broom contains alkaloids and hydroxytyramine, and should not be used except under proper supervision.

BUCHU (Barosma betulina)

Common Names: Bookoo, bucku, short-leaved buchu, buku, buchu, bucco, round buchu.

Part Used: Leaves (use the short-leaved buchu).

Medicinal Properties: Diuretic, tonic, stimulant, diaphoretic.

Description and Uses: One of the best remedies for the urinary organs. Take one capsule three times a day. It is very soothing and is a most excellent remedy when there is pain while urinating, stoppage of the urine, inflammation of the bladder, or dropsy. When used specifically for this purpose, give a cold, strong tea. DO NOT BOIL BUCHU LEAVES. When given warm, it produces perspiration, helps to reduce swelling of the prostate gland and soothes irritation of the lining membrane of the urethra. Useful in diabetes in the first stages and also for leukorrhea. When combined with equal parts of uva-ursi, it is a wonderful help for urinary problems. Take one capsule three times a day with a glass of water. Infusion: one ounce of the leaves in one pint of boiling water. Take one wineglassful three or four times a day.

BUCKBEAN (Menyanthes trifoliata)
Common Names: Marsh trefoil, water shamrock, bog bean, bitter trefoil, marsh clover, bog myrtle, bitterworm, brook bean, bean trefoil, moonflower.
Part Used: Leaves.
Medicinal Properties: Tonic, cathartic, diuretic, anthelmintic, emetic.
Description and Uses: Expels worms. When taken in large doses it acts as an emetic. Promotes digestion by increasing the production of gastric juice. An excellent remedy in stomach catarrh, rheumatism, scrofula, scurvy, intermittent fevers, jaundice, dyspepsia, liver and kidney troubles. Buckbean is available in capsule or powder form. Take one capsule three times a day or one-half teaspoonful of the powder in a glass of water three times a day.

BUCKTHORN BARK (Rhamnus frangula)
Common Names: European buckthorn, black alder

dogwood, black alder tree, alder buckthorn, black dogwood, Persian berries, European black alder, arrow wood.

Part Used: Bark, fruit.

Medicinal Properties: Purgative, diuretic, emetic, vermifuge. Fruit – purgative.

Description and Uses: Buckthorn bark is a very well-known cure for constipation. It is important to note that freshly cut bark should NOT be used: the bark should be dried for one to two years before using. It is not habit-forming. It is an effective remedy for appendicitis. Good in rheumatism, gout, dropsy, and skin diseases. Will produce profuse perspiration when taken hot. Expels worms. Take both internally and apply externally as a wash. Ointment made of buckthorn is very effective in reducing itching. Will remove warts. Good used as a fomentation or poultice.

BUGLEWEED (Lycopus virginicus)

Common Names: Sweet bugle, water bugle, gipsywort.

Part Used: Entire plant.

Medicinal Properties: Sedative, astringent, mild narcotic, tonic.

Description and Uses: The infusion of this herb is excellent for coughs. To make the infusion, use 1 ounce of the herb, cut fine, to a pint of boiling water. Let cool and take a cupful several times a day.

BURDOCK (Arctium lappa)

Common Names: Grass burdock, clotbur, bardana, burr seed, hardock, hareburr, hurr-burr, turkey burr seed, beggar's buttons, thorny burr, lappa, cocklebur.

Part Used: Roots, leaves, seeds.

Medicinal Properties: Roots – diuretic, depilatory, alterative. Leaves – maturating. Seeds – alterative, diuretic, tonic.

Description and Uses: The root is one of the best blood purifiers for syphilis and other diseases of the blood. It cleanses and eliminates impurities from the blood very rapidly. Burdock tea taken freely will heal all kinds of skin diseases, boils, and carbuncles. Increases the flow of urine. Excellent for gout, rheumatism, scrofula, canker sores, sciatica, gonorrhea, and leprosy. Wring a hot fomentation out of the tea and use on swellings. It is good to apply externally as a salve for skin eruptions, burns, wounds, swellings, and hemorrhoids. Excellent to reduce flesh.

Burdock root can be obtained either as a powder or in capsules. Take one capsule twice daily; or for powder, use half a teaspoonful twice daily in a glass of water. Make a decoction of the seeds or root, using one ounce of the herb to one and one-half pints of boiling water. Take a wineglassful three or four times a day.

BURNET (Pimpinella saxifraga)
Common Names: Burnet saxifrage, small saxifrage, pimpernel, small pimpernel, European burnet saxifrage, small burnet saxifrage.
Part Used: Root.
Medicinal Properties: Aromatic, stimulant, stomachic, pungent. carminative.
Description and Uses: It is very useful for cleansing the chest, lungs, and stomach. Will aid in expelling stones from the bladder. Good for cuts, wounds, running sores, toothache, earache, and piles. Steep a teaspoonful of the root in a cup of boiling water, let cool, strain, and drink one or two cups a day cold, a large swallow at a time. Best remedy known for sour stomach.

BUTTERNUT BARK (Juglans cinerea)
Common Names: Oilnut, oilnut bark, white walnut, lemon walnut, Kisky Thomas nut.
Part Used: Inner bark.
Medicinal Properties: Tonic, astringent, cholagogue, anthelmintic, alterative, cathartic.

Description and Uses: An excellent gentle laxative, very good for chronic constipation. Will expel worms from the intestines. Good for sluggish liver, fevers, colds, and la grippe. It is an old-fashioned remedy. As a powder, use five to ten grains or take one No.00 capsule daily.

CALAMINT (Calaminta officinalis)
Common Names: Mountain mint, basil thyme, common calamint.
Part Used: Herb.
Medicinal Properties: Expectorant, diaphoretic.
Description and Uses: Calamint is a wonderful herb to use in attacks of asthma or bronchitis. It is also good when applied to joints affected by arthritis or rheumatism or to the skin to help heal bruises and similar injuries.

CALAMUS (Acorus calamus)
Common Names: Sweet flag, grass myrtle, sweet grass, sweet root, sweet cane, sweet rush, sweet sedge, myrtle flag, sweet myrtle, sea serge.
Part Used: Root.
Medicinal Properties: Carminative, aromatic, tonic, vulnerary.
Description and Uses: Excellent for use in intermittent fevers. It is a valuable stomach remedy and is good for that purpose when mixed with other herbs. It is also helpful in preventing griping caused by other herbs. It stimulates the appetite, is good for dyspepsia, prevents fermentation and hyperacidity, and keeps the stomach fluids sweet. If the dried root is chewed, it will cause nausea in those who smoke, thereby helping to destroy the taste for tobacco. The tea is excellent when applied externally to sores, burns, and ulcers. Valuable in the treatment of scrofula. Take one capsule a day for only one week at a time without a break.
Caution: Calamus may have some toxic effects when taken internally. It is good when used externally.

CAMOMILE (Anthemis nobilis)

Common Names: Roman camomile, garden camomile, low camomile, ground apple, whig plant.

Part Used: Flowers.

Medicinal Properties: Stimulant, bitter, tonic, aromatic, emmenagogue, anodyne, antispasmodic, stomachic.

Description and Uses: An old well-known home remedy that grows freely everywhere. Was supposedly dedicated to the sun by the Egyptians because of its curative value in the treatment of ague. Everyone should gather a bag full of camomile blossoms, as they are good for many ailments. An excellent general tonic that increases the appetite and is good for dyspepsia and a weak stomach. Used in various parts of the world as a table tea. Good to regulate monthly periods. Splendid for kidneys, spleen, colds, bronchitis, bladder troubles, to expel worms, for ague, dropsy, and jaundice. The tea makes an excellent wash for sore and weak eyes and also for other open sores and wounds. Use as a poultice for pains and swellings. Intermittent and typhoid fever can be broken up in the early stages with this herb. Good in hysteria and nervous diseases. Made and used as a poultice, it will prevent gangrene. Combine with bittersweet as an ointment for bruises, sprains, callouses, or corns. *Do not use during pregnancy.* Take one capsule twice daily.

CARAWAY (Carum carvi)

Common Names: Caraway seed, caraway fruit.

Part Used: Seeds.

Medicinal Properties: Carminative, aromatic, stomachic, emmenagogue.

Description and Uses: It is very useful for colic in infants when taken in hot water or milk. It should be taken hot for colds and female troubles.

It is very good for the prevention of fermentation in the stomach and aids digestion. It strengthens and gives tone to the stomach, and helps to expel gas from the bowels. It is often used to flavor other herbs and to prevent griping. Use as a poultice for bruises.

_____

CARROT (Daucus carota)

Common Names: Garden carrot, bee's nest plant, bird's nest root, wild carrot.

Part Used: Root, seed.

Medicinal Properties: Anthelmintic, carminative, diuretic, stimulant.

Description and Uses: If carrots were used more extensively as a vegetable, they would prove of great benefit to mankind. Patients are often put on a carrot diet for a short period of time for cancer, liver, kidney, and bladder troubles. Carrots are very useful in dropsy, gravel in the bladder, painful urination, to increase the menstrual flow, and in expelling worms from the bowels. Grated carrots make an excellent poultice for ulcers, abscesses, carbuncles, scrofulous and cancerous sores, and bad wounds. The seeds of carrots, ground to powder and taken as a tea, relieve colic and increase the flow of urine. The powder may also be placed in capsules and one or two taken daily with a glass of water. Carrot blossoms, used as a tea, are a most effective remedy for dropsy and will very often effect a cure when all other means have failed.

_____

CASCARA SAGRADA (Rhamnus purshiana)

Common Names: Purshiana bark, Persian bark, sacred bark, chittem bark, bearberry, California buckthorn.

Part Used: Bark.

Medicinal Properties: Purgative, bitter tonic.

Description and Uses: One of the oldest, time-proven, and most reliable remedies for chronic constipation. It is not habit-forming. It is a good intestinal tonic. An excellent remedy for gallstones and increases the secretion of bile. Good for liver complaints; especially an enlarged liver. Mix four teaspoonfuls in a quart of boiling water, let steep for one hour, and drink one or two cupfuls a day one hour before meals or on an empty stomach. It is well sometimes to drink a cupful on retiring. Cascara sagrada is a wonderful remedy.

Among the Indians it was known as "sacred bark." It was called sacred by them because of the excellent results they obtained from its use. The writer has used this remedy for over thirty years, with gratifying results. The bark is very bitter and disagreeable to the taste of many people. It can be procured from drugstores in three and five grain chocolate-coated tablets, called extract of cascara sagrada. (Do not mistake this for Cascarets, as they are an entirely different product). Have them on hand when needed. When there is a bad taste in the mouth, or the bowels do not move as they should, take one or more of these tablets according to your needs. Take them immediately after meals, or upon retiring. An excellent remedy for children when constipated. It is also now available as a tincture. Use 15 to 30 drops.

Caution: *Fresh bark should not be used.* It should be at least one year old before using.

CATNIP (Nepeta cataria)
Common Names: Catmint, catrup, cat's-wort, field balm.
Part Used: Herb.
Medicinal Properties: Anodyne, antispasmodic, carminative, aromatic, diaphoretic, nervine.
Description and Uses: Catnip is one of the oldest household remedies. It is wonderful for very small children and infants. Use the tea as an enema for children with convulsions. Very useful in pain of any kind, spasm, gas pains, hyperacidity in the stomach, and for the prevention of griping in the bowels. A tablespoonful steeped in a pint of water and used as an enema is soothing and quieting, and very effective in convulsions, fevers, and for expelling worms in children. A high enema of catnip will relieve headaches. It is good to restore menstruation. Catnip, sweet

balm, marshmallow, and sweet weed make an excellent baby remedy. If mothers would have this on hand and use it properly, it would save them many sleepless nights and doctor's bills, and also save the baby much suffering. It is a harmless remedy and should take the place of the various soothing syrups on the market, many of which are very harmful. This wonderful remedy should be in every home. A little honey or malt honey may be added to make it palatable. Steep; NEVER BOIL CATNIP. Take internally freely.

A warm enema of catnip will help to free the flow of urine when it is blocked. This herb gets its name from the great attraction it has for cats, who like to chew on it and roll in it.

CAYENNE (Capsicum frutescens)
Common Names: Cayenne pepper, red pepper, capsicum, Spanish pepper, bird pepper, pod pepper, chillies, African pepper, chili pepper, African red pepper, cockspur pepper, American red pepper, garden pepper.

Part Used: Fruit.

Medicinal Properties: Stimulant, tonic, sialagogue, alterative, rubefacient, carminative, digestive.

Description and Uses: Red pepper is one of the most wonderful herb medicines we have. We can do many things with it that we are not able to do with any other known herb. It should never be classed with black pepper, vinegar, or mustard. These are all irritating, but red pepper is very soothing. While red pepper smarts a little, it can be put in an open wound, either in a fresh wound or an old ulcer, and it is very healing instead of irritating; but black pepper, mustard, and vinegar are irritating to an open wound and do not promote healing. Red pepper is one of the most stimulating herbs known to man. It causes no harm and has no unhealthy reaction.

It is effective when used as a poultice for rheumatism, inflammation, and pleurisy, and is also helpful if taken internally for these. For sores and wounds it also makes a good

poultice. It is a stimulant when taken internally as well as
being an antispasmodic. Good for kidneys, spleen, and pancreas. Wonderful for lockjaw. Will heal a sore, ulcerated
stomach, while black pepper, mustard, or vinegar will irritate
it. Red pepper is a specific and very effective remedy in
yellow fever, as well as other fevers, and may be taken in
capsules followed by one or more glasses of water.

It is one part of a most wonderful liniment, which may be
made as follows:

Kloss's Liniment

    2 ounces gum myrrh
    1 ounce golden seal
    1/2 ounce African red pepper (cayenne pepper)

Put this either into a quart of rubbing alcohol, or a mixture
of a pint of raspberry vinegar and a pint of water. Add the
alcohol or vinegar to the powder. Let it stand for a week or
ten days, shaking every day. This can be used wherever a
liniment is used or needed. It is very healing to wounds,
bruises, sprains, scalds, burns, and sunburns, and should be
applied freely. Wonderful results are obtained in pyorrhea by
rinsing the mouth with the liniment or applying the liniment
on both sides of the gums with a little cotton, Q-tips, or gauze.

The following paragraphs are quoted from *Standard
Guide to Non-Poisonous Herbal Medicine,* pages 52,53,95-
98.

From the Greek kapto, "I bite" – a biting plant. The best
capsicum is obtained from Africa and South America; one
province of the latter, Cayenne, giving its name to the article.
It can be produced in good quality in the Southern States,
especially those that lie beyond the southern line of Tennessee. It grows abundantly and of excellent quality in the West
Indies, where the negroes count it almost a certain remedy
for nearly all their maladies. They have no fears of fatal
effects from fevers, even the terrible and devastating yellow
fever, if they can get plenty of capsicum. They not only drink
a tea of it, but they chew and swallow the pods one after

another, as we should so many doughnuts, and never dream of it doing them any injury. Dr. Thomas, of London, who practiced a long time in the East Indies, found cayenne pepper an almost certain remedy for yellow fever, and almost every other form of human malady. There is, perhaps, no other article which produces so powerful an impression on the animal frame that is so destitute of all injurious properties. It seems almost incapable of abuse, for however great the excitement produced by it, this stimulant prevents that excitement subsiding so suddenly as to induce any great derangement of the equilibrium of the circulation. It produces the most powerful impression on the surface, yet never draws a blister; on the stomach, yet never weakens its tone. It is so diffusive in character that it never produces any local lesion, or induces permanent inflammation.

Yet its counter excitation is the most salutary kind, and ample in degree. A plaster of cayenne is more efficient in relieving internal inflammation than a fly blister ever was, yet I never knew it to produce the slightest vesication, though I have often bound it thick as a poultice on the tenderest flesh to relieve rheumatism, pleurisy, etc., which, by the aid of an emetic, an enema, and sudorifics, it is sure to do. I have thus cured with it, in a single night, cases of rheumatism that had been for years most distressing. Though severe on the tissue to which applied, it is so diffusive that it does not long derange the circulation, but, on the contrary, equalizes it. Thus it is not only stimulant, but antispasmodic, sudorific, febrile, antiinflammatory, depurating, and restorative. It is powerful to arrest hemorrhage from the mucous membranes. When the stomach is foul, a strong dose of the powder will excite vomiting and an enema of it and lobelia and slippery elm will relieve the most obstinate constipation. Taken as powder in cold water, it is sure to move not only the internal canal, but all the splanchnic viscera, as the liver, the kidneys, the spleen, and the pancreas, the mesentery, etc. This article, along with lobelia, some good astringent, such as bayberry or sumach leaves, a good bitter, a mucilage, a good sudorific and the vapor bath, must ever constitute the basis of the most effective medication.

One of the best LINIMENTS in use is prepared as follows: Boil gently for ten minutes one tablespoonful of cayenne pepper in one pint of cider vinegar. Bottle that hot, unstrained. This makes a powerfully stimulating external application for deep-seated congestions, sprains, etc.

In connection with capsicum may be mentioned the slippery elm compound, which is excellent for coughs. Cut obliquely into small pieces, about the thickness of a match, one ounce or more of slippery elm bark; add a pinch of cayenne, flavor with a slice of lemon, sweeten with sugar, and infuse in one pint of boiling water. Take this in small doses, frequently repeated. Let a consumptive patient drink a pint of this each day. It is one of the grandest remedies that can be given, as it combines both stimulating and demulcent properties. As slippery elm is mucilaginous it will roll up the mucous material troubling the patient, and pass it down through the intestines. It is also very nourishing, and possesses wonderful healing properties. For an infant's food, mix with an equal quantity of milk, and leave out the lemon and cayenne.

Cayenne is good in coughs, torpor of the kidneys, and to arrest mortification. A peculiar effect of capsicum is worth mentioning. In Mexico the people are very fond of it; and their bodies get thoroughly saturated with it, and if one of them happens to die on the prairie the vultures will not touch the body on account of its being so impregnated with the capsicum.

It is good in all forms of low diseases. The key to success in medicine is stimulation, and capsicum is the great stimulant. There are many languid people who need something to make the fire of life burn more brightly. Capsicum, not whiskey, is the thing to do it. It can be given without stint or measure. It is excellent in yellow fever, black vomit, putrefaction or decay, given frequently in small doses. It is good, also, in asthmatical asphyxia (i.e., when a person cannot get his breath) combined with lobelia in what would be called the lobelia compound. It is good in profound shock. For local application it is, or should be, the base of all stimulating liniments. It is not injurious to the skin, as is turpentine or acetic acid. It is an agent that is seldom used alone.

A CAPSICUM TINCTURE may be made as follows: Take two ounces of cayenne and macerate for ten to fourteen days in one quart of alcohol. Then strain and bottle. Keep in a warm place while macerating during cold weather.

A splendid STIMULATING LINIMENT is made as follows:

tincture of cayenne	1 quart
Castille soap	2 ounces
oil of hemlock spruce	1/2 ounce
oil of origanum	1/2 ounce
oil of cedar	1/2 ounce
oil of peppermint	1/2 ounce

Shave or scrape the soap very fine, and dissolve in one pint of water. Stir the oils into the tincture and mix with the soapy solution. A little additional oil of peppermint will greatly increase its efficacy. In a four-ounce bottle put one ounce of lobelia compound (without gum myrrh) and fill the bottle up with the stimulating liniment. Shake this well, and after application cover the affected part with a piece of warmed flannel.

The following paragraphs are quoted from *The Medicine of Nature,* by R. Swinburne Clymer, pages 69-71, 79-80, 143, 150.

Capsicum (red pepper) is the most pronounced, natural, and ideal stimulant known in the entire materia medica. It cannot be equaled by any known agent when a powerful and prolonged stimulant is needed, as in congestive chills, heart failure, and other conditions calling for quick action. The entire circulation is affected by this agent and there is no reaction. In this it stands alone as ideal.

In congested, ulcerated, or infectious sore throat it is an

excellent agent, but should be combined with myrrh to relieve and remove the morbidity.

Capsicum is antiseptic and therefore a most valuable agent as a gargle in ordinary sore throat or in diptheria.

In all diseases prostrating in their nature, whether pneumonia, pleurisy, or typhoid fever, capsicum is invaluable in the prescription as the toning agent which helps the system to throw off the disease and reestablish equilibrium.

In all acute conditions where capsicum is indicated, the call is for the maximum dose – from three to ten grains, preferably in tablet form, followed by a large drink of hot water. In chronic and sluggish conditions, the small dose frequently given is 1 to 3 grains with either hot or cold water.

Capsicum plasters are valuable in pneumonia, pleurisy and other acute congestions. Combine with lobelia and bran or hops. One hour is the maximum time to keep them applied.

As the common red pepper of table use, capsicum is well known to almost all people. None know better its virtue than the habitual drinker who considers it his best friend and never fails to use plenty of it in his hot soups when sobering up and soothing his cold and sore stomach after a prolonged spree. Common red pepper may be given safely in capsules, which take the place of tablets. In the onset of chills and colds it is the sovereign remedy. Whenever a stimulant is necessary, capsicum should have first consideration. It is indicated in low fevers and prostrating diseases. Capsicum is nonpoisonous and there is no reaction to its use. It is the only natural stimulant worthwhile considering in diarrhea and dysentery with bloody mucus, stools, and offensive breath.

The stimulant. There is no other stimulant known to medical science so natural, so certain and with less reaction following its constant use.

Capsicum is indicated in all low-grade fevers and prostrating diseases. Capsicum increases the power of all other agents, helps the digestion when taken with meals, and arouses all the secreting organs. Whenever a stimulant is indicated, capsicum may be given with the utmost safety.

Capsicum, cayenne (red pepper) is not a pepper, no more than water pepper or peppermint. Water pepper is also called smart weed, is very hot but a wonderful medicine.

The following paragraphs are quoted from Dominion Herbal College, Ltd., pp 1-2, Lesson 5.

Peppermint, well-known all over the civilized world, is very healing, will stimulate like a drink of whiskey, but there is no reaction from it, no bad aftereffects. It permanently strengthens the whole system. Red pepper does the same. There are a number of other herbs that are very hot which are God-given medicines.

Capsicum, cayenne, or red pepper is indigenous to the warmer climates, Asia, Africa, and the Southern States. The kind bearing the larger berries grows in the more northern places and is frequently used for culinary purposes.

African bird pepper is the purest and best stimulant known. It has a pungent taste, and is the most persistent heart stimulant ever known. It is exceedingly prompt in its effect. Through the circulation, its influence is manifest through the whole body. The heart first, next the arteries, then the capillaries and the nerves. We have known in cases of apoplexy a bath of hot water and mustard, with half a teaspoon of cayenne added and the feet thrust in, to give good results; the pressure being removed from the brain by the equalizing of the circulation.

The negroes of the West Indies soak the pods in water, add sugar and the juice of sour oranges, and drink freely in fevers. Capsicum has a wonderful place in inflammation. We have often been told that it would burn the lining of the stomach, and our medical, as well as lay friends, have at times shown fear at its use. We assure the student that the fear of capsicum is unfounded. We have used it freely for over a quarter of a century, and therefore feel that our experience is worth more than the opinions of those who know nothing about it experimentally.

It is useful in cramps, pains in the stomach and bowels, and sometimes in constipation will create a heat in the bowels, causing peristaltic action of parts previously contracted. In these later cases it would be well to give it in small doses in the form of warm infusion, from half to one teaspoonful to a cup of boiling water. In typhoid fever, in combination with hepatics and a little golden seal, it will sustain the portal circulation and give much more power to the hepatics used.

In quinsy and diphtheria, apply the tincture of cayenne around the neck. Then place a flannel around the neck wet with the infusion of cayenne and use the infusion internally, at the same time, freely.

A good liniment for sprains, bruises, rheumatism, and neuralgia may be made as follows:

tincture capsicum (red pepper)	2 fluid ounces
fluid extract lobelia	2 fluid ounces
oil of wormwood	1 fluid dram
oil of rosemary	1 fluid dram
oil of spearmint	1 fluid dram

In setting forth the above uses of this agent, we do not wish the student to consider it a cure-all. Such is not the case; but where a stimulant is needed of this type, it will not fail the physician. It is not used more because its value is not realized.

The following paragraphs are quoted from *The Model Botanic Guide to Health,* pages 33-35.

Capsicum is the botanical name of a large genus or family of plants which grow in various countries, such as Africa, South America, and the East and West Indies. We use only the African bird pepper, as it retains its heat longer in the system than any other, and is the best stimulant known. It has a pungent taste, which continues for a considerable length of time; when taken into the stomach it produces a pleasant sensation of warmth, which soon diffuses itself throughout the whole system, equalizing the circulation. Hence it is so useful in inflammation and all diseases which depend upon a morbid increase of blood in any particular part of the body. According to analysis, cayenne consists of albumen, pectin (a peculiar gum), starch, carbonate of lime, sesquioxide of iron, phosphate of potassium, alum, magnesium, and a reddish kind of oil. In apoplexy we have found it beneficial to put the feet in hot water and mustard, and at the same time give half a teaspoonful of cayenne pepper in a little water.

This treatment has caused a reaction, taking the pressure of the blood from the brain, and by this means saved the patients. Some may ask, "Will it produce an inflammatory action?" We say decidedly not, for there is nothing that will take away inflammation so soon. We have used it in every stage of inflammation and never without beneficial results. Mr. Price, the well-known traveler, lays it down as a positive rule of health that the warmest dishes the natives delight in are the most wholesome that strangers can use in the putrid climates of lower Arabia, Abyssinia, Syria, and Egypt. Marsden, in his history of Sumatra, remarks that cayenne pepper is one of the ingredients of the dishes of the natives. The natives of the tropical climates make free use of cayenne, and do not find it injurious.

Dr. Watkins, who visited the West Indies, says the negroes of those islands steep the pods of the cayenne in hot water, adding sugar and the juice of sour oranges, and drink the tea when sick or attacked with fever. It is very amusing to see the medical man prohibiting the use of cayenne in inflammatory diseases as pernicious, if not fatal, and yet find them recommending it in their standard works for the same diseases. Dr. Thatcher, in his dispensation, says: "There can be but little doubt that cayenne furnishes us with the purest stimulant that can be introduced in the stomach." Dr. Wright remarks that cayenne has been given for putrid sore throats in the West Indies with the most signal benefit. Paris, in his *Pharmacologia,* says that the surgeons of the French army have been in the habit of giving cayenne to the soldiers who were exhausted by fatigue. Dr. Fuller, in his prize essay on the treatment of scarlet fever, says: "Powdered cayenne made into pills with crumbs of bread and given four times a day, three or four each time, is a most valuable stimulant in the last stages of the disease, and is also good in all cases of debility, from whatever cause it may arise." Cayenne given in half teaspoonful doses, mixed with treacle and slippery elm, at night, is a valuable remedy for a cough. Bleeding of the lungs is easily checked by the use of cayenne and the vapor bath. By this means circulation is promoted in every part of the body, and consequently the pressure upon the lungs is diminished, thus affording an opportunity for a coagulum to form around the ruptured vessel.

In advocating the use of cayenne we do not wish to be understood that it will cure everything, nor do we recommend it to be taken regularly, whether a stimulant is required or not. Medicines ought to be taken only in sickness. If persons take a cold, a dose of cayenne tea will generally remove it, and by this means prevent a large amount of disease. It is an invaluable remedy in the botanic practice.

The preceding quotations on capsicum are from some of the world's foremost herbalists, and therefore are very valuable. I quote these herbalists because I know them to be Christians, and they verify my own practical experience with capsicum.

CEDRON (Simaba cedron)
Common Names: Cedron, rattlesnake's beans.
Part Used: Seeds.
Medicinal Properties: Antispasmodic, nervine, stomachic.
Description and Uses: Cedron strengthens and invigorates the entire system. It is excellent for the stomach, prevents gas and fermentation. A good remedy in intermittent fevers, spasms, convulsions, and nervous troubles. Make a strong tea of it and apply to a snake bite or a poisonous insect bite by moistening a cloth in the tea and keeping it over the bite.

Keep the area well saturated with the tea. In addition, take the tea internally, one tablespoonful four times a day. Make the infusion with one ounce of the herb in one pint of boiling water.

CELANDINE (Chelidonium majus)

Common Names: Greater celandine, garden celandine, tetterwort, jewel weed, quick-in-hand, slippers, snap weed, pale touch-me-not, slipper weed, balsam weed, weathercock, touch-me-not.

Part Used: Herb.

Medicinal Properties: Alterative, antispasmodic, caustic, diuretic, purgative.

Description and Uses: The fresh juice mixed with vinegar may be applied for removal of warts and corns. It may also be made into an ointment to be used on various skin diseases, such as ringworm, eczema, etc. When taken internally as an infusion, is good for diseases of the stomach, gallbladder, and liver. Also may be useful in asthma. Take one or two capsules daily.

Do not confuse this herb with small or lesser celandine, commonly known as pilewort.

Caution: Do not give this herb to children.

CELERY (Apium graveolens)

Common Names: Smallage, garden celery.

Part Used: Root, seed.

Medicinal Properties: Diuretic, stimulant, aromatic.

Description and Uses: Excellent for use in incontinence of urine, dropsy, and liver troubles. Produces perspiration and is a splendid tonic. Good in rheumatism, neuralgia, and nervousness. Is much used as a table relish and the ground seed for flavoring soups.

CENTAURY (Erythraea centaurium)

Common Names: Century, centory, feverwort, bitter herb, common centaury, lesser centaury.

Part Used: Herb.

Medicinal Properties: Tonic, stomachic, aromatic, cholagogue, diaphoretic, digestive, febrifuge, emetic.

Description and Uses: This is an herb that maybe used for nearly any problem. It is also good as a tonic for those who are unable to get sufficient exercise in the open air. It is used extensively for gas, colic, bloating, heartburn, dyspepsia, and constipation and aids the proper assimilation and digestion of food. If taken in too concentrated an infusion, it will produce vomiting. Lotions containing centaury have been used on the skin to remove different kinds of blemishes.

Use 2 teaspoonfuls of the herb to a cup of boiling water: let steep for 20 to 30 minutes, cool, and take a cupful every day, one swallow at a time.

CHICKWEED (Stellaria media)

Common Names: Starweed, starwort, satin flower, adder's mouth, Indian chickweed, star chickweed, tongue grass, winter weed, stitchwort.

Part Used: Herb

Medicinal Properties: Alterative, demulcent, refrigerant, mucilaginous, pectoral, resolvent, discutient.

Description and Uses: Chickweed can be used in many ways. It is considered a great nuisance by gardeners, but it can be used as a food like spinach. It may be used fresh, dried, powdered, in poultices, fomentations, or made into a salve. Excellent in all cases of bronchitis, pleurisy, coughs, colds, hoarseness, rheumatism, inflammation, or weakness of the bowels and stomach, lungs, bronchial tubes - in fact, any form of internal inflammation. It heals and soothes anything it comes in contact with.

It is one of the best remedies for external application to inflamed surfaces, skin diseases, boils, scalds, burns, inflamed or sore eyes, erysipelas, tumors, piles, cancer, swollen testes, ulcerated throat and mouth, and all kinds of wounds. Chickweed salve should be applied after bathing any external part with tea and left on as long as possible. Apply at night and leave on. Give several applications during the day if possible. It will cure burning and itching genitals. Anyone who is covered with any kind of sores should take a chickweed herb bath, and then apply the chickweed salve.

Bathe the surface with the decoction, and the swelling and inflammation will go down. In blood poisoning it should be taken internally, and a poultice applied externally. For constipation when the bowels are completely obstructed, take three heaping tablespoonfuls of the fresh herb, boil in one quart of water down to one pint. Take a cupful warm every three hours or more often until the desired results are obtained. Good for scurvy and blood disorders. For tea to be taken internally, steep a heaping teaspoonful for half an hour in a cup of boiling water. Take three or four cups a day between meals, a swallow at a time and take a cup warm upon retiring. Chickweed can also be obtained in powder or capsule form. Take one or two capsules daily as an average dose; more if needed.

CHICORY (Cichorium intybus)

Common Names: Succory, wild chicory, garden endive, garden chicory, endive

Part Used: Root.

Medicinal Properties: Tonic, laxative, diuretic.

Description and Uses: While chicory root is very well-known for its combination with coffee, its value for various remedies is not well-known.

Chicory is effective in disorders of the kidneys, liver, urinary organs, stomach, and spleen. It is good for jaundice. It is also good for settling an upset condition in the stomach, expelling the morbid matter and toning up the system. The leaves of the common garden endive (Cichorium endive) are commonly used in salads. It is available in most grocery stores.

___

CLEAVERS (Galium aparine)
Common Names: Bedstraw, clivers, coachweed, goose grass, goose's hair, grip grass, gravel grass, gosling weed, hedge-burrs, clabber grass, catchweed, milk sweet, poor robin, savoyan, scratchweed, cleaverwort, cheese rent herb

Part Used: Entire herb.

Medicinal Properties: Refrigerant, diuretic, aperient, alterative, tonic.

Description and Uses: One of the best remedies for kidney and bladder troubles, particularly burning or suppressed urine, especially when used with broom, uva ursi, buchu, and marshmallow. Makes an excellent wash for the face to clear the complexion Due to its refrigerant properties it is excellent in all cases of fever, scarlet fever, measles, and all acute diseases. Good in many skin diseases, such as cancer, scrofula, and severe cases of eczema. Also good for inflammatory stages of gonorrhea.

Excellent for stones in the bladder, scurvy, and dropsy. This herb may be used freely. Can be used like spinach. Is excellent to cleanse the blood and strengthen the liver when used in this way. Cleavers is very astringent due to its high tannin content. It should be taken for only two weeks at a time, and then skip one or two weeks. Place one ounce in one pint of hot water and simmer for 20 minutes Take one teaspoonful three times a day.

___

CLOVER (See Red Clover; White Clover)

___

COHOSH (See Black Cohosh; Blue Cohosh)

COLOMBO (Cocculus palmatus)
Common Names: Calumba, calumbo, columbo root, columba, foreign columbo, kalumb, calumba root.
Part Used: Root.
Medicinal Properties: Antiemetic, tonic, febrifuge.
Description and Uses: One of the best and purest tonics to strengthen and tone up the entire system. Useful in intermittent and remittent fevers.

Will keep the system pure and toned up in debilitating and hot swampy climates. Excellent to allay vomiting during pregnancy and can be used with good effect before and after pregnancy. Can be used for colon trouble such as cholera, chronic diarrhea, and dysentery, no matter how longstanding the disease. A splendid remedy in dyspepsia and improves the appetite. Good for rheumatism and pulmonary consumption.

COLTSFOOT (Tussilago farfara)
Common Names: Bull's foot, horsefoot, horsehoof, butterbur, British tobacco, foal's-foot, flower velure, coughwort, ginger root.
Part Used: Root, leaves.
Medicinal Properties: Emollient, demulcent, expectorant, pectoral, diaphoretic, tonic.
Description and Uses: An excellent remedy for catarrh, consumption, and all lung troubles. Very soothing to the mucous membranes. Good results are obtained when a tea is made by steeping a heaping tablespoonful in a quart of water and using as a fomentation or just moisten a cloth in the tea and apply it to the chest and throat. Excellent to relieve the chest of phlegm in all coughs, asthma, bronchitis, whooping cough, and spasmodic cough. It is good for inflammation and swelling, piles, stomach troubles, and fever. The powdered leaves sniffed up the nostrils are excellent for nasal obstruction and headache. For scrofula or scrofulous tumors, take internally, one or two capsules a day, or make a poultice

and apply externally. Coltsfoot has been much used in cough and lung medicines. It is excellent when combined with other herbs and made into a cough syrup.

Has also been used internally for diarrhea and applied externally for burns, sores, ulcers, and insect bites. Make a decoction by placing one ounce of the leaves in a quart of water and letting it boil down to a pint. Sweeten with honey and take one cupful three or four times a day.

COMFREY (Symphytum officinale)
Common Names: Blackwort, bruisewort, gum plant, healing herb, knitback, slippery root, wallwort, nipbone.
Part Used: Root.
Medicinal Properties: Demulcent, astringent, pectoral, vulnerary, mucilaginous, static, nutritive.
Description and Uses: Powerful remedy in coughs, catarrh, ulceration or inflammation of the lungs, consumption, hemorrhage and excessive expectoration in asthma and tuberculosis. Very valuable in ulceration or soreness of the kidneys, stomach, or bowels. The best remedy for bloody urine.

Apply a fomentation wrung out of the strong hot tea for bad bruises, swellings, sprains, fractures: it will greatly reduce the swelling and relieve the pain. Also use as a fomentation on boils.

A poultice of the fresh leaves is excellent for ruptures, sore breasts, fresh wounds, ulcers, burns, bruises, gangrenous sores, insect bites, and pimples. The tea taken internally is useful in scrofula, anemia, dysentery, diarrhea, leukorrhea, and female debility. Also has an excellent effect on internal sores and pains. Take one or two capsules daily for one or two weeks, then take a week's rest. Boil one ounce of the root in one quart of water and take several wineglassfuls a day as a decoction.

CORAL (Corallorhiza odontorhiza)

Common Names: Crawley, crawley root, coral root, chicken's toes, turkey claw, fever root, scaly dragon's claw.

Part Used: Root.

Medicinal Properties: Febrifuge, sudorific, sedative, diaphoretic.

Description and Uses: A most powerful and effective remedy in skin diseases of all kinds, scrofula, scurvy, boils, tumors, fevers, acute erysipelas, cramps, pleurisy, night sweats, and is highly recommended for cancer. Very useful for enlarged veins. Dip a cloth in the tea and apply to boils and tumors. Will produce profuse perspiration without exciting the system. Especially good in low grade fever. Valuable in typhus and inflammatory diseases. Excellent combined with blue cohosh for scanty or painful menstruation. It is available in tincture form. Follow the instructions on the label.

CORIANDER (Coriandrum sativum)

Common Names: Coriander seed.

Part Used: Seed.

Medicinal Properties: Aromatic, stomachic, cordial, pungent, carminative.

Description and Uses: Coriander is a good stomach tonic and very strengthening to the heart. Will allay griping caused by other laxatives and expel wind from the bowels. Good for flavoring other unpleasant-tasting herbs. You may take one or two capsules daily or 5 to 15 drops of the fluid extract in water.

CORN SILK (Zea mays)

Common Names: Corn, Indian corn, maize jagnog, Turkish corn.

Part Used: Fresh or dried flower pistils.

Medicinal Properties: Anodyne, diuretic, demulcent, alterative, lithotriptic.

Description and Uses: Corn silk is one of the best remedies for kidney, bladder, and prostate troubles. Especially useful for pain or burning during urination and for difficulty in starting urination. May also be useful in helping to prevent bedwetting. Infuse two ounces of the herb in one pint of boiling water and drink several wineglassfuls a day.

CUBEB BERRIES (Piper cubeba)
Common Names: Java pepper, cubebs, tailed cubebs, tailed pepper.
Part Used: Dried unripe berries.
Medicinal Properties: Aromatic, purgative, stimulant, diuretic, antisyphilitic, carminative, stomachic.
Description and Uses: Is excellent in chronic bladder troubles, burning urine, leukorrhea, gonorrhea, bronchial troubles, cough, colic. Gives tone to the stomach and bowels. Heretofore has been used largely for seasoning soups. Increases the flow of urine. Of the fluid extract, take one-fourth to one teaspoonful in a glass of water.

DANDELION (Taraxacum officinale)
Common Names: Lion's tooth, swine snout, puff ball, wild endive, priest's crown, white endive.
Part Used: Root, leaves.
Medicinal Properties: Hepatic, aperient, diuretic, depurative, tonic, stomachic.
Description and Uses: Young dandelion leaves have been used in much the same way as spinach or in fresh green salads. Dandelion contains twenty-eight parts sodium. The natural nutritive salts purify the blood and help to neutralize the acids in the blood. Anemia is caused by a deficiency of proper nutrients in the blood and really has little to do with the quantity of blood. Dandelion is one of the old well-known remedies. The root is used to increase the flow of urine in liver problems. It is slightly laxative. It is a splendid remedy for jaundice and skin diseases, scurvy, scrofula, and eczema.

Useful in all kinds of kidney troubles, diabetes, dropsy, inflammation of the bowels, and fever.

Has a beneficial effect on the female organs. Increases the activity of the liver, pancreas, and spleen, especially in enlargement of the liver and spleen. Promotes bile formation. The roasted, ground roots make an excellent substitute for coffee and are especially good in cases of dyspepsia and rheumatism. If you use the capsules, take one three times a day.

————

DILL (Anethum graveolens)
Common Names: Garden dill, dilly, dill seed, dill fruit.
Part Used: Seed.
Medicinal Properties: Stomachic, aromatic, stimulant, carminative, diaphoretic.
Description and Uses: Dill tea is an excellent old-fashioned remedy for upset stomach and dyspepsia. It helps prevent gas and fermentation in the intestines. It stimulates the appetite. It is very quieting to the nerves and useful in swellings and pains. It helps to stop hiccoughs. The seeds may be chewed in cases of bad breath.

Dill seeds have been used to flavor other foods. The leaves and seeds have been used in preparing pickles, but pickles should never be introduced into the stomach.

————

ECHINACEA (Echinacea angustifolia)
Common Names: Sampson root, purple cone flower, black Sampson, red sunflower.
Part Used: Root.
Medicinal Properties: Alterative, antiseptic, tonic, depurative, maturating, febrifuge.
Description and Uses: An excellent blood cleanser. Used for blood poisoning, fevers, carbuncles, acne, eczema, boils, peritonitis, syphilitic conditions, bites and stings of poisonous insects or snakes, erysipelas, gangrenous conditions, diphtheria, tonsillitis, sores, infections, wounds.

Use as a gargle for sore throat. Combined with myrrh, it is an excellent remedy for all of these purposes. It acts powerfully to cleanse the morbid matter from the stomach and to expel poisons, toxins, pus, or abscess formations. Combined with myrrh, it is also excellent for typhoid and other fevers. In severe cases use two capsules four times a day or 10 to 25 drops of the tincture every two hours in water.

ELECAMPANE (Inula helenium)
Common Names: Scabwort, elfwort, horseheal, horse-elder.
Part Used: Root.
Medicinal Properties: Diaphoretic, diuretic, expectorant, aromatic, stimulant, stomachic, astringent, and tonic.
Description and Uses: Useful in coughs, asthma, and bronchitis. When combined with echinacea, is an excellent remedy in tuberculosis. It is a stimulant and tonic to the mucous membranes. Warms and strengthens the lungs and promotes expectoration. A tea of elecampane is useful in whooping cough. It strengthens, cleanses, and tones up the mucous membranes of the lungs and stomach. It can also be used in urinary retention, kidney and bladder stones, and delayed menstruation. Take one capsule three times a day. Liquid extract; one-half to one teaspoonful.

FENNEL (Foeniculum vulgare)
Common Names: Large fennel, wild fennel, sweet fennel.
Part Used: Seed, leaves.
Medicinal Properties: Stomachic, carminative, pectoral, diuretic, diaphoretic, aromatic.
Description and Uses: Fennel is an old reliable household remedy and is also used as a culinary herb. It is good for flavoring foods and other medicines. The tea makes an excellent eye wash. Fennel is one of the thoroughly tried remedies for gas, acid stomach, gout, cramps, colic, and

spasms. Ground fennel sprinkled on food will prevent gas in the stomach and bowels. It is an excellent remedy for colic in small children. For this use, the herb should be steeped and given in small doses every half hour until the infant or child is relieved. Fennel seed ground and made into a tea is good for snake bites, insect bites, or food poisoning. It is good in cases of jaundice when the liver is obstructed. Excellent for obesity. Increases the flow of urine and also increases the menstrual flow. Fennel oil may be rubbed over painful joints to relieve pain and may also be added to gargles for hoarseness and sore throat. Available in capsule or powder form. Take one or two capsules daily.

***

FENUGREEK (Trigonella foenum-graecum)
Common Names: Foenugreek seed.
Part Used: Seeds.
Medicinal Properties: Mucilaginous, emollient, febrifuge, restorative.

Description and Uses: Excellent when made into a poultice and used on wounds and inflammations. Grind the seed, mix it with powdered charcoal, and make it into a thick paste. The charcoal will make the poultice more effective. Treating ulcers and swellings in this manner will prevent blood poisoning. The tea is an excellent gargle for sore throat and will help clear the mucous from the bronchial passages. The seed is jelly-like when moistened and has a very cooling and healing effect on the bowels, as well as providing lubrication. The tea is excellent in fevers. The seeds boiled in soybean or nut milk are very nourishing.

***

FEVERFEW (Chrysanthemum parthenium)
Common Names: Featherfew, featherfoil, febrifuge plant.
Part Used: The herb.
Medicinal Properties: Aperient, carminative, purgative, tonic, emmenagogue.

Description and Uses: Feverfew is good for gas, bloating and worms. It promotes the onset of the menstrual period. Is good to treat hysteria and alcoholism with delirium tremens. The flowers act as a purgative. As an infusion, use 1 ounce of the herb to a pint of boiling water and take frequently, a teaspoonful at a time. Take 10 to 30 drops of the tincture in a glass of water every four hours as needed.

FIGWORT (Scrophularia nodosa)
Common Names: Scrofula plant, throatwort, rosenoble, carpenter's square, figwort root, heal-all, kernelwort.
Part Used: Entire plant.
Medicinal Properties: Diuretic, depurative, anodyne, exanthematous.
Description and Uses: As can be seen from one of the common names of this herb, scrofula plant, it is an excellent remedy to use for all skin eruptions, abscesses, boils, eczema, scabies, bruises, wounds, etc. A poultice should be made using the leaves, as well as drinking the infusion several times a day. Use one heaping teaspoonful of the herb to a cup of boiling water, let cool, and drink one to two cups a day. The liquid extract may also be used. Follow the directions on the bottle.

FIREWEED (Erechtites hieracifolia)
Common Names: Pilewort, various leaved fleabane.
Part Used: Entire plant.
Medicinal Properties: Astringent, tonic, emetic, alterative.
Description and Uses: Is strongly astringent and therefore most excellent in diseases of the mucous membranes, colon troubles, cholera, and dysentery. Will quickly relieve pain in these conditions. Is almost a specific for piles. Very effective in children for summer diarrhea. It gives prompt relief when taken very hot. Excellent remedy for fevers and

as a tonic and blood purifier. Take for only one week at a time. Take the capsules with a swallow of milk.

Steep a heaping teaspoonful in a cup of boiling water for 30 minutes. When cool, drink one to two cups a day, one swallow at a time.

FIT ROOT (Monotropa uniflora)

Common Names: Ice plant, Indian pipe, fit root plant, pipe plant, Dutchman's-pipe, bird's nest plant, ova ova, bird's nest, corpse plant, nest root, convulsion weed.

Part Used: Root.

Medicinal Properties: Antispasmodic, nervine, tonic, sedative, febrifuge.

Description and Uses: Is splendid in all kinds of fevers. Takes the place of quinine and opium. An excellent remedy for restlessness, fainting, nervous irritability, muscle spasm, and convulsions. Should be used in place of opium and quinine. It will cure intermittent and remittent fevers. Oh, why will not people use this wonderful remedy in place of poisonous drugs? It is efficient and harmless. A teaspoonful of fit root and fennel seed, steeped in a pint of boiling water for twenty minutes, is an excellent douche for inflammation of the vagina and uterus, also good used as a wash for sore eyes. A valuable remedy for epilepsy and lockjaw in children.

FLAXSEED (Linum usitatissimum)

Common Names: Linseed, common flax, winterlien, lint bells.

Part Used: Ripe seed.

Medicinal Properties: Demulcent, pectoral, maturating, mucilaginous, emollient.

Description and Uses: This is the common flaxseed with which almost everyone is familiar. The ground seed, when mixed with boiling water, makes a thick mush that is excellent for use in poultices. Any herb may be added for this purpose, such as smartweed, elm bark, granulated hops, mullein, or any of the other herbs recommended for use in poultices. These herbs mixed and used as a poultice with flaxseed make one of the best poultices for all kinds of old sores, boils, carbuncles, inflammations, and tumors. Charcoal is also good to mix with flaxseed. The oil made from crushing the flaxseed is good for coughs, asthma, and pleurisy, and has been used externally as an application for burns, sores, scalds, etc.

Place one teaspoonful of the seed in a cup of boiling water, let cool, and take one or two mouthfuls three times a day.

FLEABANE (Erigeron canadense)
Common Names: Canada fleabane, horse tail, cow's tail, horseweed, pride weed, colt's tail, mare's tail, scabious, blood staunch, butter weed, bitter weed.
Part Used: Leaves or entire plant.
Medicinal Properties: Styptic, astringent, diuretic, tonic.
Description and Uses: Excellent for cholera, dysentery, and summer complaint, especially for children, when all other remedies fail. In these afflictions, use as an enema. Steep a teaspoonful in a quart of boiling water for twenty minutes; use hot, about 112° to 115°F. This is an excellent remedy for all colon troubles. It can be improved by using equal parts of white oak bark, wild alum root, and catnip. Taken internally, it is very reliable for bladder troubles, burning urine, and hemorrhages from the bowels and uterus. Good for tuberculosis.

FROSTWORT - See Rock Rose.

GENTIAN ROOT (Gentiana lutea)
Common Names: Bitterroot, bitterwort, gentian, yellow gentian, pale gentian, felwort.
Part Used: Root, leaves.

Medicinal Properties: Stomachic, tonic, anthelmintic, antibilious.

Description and Uses: An excellent and reliable tonic. Purifies the blood. Good for liver complaints and dysentery. Most effective for jaundice. Excellent for the spleen. Gentian root will improve the appetite and strengthen the digestive organs. It is especially good for gastritis, indigestion, heartburn, and stomach aches. When used for these conditions, gentian should be taken thirty to sixty minutes before meals.

It increases the circulation, benefits the female organs, and invigorates the entire system. Useful in fevers, colds, gout, convulsions, scrofula, and dyspepsia. It will expel worms. Excellent in suppressed menstruation and scanty urine. Because of its bitterness, it is better to combine gentian root with some aromatic herb such as a small amount of licorice.

It is more effective than quinine. Allays poison from mad dog, insect, and snake bites. Take one-fourth to one-half teaspoonful of the powder in a cup of water three times a day 30 minutes before meals.

GINGER (Zingiber officinale)

Common Names: Black ginger, race ginger, African ginger.

Part Used: Root.

Medicinal Properties: Stimulant, pungent, carminative, aromatic, sialagogue, condiment, diaphoretic.

Description and Uses: When taken hot, ginger is excellent in cases of suppressed menstruation. Chewing a little of the root stimulates the salivary glands and is very useful in paralysis of the tongue and is also good for sore throats. Prevents griping and is good for diarrhea, colds, la grippe, chronic bronchitis, coughs, dyspepsia, gas and fermentation, cholera, gout, and nausea when combined with stronger laxative herbs. Produces sweat when taken hot.

GINSENG (Panax quinquefolia)

Common Names: Five-fingers root, American ginseng, ninsin, red berry, garantogen, sang.

Part Used: Root.

Medicinal Properties: Demulcent, stomachic, mild stimulant, tonic.

Description and Uses: The word "panax" in the botanical name means "all-healing". Ginseng is very commonly used in hot, moist climates as a preventive against all manner of illnesses, and is also used in severe diseases of all types. Promotes appetite and is useful in digestive disturbances. Flavored with any flavoring you like, ginseng makes an agreeable and very effective drink for colds, chest troubles, and coughs.

If taken when hot, it will produce perspiration. It is also good for stomach troubles and constipation. Has been used frequently in lung troubles and inflammation of the urinary tract. Ginseng has been used for thousands of years in China to treat all kinds of illnesses and is held in high regard by the Chinese as an aphrodisiac. A good systemic tonic, but don't use it if you have high blood pressure. Take one capsule a day, and adjust to fit your needs. Of the powder, take one No.00 capsule or 15 grains in water after each meal.

GOLDEN SEAL (Hydrastis canadensis)

Common Names: Yellow paint root, orange root, yellow puccoon, ground raspberry, eye root, yellow Indian plant, tumeric root, Ohio curcuma, eye balm, yellow eye, jaundice root.

Part Used: Root.

Medicinal Properties: Laxative, tonic, alterative, detergent, opthalmicum, antiperiodic, aperient, diuretic, antiseptic, deobstruent.

Description and Uses: This is one of the most wonderful remedies in the entire herb kingdom. When one considers all that can be accomplished by its use and what it actually will do, it does seem like a real cure-all. It is especially valuable in all diseased states of the digestive system.

It is a wonderful remedy for all stomach disorders and acute inflammations. The wild plant is nearly extinct in North America, but it is being cultivated. It is one of the best substitutes for quinine, and is a most excellent remedy for colds, la grippe, and all kinds of stomach and liver troubles. It exerts a special influence on all the mucous membranes and tissues with which it comes in contact. For open sores, inflammations, eczema, ringworm, erysipelas, or any skin disease, golden seal excels. Golden seal tea is made by steeping one teaspoonful in a pint of boiling water for twenty minutes. Use this tea as a wash. Then after the area is thoroughly clean, sprinkle on some of the powdered root and cover. It is beneficial to also use hydrogen peroxide for cleansing the area.

Taken in small but frequent doses, it will allay nausea during pregnancy. Steep a teaspoonful in a pint of boiling water for twenty minutes, stir well, let settle, and pour off the liquid. Take six tablespoonfuls a day. It equalizes the circulation and, when combined with skullcap and red pepper (cayenne), will greatly relieve and strengthen the heart. It has no superior when combined with myrrh, one part golden seal to one-fourth part myrrh, for an ulcerated stomach or duodenum or dyspepsia, and is especially good for enlarged tonsils and sores in the mouth. Smoker's sores, caused by holding a pipe in the mouth, will heal after just a few applications of the powder to the sore. I have used it in a number of cases that were called "skin cancers" with excellent results. If the sore continues to enlarge, however, proper medical advice should be sought.

It is an excellent remedy for diphtheria, tonsillitis, and other serious throat troubles, and has a good effect when combined with a little myrrh and cayenne. Excellent for chronic catarrh of the intestines and all catarrhal conditions. Will improve the appetite and aid digestion.

Combined with skullcap and hops, it is a very fine tonic for spinal nerves and is very good in spinal meningitis. Very useful in all skin eruptions, scarlet fever, and smallpox.

To cure pyorrhea or sore gums, put a little of the tea in a cup, dip a toothbrush in it, and thoroughly brush the teeth and gums. The results will be most satisfactory. In any nose trouble, pour some tea in the hollow of the hand and snuff it up the nose. Very useful in typhoid fever, gonorrhea, leukorrhea, and syphilis. For bladder troubles, it should be introduced into the bladder through a catheter immediately after the bladder has been emptied and retained as long as possible, repeating two or three times a day. I do not recommend that individuals do this themselves unless experienced. Have a physician or nurse inject it for you through a sterile rubber catheter.

Golden seal combined with alum root, taken internally, is an excellent remedy for bowel and bladder troubles, Use two parts of golden seal and one part of wild alum. This is a good laxative. Good for piles, hemorrhoids, and prostate trouble. When combined with equal parts of red clover blossoms, yellow dock, and dandelion, it has a wonderful effect on the gallbladder, liver, pancreas, spleen, and kidneys. Combined with peach leaves, queen of the meadow, cleavers, and corn silk, it is a reliable aid for Bright's disease and diabetes.

Golden seal is excellent for the eyes. The following is the way I use it for my eyes: steep one small teaspoonful of golden seal and one of boric acid in a pint of boiling water, stir thoroughly, let cool, and pour liquid off. Put a tablespoonful of this liquid in a half cup of water. Bathe the eyes with this, using an eye cup, or drop it in with an eye dropper.

Golden seal may be taken in different ways, and in all cases previously given where it is suggested to combine it with others, it may be used alone. Take one-fourth teaspoonful of golden seal dissolved in a glass of hot water immediately upon arising, and one hour before the noon and evening meals. Or you may steep a teaspoonful in a pint of boiling water, stir thoroughly, let cool, pour the liquid off and take a tablespoonful four to six times a day. Children should take less of all doses according to age.

There are many remedies advertised as containing golden seal; but the fact is that the herb is very expensive. Usually there is so little golden seal in commercial preparations that it does very little good.

Chronic catarrh (inflammation with a discharge) of the intestines, even to the extent of ulceration, is greatly benefitted by golden seal. Golden seal is effective in treating hemorrhage from the rectum and will heal ulcerations of the mucous lining in this area. It is a remedy for chronic and intermittent malaria or enlarged spleen caused by malaria.

From the above it will be seen how applicable golden seal is in all catarrhal conditions, whether of the throat, nasal passages, bronchial tubes, intestines, stomach, bladder, or wherever there is a lining of mucous membrane. It kills and neutralizes many poisons. Take one or two capsules daily. Don't take too much as golden seal may be quite strong.

Do not take either during pregnancy or continuously for a long period of time without some periods of rest.

GOLD THREAD (Coptis trifolia)
Common Names: Yellow root, mouth root, canker root.
Part Used: Root.
Medicinal Properties: Tonic.
Description and Uses: Excellent for digestion. A well-tried remedy for ulcers and canker sores in the mouth and for sore throat when used as a gargle. Has also been used in ulcers of the stomach, as well as inflammation of the stomach and in dyspepsia.

Effective in destroying the desire for strong drinks. Especially beneficial and effective when used in combination with golden seal in ulcers and cancerous afflictions of the stomach.

GRAVE ROOT - See Queen of the Meadow.

HAWTHORN (Crataegus oxyacantha)
Common Names: English hawthorn, May bush, May tree, quick-set, thorn-apple tree, whitethorn, haw.
Part Used: Flowers, dried berries.
Medicinal Properties: Antispasmodic, sedative, tonic.
Description and Uses: This herb is very good when treating either high or low blood pressure by strengthening the action of the heart. Helps many blood pressure problems. The tea is good for nervous tension and sleeplessness. Take one or two capsules daily. Make an infusion by steeping one teaspoonful of the flowers in one-half cup of water. Take one or two cups a day, taking only a swallow at a time. May be sweetened with honey if desired.

HENNA (Lawsonia inermis)
Common Names: Jamaica mignonette, Egyptian privet, alcanna, henna plant.
Part Used: Leaves, root.
Medicinal Properties: Astringent.
Description and Uses: The leaves can be used internally or externally for jaundice, leprosy, and other skin problems. It is occasionally used for headaches and a tea made from the leaves is useful as a gargle for sore throat. The bark is used as a dye.

HOLY THISTLE (Cnicus benedicta)
Common Names: Saint Benedict thistle, blessed thistle, spotted thistle, cardin, bitter thistle, blessed cardus, holy thistle.
Part Used: Herb.
Medicinal Properties: Diaphoretic, emetic, tonic, stimulant, febrifuge.
Description and Uses: This plant has very great power in the purification and circulation of the blood. It is such a good blood purifier that drinking a cup of thistle tea twice a day will cure chronic headaches. Some have called it "blessed thistle" because of its excellent qualities.

About two ounces of the dried plant simmered in a quart of water for two hours makes a tea satisfactory for most purposes. This tea is best taken at bedtime as a preventive of disease and it will cause profuse perspiration. The tea can be used for stomach and digestive problems, as well as for gas in the intestines, constipation, and liver troubles.

Caution should be used not to make the tea too strong as it may cause vomiting. Holy thistle is a plant that has been used for centuries. It is very good combined with any of the dock roots (red dock, yellow dock, or burdock).

It is very effective for dropsy, strengthens the heart, and is good for the liver, lungs, and kidneys. It is a good tonic for girls entering womanhood. It is claimed that the warm tea given to mothers will produce a good supply of milk.

HOPS (Humulus lupulus)
Part Used: Flowers.
Medicinal Properties: Febrifuge, tonic, nervine, diuretic, anodyne, hypnotic, anthelmintic, sedative.
Description and Uses: Hops is an old-fashioned and very useful remedy. An excellent nervine. Will produce sleep when nothing else will. Two or three cups should be taken hot. Valuable in delirium tremens. Is a good remedy for toothache, earache, neuralgia, and like ailments. Will tone up the liver, increase the flow of urine and bile, and is good for excessive sexual desires and gonorrhea. Put a tablespoonful in a pint of water and simmer for ten minutes. Drink a half pint morning and evening. A pillow stuffed with hops has long been used to produce sleep and is very effective. Good in diseases of the chest and throat. Hop poultices are very effective for inflammation, boils, tumors, painful swellings, and old ulcers.

HOREHOUND (Marrubium vulgare)
Common Names: White horehound, hoarhound, marrubium.

Part Used: Plant.

Medicinal Properties: Pectoral, aromatic, diaphoretic, tonic, expectorant, diuretic, hepatic, stimulant.

Description and Uses: Horehound will produce profuse perspiration when taken hot. Taken in large doses, it is a laxative. When taken cold, it is good for dyspepsia, jaundice, asthma, hysteria, and will expel worms. Very useful in chronic sore throat, coughs, consumption, and all pulmonary infections. If the menses stop abnormally, it will bring them back.

Horehound is one of the old-fashioned remedies and should be in every home ready for immediate use. Horehound syrup is excellent for coughs, colds, asthma, and difficult breathing. For children with coughs or croup, steep a heaping tablespoonful in a pint of boiling water for twenty minutes; strain, add honey, and let them drink it freely. Horehound is one of the bitter herbs that the Jews eat at Passover time, the others being nettle, horseradish, coriander, and lettuce.

———————

HYDRANGEA (Hydrangea aborescens)

Common Names: Wild hydrangea, seven barks.

Part Used: Leaves, root.

Medicinal Properties: Root–diuretic, lithontryptic. Leaves–tonic, diuretic, sialagogue, cathartic.

Description and Uses: This is an old remedy that is very valuable in bladder troubles. It will remove and also help prevent the formation of bladder stones and gravel; will ease the pains caused by the stones. Will relieve backache caused by kidney troubles. Good for chronic rheumatism, paralysis, scurvy, and dropsy. The hydrangea root has been used for a long time as a mild diuretic. This herb acts differently in different people.

In some it may act as a laxative. Therefore, it is better to start with a smaller dose and increase slowly as needed. The average dose is two capsules daily. To make tea, infuse one ounce of the root in one pint of boiling water and take in wineglass doses, either hot or cold.

HYSSOP (Hyssopus officinalis)
Part Used: Entire plant.

Medicinal Properties: Anthelmintic, aromatic, aperient, carminative, expectorant, febrifuge, pectoral, stimulant, sudorific.

Description and Uses: Hyssop is an old remedy recorded even in Bible times. David knew the benefits to be derived from its use. He drew the most wonderful lessons from it, which he used in showing the cleansing of the body from sin, for he said, "Purge me with hyssop, and I shall be clean; wash me, and I shall be whiter than snow" (Psalms 51:7). Hyssop, in connection with the proper use of water and deep breathing, is a most wonderful body cleanser.

Valuable in quinsy, asthma, colds, coughs, and all lung afflictions. Loosens phlegm in the lungs and throat. Is excellent for children's and infant's diseases, such as sore throat and quinsy. Can be applied as a compress and used as a gargle. In fevers, give a glassful every hour of a tea made by simmering a tablespoonful of the herb in a pint of boiling water for ten minutes. It will start perspiration, relieve the kidneys and bladder, and is slightly laxative. Hyssop increases the circulation of the blood and will reduce blood pressure. Excellent blood regulator and is a fine tonic when the system is in a weakened condition. It is excellent for scrofula, gravel in the bladder, various stomach troubles, jaundice, dropsy, and for the spleen. It has a splendid effect on the mucous lining of the stomach and bowels. It is good for coughs and shortness of breath.

A fine remedy for epilepsy in connection with other hygienic measures. It will expel worms. The leaves, applied to inflammations and bruises, will remove the pain and discoloration. Effective for insect stings and bites. Kills body lice.

For use as a poultice, soak the herb fifteen minutes in

boiling water and place in a cloth. Hyssop is good for all kinds of fevers. Hyssop tea is an excellent remedy for eye trouble. It should be used in an eye cup.

For general use, steep a heaping teaspoonful in a cup of boiling water for twenty minutes. Take from one to three cups a day, a large swallow at a time. Children less according to age. Don't use for longer than two weeks without a break.

INDIAN HEMP (Pilocorpus selloanus)
Part Used: Leaves and root
Medicinal Properties: Same as Jaborandi (see below).

INDIAN PIPE (See Fit Root)

JABORANDI (Pilocarpus microphyllus)
Part Used: Leaves.
Medicinal Properties: Stimulant, expectorant, sialagogue, antivenomous, diaphoretic.
Description and Uses: This is excellent for breaking up colds, for rheumatism, asthma, influenza and Bright's disease. It causes profuse perspiration. Effective in various fevers, in diabetes, dropsy, pleurisy, catarrh, and jaundice. An excellent remedy for mumps, taken internally as a tea, and applied externally as a fomentation or poultice to reduce the swelling. Fold the cloth three or four thicknesses and dip in the hot tea and apply. Very effective in asthma and diphtheria. It will stop hiccoughs. Excellent to stimulate the growth of the hair. Dip the fingers in tea made of the leaves several times a day and massage the scalp thoroughly.

Infuse one ounce of the leaves in one pint of boiling water and take a wineglassful or less as needed.

JUNIPER (Juniperus communis)
Common Names: Juniper bush, Juniper bark.

Part Used: Berries.

Medicinal Properties: Diuretic, carminative, tonic, antiseptic, stomachic.

Description and Uses: The tea is very effective for kidney, prostate and bladder trouble, gleet, leukorrhea, gonorrhea, digestive diseases, and dropsy. For leukorrhea, it may be combined with other herbs and used as a douche. For most purposes, Juniper berries are most effective when used in combination with such herbs as broom, uva ursi, cleavers, and buchu.

The dried berries are excellent as a preventive of disease, and should be chewed or used as a strong tea to gargle the throat when exposed to contagious diseases.

When Juniper oil is placed in a hot vapor bath, it is useful to inhale the steam for respiratory infections, colds, bronchitis, etc. The pure oil should not be rubbed on the skin as it can be very irritating and cause blisters. It is not recommended for pregnant women and should not be taken in large doses or over a prolonged period of time because of its possible irritating effect on the bladder and kidneys. Take one or two cups of the tea a day, a mouthful at a time, for one week.

LAVENDER (Lavandula vera)

Common Names: Garden lavender, spike lavender, common lavender.

Part Used: Plant.

Medicinal Properties: Stimulant, aromatic, fragrant, carminative.

Description and Uses: A tea steeped from the flowers is tonic, prevents fainting, and allays nausea. Excellent when combined with other herbs to disguise their taste. The flowers are also used in making perfumes. The dried flowers and leaves are used to put in drawers and linen closets.

Sometimes used to keep moths from clothing and furs. Leaves are used as a culinary herb for seasoning. Not used very often as a medicine nowadays.

LICORICE (Glycyrrhiza glabra)
Common Names: Sweetwood, licorice root.
Part Used: Root.
Medicinal Properties: Laxative, tonic, expectorant, demulcent, pectoral, emollient.
Description and Uses: Licorice is primarily used for lung and throat problems. It is useful in coughs, bronchitis, congestion, etc. It was used as a treatment for coughs as long ago as the third century B.C. It is frequently added to other herbal combinations to make them more palatable and for its demulcent action. Acts as a mild laxative. A decoction of one teaspoonful of the root in one cup of water is a good strength to use for children. A mixture of licorice, wild cherry, and flaxseed makes a wonderful cough syrup. It is available as a powder or in capsules.
Caution: Do not take licorice if you have high blood pressure.

LILY OF THE VALLEY (Convallaria majalis)
Common Names: May lily, May bells, convallaria, conval lily.
Part Used: Entire plant.
Medicinal Properties: Diuretic, cardiac, tonic, laxative, mucilaginous.
Description and Uses: Very quieting to the heart and good for the heart generally. Useful in epilepsy, dizziness, and convulsions of all kinds.
Good for palsy and apoplexy. Strengthens the brain and makes the thoughts clearer. Extremely useful in dropsy. Large doses may cause nausea vomiting and diarrhea.
Caution: Lily of the Valley has an action on the heart similar to digitalis (foxglove) and SHOULD NOT BE USED WITHOUT PROPER SUPERVISION.

LOBELIA (Lobeloa Inflata)
Common Names: Indian tobacco, bladderpod, wild

tobacco, emetic herb, emetic weed, lobelia herb, puke weed, asthma weed, rag root, eye-bright, vomit wort.

Part Used: Entire plant.

Medicinal Properties: Emetic, expectorant, diuretic, nervine, diaphoretic.

Description and Uses: Lobelia is one of the most extensively used herbs and is used chiefly as an emetic or in pulmonary complaints such as bronchitis, croup, whooping cough, asthma, etc., antispasmodic, stimulant.

Caution: Lobelia may have some toxic effects and should not be taken internally without proper consultation. It is safe if used externally.

Lobelia is the most powerful relaxant known among the herbs that have no harmful effects. Lobelia acts differently upon different people, but it will not hurt anyone. It makes the pulse fuller and slower in cases of inflammation and fever. Lobelia reduces palpitation of the heart. It is fine in the treatment of all fevers and in pneumonia, meningitis, pleurisy, hepatitis, peritonitis, periostitis, and nephritis. Lobelia alone cannot cure, but it is very beneficial if given in connection with other measures, such as an enema of catnip infusion morning and evening. The enema should be given even if the patient is delirious. It will relieve the brain.

Pleurisy root is a specific remedy for pleurisy, and it is also excellent if combined with lobelia for its relaxing properties.

The use of lobelia in fevers is superior to any other remedy. It is excellent for very nervous patients. Poultices or hot fomentations of lobelia are good in external inflammations, such as rheumatism. It is excellent to add lobelia to poultices for abscesses, boils, and carbuncles. Use one-third lobelia to two-thirds slippery elm bark or the same proportion to any other herb you are using.

While lobelia is an excellent emetic, it is a strange fact that when given in small doses for an irritated stomach it will stop vomiting. In cases of asthma, give a lobelia pack, followed the next morning by an emetic. The pack will loosen the waste material and it will be cast out with the emetic. In bad cases where the liver is affected and the skin yellow, combine equal parts of pleurisy root, catnip, and bitterroot.

Steep a teaspoonful in a cup of boiling water. Give two tablespoonfuls every two hours hot. For hydrophobia (rabies), steep a tablespoonful of lobelia in a pint of boiling water, drinking as much as possible to induce vomiting: this will clean the stomach out. Then give a high enema. This treatment should be given immediately after the person is attacked.

Lobelia is excellent for whooping cough. (See the paragraphs on whooping cough in Chapter 7 of this Section and in Section III.) There is nothing that will as quickly clear the air passages of the lungs as lobelia. A tincture, made as follows, will stop difficult breathing and clear the air passages of the lungs if taken a tablespoonful at a time.

lobelia herb	2 ounces
crushed lobelia seed	2 ounces
apple vinegar	1 pint

Soak for two weeks in a well-stoppered bottle, shaking every day. Then strain, and it is ready for use. This is also good used as an external application, rubbing between the shoulders and chest in asthma. A lobelia poultice is excellent for sprains, felons, bruises, ringworm, erysipelas, stings of insects, and poison ivy.

The following paragraphs are quoted from *The Medicines of Nature,* pages 65-69, and are the opinions of Drs. Thompson, Scudder, Lyle, Greer, Stephens, and other physicians.

LOBELIA INFLATA The herb and seeds of this plant are largely used by all herbal practitioners. It is employed in quite a number of cases and has won a richly deserved place in the annals of herbal writers. To Dr. Samuel Thompson is due the credit of first bringing this article into real use. It had, no doubt, been used to produce emesis in some localities previously, but its great uses were made known by him.

Now for the uses of this plant. The herb and seed have

similar properties, the seed, however, being much the stronger. In infusing the seeds, it is best to crush them. Both herb and seed contain a volatile oil, and if the seed is kept in paper, some of the oil will be absorbed by the paper.

Lobelia is a most efficient relaxant, influencing mucous, serous, nervous, and muscular structures. *It is a good rule to always give a stimulant before administering lobelia, or to combine a stimulant with it.*

It is used in coughs, bronchitis, asthma, whooping cough, pneumonia, hysteria, convulsions, suspended animation, tetanus, febrile troubles, etc.

It may be used in substance, i.e., the powdered herb or seed, in fluid extract, acid tincture, infusion, decoction, pills or capsules, in syrup, by enema, and in poultices.

We have used the acid tincture of lobelia for nearly forty years and have had splendid results. Dr. H. Nowell reports that forty years ago he was asked to try to help a case of asthma in a patient where the regulars, after consultation, had declared the patient's cough could not be stopped.

To stop the cough, they declared, would stop the patient. The case was a woman forty years of age, and at the time was seven months pregnant with her first baby. The asthmatic spasms were most trying, the patient being unable to lie in bed, and she would tear at the throat, fighting for breath, and both she and her husband begged of their doctor to stop the cough.

They were told that nothing could be done until after the child was born. The husband was given a one-ounce bottle of the acid tincture of lobelia and instructed that a teaspoonful be given when the spasm came on, with instructions to give a second teaspoonful ten minutes later... if necessary.

The next morning, upon inquiry as to the patient, he (the doctor) was told that almost immediately after taking the first dose the patient brought up long, thick masses of phlegm from the lungs the size of a man's fist. No further dose was taken and the patient has never had a trace of asthma or any chest trouble since.

We quote here the statement of Dr. Butler: "It has been my misfortune to be an asthmatic for about ten years, and I have made trial of a variety of the usual remedies with very little benefit. The last time I had an attack it was the worst I ever experienced. It continued for eight weeks. My breathing was so difficult that I took a tablespoonful of the acid tincture of lobelia, and in about three or four minutes my breathing was as free as it ever was. I took another in ten minutes, after which I took a third, which I felt through every part of my body, even to the ends of my toes, and since that time I have enjoyed as good health as before the first attack."

We have also used the acid tincture as an external application, rubbing it between the shoulders and on the chest in asthma and have found it most helpful. Dr. H. Nowell uses this regularly in this manner and has had some surprising results in cases where the breathing has been most difficult. Dr. Nowell's method of making the acid tincture is as follows:

lobelia herb	2 ounces
lobelia seed (crushed)	2 ounces
best malt vinegar	1 pint

Macerate (these ingredients) in a closely stoppered bottle for ten days to two weeks, shaking every day. Strain off and bottle for use. This is the formula he has used for nearly thirty years.

Another formula for the acid tincture of lobelia is as follows:

lobelia seed (crushed)	2 ounces
lobelia herb	1/2 ounce
cayenne	1 teaspoonful

Macerate ten days in one pint of malt vinegar, shaking well daily. Strain and bottle for use.

Another extremely useful acid tincture of lobelia is made

by using raspberry vinegar instead of the plain malt vinegar. For the benefit of those who may not know, we give herewith a formula for raspberry vinegar, which we always use ourselves. We strongly advise the reader to make his own; he is then sure of having a pure article.

Raspberry Vinegar: Bruise two quarts of raspberries. Add two quarts of best malt vinegar, stand for two days, then strain off the liquor, and to each quart of liquid add twelve ounces of good sugar (loaf sugar, if obtainable). Bring to a boil and remove the scum as it rises. The longer it boils the thicker the syrup becomes.

Allow to cool and bottle for use. Keep in a dry place. This makes an excellent raspberry vinegar, is useful to add to some cough syrups, and makes a pleasant drink, with water added.

The acid tincture can be added to horehound, hyssop, sage or other teas, or may be added to the composition tea in doses of a teaspoonful to a cupful of the herb tea for cough, asthma, colds, etc. It is also extremely useful as an emetic when one feels that the stomach should be thoroughly cleansed....

Antispasmodic tincture or third preparation: What is known among the herbal practitioners as antispasmodic tincture, or the third preparation of lobelia, is a most effective compound. It is useful in many violent cases such as epilepsy, convulsions, lockjaw, delirium tremens, fainting, hysteria, cramps, suspended animation, etc. We give below what we believe to be two of the best compounds that can be made.

Antispasmodic tincture:
    One ounce each of
    lobelia seed
    crushed skullcap
    skull cabbage, root
    gum myrrh
    black cohosh
    One-half ounce of cayenne

Infuse for one week in one pint of rectified spirits of wine

(alcohol) in a closely corked vessel. Shake well once daily.
It is well if possible to have a somewhat wide neck on the
bottle. After one week, strain and press out the clear liquid,
when it is ready for use. We assure the reader that we have
used this very formula with remarkable results. We have
given just a drop or two on the tip of the finger, thrusting the
finger into the mouth of a baby in convulsions, and in less
time than it takes to write this statement the convulsions have
ceased.

We have seen a man rolling in agony and moaning with
pain and have given one teaspoonful of antispasmodic tincture in half a cup of sweetened warm water and had the
patient drink the whole, warm: we affirm that within fifteen
seconds all traces of cramps and spasm had gone.

Dr. H. Nowell has poured a teaspoonful of the antispasmodic tincture, full strength, between the clenched teeth of
a case of lockjaw and before a second teaspoonful could be
poured from the bottle the locked jaws had relaxed and the
patient asked, "My God! What have you done?" It traverses
the system with most remarkable rapidity, and we verily
believe that in cases of suspended animation, locked jaws,
spasms, and cramps it stands unequalled in the whole realm
of therapeutic agents.

The formula of the late Mr. Hool, of Lancashire, in making
his antispasmodic tincture, is as follows:

> One-half ounce each, powdered of
> lobelia herb
> lobelia seed
> skullcap
> valerian
> skunk cabbage
> gum myrrh
> cayenne

Place in a bottle with one and a half pints of rectified spirits
of wine (pure alcohol, called also spirit vini rect. and written

S.V.R.)....cork well and shake once daily for fourteen days. Filter through white blotting paper and bottle for use.

We quote from Mr. Hool's latest writings, knowing of his wonderful work and integrity of character. He said: "The above tincture will be found superior to any other single agent, as its purely innocuous character renders it a safe and reliable remedy for patients of all ages. In...mucus and spasmodic croup the tincture must be administered promptly and in full teaspoonful doses in warm water and repeated at intervals of every ten or fifteen minutes until free vomiting ensues, as it is necessary in all such cases to induce complete relaxation of the system, by means of full emetic doses repeated at suitable intervals.

"Where the case is very severe or the tincture is difficult to administer, as in the case of infants, it should be rubbed well into the neck, chest, and between the shoulders at the same time. Two or three drops of the tincture in a raw state should be placed in the mouth and washed down with teaspoonful doses of warm water and the patient kept warm in bed. In all such cases relief will be experienced in a few minutes, and by repeating the same treatment every one or two hours a cure will soon be effected and the patient brought to a state of convalescence.

"But how is the result brought about? The properties of the lobelia, by immediate action on the muscular and mucous parts of the esophagus, glottis, larynx, windpipe and bronchial tubes, cause immediate relaxation; the parts previously contracted are made to expand and breathing is made easier. The properties of the cayenne pepper warm and stimulate the blood, allay the inflammation of the parts, cause better secretions and action of the mucous membranes.

"The skullcap and valerian being nervines, allay the irritation of the nerves and prevent too much straining and excitement and by that means prevent rupture of the small vessels, while the action of the properties of the skunk cabbage and gum myrrh is to keep canker away and to brace up the system."

As we feel the above writer, Mr. Hool, is absolutely reliable, we quote further from his writing found in Lesson 26, Dominion Herbal College, Ltd., regarding his method of treating, as follows.

Scarlet Fever and Other Febrile Conditions. "In typhoid, typhus, spotted black or slow fever, and especially malignant scarlet fever, its (antispasmodic tincture) value cannot be half told. I have seen in my time some of the worst cases of scarlet fever cured by the following simple treatment, even when death seemed to have set in and there has been no apparent hope of recovery. I have gone into such cases and caused to be administered one teaspoonful of the antispasmodic tincture of lobelia in a little water made warm, and given every half hour until the patient seemed easier. Then make up a good fire in the room, have clean underclothing warm and ready to put on.

"Then get two quarts of hot water and one quart of the best malt vinegar. Mix the water and vinegar together, bring the patient near the fire and wash the body all over with the vinegar and water and wipe dry. Put the clean clothing on and clean sheets on the bed. Put the patient back in bed and give a teaspoonful of the preparation (antispasmodic tincture) in warm tea (herbal tea) or warm water every two hours afterwards, taking care to wash with vinegar and warm water every day and Hey Preste, the patient will be on the highway to recovery. I have treated some scores of cases of scarlet fever in the above way, and never lost a single case by death."

We have thus quoted extensively because we personally know of the long life work, the labor of love, and the remarkable success of this noble-hearted man. We have used the acid tincture and the antispasmodic tincture in our practice and commend all that has been said to the careful study of the nature cure physician.

In rheumatic fever, the antispasmodic tincture will generally work wonders with the patient. Proceed as follows: Rub the whole body from neck to toes with the tincture, and if the case is bad, such as a patient who cannot sit up or move arms or legs, give a teaspoonful of the tincture in a little hot water, every half hour until free perspiration ensues.

Keep the patient in bed and allow him to cool down, then wash the whole body down with vinegar and hot water. After this, give the tincture in teaspoonful doses in hot water every two hours for one day, then every three hours for a few days. If the case demands it, also use a little for rubbing as needed. Sponge down daily with the hot water and vinegar. If this course is followed, the practitioner will find both himself and his patient surprised at the speedy recovery the case will make.

Finally, we believe that lobelia is one of the finest remedies a kind Providence has blessed mankind with. (Dominion Herbal College, Ltd. Lesson 26, 1962.)

The following paragraphs are quoted from *The Model Botanic Guide to Health,* pages 35-37.

Lobelia inflata is one of the most valuable herbs used in the botanic practice. Much has been written as to whether this herb is a poison or not. Practical experience - which is far better than theory - has proved that it is as harmless as milk, and instead of being a poison, it is an antidote to poison. The analysis of its chemical constituents shows it to contain an alkaloid lobelina and an acid lobelic acid, resin, wax, and gum; the seeds contain in addition about 30 percent of fixed oil. We have attended cases where poison had been given in mistake, and lobelia has had the desired effect of discharging the contents of the stomach. Medical men are often deluded by giving heed to mere opinions instead of noticing facts; but men who have divested themselves of that which has been taught them in medical schools have discovered truth from error.

We have prescribed the acid tincture of lobelia inflata for whooping cough with striking success. There is no other medicine that so effectually frees the air passages of the lungs of their viscid secretions.

As an emetic, we are satisfied that it is as kind and destitute of all hazard as ipecacuanha, though it is more efficient; and we consider it one of the best remedies in the whole materia medica: and are confident–the old women's stories in the books, (meaning the medical school books) to the contrary notwithstanding–that lobelia is a valuable, a safe, and sufficiently gentle article of medicine; and we think the time will come when it will be much better appreciated. Little, however, of its value, can be specified within the compass of a single sheet of paper. We not only give it to our patients, but take it ourselves whenever we have the occasion for an emetic. We can assure the public that it can be used without apprehension or danger; we have given it to infants a few months old. It tends to remove obstructions from every part of the system, and is felt even to the ends of the toes; it not only cleanses the stomach, but exercises a beneficial influence over every part of the body; it is very diffusable, however, and requires to be used with cayenne or some other permanent stimulant. The effects of lobelia may be compared to a fire made of shavings, which will soon go out unless other fuel be added; cayenne therefore, maybe said to keep alive the blaze which the lobelia has kindled. We can bear testimony that it is harmless when given in a proper manner; we never saw any evil effect, and our experience should be worth something when we say that we have sold in our practice upwards of one hundred pounds weight per year for seventy years past, which, according to the notions of some medical men, would have been sufficient to poison one-half the population of England. There is no other medicine that is half so effective as lobelia in removing the tough, hard, and ropy phlegm from asthmatic and consumptive persons. It is an indispensable medicine in fevers, bilious, and longstanding chronic complaints. We have used it for deafness with good results. It is also useful in poultices to assist suppuration. There are some writers who state that it will cure hydrophobia, if taken inwardly and applied externally as well. The medical qualities of this invaluable herb are so multifarious that a large treatise might well be written on its curative powers. Suffice it, however, to say that it is a general corrector of the whole system, innocent in its nature, and moving with the general spirits. In healthy systems it will be silent and harmless. It is fully as well calculated to remove the cause of disease as food is to remove hunger; and it clears away all obstructions in the circulation regardless of the nature of the disease.

There are untold mysteries not yet uncovered, hidden in the nonpoisonous herbs.

I do thank God for the good herbal colleges we have today, which we did not have when I was a young man.

There are a number of herbs with which you can do miracles. I will mention some of them: skullcap, golden seal, myrrh, yarrow, milkweed, fennel, cubeb berries, chickweed, aloes, mandrake, calamus root, dandelion root, blueberry leaves, tansy, yellow dock, burdock root, lobelia, coltsfoot, palmetto berries, hyssop, cayenne, sage, catnip, peppermint, echinacea, and witch hazel.

Lobelia possesses most wonderful properties; it is a perfectly harmless relaxant. It loosens disease and opens the way for its elimination from the body. Its action is quick and more effective than radium, and lobelia leaves no bad aftereffects, while radium does. Shun the taking of radium as you would a rattlesnake.

Nonpoisonous herbs will do everything for which the allopath gives radium, mercury, strychnine and all the other poisonous drugs; and nonpoisonous herbs do not leave any bad aftereffects. (Editor's note: Strychnine, mercury, radium, and other heavy metals are no longer used for treatment by allopathic physicians as they were when this book was first published.)

LUNGWORT (Pulmonaria officinalis)
Common Names: Spotted lungwort, maple lungwort, Jerusalem cowslip, Jerusalem sage, spotted comfrey, oak lungs, lungmoss.

Part Used: Entire plant.

Medicinal Properties: Expectorant, demulcent, pectoral, mucilaginous.

Description and Uses: Lungwort is a most valuable remedy for coughs, influenza, catarrh, colds, la grippe, lung troubles, bleeding lungs, and all bronchial troubles. It decreases the flow of menses when excessive. Use to wash ulcers and sores of all kinds. Take one-half to one teaspoonful of the liquid extract in a cup of water daily.

MANDRAKE (Podophyllum peltatum)

Common Names: Hog apple, May apple, American mandrake, Indian apple, duck's foot, ground lemon, wild lemon, racoonberry.

Part Used: Root.

Medicinal Properties: Antibilious, cathartic, emetic, diaphoretic, cholagogue, alterative, resolvent, vermifuge, deobstruent.

Description and Uses: Excellent regulator for liver and bowels. In chronic liver diseases it has no equal. Valuable in jaundice, bilious, or intermittent fever. Good physic; is often combined with senna leaves. It is very beneficial in uterine diseases. It acts powerfully upon all the tissues of the body. Use wherever a powerful cathartic is required.

Small doses given frequently should be used in order to prevent severe purgative action. Steep a teaspoonful in a pint of boiling water and take a teaspoonful of this tea at a time. Children less according to age. Take one capsule a day for no longer than one week at a time.

Caution: Mandrake is a potent herb; *it should be taken with care.*

Other herbs can give the same results and are much safer to use.

MARJORAM (Majorana hortensis)

Common Names: Sweet marjoram, knotted marjoram.

Part Used: Entire plant.

Medicinal Properties: Aromatic, tonic, condiment, emmenagogue.

Description and Uses: This is a good tonic. Very effective in combination with camomile and gentian. Excellent for sour stomach, loss of appetite, cough, consumption, eruptive diseases, suppressed menstruation, to increase the flow of urine, for poisonous insect bites and snake bites, dropsy, scurvy, itch, jaundice, toothache, headache, and indigestion. Taken hot, it produces perspiration. This herb is not commonly used in medicine, but is largely used in cooking as a seasoning agent. The dose is one to two capsules daily.

MARSHMALLOW (Althaea officinalis)

Common Names: Althea, sweet weed, wymote, mortification root, mallards, Schloss tea.

Part Used: Root, leaves.

Medicinal Properties: Diuretic, demulcent, mucilaginous, emollient.

Description and Uses: As a poultice it is excellent for sore or inflamed parts since it is very soothing and lubricating. For lung troubles, hoarseness, cough, bronchitis, diarrhea, or dysentery, put a teaspoonful in a cup of water, simmer for ten minutes, let stand until cool. Drink one to two cupfuls a day, a large mouthful at a time. For irritation of the vagina, use as a douche, and also take internally. One to two capsules a day is an average dose. The tea is also good to bathe sore, inflamed eyes. Very soothing and healing to any inflamed condition of the bowels. Valuable in pneumonia, strangury (slow and painful discharge of the urine), gravel, and all kidney diseases. The root is sometimes used to increase milk in nursing mothers.

MASTERWORT (Heracleum lanatum)

Common Names: Madnep, cow cabbage, cow parsnip, youthwort, hogweed, madness, wooly parsnip.

Part Used: Root, seed.

Medicinal Properties: Carminative, stimulant, antispasmodic.

Description and Uses: A useful remedy for colds, fevers, increasing the flow of urine, gravel in kidneys, colic, scanty menstruation with painful cramps, dyspepsia, dropsy, epilepsy, spasms, asthma, palsy, and apoplexy. Will expel gas from the bowels. Good as a wash for sores and ulcers. Available as a fluid extract. Take one to two teaspoonfuls in a cup of water.

MILKWEED (Asclepias syriaca)

Common Names: Milkweed root, silkweed, silky swallow wort, cottonweed, Virginia silk.

Part Used: Root.

Medicinal Properties: Emetic, purgative, alterative, diuretic, tonic.

Description and Uses: This is the cotton milkweed with which almost everyone is familiar. A splendid remedy for female complaints, bowel, and kidney troubles. It increases the flow of urine and is therefore good for dropsy. Also good for asthma, stomach troubles, and scrofulous conditions of the bladder.

It is often used in place of lobelia. It is a very effective remedy for gallstones. Take equal parts of milkweed and marshmallow, steep a teaspoonful in a cup of boiling water; take three cups daily and one hot upon retiring. Children less according to age. Fomentations applied to the liver after the liver has been thoroughly massaged are very effective. The boiled roots taste similar to asparagus. Caution should be exercised in using milkweed since it may be poisonous, especially when used in large doses and particularly in children. Follow the directions carefully and take no more than is necessary.

MINT (Monarda punctata)
Common Names: Horsemint, American horsemint, monarda.
Part Used: Leaves, tops.
Medicinal Properties: Stimulant, carminative, sudorific, diuretic, emmenagogue.
Description and Uses: Very quieting and soothing. Eases pain. Excellent for suppressed urine, nausea and vomiting, gas in the stomach and intestinal tract, decreased menstrual flow, rheumatism, diarrhea, and other digestive problems. Take 10 to 30 drops of the tincture daily in a glass of water.

MISTLETOE (Viscum album)
Common Names: Birdlime, all-heal, European mistletoe, devil's fuge.
Part Used: Leaves, young twigs.
Medicinal Properties: Nervine, antispasmodic, cardiac, tonic, narcotic.
Description and Uses: This is a different plant from American mistletoe, Phoradendron flavescens. It is a fine nervine, effective in epilepsy, convulsions, hysteria, delirium, and St. Vitus dance. Persons with heart trouble should be careful when using mistletoe, particularly in large doses. It raises the blood pressure and speeds up the pulse. Use only one teaspoonful to a pint of boiling water.
Caution: The berries are poisonous and should not be eaten. Large doses have an adverse effect on the heart. Take this herb with care and preferably under proper supervision.

MOTHERWORT (Leonurus cardiaca)
Common Names: Lion's tail, lion's ear, throwwort.
Part Used: Entire plant.
Medicinal Properties: Antispasmodic, nervine, emmenagogue, laxative, hepatic, tonic.
Description and Uses: Motherwort is very well-

known and is used with excellent results to promote the
menstrual flow. It is also useful in other female troubles. It
should be taken warm. It is very useful in nervous complaints, fainting, heart flutters, cramps, convulsions, hysteria,
delirium, and sleeplessness. Good for liver infectious and
suppressed urine. A hot fomentation wrung out of the strong
tea will relieve cramps and pain due to painful menstruation.
A remedy for colds, particularly chest colds. Kills worms.
Has an excellent effect if taken during pregnancy. Steep one
teaspoonful of the herb leaves in one-half cup of water. Take
one cup a day, using only a swallow at a time, when using
the tincture, take one-half tsp. three times daily in a glass of
water.

MUGWORT (Artemisia vulgaris)

Common Names: Common mugwort, sailor's tobacco,
felon herb.

Part Used: Entire plant.

Medicinal Properties: Emmenagogue, laxative, diaphoretic.

Description and Uses: Splendid for female complaints
when combined with marigold flower and some of the herbs
recommended in Section III under menstruation. Take a
heaping teaspoonful to a cup of boiling water. Steep twenty
minutes, and drink one to three cups a day as needed. The
leaves and flowers are full of virtue.

It is a safe and excellent medicine for female complaints
and for suppressed menstruation. Steep a tablespoonful in a
pint of water twenty minutes and drink two or three cups a
day a few days before the monthly period is expected.
Mugwort is very useful in overcoming inflammatory swellings, gravel and stones in the kidneys and bladder, to increase
the flow of urine, and for fevers and gout. After using a
poultice of chickweed or slippery elm, thoroughly bathe the
affected part for some time with the hot tea, made by steeping
a tablespoonful of mugwort to a pint of boiling water for
twenty minutes. Bruises, whitlows (felons), abscesses, car-

buncles, and sometimes even tumors will yield to this treatment if it is continued. Good for rheumatism and gout. Acute
pain in the bowels and stomach can quickly be relieved by
drinking the warm infusion and applying hot fomentations
wrung out of the boiling infusion.

MULLEIN (Verbascum thapsus)

Common Names: Velvet plant, white mullein, verbascum flowers, woolen blanket herb, bullock's lungwort,
flannel flower, shepherd's club, hare's beard, pig taper, cow's
lungwort.

Part Used: Leaves, flower, roots.

Medicinal Properties: Anodyne, diuretic, demulcent,
antispasmodic, vulnerary, astringent, emollient, pectoral.

Description and Uses: This is one of the old household
herbs we have used from childhood. The root has been
successfully used for many years in asthma. For this purpose,
burn the root and inhale the fumes. A tea of the leaves is very
valuable in asthma, croup, bronchitis, all lung afflictions,
bleeding from the lungs, difficult breathing, and hay fever.

The tea is good as a throat gargle, for toothache, and for
washing open sores. A tea made from the flowers will induce
sleep, relieve pain, and in large doses act as a laxative. The
freshly crushed flowers will remove warts. Fomentations
wrung from hot tea made from the leaves are helpful for
inflamed piles, ulcers, tumors, mumps, acute inflammation
of the tonsils, and sore throat. Fomentations are excellent in
any glandular swelling.

This is a splendid remedy when taken internally for
dropsy, catarrh, or swollen joints. Boil one ounce of mullein
for a few minutes in a pint of boiling water or milk (soybean
milk is preferred) and take a half teacupful after each bowel
movement for dysentery, diarrhea, and bleeding from the
bowels. For swollen testicles or scrotum, apply fomentations
for one hour three or four times a day wrung out of the tea,
made by simmering one ounce of mullein and one ounce of

sanicle herb in two quarts of water for fifteen minutes. These fomentations are good for any kind of swelling or bad sores. Excellent pain killer without being habit-forming. Helps to calm the nerves.

MUSTARD (Sinapsis alba)
Common Names: White mustard seed, yellow mustard, kedlock, yellow mustard seed, white mustard.
Part Used: Seeds.
Medicinal Properties: Pungent, laxative, stimulant, condiment, emetic, irritant, digestive.
Description and Uses: This is the common yellow ground mustard that is used so much in food, even though it is harmful when used in this way.

Mustard is an old-fashioned remedy used to produce vomiting. Steep a teaspoonful of mustard in a large cup of boiling water, stir well, let cool to lukewarm, drink all at one time. If this does not produce vomiting, tickle the back of the throat with the finger. Mustard is excellent when put in a foot bath to draw the blood to the lower part of the body in congestion of the lungs or head. It is excellent to use in a poultice for pneumonia, bronchitis, and other diseases of the respiratory tract.

Mustard plaster is also excellent applied over the kidneys in irritation of the kidneys. A good mustard plaster is made as follows: one part mustard and four parts whole wheat flour. Make into a paste by mixing with warm water. Have it thick enough to nicely spread on a piece of cloth. If the mustard is very strong, be careful not to blister the skin. When the burning becomes too uncomfortable, the mustard plaster should be removed.

After it is removed, be sure to thoroughly cleanse the skin, making sure that no mustard remains. If you wish to leave the plaster on for a longer time, it can be made weaker. If you mix the mustard and flour with the whites of eggs in place of water it will not blister the skin.

MYRRH (Balsamodendron myrrha)
Common Names: Gum myrrh tree.
Part Used: Powdered gum, resin.
Medicinal Properties: Antiseptic, stimulant, tonic, expectorant, vulnerary, emmenagogue.

Description and Uses: An ancient Bible remedy, still in use today and one of the best, it is valuable as a tonic and stimulant for bronchial and lung diseases. Excellent for pyorrhea, as it is antiseptic and very healing.

Brush the teeth with the powder. Thoroughly rinse the mouth and bathe the gums with the tea. For use as a gargle and mouthwash, steep a teaspoonful of myrrh and one of boric acid in a pint of boiling water. Let stand for one-half hour, pour off the clear liquid and use. Cures halitosis (bad breath) when taken internally. Take a small teaspoonful of powdered myrrh and one of golden seal to a pint of boiling water. Steep a few minutes, pour off the clear liquid, and take teaspoonful doses five or six times a day. It is also an excellent remedy for ulcers, piles, hemorrhoids, and for bathing bedsores or any sores on the body. Made into an ointment with equal parts of golden seal, it is an excellent infection for piles and hemorrhoids; or the tea can be used for these conditions as a wash. After thoroughly washing sores, ulcers, etc., with the tea, sprinkle a little of the powder on the sore. Charcoal moistened with this tea and applied to old ulcers and sores is healing. Is also effective for gangrene. This is also an excellent remedy for diphtheria, ulcerated throat, and sores in the mouth. Use for cough, asthma, tuberculosis, and all chest affections, as it diminishes the mucus discharge.

NETTLE (Urtica dioica)
Common Names: Common stinging nettle, stinging nettle, common nettle.
Part Used: Entire plant.
Medicinal Properties: Pectoral, diuretic, astringent, tonic, styptic, rubefacient.

Description and Uses: This herb will help prevent scrofula. It is an excellent remedy for kidney trouble. It will expel gravel from the bladder and increase the flow of urine. Splendid for neuralgia. A poultice of the green steeped leaves will relieve pain; however, such a poultice will raise blisters if kept on too long. The tea increases the menstrual flow. It will kill and expel worms. For diarrhea, dysentery, piles, hemorrhages, hemorrhoids, gravel, or inflammation of the kidneys, make a decoction using a teaspoonful to a cup of water and simmer for ten minutes. For chronic rheumatism, take the bruised leaves and rub on the skin. Excellent for reducing in combination with seawrack. Tea made from the root will cure dropsy in the first stages and will stop hemorrhage from the urinary organs, lungs, intestines, nose, and stomach. The boiled leaves applied externally will stop bleeding almost immediately. Nettle tea is good for fever, colds, and la grippe. It is an old-fashioned remedy for backache.

Very fine for eczema. Tea made from the leaves of the nettle will expel phlegm from the lungs and stomach and will clean out the urinary passages.

An infusion of one ounce of the herb or seed in one pint of boiling water is taken in wineglassful doses. The dose of the fluid extract is one-half to one teaspoonful.

Nettle tea is an excellent hair tonic and will bring back the natural color of the hair. Use as the last rinse when shampooing. Make a cup of the tea by steeping a teaspoonful in a cup of boiling water for thirty minutes. Dip the fingers in and thoroughly massage the scalp. This will cure dandruff. It is well to boil the leaves in vinegar for this purpose.

In the summer when you can get the green leaves, cook them like spinach. They are a splendid blood purifier. Nettle is a weed people generally dislike because when they touch it, it stings the hands, but they do not know the wonderful medicinal properties it contains. The nettle plant should be handled with care because of the small sharp spurs that can cause a severe local irritation and pain when touching the skin. Old plants may cause kidney damage if eaten without being cooked.

"Tender-handed grasp the nettle
And it stings you for your pains.
Grasp it like a man of mettle
And it soft as silk remains."

NUTMEG (Myristica fragrans)

Common Names: Nutmeg flower, black caraway, flower seed, black cumin, nigella seed, bishop's wort, small fennel flower.

Part Used: Seeds.

Medicinal Properties: Carminative, expectorant, deobstruent, sialagogue, emmenagogue, aromatic.

Description and Uses: Nutmeg is commonly used for seasoning foods. It helps prevent gas and fermentation in the intestinal tract. It improves the appetite and digestion and is good in nausea and vomiting. It is mildly hallucinogenic. Nutmeg is no longer commonly used for medicinal purposes as there are other less toxic herbs having greater effect on the system. Serious symptoms of poisoning can result from eating only a few of the nutmegs.

OREGON GRAPE - See Wild Oregon Grape.

ORIGANUM (Origanum vulgare)

Common Names: Wild marjoram, winter marjoram, mountain mint, winter sweet, oregano.

Part Used: Entire plant.

Medicinal Properties: Aromatic, pungent, stomachic, tonic, stimulant, emmenagogue, carminative, diaphoretic.

Description and Uses: Very strengthening to the stomach and increases the appetite. Excellent for relieving sour stomach. Excellent in tuberculosis and severe cough. Good in suppressed urine, suppressed menstruation, dropsy, yellow jaundice, scurvy, and itch. The extracted juice is excellent for deafness or pain and noise in the ears. Drop a few drops in the ear whenever necessary. The oil dropped in the hollow of an aching tooth will stop the pain. Will expel gas from the stomach and bowels.

Very helpful in dyspepsia. Good for rheumatism, colic, nausea, and neuralgia. A poultice made from this herb is very beneficial for painful swellings, sprains, felons, boils, and carbuncles. It is an excellent medicine in nervous persons. Good to use in salves and liniments. It is excellent for a sore throat when applied as a heating compress. Steep a heaping tablespoonful in a pint of boiling water for thirty minutes. Dip a cloth in this hot tea, apply to the neck, binding snugly with a dry cloth.

It is well to cover the compress with oiled silk or a piece of plastic, which will keep it moist. For general use, steep a teaspoonful to a cup of boiling water for twenty minutes; drink cold one or two cupfuls a day, one hour before meals. Children less according to age.

PARSLEY (Petroselinum sativum)
Common Names: Garden parsley, rock parsley, common parsley, march.
Part Used: Leaves, root, seeds.
Medicinal Properties: Diuretic, aperient, expectorant, carminative.

Juice–antiperiodic. Seeds–febrifuge, emmenagogue.
Description and Uses: Parsley is a member of the carrot family. It has largely been ignored in the past, when a sprig or two was used to decorate a salad or other dish. Lately it is being used more frequently as a food, as it is very rich in iron and vitamin C. It contains more calcium, potassium and phosphorus than the same amount of spinach and may actually have up to 30,000 I.U. of vitamin A in each ounce.

Parsley is used chiefly for its diuretic effect and to promote menstruation. The roots or leaves are one of the most excellent remedies for difficult urination, dropsy, jaundice, fevers, stones or gravel in the urinary tracts, obstructions of the liver and spleen, strangury, syphilis, and gonorrhea. Also excellent for cancer and should be classed among the preventive herbs. Simmer a tablespoonful to a pint of boiling water for ten minutes, let stand, strain, and drink one to three cups a day, a large swallow at a time, more or less, as needed. For painful or scanty menstruation it is well to combine the leaves with equal parts of buchu, black haw, and cramp bark. One of the most excellent remedies for gallbladder, it also helps to expel gallstones.

A hot fomentation wrung out of the tea and applied to insect bites and stings will cure them. Use a tablespoonful of the leaves to a cup of boiling water, and steep twenty minutes. Parsley is rich in potassium. A poultice of the bruised leaves is excellent for swollen glands, swollen breasts, or to dry up milk. A tea made of the crushed seeds, a teaspoonful to the cup, steeped, strained, and applied to the hair will kill vermin.

Parsley should be used freely in salads, soups, and slaws for its beneficial results. *Do not use parsley if you have a kidney infection.*

PENNYROYAL (Hedeoma pulegioides)
Common Names: Tickweed, squaw mint, stinking balm, thickweed, American pennyroyal, mock pennyroyal, mosquito plant, squaw balm.

Part Used: Entire plant, oil.

Medicinal Properties: Sudorific, carminative, emmenagogue, stimulant, diaphoretic, aromatic, sedative.

Description and Uses: it is excellent in burning fevers and will promote perspiration when taken hot. Excellent remedy for toothache, gout, leprosy, colds, consumption, phlegm in the chest and lungs, jaundice, dropsy, cramps, convulsions, headache, ulcers, sores in mouth, insect and snake bites, itch, intestinal pains, colic, and griping. If troubled with suppressed or scanty menstruation, take one or two cupfuls hot at bedtime along with a hot foot bath, several days before menstruation is expected.

It will relieve nausea, but SHOULD NOT BE TAKEN DURING PREGNANCY. Good as a poultice and wash for bruises or black eyes. Good for nervousness and hysteria. Useful for skin diseases and the oil is an excellent insect repellent. Take one or two cups a day or use one-half tea-spoonful of the powder in a cup of hot water.

PEPPERMINT (Mentha piperita)

Common Names: Brandy mint, balm mint, curled mint, lamb mint.

Part Used: Leaves, oil.

Medicinal Properties: Aromatic, stimulant, stomachic, carminative, rubefacient.

Description and Uses: This is one of the oldest household remedies and should be in every garden as it grows very prolifically. Excellent remedy for chills, colic, fevers, dizziness, flatulence, nausea, vomiting, diarrhea, dysentery, cholera, heart trouble, palpitation of the heart, influenza, la grippe, and hysteria. Applied externally, it is good for rheumatism, neuralgia, and headache. Peppermint enemas are excellent for cholera and colon troubles. It is especially useful for convulsions and spasms in infants.

Peppermint is a general stimulant. A strong cup of peppermint tea will act more powerfully on the system than any liquor stimulant, quickly diffusing itself through the system and bringing back to the body its natural warmth and glow without the usual tendency to relapse. It is good in cases of sudden fainting or dizziness with extreme coldness and pale countenance. Useful for griping pains caused by eating unripe fruit or irritating foods.

Do not drink coffee and tea, which are harmful. Coffee weakens the heart muscle. Peppermint tea is delicious and strengthens your heart muscle. Coffee hinders digestion, is a cause of constipation, and poisons the body. Peppermint tea cleanses and strengthens the entire body. Give it a fair trial and see how much better you feel when you leave off coffee and tea and drink peppermint tea.

Instead of using aspirin or some other harmful drug for headaches, take a cup of peppermint tea as strong as you like it, lie down for a little while, and see what a good effect it has on you. If need be, drink two or three cups, so that enough gets into the system to help you. You will not be disappointed. It strengthens the nerves, instead of weakening them as aspirin and other drugs do.

If the tea is not at hand, take some of the leaves and chew them up until you can swallow them easily. This will start your food digesting and assist the entire body in doing its work more normally. Use one ounce of the herb in a pint of boiling water and sweeten with some honey if desired.

Take in doses of one wineglassful. You may also use 5 to 15 drops of the liquid extract in a cup of water.

PILEWORT (See Fireweed)

PIMPERNEL (See Burnet)

PIPSISSEWA (Chimaphila umbellata)
Common Names: Prince's pine, ground holly, false wintergreen, rheumatism weed, bitter wintergreen, king's cure.

Part Used: Entire plant, leaves.

Medicinal Properties: Diuretic, tonic, alterative, astringent, diaphoretic.

Description and Uses: A good herb to use in kidney diseases and infections.

One of the great advantages of this herb is its almost total lack of irritating side effects. It has been reported to dissolve small stones in the bladder. A poultice may be made from the leaves and applied to the skin for ulcers, sores, bruises, blisters, etc.

Make an infusion of 1 ounce of the herb in 1 pint of boiling water; drink cold one or two cupfuls a day, a swallow at a time. Use 5 to 15 drops of the tincture. Follow the directions as given on the bottle.

PLANTAIN (Plantago major)

Common Names: Waybread, round-leaved plantain, Englishman's foot, common plantain, ribwort, ripple grass, snake weed.

Part Used: Entire plant.

Medicinal Properties: Alterative, diuretic, antisyphilitic, antiseptic, astringent, deobstruent, styptic, vulnerary.

Description and Uses: Plantain is an old-fashioned herb. The Indians used it to great advantage. It grows practically all over the United States.

Every family should gather some and have it ready for use. It has wonderful properties and many uses. There are two kinds of plantain – narrow and wide leaf. Both are good. The whole plant should be used.

Plantain has a soothing, cooling, and healing effect on sores and ulcers. The fresh leaves, when pounded into a paste and applied to wounds, will check the bleeding. They may also be rubbed directly onto insect bites and stings. It is extremely useful in erysipelas, eczema, burns, and scalds. Make a strong tea and apply to the affected parts, using frequently in bad cases.

For piles and hemorrhoids, make a strong tea with an ounce of granulated plantain to a pint of boiling water. Let steep for twenty to thirty minutes.

For hemorrhoids, inject one tablespoonful of this tea three or four times a day at least, and especially after each stool, using more frequently in bad cases. Apply externally with a soft gauze or cotton as needed. A saturated piece of gauze may be kept on the piles by using a belt or band around the body to which has been attached a narrow strip of cloth for holding the saturated gauze against the piles. An ointment for piles may be made by boiling slowly for about two hours two ounces of granulated plantain in one pint of soybean oil, peanut oil, or any other soluble oil.

For use in leukorrhea, make a strong tea and use as a douche.

For diarrhea, kidney, and bladder trouble, aching in the lumbar region, and bedwetting, plantain is wonderful. Make a tea by using one teaspoonful of granulated herbs in one cup of boiling water. Let steep for twenty or thirty minutes. If powdered herbs are used, place one small teaspoonful in a cup of hot water. Let stand about fifteen or twenty minutes. Drink a cupful of this tea four or five times a day until relief is obtained.

For use in tuberculosis and syphilis, use both internally and externally.

The green leaves give wonderful relief if mashed up and applied as a poultice to any part of the body stung by poisonous insects, or to snake bites, boils, carbuncles, and tumors.

Plantain tea will ease pain in the bowels. It will help clear the head of mucus and slows all manner of flowings, even excessive menstruation. The plantain seed is good for dropsy, by making a tea of one teaspoonful to a cup of boiling water. The roots, beaten into powder, are good for toothache. A tea made with distilled water is good for inflamed eyes. The tea kills worms in the stomach and bowels. Equal parts of plantain and yellow dock make a very excellent wash for itch, ringworms, and all running sores. Plantain is excellent for healing fresh or old wounds or sores, either internal or external.

PLEURISY ROOT (Asclepias tuberosa)
Common Names: Butterfly weed, wind root, Canada root, silkweed, orange swallow wort, tuber root, white root, flux root, asclepias.

Part Used: Root.

Medicinal Properties: Expectorant, carminative, tonic, diuretic, diaphoretic, relaxant, antispasmodic.

Description and Uses: As the name suggests, this herb is very valuable in pleurisy. It eases the pain, which helps to make breathing easier. It is excellent for breaking up colds as well as for asthma and all bronchial and pulmonary complaints. Very useful in scarlet fever, rheumatic fever, bilious fever, typhus, all burning fevers, and measles. Good for suppressed menstruation and acute dysentery.

Treatment of pleurisy: Steep a teaspoonful of powdered pleurisy root in a cup of boiling water for forty-five minutes, strain, and take two tablespoonfuls every two hours – more often if necessary. Apply a cold compress to the affected part, covering well with a flannel. Give a high enema of pleurisy root. Using a tablespoonful to a quart of boiling water, let steep, and use at about 112°F. It also acts as a tonic for the kidneys.

POKE ROOT (Phytolacca decandra)

Common Names: Red weed, red ink plant, poke weed, garget, pigeon berry, scoke, coakum, Virginia polk, pocan bush, American nightshade, red ink berries.

Part Used: Root, leaves, berries.

Medicinal Properties: Alterative, resolvent, deobstruent, detergent, antisyphilitic, antiscorbutic, cathartic.

Description and Uses: Caution: *Do not eat this plant raw or inadequately cooked. Poke root should be boiled before eating and the water drained off and discarded; boil it again in fresh water and drain off the water again. It may then be eaten.*

The tender leaves are excellent as greens for the dinner table, especially in the early spring. They are eaten by many people for the purpose of toning up the whole system. The green root of poke is a most useful agent. Very good in enlargement of the glands, particularly the thyroid gland.

Very good for hard liver, biliousness, inflammation of the kidneys, enlarged lymphatic glands. It is effective in goitre, either taken internally or applied as a poultice or liniment. Excellent in skin diseases, scrofula, and eczema. If a tea is made of the root and applied to the skin, it will cure itching.

Poke root makes a good poultice for caked breasts. It has also been used as an aid in advanced cancer of the breast as a poultice. First, grind fine the fresh root. Roll this out to make a plaster to cover the breast completely, cutting out a hole for the nipple. Use a piece of cheese cloth or other thin material to put this on the breast, and once daily moisten the poultice with poke root tea, made fresh each time. Do this for three days, putting on a fresh poultice daily, and continuing the treatment for fifteen days. The skin will be covered with little sores with pus. In about four to six weeks the hardness should then leave the breast. Then cleanse the skin thoroughly and cover with boric acid powder, and allow the entire surface to become dry. In about ten days the sores will be completely healed.

Care should be taken in using roots that are insufficiently cooked or fresh.

Caution: The seeds, which are present in the berries, are poisonous and should not be eaten.

PSYLLIUM (Plantago psyllium)

Common Names: Branching plantain, flea seed, flea-wort, spogel.

Part Used: Seeds.

Medicinal Properties: Demulcent, purgative, detergent.

Description and Uses: Psyllium assists greatly in cases of colitis, anal fissures or ulcers, and hemorrhoids by relieving the stress occasioned during difficult evacuation of the bowel. It relieves autointoxication, the cause of many diseases, by cleansing the intestines and removing the putrefactive toxins. Psyllium, being a purely vegetable product, causes no harmful effects, either physiological or chemical. It is superior to emulsions, oils, and agar compounds, which are widely known and used. For adults, take two teaspoonfuls after meals, or an hour before meals in a glass of water, warm water being preferred. For children the dose is one-half to one teaspoonful after meals. Vary the dose according to the individual needs.

When soaked in water or any liquid, the seeds swell into a jelly-like mass that lubricates the intestines and stimulates the normal muscular activity without causing cramps and griping in the bowels. Psyllium could really be called a colon broom, as it cleans out the colon. Some psyllium preparations come with natural flavors, such as lemon, which makes it easier for children to take.

QUEEN OF THE MEADOW (Eupatorium purpureum)
Common Names: Grave root, kidney root, joe-pye weed, purple boneset, trumpet weed.
Part Used: Root, whole herb.
Medicinal Properties: Diuretic, stimulant, tonic, astringent, relaxant.
Description and Uses: This is a good remedy for gravel in the bladder, chronic urinary and kidney disorders, dropsy, neuralgia, and all such ailments. Excellent for rheumatism. Very soothing and will relax the nerves. Increases the flow of urine. Wonderful remedy when combined with uva ursi, marshmallow, blue cohosh, and lily root for female troubles, bladder and kidney infections, diabetes, and Bright's disease. As a tincture, take 5 to 15 drops in a cup of water.

RAGWORT (Senecio aureus)
Common Names: Uncum root, waw weed, uncum, liferoot, liferoot plant, false valerian, golden sececio, cough weed, squaw weed, female regulator, cocash weed, ragweed, staggerwort, St. James wort.

Part Used: Entire plant.

Medicinal Properties: Expectorant, diaphoretic, febrifuge, emmenagogue, pectoral, tonic.

Description and Uses: Has a very powerful influence upon the female organs. Combined with white pond lily, it is one of the most certain and safe cures known for severe cases of leukorrhea, and also for suppressed menstruation.

Good in all urinary diseases and gravel. Useful for rheumatism, sciatica, joint pains, coughs, and colds. As a fluid extract, take one-half to one teaspoonful in a cup of water.

RED CLOVER (Trifolium pratense)

Common Names: Wild clover, cleaver grass, marl grass, cow grass, trefoil, purple clover.

Part Used: Flowers.

Medicinal Properties: Depurative, detergent, alterative, mild stimulant.

Description and Uses: Red clover is one of God's greatest blessings to man. Very pleasant to take and a wonderful blood purifier. Combined with equal parts of blue violet, burdock, yellow dock, dandelion root, rock rose, and golden seal, it is a great help in treating cancerous growths, leprosy, and pellagra. Learn to use this God-given remedy effectively. Used without other herbs, it is good for cancer of the stomach, whooping cough, and various spasms. The warm tea is very soothing to the nerves. I have used red clover blossoms for many years with excellent results. When I was a boy, my parents had me gather it for their postmaster, who had a serious cancer. He lived to be an old man, without an operation.

Red clover blossoms were also one of Mrs. E. G. White's home remedies. Mrs. White, mentioned earlier in this book, wrote several books on health and good diet. Red clover is effective in bronchial troubles and whooping cough.

It is healing to fresh wounds as well as old ulcers and makes an excellent healing salve. Red clover is splendid for syphilis. A good prescription is the following.

1 ounce red clover
1 ounce burdock seed
2 ounces wild Oregon grape
1/2 ounce bloodroot

Use the granulated herbs, mixing them well in one pint of hot water and one pint of hot apple cider. Cover and let stand for two hours. The dose is one wineglassful four times a day.

Red clover is exceedingly good for cancer on any part of the body. If in the throat, make a strong tea and gargle four or five times a day, swallowing some of the tea. If in the stomach, drink four or more cups of red clover tea a day on an empty stomach. If there are sores on the outside of any part of the body, bathe them freely with the tea. If in the rectum, inject with a syringe, five or six times a day. If in the uterus, inject with a bulb syringe, holding the vagina closed after the syringe is inserted so the tea will be forced well around the head of the womb. This should be held in for several minutes before expelling.

Every family should have a good supply of red clover blossoms. Gather them in the summer when in full bloom and dry them in the shade on paper. Put them in paper bags when dry and hang in a dry place. Use this tea in place of tea and coffee and you will have splendid results. Use it freely. It can be taken in place of water. If used as a capsule, take one or two, three times a day.

———

RED PEPPER – See Cayenne

———

RED RASPBERRY (Rubus strigosus)
Common Names: Wild red raspberry, reapberry.
Part Used: Leaves, berries.
Medicinal Properties: Leaves – antiemetic, astringent, purgative, stomachic, parturient, tonic, stimulant, alterative. Fruit – laxative, esculent, antacid, parturient.
Description and Uses: Will heal canker sores that

develop on mucous membranes. Take one cup of tea every hour until the canker sores disappear.

During this time, eat no food but drink only juice. The tea has been reported to speed up delivery as well as easing labor pains. Excellent for dysentery and diarrhea, especially in infants. It decreases the menstrual flow without abruptly stopping it. Good to combine in such cases with prickly ash, blue cohosh, wild yam, and cinnamon. Is very soothing and does not excite. Will allay nausea. When the bowels are greatly relaxed, use in place of coffee or tea. Good for intestinal problems in children.

To make red raspberry tea, take one ounce of the dried herb or one handful of fresh leaves and pour over them a pint of boiling hot water.

Cover and let steep for fifteen to twenty minutes. Then strain and drink one or two cups a day. A little honey may be added if desired. The leaves are available in powder form also.

RED ROOT (Ceanothus americanus)

Common Names: New Jersey tea, Walpole tea, wild snow ball, Jersey tea, mountain sweet, New Jersey tea tree, bobea.

Part Used: Root.

Medicinal Properties: Astringent, expectorant, sedative.

Description and Uses: This is one of the most wonderful remedies for any spleen trouble: it has a direct action on the spleen. It is also good in dysentery, asthma, chronic bronchitis, whooping cough, and tuberculosis, and is a splendid wash for a sore mouth during fevers and for canker sores in the mouth or throat. Gargling with a strong tea every two hours will reduce sore, swollen tonsils. If tonsils are very sore and swollen, make a swab and work around good and then gargle. It will reduce very badly enlarged tonsils, and the trouble will rarely recur. Excellent for piles or hemorrhoids. Inject the strong tea often.

It is effective in spasms, also is very effective in syphilis and gonorrhea. When combined with fringe tree and golden seal, it is good for sick headache, acute indigestion, and nausea due to poor activity of the liver. Use one teaspoonful of the granulated red root to a pint of boiling water. Steep for twenty or thirty minutes. Drink one cupful of this tea before each meal and before going to bed. If the powdered herb is used, take half a teaspoonful in a cup of hot or cold water, an hour before each meal and before going to bed. If capsules are used, take one No.00 capsule before meals and also at bedtime.

Red root is also an excellent remedy in diabetes and is commonly used in asthma, bronchitis, and other lung infections.

RHUBARB (Rheum palmatum)
Common Names: Turkey rhubarb, Chinese rhubarb.
Part Used: Root.
Medicinal Properties: Vulnerary, tonic, stomachic, purgative, astringent, aperient.
Description and Uses: Rhubarb is an old-fashioned remedy and is very useful in small doses for diarrhea and dysentery in adults and children. In larger doses, it is an excellent laxative for infants, as it is very mild and tonic. Excellent to increase the muscular action of the bowels and for use in stomach troubles. Will relieve headache. It stimulates the gallbladder, thereby causing the ejection of bilious material. Excellent for scrofulous children with distended abdomens. Good for the liver. Cleanses and tones the bowels. Rhubarb is very high in oxalates and therefore should not be used by those who develop kidney stones. NEVER EAT THE LEAVES, which are poisonous. Available as the powdered root or as a tincture, 10 to 20 drops in water.

ROCK ROSE (Helianthemum canadense)

Common Names: Frostwort, frost weed, frost plant, sun rose, scrofula plant.

Part Used: Oil from the herb.

Medicinal Properties: Aromatic, tonic, alterative, astringent.

Description and Uses: It is a valuable remedy for scrofula and has long been used for this purpose. Simmer a teaspoonful of the herb in a cup of water for ten minutes. Cool, strain, and take from four to six large swallows. A poultice made from the leaves is good for scrofulous tumors and ulcers. Excellent gargle for sore throat and scarlatina. Good for diarrhea, syphilis, and gonorrhea. Helpful in treating some forms of cancer.

ROSEMARY (Rosemarinus officinalis)

Common Names: Garden rosemary, rosemary plant.

Part Used: Leaves, flowers.

Medicinal Properties: Stimulant, antispasmodic, emmenagogue, tonic, astringent, diaphoretic, carminative, nervine, aromatic, cephalic.

Description and Uses: An old-fashioned remedy for colds, colic, and nervous conditions. Very good in headaches caused by nervousness. Should be taken warm for these complaints. Good as a wash for mouth, gums, halitosis (foul breath), and sore throat. Is useful for female complaints. The leaves are used for flavoring. The oil is used as a perfume for ointments and liniments. This is an excellent ingredient for shampoos and is reported to prevent premature baldness. Rosemary is helpful in some cases of mental disturbance. It aids digestion, cough, consumption, and strengthens the eyes.

RUE (Ruta graveolens)

Common Names: Herb of grace, garden rue, countryman's treacle.

Part Used: Entire plant.

Medicinal Properties: Aromatic, pungent, tonic, emmenagogue, stimulant, antispasmodic.

Description and Uses: This is one of the herbs that have been used from time immemorial. It was used by the priests in ancient times, and even in Christ's time it was a well-known herb, widely used by the people. It has been much used by Germans and other nationalities since then. This herb should be in every garden. Rue is very much like hyssop as a fine remedy for the many ills of humanity. It will relieve congestion of the uterus, lending a very stimulating and tonic effect. Excellent in suppressed menstruation.

Steep a tablespoonful in a pint of boiling water for half an hour. DO NOT BOIL. Strain, drink warm, a teacupful every two to four hours. Also good for painful menstruation. Excellent remedy for stomach trouble, cramps in the bowels, nervousness, hysteria, spasms, convulsions, will expel worms, relieve pain in the head, confusion, and dizziness. Excellent for colic and convulsions in children. A poultice of rue is good for sciatica, pain in the joints, and gout. It resists poison.

Caution: DO NOT BOIL RUE. DO NOT USE IF PREGNANT. DO NOT USE IN LARGE DOSES.

SAFFRON (Crocus sativus)

Common Names: Dyer's saffron, saffron seed, American saffron, thistle saffron, false saffron, bastard saffron, parrot's corn, safflower.

Part Used: Flower, seeds.

Medicinal Properties: Laxative, emmenagogue, condiment, carminative, sudorific, diuretic, diaphoretic. Seed: aromatic, laxative, diuretic.

Description and Uses: Saffron is one of the old-fashioned remedies. One of the most reliable in measles, all skin diseases, and scarlet fever. Will produce profuse perspiration when taken hot; therefore, it is very useful in colds and la grippe, also in regulating and increasing the menstrual flow, especially when checked by cold. It is available as a tincture, but is quite expensive. Take 5 to 15 drops in water.

As a culinary herb, it is used for food coloring.

SAGE (Salvia officinalis)

Common Names: Garden sage, red sage, purple top sage.

Part Used: Leaves.

Medicinal Properties: Sudorific, astringent, expectorant, tonic, aromatic, antispasmodic, nervine, vermifuge, emmenagogue, diuretic, stimulant, diaphoretic, stomachic, antiseptic.

Description and Uses: Sage is a wonderful remedy for many diseases. It could almost be called a "cure-all." It might be said that you could never go amiss if you take sage.

Sage is a well-known seasoning for roasts, soups, etc.

A strong sage tea is an excellent gargle for tonsillitis or ulcers in the throat or mouth. It can be mixed with a little lemon or honey. This tea, drunk cold during the day, will prevent night sweats. For quinsy, use the tea externally and also as a gargle for the throat. One of the best remedies for stomach troubles, dyspepsia, biliousness, gas in the stomach, and bowels. Will expel worms in adults and children. Also used in liver and kidney troubles. Will stop bleeding of wounds and is very cleansing to old ulcers and sores. Wounds of any kind will heal more rapidly when washed with sage tea. Good when used in a poultice for inflammation of all kinds; very useful for typhoid and scarlet fever, measles, and smallpox. It is very soothing in nervous troubles and will relieve headaches. Good in high fevers of all kinds. A most effective hair tonic. Will make hair grow if the roots have not been destroyed. Will remove dandruff. Is a good substitute for quinine. For all kinds of lung trouble, colds, influenza, asthma, coughs, bronchitis, or pneumonia, first take a high enema; next take a big dose of body cleanser or laxative.

Then go to bed and take three, four, or five cups of hot sage tea at short intervals – say a half hour apart. This will cause free perspiration, make the whole body active, produce a strong circulation, and will throw off the infection. Fine remedy for female troubles. Will increase menstruation when too scanty and check it when profuse.

The American people would do well if they would use sage instead of tea and coffee. The Chinese make fun of the American people because they buy the tea for their drink and pay a big price for it, while the Chinese buy sage from America for a small price and drink that for their tea, which is a most wonderful remedy. The Chinese know that the sage tea will keep them well while the tea that we buy from the Chinese makes the American people sick. Sage tea is very soothing and quieting to the nerves, while the tea that we buy from China is a great cause of nervousness and headache. When weaning a child, or when it is desired that the milk should cease in the breast in case of sickness or for some other reason, sage tea drunk cold will cause the flow of milk in the breasts to cease.

For any throat trouble, red root or wood betony, half-and-half, can be added to the sage. The tea should not be boiled, but just steeped. It should be kept covered while steeping. The ordinary dose is a heaping teaspoonful to a cup of hot water. Let it steep twenty or thirty minutes. Then strain and drink three or four cups a day, one hour before meals and upon retiring, more or less as the case requires. Children less according to age. *Never steep herbs in aluminum containers.*

SANICLE (Sanicula marilandica)
Common Names: Black sanicle, black snake root, wood sanicle, sanicle root, American sanicle, pool root, butterwort.
Part Used: Root, leaves.
Medicinal Properties: Vulnerary, astringent, alterative, expectorant, discutient, depurative.

Description and Uses: Sanicle has powerful medicinal properties and many uses. This is one of the herbs that could well be called a "cure-all," because it possesses powerful cleansing and healing properties. Both the leaves and roots are used.

It is a powerful herb that heals both internal and external wounds and tumors. Use a heaping teaspoonful of the granulated herb to a cup of water. Let it steep for twenty or thirty minutes. Drink five or six cups a day. When using the powder, use a good half-teaspoonful to a cup of hot or cold water.

It will help to check excessive menstruation. It is also good to reduce hemorrhage from the lungs, bowels, and kidneys. It will stop pain in the bowels. It is excellent in gonorrhea and syphilis, as it is strong enough to cleanse the body of mucous and poisonous waste matter. It is very healing for sores in the mouth, for sore throat, quinsy, and to cleanse the throat of mucus when the strong tea is used as a gargle. It is very healing to ulcers in the stomach and is an effective remedy for the dreadful disease, consumption (tuberculosis). The following combination is very effective:

2 ounces sanicle
1 ounce marshmallow root
1 ounce mullein herb
1 ounce golden seal
1/2 ounce myrrh

Of this mixture, take a heaping teaspoonful to a cup of boiling water. Let steep twenty or thirty minutes, and drink one cupful an hour before each meal and before going to bed.

If powdered herbs are used, make a mixture using the same proportions and take a small half-teaspoonful to a cup of hot or cold water. For external use, make a strong tea and bathe the affected parts four or five times a day.

In scurvy, erysipelas, scald head, tetters, and rashes, it is effective used externally.

SARSAPARILLA (Smilax officinalis)

Common Names: Jamaica sarsaparilla, guay-quill sarsaparilla, red sarsaparilla.

Part Used: Root.

Medicinal Properties: Alterative, diuretic, demulcent, antisyphilitic, stimulant, antiscorbutic.

Description and Uses: Very useful in rheumatism, gout, skin eruptions, tetters, ringworm, scrofula, and psoriasis. An excellent antidote after taking a deadly poison. Drink copiously after thoroughly cleaning out the stomach with an emetic. Excellent for internal inflammations, colds, catarrh, and fever. Will increase the flow of urine. Good eyewash. Will promote profuse perspiration when taken hot. Powerful to expel gas from the stomach and bowels. One of the best herbs to use for infants infected with venereal disease. But since it was first used for syphilis by the Spaniards several centuries ago, experience has taught us that it is not a sure remedy for this disease in either children or adults. Wash the local pustules or sores with a tea made of the root, and administer inwardly by mixing the powdered root with their food. An excellent blood purifier. Take only for two weeks out of every three. If the tincture is used, take 25 to 50 drops in water twice a day.

———

SASSAFRAS (Sassafras officinale)

Common Names: Ague tree, saxifrax, cinnamon wood, saloip.

Part Used: Bark of the root.

Medicinal Properties: Aromatic, stimulant, alterative, diaphoretic, diuretic.

Description and Uses: Sassafras is often called a spring medicine to purify the blood and cleanse the entire system. Good to flavor other herbs that have a disagreeable taste, and commonly used in combination with other blood-purifying herbs. Useful as a tonic for stomach and bowels.

Will relieve gas and colic. Taken warm, it is an excellent remedy for spasms. Valuable in all skin diseases and eruptions. Good wash for inflamed eyes. Good for kidneys, bladder, chest, and throat troubles. Oil of sassafras is excellent for toothache. Good in varicose ulcers as a wash externally and also when taken internally. Take for no more than a week at a time. As a tincture, use 10 to 20 drops in water.

SAW PALMETTO BERRIES (Serenoa serrulata)
Common Names: Pan palm, dwarf palmetto.
Part Used: Berries.
Medicinal Properties: Antiseptic, sedative, cardiac, tonic, diuretic.
Description and Uses: A very useful article in asthma and all kinds of throat troubles, colds, bronchitis, la grippe, whooping cough, and when the throat is irritated and painful. Especially useful when there is excessive mucous discharge from the sinuses and nose. Valuable in all diseases of the reproductive organs, ovaries, prostate, testes, etc. Very useful in Bright's disease and diabetes. Excellent as a general tonic to regain strength and weight following a debilitating illness. Thought by some to be an aphrodisiac. Excellent to use in diseases of the prostate gland. Available as capsules or as a tincture, 20 to 40 drops in water daily.

SEAWRACK (Fucus vesiculosus)
Common Names: Bladder fucus, seaweed, bladder wrack, sea oak, kelpware, black tany, cutweed.
Part Used: Entire plant.
Medicinal Properties: Alterative, diuretic.
Description and Uses: The best remedy for obesity. Good in all glandular afflictions, goiter, and scrofula. Has an excellent effect on the kidneys. Steep a heaping teaspoonful to a cup of boiling water for thirty minutes. Drink three or four cups a day an hour before meals, and one hot upon retiring.

SELF-HEAL (Prunella vulgaris)
Common Names: Wound wort, all heal, heal all, Hercules wound wort, brownwort, sickle wort, blue curls, panay, hook heal, hood weed, carpenter's herb.
Part Used: Entire plant.
Medicinal Properties: Pungent, tonic, antispasmodic, vermifuge, diuretic, astringent, styptic, vulnerary.
Description and Uses: Excellent for epilepsy, convulsions, falling sickness, and obstructed liver. Especially useful for internal and external wounds.

For internal wounds, take the tea. Use as a poultice and as a wash in all external wounds and sores. Will stop bleeding. Also very cleansing. Will cleanse and heal ulcers of the mouth. An old Italian proverb says: "He that hath self-heal and sanicle needs no other physician." Make an infusion of one ounce of the herb to a pint of boiling water. Take one wineglass full several times a day.

SENNA (Cassia marilandica)
Common Names: American senna, locust plant, wild senna.
Part Used: Leaves.
Medicinal Properties: Laxative, vermifuge, diuretic.
Description and Uses: Senna is a valuable, effective laxative. It sometimes causes griping; therefore it should be combined with an aromatic herb. Some of the many common aromatic herbs are goldenrod, mint, rosemary, anise, balm, allspice, buchu, coriander, lavender, and pennyroyal. Excellent for worms, biliousness, halitosis (bad breath), and bad taste in the mouth. Most effective for worms when combined with other herbs that are also indicated for worms. Steep two ounces in a pint of boiling water with one teaspoon of ginger for 30 to 60 minutes, strain, and drink a wineglassful, more or less according to needs.

SHEPHERD'S PURSE (Capsella bursa-pastoris)

Common Names: Cocowort, shepherd's heart, pickpocket, toywort, pick purse, St. James' weed, St. James' wort, St. Anthony's fire, pepper grass, shepherd's sprout, mother's heart, case wort, permacety.

Part Used: Entire plant.

Medicinal Properties: Astringent, detergent, vulnerary, diuretic, styptic.

Description and Uses: Most excellent in cases of hemorrhage after child birth, and all other internal hemorrhages. Has been successful in such cases when all other remedies have failed. Good for bleeding from the lungs. One of the best remedies to check profuse menstruation. Excellent in fever, kidney complaints, bleeding piles, and hemorrhoids. Steep a heaping teaspoonful to a cup of boiling water for thirty minutes, and drink cold, not more than two cupfuls a day, a large mouthful at a time. Is also an excellent remedy for diarrhea.

Nearly every wheat field is full of this herb. It grows over the entire United States. When you chew the green grass, it has a very pleasant peppery taste.

SKULLCAP (Scutellaria lateriflora)

Common Names: Scullcap, blue skullcap, blue pimpernel, hoodwart, hooded willow herb, side-flowering skullcap, mad dogweed, mad weed, helmet flower, American skullcap.

Part Used: Entire plant.

Medicinal Properties: Antispasmodic, nervine, tonic, diuretic.

Description and Uses: It is one of the best nerve tonics we have and is often combined with other herbs whenever diseases of the nervous system are present. Very quieting and soothing to the nerves of people who are easily excited. For those with delirium tremens, it will produce sleep. Good in neuralgia, aches, and pains. Useful in St. Vitus' dance, shaking palsy, convulsions, fits, rheumatism, hydrophobia, epilepsy, and bites of poisonous insects and snakes. Splendid to suppress excessive sexual desire.

The following combination is a positive remedy for wakefulness: equal parts skullcap, nerve root, hops, catnip, and black cohosh. Take a tablespoonful of each, mix together, and use a heaping teaspoonful to a cup of boiling water. This combination is very useful in aiding a morphine addict to sleep. As a substitute for quinine, skullcap is more effective and is not as harmful.

SKUNK CABBAGE (Symplocarpus foetidus)
Common Names: Meadow cabbage, skunk weed, collard, stinking poke, fetid hellebore, polecat weed, swamp cabbage.

Part Used: Root, seed.

Medicinal Properties: Sudorific, expectorant, pectoral, antispasmodic, stimulant, diaphoretic.

Description and Uses: One of the old-fashioned, well-known remedies. Very reliable in tuberculosis, chronic catarrh, all bronchial and lung infections, whooping cough, spasmodic asthma, hay fever and pleurisy. Excellent remedy in chronic rheumatism, nervous troubles, dysentery, spasms, convulsions, dropsy, hysteria, epilepsy, and for use during pregnancy. When made into an ointment, it greatly relieves the pain of all external tumors and sores.

SMARTWEED – See Water Pepper

SOLOMON'S SEAL (Polygonatum multiflorum)
Common Names: Dropberry, sealwort, seal root.

Part Used: Root.

Medicinal Properties: Tonic, expectorant, astringent, mucilaginous.

Description and Uses: A fine remedy for all kinds of female troubles. Excellent as a wash for poison ivy, erysipelas, and other sores on the body. Will allay pain and heal piles. Inject four or five tablespoonfuls of the tea several times a day into the rectum. Take internally the same as other tea for neuralgia. Use one ounce of the cut herb in a cup of hot water. Solomon's seal makes an excellent poultice for external inflammations, wounds and piles.

SORREL (Rumex acetosa)
Common Names: Common field sorrel, red top sorrel, garden sorrel, meadow sorrel, sourgrass.
Part Used: Leaves, root.
Medicinal Properties: Diuretic, antiscorbutic, refrigerant, vermifuge.
Description and Uses: The leaves are used like greens, as spinach, and are very high in life-giving properties.

It kills putrefaction in the blood, expels worms, and is warming to the heart. The root boiled is good for profuse menstruation or stomach hemorrhage. Also expels gravel from the kidneys, and is good in jaundice. A tea made from the flowers is good for internal ulcers, scurvy, scrofula, and all skin diseases. Steep one ounce of the cut herb in a cup of hot water. A sorrel poultice is excellent for cancer, boils, and tumors. As a cold drink, it is good to reduce fevers.

The leaves eaten as a salad in the spring are an excellent preventive for scurvy.

SPEARMINT (Mentha viridis)
Common Names: Mint, peamint, mackerel mint.
Part Used: Entire plant.
Medicinal Properties: Antispasmodic, aromatic, diuretic, diaphoretic, carminative.
Description and Uses: A highly esteemed remedy for colic, gas in the stomach and bowels, nausea and vomiting, dyspepsia, spasms, and dropsy. It will relieve suppressed, painful, or scalding urine, and is also good for gravel in the bladder. Locally applied, it is excellent for piles and hemorrhoids. For this purpose, inject a small amount into the rectum several times a day with a soft-tipped syringe. Good

in inflammation of the kidneys and bladder. Excellent for treating vomiting during pregnancy. Very good to quiet and soothe the stomach after an emetic. Very soothing and quieting to the nerves. NEVER BOIL SPEARMINT. Is added to many compounds for its pleasing taste. No home should be without this excellent home remedy. (See also preceding paragraph on Peppermint.) An infusion of one ounce in a pint of boiling water can be taken in doses of a wineglassful as needed.

SPIKENARD (Aralia racemosa)
Common Names: American spikenard, Indian root, pettymorrel, life-of-man, spignet, Indian aralia bark, nard.

Part Used: Root.

Medicinal Properties: Pectoral, diaphoretic, stimulant, alterative, balsamic.

Description and Uses: One of the old-fashioned remedies. It makes childbirth easier and shortens the length of labor. Take the tea for some time before labor. It is an excellent blood purifier. For use in treating venereal diseases, combine spikenard with the following: equal parts of dandelion, burdock, and yellow dock. Flavor with one of the following by using an equal part: catnip, peppermint, wintergreen, or sassafras. Good in all skin diseases, pimples, or eruptions. Very useful in coughs, colds, and all chest infections. As an infusion use one-half ounce of the herb in a pint of boiling water. Take in wineglass doses.

SQUAW VINE (Mitchella repens)
Common Names: Partridgeberry, checkerberry, deerberry, winter clover, twin-berry, one-berry, hive vine, one-berry leaves, squawberry.

Part Used: Entire plant.

Medicinal Properties: Diuretic, astringent, tonic, alterative, parturient.

Description and Uses: This herb was very highly

esteemed by the Indian women. It is an excellent medicine to take during the last few weeks of pregnancy and will make childbirth much easier. It is better than red raspberry leaves, but it is good to combine the two. Good in scanty or painful menstruation. An excellent wash for sore eyes in infants. For this purpose combine with equal parts of raspberry leaves and witch hazel leaves. If the witch hazel leaves cannot be secured, use wild strawberry leaves. This is also an excellent injection for mild leukorrhea, dysentery, and gonorrhea. This herb is good for gravel, urinary troubles, uterine troubles, female complaints, and increases the menstrual flow. A strong tea made from the berries is good to bathe sore nipples. Add a little olive oil or cream.

Stir thoroughly and apply. As a decoction, use two ounces in one pint of water and take in wineglass doses. As a tincture, 5 to 10 drops three times a day.

STAR GRASS (Aletris farinosa)
Common Names: Ague grass, bitter grass, blazing star, colic root, mealy starwort, star root, true unicorn root.
Part Used: Rootstock (rhizome).
Medicinal Properties: Tonic, stomachic.
Description and Uses: *Be sure to use only the dried rootstock.* The fresh rootstock is toxic and should never be used. Star grass is an excellent female tonic and is used in painful menstruation. It is also useful in digestive trouble, colic, and gas.

Small doses only should be used. Boil a teaspoonful of the dried rootstock in a cup of water; let cool and drink no more than a cup a day, taking only a small mouthful at a time. Fifteen to thirty drops of the tincture in hot water can be taken daily for menstrual problems.

ST. JOHN'S WORT (Hypericum perforatum)
Common Names: Johnswort, goat weed, amber, Klâmath weed.

Part Used: Tops, flowers.

Medicinal Properties: Aromatic, nervine, astringent, resolvent, sedative, diuretic, vulnerary.

Description and Uses: Powerful as a blood purifier. Very good for tumors and boils, as well as for chronic uterine troubles, pains following childbirth, suppressed urine, diarrhea, dysentery, and jaundice. Will correct irregular menstruation. Good in hysteria and nervous afflictions. Excellent for pus in the urine. Good used externally as fomentations or as an ointment for caked breasts, all wounds, ulcers, and old sores. Will correct bed-wetting in children when proper diet is given. The seeds steeped in boiling water will expel congealed blood from the stomach. For this purpose, use a heaping teaspoonful of the seeds to a cup of boiling water and take a mouthful several times a day.

Caution: May be toxic. Use with care under competent medical supervision.

STRAWBERRY (Fragaria vesca)

Common Names: Mountain strawberry, pineapple strawberry, wood strawberry, common strawberry, wild strawberry.

Part Used: Leaves.

Medicinal Properties: Astringent, tonic, diuretic.

Description and Uses: This is the common, well-known strawberry leaf that is in every garden. All should become thoroughly acquainted with the medicinal properties and value of strawberry leaves. If a tea made of the leaves were used in place of tea and coffee, it would prove a blessing. It tones up the appetite and the entire system generally. It is good for various bowel troubles and cleanses the stomach. It is an excellent remedy for diarrhea in children. Good for eczema used internally and as a wash externally. Will prevent night sweats. Very useful in diarrhea, dysentery, and weakness of the intestines. Should be taken internally and also used as an enema. Take one or two tablespoonfuls as an infusion.

SUMACH BERRIES (Rhus glabra)
Common Names: Scarlet sumach, smooth sumach, dwarf sumach, upland sumach, Pennsylvania sumach, sleek sumach, mountain sumach.

Part Used: Bark, leaves, berries.

Medicinal Properties: Bark and leaves – tonic, astringent, alterative, antiseptic. Berries – diuretic, refrigerant, emmenagogue, diaphoretic, cephalic.

Description and Uses: A valuable treatment to try in gonorrhea and syphilis when others have failed is the following: equal parts sumach berries and bark, white pine bark, and slippery elm. This tea is very cleansing to the system, and is very useful in leukorrhea, scrofula, and for inward sores and wounds. A tea of sumach berries alone is excellent for bowel complaints, diabetes, and all kinds of fevers; and for sores in the mouth there is no superior. Use also as a gargle and mouthwash. As a tincture take 5 to 15 drops in water two times a day.

SUMMER SAVORY (Satureja hortensis)
Common Names: Savory, bean herb.

Part Used: Entire plant.

Medicinal Properties: Aromatic, stimulant, carminative, condiment, emmenagogue, aphrodisiac.

Description and Uses: The tea is a specific remedy for eliminating gas from the stomach and the intestines. Taken warm it is excellent for suppressed menstruation. The tea is also very useful for colds and when used as a gargle it is good for sore throats. It is helpful in diarrhea. The oil dropped onto a tooth will relieve toothache.

As a culinary herb, the leaves are used for flavoring, usually combined with sage.

SWEET BALM (See Balm)

TANSY (Tanacetum vulgare)

Common Names: Hindheel, common tansy, bitter buttons, parsley fern, ginger plant, golden buttons, bachelor's buttons.

Part Used: Entire plant.

Medicinal Properties: Aromatic, tonic, emmenagogue, diaphoretic, vulnerary, anthelmintic. Seeds – vermifuge.

Description and Uses: Tansy was used for thousands of years, until about the midnineteenth century, as an embalming agent. Tansy was also found useful as an insect repellent when placed on the floors or walls of houses.

It is an old well-known family remedy used to tone up the system and soothe the bowels. It is excellent taken hot for colds, fevers, la grippe, and ague.

Good for dyspepsia. One of the best remedies to promote menstruation. Tansy seed will expel worms. Useful in hysteria, jaundice, dropsy, worms, and kidney troubles. Strengthens weak veins. Hot fomentations wrung out of tansy tea are excellent for swellings, tumors, inflammations, bruises, freckles, sunburn, leukorrhea, sciatica, toothache, and inflamed eyes. Good in heart trouble. Will check palpitation of the heart in a very short time. Tansy should be taken in moderate doses only.

AN OVERDOSE MAY PROVE FATAL.

Use one-half to one teaspoonful of the fluid extract or infuse one ounce to one pint of boiling water and take a wineglass-full one to three times a day.

THYME (Thymus vulgaris)

Common Names: Common garden thyme, mother of thyme.

Part Used: Entire plant.

Medicinal Properties: Tonic, carminative, emmenagogue, resolvent, antispasmodic, antiseptic.

Description and Uses: One of the old-time household remedies. Usually used in combination with other herbs.

Excellent taken hot for suppressed menstruation. Good in fevers. Will produce profuse perspiration when taken hot. A reliable nervine and excellent for relief of nightmares. Valuable in whooping cough, asthma, and lung troubles. For small children, give small and frequent doses. Good remedy for weak stomach, dyspepsia, gas, griping, cramps in the stomach, and diarrhea. Better taken cold for these purposes. Will relieve headache and acts as a mood elevator. Use one ounce of the dry herb to one pint of boiling water. Take two tablespoonfuls two times a day.

Use sparingly. Do not make a habit of using thyme.

TURKEY CORN (Dicentra canadensis)
Common Names: Wild turkey pea, staggerweed, dielytra, turkey pea, squirrel corn, choice dielytra.
Part Used: Root.
Medicinal Properties: Tonic, alterative, diuretic, antisyphilitic.
Description and Uses: An excellent remedy in syphilis, scrofula, and all skin diseases. For boils, it is most effective when used in combination with hot baths and salt glows. An excellent tonic in all enfeebled conditions. One of the most valuable alteratives in the herbal kingdom. Take as a tea like other herbs.

TWIN LEAF (Jeffersonia diphylla)
Common Names: Ground squirrel pea, rheumatism root, helmet pod, yellow root, twin leaf root.
Part Used: Root.
Medicinal Properties: Diuretic, alterative, antisyphilitic, antirheumatic, antispasmodic, tonic.
Description and Uses: Very useful in chronic rheumatism, nervous, and spasmodic afflictions. Very successful in neuralgia, cramps, and syphilis. Splendid gargle for throat troubles. Fine in scarlet fever, scarlatina, and indolent ulcers. A poultice or hot fomentation made out of the strong tea, will

relieve pain anywhere in the body. In severe pains, take hot internally. Steep a teaspoonful in a cup of boiling water for thirty minutes; simmer ten minutes, then strain and drink one cupful. Follow with small frequent doses.

UVA-URSI (Arctostaphylos uva-ursi)
Common Names: Bearberry, upland cranberry, universe vine, mountain cranberry, mountain box, wild cranberry, bear's grape, kinnpikinnick, mealberry, sagackhomi, red bearberry, arberry.
Part Used: Leaves.
Medicinal Properties: Diuretic, astringent, tonic, mucilaginous.
Description and Uses: Very useful in diabetes, Bright's disease, and all kidney and bladder troubles. Good when there is mucous discharge from the bladder with pus and blood. Excellent remedy for dysentery, piles, hemorrhoids, excessive menstruation, and for spleen, liver, and pancreas problems. Excellent in gonorrhea, ulceration in the mouth of the womb, and other female troubles. Take internally and use also as a douche. Steep a heaping teaspoonful in a pint of boiling water thirty minutes and drink one-half cupful every four hours. Also comes in capsules; one to two daily. When combined with an equal amount of buchu, uva ursi makes an excellent treatment for kidney and bladder troubles.

VALERIAN (Valeriana officinalis)
Common Names: English valerian, German valerian, great wild valerian, Vermont valerian, vandal root, all-heal, setwall, American English valerian (grown in U.S.).
Part Used: Root.
Medicinal Properties: Aromatic, stimulant, tonic, anodyne, antispasmodic, nervine, emmenagogue.
Description and Uses: Excellent nerve tonic – very quieting and soothing.

Useful in hysteria. Will promote menstruation when taken
hot. Useful in colic, low fevers, to break up colds, and also
for gravel in the bladder. Healing for stomach ulcers and very
good for prevention of fermentation and gas. The tea is very
healing when applied to sores and pimples externally, and
must also be taken internally at the same time. Relieves
palpitation of the heart. DO NOT BOIL THE ROOT. Poisoning may result if large amounts of the tea are taken for more
than two to three weeks. As a tincture use one to two
teaspoonfuls in a glass of water. When used in capsule form,
take one or two a day.

VERVAIN (Verbena officinalis)

Common Names: American vervain, wild hyssop, blue
vervain, false vervain, simpler's joy, traveler's joy, Indian
hyssop, purvain.

Part Used: Entire plant.

Medicinal Properties: Tonic, sudorific, expectorant,
vulnerary, emetic, nervine, emmenagogue, vermifuge.

Description and Uses: Vervain is one of the most
wonderful gifts of God for the healing of diseases. This herb
should be in every home ready for use immediately when
needed. Very powerful to produce profuse perspiration. Excellent in fevers. Will often cure colds overnight. Take a
warm cup of vervain tea often. An excellent remedy in
whooping cough, pneumonia, consumption, asthma, ague,
and will expel phlegm from the throat and chest. In fevers,
take a cup of the hot tea every hour. Good in all female
troubles. Will increase menstrual flow. Also good in scrofula
and skin diseases. Will often expel worms when everything
else fails. Take freely until the worms pass. Very useful in
nervousness, delirium, epilepsy, insanity, sleeplessness, and
nervous headache. Will tone up the system during convalescence from heart diseases. Will remove obstruction in the
bowels, colon, and bladder. Good in stomach troubles, shortness of breath, and wheezing. Used in combination with

equal parts of smartweed and peppermint leaves. Is excellent for appendicitis. In fevers, use in combination with boneset, willow bark, or water pepper. The tea is very healing when applied to external sores. Much better than quinine for the purposes for which quinine is used. Take one-half to one teaspoonful of the fluid extract in water.

VIOLET (Viola odorata)
Common Names: Sweet violet, common blue violet.
Part Used: Entire plant.
Medicinal Properties: Mucilaginous, laxative, emetic, alterative, antiseptic.
Description and Uses: As a tea, violet leaves are used as a blood purifier. Violet leaves are very effective in healing and give prompt relief in internal ulcers. They have been used as a treatment for cancer. Use externally for this purpose as a poultice and take the tea internally. For cancerous growths and other skin diseases, violet is especially beneficial when combined with red clover and vervain. Violet is a successful remedy in gout, coughs, colds, sores, sore throat, ulcers, scrofula, syphilis, bronchitis, and difficult breathing due to gas and morbid matter in the stomach and bowels. Violet is wonderful for nervousness or general debility when combined with nerve root, skullcap, or black cohosh. Relieves severe headache and congestion in the head. Very effective for whooping cough.

VIRGIN'S BOWER (Clematis virginiana)
Common Names: Common virgin's bower, traveler's joy.
Part Used: Leaves, flowers.
Medicinal Properties: Stimulant, diuretic, sudorific, vesicant.
Description and Uses: Will relieve severe headaches. Combine with other herbs in poultices for cancer, ulcers, and bed sores. Combine with other herbs in ointments for cancer,

itching, and ulcers. For internal use, steep a heaping tea-spoonful in a cup of boiling water for thirty minutes, strain, take a tablespoonful four to six times a day.

WAHOO (Euonymus atropurpureus)
Common Names: Whahow, wauhoo, Indian root, Indian arrow, Indian arrow wood, burning bush, bitter ash, arrow wood, spindle tree, strawberry tree, pegwood.

Part Used: Bark, bark of the root.

Medicinal Properties: Tonic, laxative, expectorant, diuretic, alterative.

Description and Uses: A splendid laxative. Excellent in chest and lung infections. Useful in fevers, malaria, dyspepsia, liver disorders, pancreas and spleen troubles. Good remedy for dropsy. Steep a small teaspoonful in a cup of boiling water for thirty minutes. Take two or three cups a day, an hour before meals. Better than quinine.

Caution: Using too much wahoo bark may result in a severe purgative action.

Be careful not to use too much and use only under proper supervision.

WATER PEPPER (Polygonum punctatum)
Common Names: Smartweed, American water pepper, water smartweed, pepperwort, culrage.

Part Used: Entire plant.

Medicinal Properties: Astringent, diaphoretic, tonic, stimulant, emmenagogue, antiseptic.

Description and Uses: Useful remedy for scanty menstruation, all womb troubles, gravel in the bladder, colds, coughs, bowel complaints, and kidney troubles. Can be used internally and externally. A poultice made of charcoal and moistened with water pepper tea is an excellent remedy for pain in the bowels and ulcers; is one of the best known remedies for this purpose. Also take the tea internally. Give high enemas, fruit juice, and liquid diet for a few days. A most wonderful remedy in appendicitis.

For cholera, the tea should be used as an enema. A fomentation should also be wrung out of the hot tea and applied over the abdomen. Use the tea as a wash in erysipelas and for sore nipples in nursing mothers.

WHITE CLOVER (Trifolium repens)
Common Names: White shamrock, shamrock.
Part Used: Blossoms.
Medicinal Properties: Depurative, detergent.
Description and Uses: Common white clover blossoms are an old-fashioned remedy to cleanse the system. A very fine blood purifier, especially in boils, ulcers, and other skin diseases. A strong tea of white clover blossoms is very healing to sores when applied externally. Equal parts of white clover and yellow dock make an excellent salve. May be used the same as red clover.

WHITE POND LILY (Nymphaea odorata)
Common Names: White water lily, sweet-scented pond lily, sweet-scented water lily, toad lily, pond lily, water lily, cow cabbage, sweet water lily, water cabbage.
Part Used: Root.
Medicinal Properties: Deobstruent, astringent, vulnerary, discutient, demulcent, antiseptic.
Description and Uses: This is one of the old-fashioned home remedies. Very astringent. Use as a douche in leukorrhea. Take internally for leukorrhea, diarrhea, bowel complaints, scrofula. Excellent remedy in mucous troubles and inflamed tissues in various parts of the body and also for bronchial troubles. Very effective in dropsy, kidney troubles, catarrh of the bladder, or irritation of the prostate. Excellent for infant bowel troubles. Very healing to inflamed gums. In making poultices for painful swellings, boils, ulcers, etc., mix the ingredients with a strong tea of this herb. Valuable as a gargle for sore throat. The leaves are very healing to

wounds and cuts. Apply the powder, combined with flaxseed, as a poultice.

_____

WILD OREGON GRAPE (Berberis aquifolium)
Common Names: Oregon grape, holly-leaved barberry, mahonia, California barberry, mountain grape.
Part Used: Root.
Medicinal Properties: Tonic, alterative.
Description and Uses: Useful in liver and kidney troubles, rheumatism, constipation, leukorrhea, and uterine diseases. Is a good blood purifier and useful in scrofulous and chronic skin diseases such as psoriasis, eczema.

The medicinal uses of this plant are nearly identical to Barberry (Berberis vulgaris).

_____

WILD YAM (Dioscorea villosa)
Common Names: Colic root, China root, yuma, devil's bones.
Part Used: Root.
Medicinal Properties: Antispasmodic, antibilious, diaphoretic, hepatic.
Description and Uses: Very relaxing and soothing to the nerves. Useful in all cases of nervous excitement. Will expel gas from the stomach and bowels. Good in cholera. Useful in neuralgia of any part. Excellent for pains in the urinary tract. One of the best herbs for general pain during pregnancy. Take during the whole period of pregnancy. Will allay nausea in small frequent doses, but may cause vomiting if taken in large amounts. Combined with ginger, it will greatly help in preventing miscarriage. Use a teaspoonful of wild yam and one-fourth teaspoonful of ginger. Also good to combine with squaw vine for use during pregnancy. Valuable in ailments of the liver, spasms, and rheumatic pains. Steep a heaping teaspoonful in a cup of boiling water thirty minutes. Drink one to three cupfuls a day cold, a large swallow at a time.

WINTERGREEN (Gaultheria procumbens)

Common Names: Spring wintergreen, Canada tea, partridge berry, checkerberry, boxberry, wax cluster, spice berry, mountain tea, deerberry, spicy wintergreen, aromatic wintergreen, chink, ground berry, grouse berry, red pollom, redberry tea, hillberry, ivory plum.

Part Used: Leaves.

Medicinal Properties: Stimulant, antiseptic, astringent, diuretic, emmenagogue, aromatic.

Description and Uses: This is an old-fashioned remedy. Taken in small frequent doses it will stimulate stomach, heart, and respiration. Useful in chronic inflammatory rheumatism, also rheumatic fever, sciatica, diabetes, all bladder troubles, scrofula, and skin diseases. Valuable in colic and gas in the bowels. Helpful in dropsy, gonorrhea, stomach trouble, and obstruction in the bowels.

The oil of the wintergreen is used internally and externally. It is very useful in liniments.

Used as a poultice, it is good for boils, swellings, ulcers, felons, and inflammation. A douche of the tea is excellent in whites and leukorrhea. The tea is also very beneficial as a gargle for sore throat and mouth. Good wash for sore eyes.

———————

WITCH HAZEL (Hamamelis virginiana)

Common Names: Winter bloom, striped alder, spotted alder, hazelnut, snapping hazel, pistachio, tobacco wood.

Part Used: Bark, leaves.

Medicinal Properties: Astringent, tonic, antiphlogistic, sedative, styptic.

Description and Uses: This is an old-fashioned remedy and is very valuable for stopping either internal or external bleeding. Also good in the treatment of piles. I have used witch hazel for over thirty years with most remarkable results. It is unsurpassed for stopping excessive menstruation, hemorrhages from the lungs, stomach, uterus, and bowels. Very useful in diarrhea when taken internally and as an enema. In nosebleed, snuff the tea up the nose. For piles or diarrhea, inject a teaspoonful into the rectum several times a day and after each stool. Excellent local application in gonorrhea. Will restore perfect circulation. As a poultice or wash it is excellent for painful tumors, all external inflammations, bed sores, and sore and inflamed eyes. Excellent gargle in throat troubles. In gonorrhea, leukorrhea, and whites, give as a douche. For use internally, steep a heaping teaspoonful in a cup of boiling water thirty minutes. Take one or more cupfuls during the day as needed, a large mouthful at a time. Children less according to age. *Do not drink witch hazel purchased from the drug store; it contains an alcohol that is not intended to be used internally.*

WOOD BETONY (Betonica officinalis)
Common Names: Lousewort, betony, bishop's wort.
Part Used: Leaves.
Medicinal Properties: Aperient, stomachic, nervine, tonic, aromatic, antiscorbutic.
Description and Uses: Excellent for the stomach. Mildly stimulating to the heart. Unsurpassed for headache, neuralgia, pains in the head or face, heartburn, indigestion, cramps in the stomach, jaundice, palsy, convulsions, gout, colic, pains, all bilious and nervous complaints, dropsy, colds, la grippe, tuberculosis, worms, delirium, poisonous snake and insect bites. Opens obstructions of the liver and spleen. More effective than quinine. Today this herb is not commonly used as a medicine.
Formula: two parts wood betony, one part skullcap, one part calamus root. Use as an infusion, one to two teaspoonfuls to a cup of water. Take one or two cups a day.

WOOD SAGE (Teucrium scorodonia)
Common Names: Garlic sage.
Part Used: Entire plant.

Medicinal Properties: Tonic, vermifuge, alterative, diuretic, slightly diaphoretic.

Description and Uses: Stimulates the appetite. When combined with chickweed it is a good external wash to cleanse old sores, indolent ulcers, swellings, and boils. As a poultice for cancer and tumors, it should be combined with comfrey and ragwort. This will often assist in effecting a cure. It is very useful in palsy, quinsy, sore throat, colds, fevers, kidney and bladder troubles. Increases the flow of urine and also the menstrual flow. This may be purchased as a fluid extract. Use one-half to one teaspoonful daily.

WORMWOOD (Artemisia absinthium)

Common Names: Absinthium, green ginger, absinthe, old woman.

Part Used: Entire plant.

Medicinal Properties: Aromatic, tonic, antiseptic, febrifuge.

Description and Uses: An old and good remedy for bilious and liver troubles, jaundice, and intermittent fevers. Excellent appetizer. Will expel worms. Good in chronic diarrhea and leukorrhea. Good in poor digestion or lack of appetite. The oil of wormwood is an excellent ingredient to put in liniments for use in sprains, bruises, lumbago, etc.

Fomentations wrung out of the hot tea are excellent for use in rheumatism, swellings, and sprains.

For internal use, steep a heaping teaspoonful in a cup of boiling water for thirty minutes. Drink one cup a day, a large swallow at a time. Children less according to age.

Caution: Follow the directions carefully and do not take larger doses, as wormwood can be poisonous.

ADDENDUM: Wormwood is the principal herb used in absinthe, a bitter, aromatic, alcoholic drink that was very popular in Italy, France, and Switzerland during the nineteenth century. Because of the addictive nature of wormwood, however, and the frequent side effects when absinthe

was used to excess – dizziness, seizures, stupor, delirium,
hallucinations, and even death – it has now been banned in
nearly every country of the world.

YARROW (Achillea millefolium)

Common Names: Milfoil, noble yarrow, nosebleed,
millefolium, ladies' mantle, thousand leaf, old man's pepper,
thousand seal, soldier's woundwort.

Part Used: Entire plant.

Medicinal Properties: Astringent, tonic, alterative, diuretic, vulnerary, diaphoretic.

Description and Uses: I have used yarrow very extensively as it grows abundantly in the northern part of Wisconsin where I was born and reared. It also grows in many other
parts of the United States.

Excellent for hemorrhages and bleeding from the lungs. If
taken freely at the beginning of a cold, with other simple
remedies, it will break it up in twenty-four hours. A fine
remedy in all kinds of fevers when taken hot. It will open the
pores to release toxins, raise the temperature, and increase
the circulation. It is a most effective remedy for suppressed
urine, scanty urine and where there is mucous discharge from
the bladder. An ointment of yarrow will cure old wounds,
ulcers, and fistulas. Excellent douche for leukorrhea. Very
useful in measles, smallpox, and chicken pox. Good for
dyspepsia and hemorrhages from the lungs and bowels.

Where there is a bad condition of piles or hemorrhoids,
take a cleansing enema and a yarrow enema each day. If there
is much pain, have the water at 112° to 115°F. Yarrow has a
very healing and soothing effect on the mucous membranes.
Also inject two tablespoonfuls several times a day and after
each stool. It is a very successful remedy in typhoid fever. It
is good for diarrhea and dysentery in both infants and adults.
For very small infants, inject a cupful or more according to
age. Successful in female troubles and in womb troubles.
Good for expelling gas from the stomach and intestines. Very

useful in diabetes and Bright's disease. Yarrow is more effective than quinine. For fevers, drink hot yarrow tea. Steep a heaping teaspoonful in a cup of boiling water for thirty minutes. Drink three or four cups a day an hour before meals, and one upon retiring. It must be given warm to be effective.

YELLOW DOCK (Rumex crispus)
Common Names: Sour dock, curled dock, narrow dock, garden patience, rumex.
Part Used: Root.
Medicinal Properties: Alterative, tonic, depurative, astringent, antiscorbutic, detergent.
Description and Uses: Tones up the entire system and is an excellent and effective remedy for the following: impure blood, eruptive skin diseases, scrofula, glandular tumors, swellings, leprosy, cancer, ulcerated eyelids, syphilis, and running ears. Makes a valuable ointment for itch and sores. For glandular tumors and swellings, apply fomentations wrung from the hot tea. Most wonderful blood purifier. Yellow dock is high in tannin content and should be taken only every other week. As a capsule, one a day. As a decoction, one teaspoonful in a cup of water, one to two cups a day.

YERBA SANTA (Eriodictyon glutinosum)
Common Names: Consumptive's weed, gum plant, bear's weed, mountain balm, tar weed.
Part Used: Leaves.
Medicinal Properties: Tonic, expectorant, aromatic.
Description and Uses: This is a well-tried and much-used remedy in laryngitis, chronic bronchitis, asthma, and various catarrhal lung ailments. Effective when there is excessive discharge from the nose. Good in rheumatism. Can be applied as a poultice for sores, insect bites, sprains, and bruises.

6

MEDICINAL TREES

When I study the herbs, flowers, roots, bark, and leaves of the trees and see the wonderful medicinal properties they contain and the marvelous benefits that are derived from their use, I feel that the word "wonderful" is inadequate to express the real truth. The phrase, "the mighty miracle-working power of God" is none too strong. If you had seen the things that have actually been done by using these herbs in connection with other hygienic measures, you would not think for one moment that these statements are overdrawn. As I go out into the woods and see the lofty trees, I feel like taking my hat off in reverence to God, for not only do these trees have wonderful medicinal properties for the healing of man, but they also provide wood for building houses in which to live, furnish fuel with which to cook our food and for heat to keep us warm.

Following is a list of trees that are valuable for medicine. They are arranged in alphabetical order.

ACACIA (Acacia senegal)
Common Names: Gum arabic, gum acacia, cape gum, Egyptian thorn, India gum tree, gum Arabic tree, bablah pods, acacia bambolah.
Part Used: Gum.
Medicinal Properties: Demulcent, mucilaginous.
Description and Uses: The gum, which exudes naturally from the acacia tree, is made into a mucilage with boiling water. In this form it acts as a demulcent and provides a soothing protective coat over the lining of the respiratory, gastrointestinal, and urinary tracts.

Used in poultices or applied externally, it retains warmth

and moisture, thus proving relaxing. It absorbs discharges and is excellent to use with the powdered herbs for poultices. Taken internally, it lubricates mucous membranes, and is soothing in conditions such as inflammation of the stomach, bowels, uterus, and vagina.

ALDER (Alnus Glutinosa)
Common Names: European alder, winterberry, feverbush.
Part Used: Leaves, bark.
Medicinal Properties: Astringent, emetic, hemostatic, mucilaginous, tonic.
Description and Uses: Both the leaves and the bark of the alder tree are used. Use the leaves when you can get them. They are very useful for swellings of all kinds. When you can get the green leaves, crush them and lay them on painful swellings. They will relieve the pain and reduce the swelling. The green or dry leaves made into a poultice will allay inflammation in a swollen and painful breast. Take a heaping tablespoonful of crushed alder leaves to a pint of boiling water. Let steep for half an hour. If used for a poultice, use just enough water so the leaves are moist. The fresh leaves are excellent for burning and aching feet when laid in the shoes under the bare feet. Also good for the feet is to bathe them in a strong tea made of crushed, fresh alder leaves. The fresh alder bark will cause vomiting. A decoction made from the dry bark is excellent as a gargle to use for sore throats. Culpepper, the famous English herbalist, states: "The said leaves gathered while the morning dew is on them, and brought into a chamber troubled with fleas, will gather them there unto, which being suitably cast out, will rid the chamber of these troublesome fellows."

APPLE TREE (Pyrus Malus)
Common Names: Apple tree
Part Used: Fruit, bark.

Medicinal Properties: Fruit – diuretic, laxative. Bark – tonic, febrifuge.

Description and Uses: Tea made from apple tree bark is an old fashioned remedy. It is most useful for gravel in the bladder, as a tonic, for biliousness and intermittent fever. When taken hot it induces perspiration. It has been used for suppressed menstruation, to help digestion, nausea, vomiting, liver, spleen, kidneys, griping in the bowels, dysentery, boils, insect stings, rabid dog bites, and toothache.

The apple tree itself has medicinal properties, being rich in potassium, sodium, magnesium, and iron salts, which contribute to the building of blood and bone. It is rightly called the King of Fruits. Persons who have too much acid should select sweet apples, which have little acid, and those who have not enough acid can eat sour apples. Old people and very small babies can eat a mellow apple if it is scraped, and do well on it. Apples are very high in food value and life-giving properties. They should not be eaten between meals but one can make an entire meal of them. If you have good teeth, eat the peeling, core, and seeds and chew them thoroughly. An apple is especially good for diabetes and is also excellent for the liver and kidneys, as well as being beneficial in hyperacidity. An exclusive apple diet for a while would prove of great benefit to the system. If anyone would drink a glass of good apple juice an hour before each meal it would prove of great benefit, but it must be made from good sound apples. The ordinary apple cider is not fit to be used.

BALM OF GILEAD (Populus candicans)
Common Names: Balsam poplar, American balm of Gilead, balm of Gilead buds, Mecca balsam.

Part Used: Buds, bark, leaves.

Medicinal Properties: Bark – stimulant, tonic, diuretic, antiscorbutic. Buds – balsamic, vulnerary.

Description and Uses: The beautiful Balm of Gilead tree which we admire so much for its wonderful fragrance, contains excellent properties in its bark and leaves for coughs, colds, lung troubles, kidney, and urinary troubles.

When the buds are boiled in olive oil, cocoa fat, or some other good oil, they make an excellent salve that is especially good for the healing or soothing of inflamed parts, the healing of fresh cuts, wounds, or bruises, and for the healing of bed sores. The buds and bark are also excellent for scurvy, as a stimulating tonic and to increase the flow of urine.

The buds are very valuable for dry asthma, coughs, and colds, and as a gargle for sore throat. When I was a child we gathered the buds before the leaves appeared and made a balm of Gilead tea of them, which could be used as a gargle for various throat troubles. Add an equal part of any one of the following herbs to add to this tea's efficiency: chickweed, coltsfoot, horehound, hyssop, licorice, lobelia, ragwort, anise, or red sage.

BALSAM (Myroxylon pereirae)
Common Names: Balsam of Peru
Part Used: Balsam, twigs, bark.
Medicinal Properties: Tonic, expectorant, exanthematous, herpatic.
Description and Uses: The balsam evergreen tree, which we use for Christmas trees and which develops big blisters on the outside of the bark, is filled with a very wonderful medicine called balsam fir. This liquid exudes from the bark of the tree after it has been injured. It is useful in all chronic mucous afflictions, catarrh, leukorrhea, as well as diarrhea and dysentery. It is useful externally in ulcers, wounds, ringworm, eczema, and other skin infections. The twigs and the bark have wonderful medicinal properties that are good for rheumatism, kidney trouble, gleet, inflammation of the bladder, and urinary complaints.

BAY – See Laurel.

BEECH (Fagus ferruginea)

Common Names: American beech, beech tree, beechnut tree.

Part Used: Bark, leaves.

Medicinal Properties: Tonic, astringent, antiseptic.

Description and Uses: The common beech tree is a valuable tree that is admired both as a shade tree and for its delicious nuts. Its leaves and bark contain wonderful medicinal properties for stomach troubles, ulcers, liver, kidneys, bladder, diabetes, and to improve the appetite. It is also an excellent tonic. It is good to take once in a while to clean and tone up the system.

The leaves are astringent and soothing to the nerves and stomach. They are very useful in swellings and soothing to sores and wounds for both man and beast. They are cooling and healing. Make a tea by taking a heaping teaspoonful to the cup of boiling water and let steep one-half hour. Bathe sores of all kinds freely and often: this tea is antiseptic and will make old sores clean and heal them if bathed often. Take three or four cups a day: be sure to take one cup before each meal and one upon retiring. It is a fine help for diabetes.

BIRCH (Betula lenta)

Common Names: Black birch, cherry birch, sweet birch, mahogany birch, mountain mahogany, spice birch.

Part Used: Inner bark and small twigs.

Medicinal Properties: Aromatic, stimulant, diaphoretic, anthelmintic.

Description and Uses: This is the common birch tree. The bark and little twigs of the birch tree have a splendid flavor similar to that of the wintergreen. We used to gather it and use it with wintergreen and spikenard in making a health drink. It has wonderful medicinal properties for bowel troubles, rheumatism, gout, and to expel worms. The tea makes a good wash for canker sores in the mouth. It is excellent for use in diarrhea, dysentery, and cholera infantum, given as an injection and taken internally. It is good for stones in the kidneys and bladder. It will purify the blood and give excellent results for boils and sores when taken internally and applied externally. The tea has a very pleasant taste and makes an excellent drink in place of water for a time. It is used in making root beer.

BLACK WILLOW (Salix nigra)
Common Names: Pussy willow, catkin's willow.
Part Used: Bark, buds.
Medicinal Properties: Bark – anodyne, antiseptic, astringent, antiperiodic, tonic, febrifuge. Buds – anti-aphrodisiac.
Description and Uses: A decoction of willow bark is a great aid in reducing fever and relieving pain. Willow bark is also good for the treatment of joint pains and to reduce inflammation and swelling. The decoction can also be used for sores in the mouth and as a gargle for sore throat. The decoction is made by soaking one to three teaspoonfuls of the bark in a cup of water for two or three hours and then bringing the water to a boil. A mouthful at a time should be taken to a total amount of about a cup a day. If you prefer the capsules, take one a day.

Black willow exerts a good influence on the sex organs, as in cases of incontinence, excessive sexual desire, and acute gonorrhea. When combined with saw palmetto berries or skullcap, it is good for nocturnal emissions.

BUTTERNUT (Juglans cinerea)
Common Names: Lemon walnut, oil nut, white walnut.
Part Used: Bark, leaves, roots.
Medicinal Properties: Tonic, cathartic, anthelmintic, nervine.
Description and Uses: Butternut is a tonic and a splendid laxative. It is soothing to the system and will expel worms from the intestines. It is an excellent remedy for chronic constipation and is good for fevers, colds, and influ-

enza. It is a splendid liver remedy. The nuts are good for food and are high in fat and minerals. Available in powder form and also as a fluid extract; use one to two teaspoonsfuls daily in a glass of water.

CHERRY – See Wild Black Cherry.

CHESTNUT (Castanea dentata)
Common Names: Sweet chestnut, Spanish chestnut, American chestnut.
Part Used: Inner bark, leaves.
Medicinal Properties: Tonic, astringent.
Description and Uses: The inner bark and leaves of the chestnut tree are used for their medicinal properties and the nuts are used for food. They are low in protein, high in carbohydrates and starch, and contain minerals such as phosphate of potash, magnesium, and some sodium and iron.

The leaves of the chestnut tree are excellent for the control of severe coughing, whooping cough, and other irritations in the respiratory tract. A tablespoonful of the infusion should be given three or four times a day.

CINCHONA (Cinchona calisaya)
Common Names: Peruvian bark, Jesuits bark, cinchona bark, yellow Peruvian bark, yellow bark, jacket bark, yellow cinchona.
Part Used: Bark.
Medicinal Properties: Antiperiodic, febrifuge, tonic, astringent, aperient.
Description and Uses: Cinchona bark is probably best known because it is the source of quinine, which is used to treat malaria. It is also good when taken in smaller doses as a general tonic and is used in the treatment of debility, dyspepsia, and neuralgia. As is well known, quinine often causes deafness, but this bark used in its natural state is

harmless. It exerts an excellent influence on the entire nervous system. In fevers, drink the tea freely. It is useful in epilepsy, female debility, aids digestion, and since it has a healing influence on the lungs, it is therefore useful in cases of pneumonia. Since cinchona bark causes contraction of the uterus, *it should not be used during pregnancy.* Cinchona bark should be used only in small doses and under supervision when possible.

CINNAMON (Cinnamonum zeylanicum)

Part Used: Bark, oil obtained from bark and leaves.

Medicinal Properties: Aromatic, astringent, stimulant, carminative.

Description and Uses: The wonderful cinnamon tree contains many remarkable properties, besides its delicious flavor. The powdered bark is stimulating and prevents gas and sour stomach. It warms up the stomach, expels gas from the stomach and bowels, and is somewhat laxative. Cinnamon is somewhat astringent and therefore is good in diarrhea as well as for nausea and vomiting. It is sometimes combined with other herbs to prevent griping and to give them a better flavor.

Dose: take a rounded teaspoonful of cinnamon to a cup of boiling water, stir it and drink while hot. Drink a small portion at a time, four or five times a day, or drink a cup as needed for griping and pain in the bowels. Use one-fourth teaspoon to a cup of other herbs to flavor them. Put it in with the herbs when you make the tea.

CYPRESS (Cupressus sempervirens)

Part Used: Cones, nuts.

Medicinal Properties: Astringent, styptic.

Description and Uses: The cones and nuts of the cypress tree are astringent and will stop bleeding of all kinds. For internal use, make a tea by placing a few of the cones in some water and simmering slowly for ten minutes. Take in small doses: two tablespoonfuls may be taken every two hours. In bad cases of diarrhea this tea is very effective. It will stop bleeding and hemorrhage from the lungs and stomach. It is very useful for treating bleeding piles, bloody diarrhea, and also dysentery. Use a little as a douche for excessive menstruation. Cypress tea is also good for pyorrhea and bleeding gums when the teeth are loose. Rinse the mouth with the tea.

ELDER (Sambucus canadensis)

Common Names: Sweet elder, American elder, rob elder, elder flowers, black elder, common elder, elderberry.

Part Used: Flowers, leaves, bark, roots, berries.

Medicinal Properties: Bark – emetic, cathartic. Flowers – diaphoretic, diuretic, exanthematous, alterative, emollient, discutient, rubrifacient, stimulant.

Description and Uses: The elder tree is an old-fashioned home remedy and is found in nearly all old people's gardens. The entire tree has marvelous medicinal properties. While some shrubs, trees, or plants have only one part which is useful, all parts of the elder – the flowers, berries, leaves, bark, and roots – are useful.

Tea made from the flowers is excellent for twitching eyelids and inflammation of the eyes. It is stimulating, a good tonic, and blood purifier. It increases the flow of urine, is cooling, good for building up the system, and is very useful in liver and kidney diseases. A splendid remedy for children's diseases such as liver derangements, erysipelas, etc.

In skin diseases the sores should be washed with the tea, and the tea should also be taken internally. It is very useful for headaches due to colds, palsy, rheumatism, scrofula, syphilis, and epilepsy. It is somewhat laxative and a wonderful remedy for dropsy as well as being useful in constipation; very good in fever and many chronic diseases; makes an excellent poultice for tumors and various swellings. The dry berries made into a tea are an excellent remedy for cholera, diarrhea, and summer complaint. It can be taken freely without harm. It is good for influenza when combined with peppermint. Made into an ointment, elder is valuable in burns, scalds, and all skin diseases.

Caution should be excercised when using elder, as poisoning may result if the fresh plant is used. The cooked berries are harmless and are frequently used to make jam or pies.

EUCALYPTUS (Eucalyptus globulus)
Common Names: Bluegum tree.
Part Used: Leaves, bark.
Medicinal Properties: Antiseptic, stimulant, expectorant, antispasmodic.
Description and Uses: The wonderful eucalyptus tree, from which eucalyptus oil is made, has a wide range of uses. The leaves and bark are very useful in fevers, acute and chronic bronchitis in its various forms, asthma, and similar ailments. The oil made from the leaves may be inhaled for asthma, diphtheria, or sore throat. The antiseptic properties make it useful for use on wounds and ulcers. When used in this way, one ounce should be added to a pint of warm water. The oil may also be applied externally to the neck and chest for cough, croup, and sore throat.

FIG (Ficus carica)
Part Used: Fruit, leaves.
Medicinal Properties: Laxative, demulcent, emollient, nutritive.
Description and Uses: The fig tree is one of our most wonderful trees. It has many valuable medicinal properties. Both the leaves and the fruit are used. Split open the fresh ripe fruit and lay it on a boil or a carbuncle and it will give great relief. Mildly laxative, figs are also one of the most delicious fruits.

When the fruit is broken off the tree before it is ripe, a milk escapes that has wonderful healing properties. It may be put on sores and boils. If this milk is put freely on warts, it removes them.

The leaves boiled in Crisco make an excellent ointment.

Fig leaf tea is excellent to wash old sores. Where the flesh has turned black from bruises or blows, bathing with the warm tea stimulates the circulation and carries away the discoloration. *Because of the presence of psoralens in fig leaf tea, do not go into the sun after applying the tea to your skin, as it will cause a severe sunburn.* Snuff the tea up the nose when there are difficulties and pain in the nostrils. The tea is also good dropped in the ear for pain, but it must be lukewarm. It is also very excellent for treating bites of poisonous insects and is good for a mouthwash and gargle, for hoarseness, sore throat, and bad breath. Fig tea is good for any kind of lung trouble, such as asthma and bronchitis and is a splendid medicine for dropsy, spasms, and convulsions. To make fig leaf tea, steep one heaping teaspoonful (cut fine) in a cup of boiling water. Drink three or four cups a day, one hour before meals. Sometimes the results are better if taken five or six times a day in wineglassful doses.

A syrup made of figs makes a very excellent cough medicine. It can be used alone or with a little lemon added. Take a pound of figs, cut them up, and put them in a quart of water. Simmer for a few minutes; then put them in a cheesecloth and squeeze out all the juice possible; add the juice of two lemons and a little honey if desired. This makes an excellent cough remedy.

FIR TREE – See Spruce.

FRINGE TREE (Chionanthus virginica)
Common Names: Old man's beard, graybeard tree, poison ash, snowflower, white fringe, snowdrop tree.
Part Used: Bark.
Medicinal Properties: Tonic, diuretic, febrifuge, aperient.
Description and Uses: A preparation of the bark is a

good blood purifier and general tonic. It reduces fever, acts as a gentle cathartic, and is good for the kidneys.

Fringe tree bark is also very good for all liver troubles, bilious fevers, jaundice, gall bladder, colic, and gallstones. Externally, the bark may be made into a poultice and used on wounds and sores. When taken internally, one teaspoonful of the bark should be boiled in one cup of water. One cup of this decoction should be taken daily for these problems.

GUM ARABIC – See Acacia.

HEMLOCK (Tsuga canadensis)
Common Names: Canada pitch tree, hemlock tree, hemlock gum tree, hemlock pitch tree, weeping spruce, pine tops, tanner's bark, hemlock bark, hemlock leaves.
Part Used: Inner bark, leaves.
Medicinal Properties: Diaphoretic, astringent, diuretic.
Description and Uses: This is the common hemlock tree, one of the old home remedies. The leaves can also be used, but should not be taken during pregnancy. This is the same kind of bark that tanners use in making shoe leather. The bark can be used to make a tea that is a very valuable remedy for a number of ailments. When I was a child I used to gather little hemlock twigs for my father for various purposes. It is a wonderful astringent and can be used both internally and externally. For external use, simmer a teaspoonful in a cup of water for ten minutes. For internal use, steep a teaspoonful of inner bark or twigs in a cup of boiling water. It is better to take smaller doses more often. Hemlock bark tea is an ideal remedy for canker sores in the mouth and it can be used as a gargle and mouthwash. It can also be used in dropsy with splendid success, as it increases the flow of urine; has a healing effect on the kidneys and bladder; and is good for gravel in the urinary passages. This tea may be used as a douche for leukorrhea; is good for uterine troubles; and

is a splendid remedy when used as an enema for colon trouble and diarrhea. Good when applied externally as a wash for gangrene, old sores, and ulcers. The powdered bark is excellent when used in shoes or stockings for sore, tender, or sweaty feet.

HICKORY (Carya ovata)
Part Used: Inner bark, leaves.
Medicinal Properties: Laxative, depuritive, detergent.
Description and Uses: The hickory is a well-known tree noted for its strength and the toughness of its wood, which is used for making ax handles and wheels of vehicles of various kinds and many other things where a strong wood is needed.

The inner bark and leaves have medicinal properties. They are laxative, useful in purifying the system, good for washing ulcers and sores, for diarrhea, and kindred troubles. Very useful in colitis. Take a heaping tablespoonful to a quart of boiling water, let simmer fifteen minutes, strain off, and use as an enema.

To take internally, use one teaspoonful of the granulated bark or leaves to one cup of boiling water. Let simmer thirty minutes, strain off, and drink from one to three cups a day.

IRONWOOD (Ostrya virginica)
Common Names: Lever wood, hop hornbeam.
Part Used: Inner bark, inner red wood.
Medicinal Properties: Tonic, depuritive.
Description and Uses: The ironwood tree, also called lever wood, has a number of splendid medical properties. Use the inner bark and the inner red wood of the tree. In order to use the bark or inner red wood, you must shave it or cut it up into small chips and boil them for fifteen or twenty minutes. A good time to gather the bark is in the latter part of the summer. It is a good tonic and a splendid blood purifier, and is very beneficial to the stomach. It is good for use in

dyspepsia, neuralgia, fever, ague, scrofula, and as a nerve tonic.

———————

JUNIPER (Juniperus communis)
Part Used: Berries, new twigs.
Medicinal Properties: Diuretic, tonic, carminative, antiseptic, stomachic.
Description and Uses: The juniper tree yields berries that are a most wonderful medicine. I used to gather these berries when just a young lad.

For kidney and urinary troubles, take one heaping teaspoonful of juniper berries, granulated or chopped up, or the whole berry, one teaspoonful of granulated peach leaves, and one teaspoonful of marshmallow. Mix together.

Use one heaping teaspoonful to the cup of boiling water and let steep. Drink from one to three cups a day, more or less as needed; children according to age. It is important to remember that large doses or prolonged use may irritate the kidneys, so it should be used with caution if you have a kidney infection. It is also NOT recommended for pregnant women.

The tea of the juniper is very cleansing to the system and, combined as above, makes a most excellent medicine. The juniper berries alone, made into a strong tea by using two teaspoonfuls to a cup of boiling water, make an excellent wash for the bites of poisonous insects, snakes, dogs, and bee stings.

Another tea made from the berries alone, but using only ONE teaspoonful to the cup of water, is an excellent stomach medicine, expelling the wind from the stomach and bowels, and can safely be used in cases of colic. It is a very effective remedy for coughs, shortness of breath, consumption, pain in the bowels, cramps, and convulsions. It is wonderful for women when their time of delivery has come. It is also a good brain medicine.

Combining equal parts with rue makes an excellent remedy for any kind of head trouble. It is soothing and strength-ening to the nerves and it also helps the vision. In fact, it strengthens the nerves throughout the whole body. It is good for gout, sciatica, rheumatism, or pain in any part of the body. It is also very good combined with gentian and calamus. Juniper tea is excellent as a remedy for the gums and to gargle with. It also checks bleeding in hemorrhoids or piles, and it is good for worms in both children and adults.

The ashes of the wood, a teaspoonful to the pint of boiling water, is a splendid remedy when used as a wash for itch, scabs on any part of the body, or the sores of leprosy. The berries are good for convulsions. They make a good medicine for palsy. Take equal parts of prickly ash, juniper berries, and calamus root; if constipated, add buckthorn bark. Make an infusion using one ounce of the combined herbs to a pint of boiling water.

LAUREL (Laurus nobilis)
Common Names: Bay tree, sweet bay, noble laurel, Roman laurel, bay laurel, Indian bay.

Part Used: Bark, berries, leaves.

Medicinal Properties: Carminative, aromatic, stomachic, astringent, digestive.

Description and Uses: The bark, leaves, and berries of the bay tree are used. The bark is slightly astringent and is highly recommended for stones in the kidneys and bladder. It is a splendid remedy for the pancreas, spleen, and various liver troubles.

A strong tea made from the berries, taken both internally and applied externally, is very effective for all poisonous insect bites, snake bites, and stings of wasps. This is also an excellent tea to take during epidemics of contagious diseases such as smallpox, typhoid fever, measles, diphtheria, taken both internally and used as a gargle; very efficient in tonsillitis, sore throat, and nose troubles, and various lung troubles.

The berries are very helpful in suppressed menstruation

and womb troubles. The berries are also very helpful during childbirth if taken when the time of delivery is at hand, and they also help in expelling the afterbirth.

Tea made from the berries is an excellent remedy in colds, influenza, and fever. It helps to clear out the brain, the eyes, and the lungs, or any other part of the body. It is a regular cleanser and a very good remedy for chronic coughs, consumption, and asthma when there is shortness of breath. It will destroy worms in the body; helps to increase the flow of urine, and is an excellent tea for those troubled with fermentation and gas in the stomach and bowels.

Make a tea of the leaves, bark, or berries for adding to a sitz bath, as it is very excellent for any bladder or uterine troubles, or pain in the bowels. When the soft palate hangs down and is inflamed, a gargle made from a tea of the berries, leaves, or bark will make it shrink to normal size. A strong tea made of the berries or the oil of the berries is most excellent when applied to rheumatic or arthritic joints and is good for nerve troubles or pain in the bowels or womb; good for any kind of cramps or pain in the chest, or numbness in any part of the body. The oil is an excellent remedy for itch, eczema, or bruises. After receiving a blow, when the flesh becomes black, it will help to congeal the blood and return the skin color to normal. It is also good for other black or brown spots on the flesh, and is excellent for sunburn. The berries, bark, and leaves are a most wonderful remedy for many troubles. Take a heaping teaspoonful of the granulated bark from the roots in a cup of boiling water. Let it steep for one-half hour and drink from one to three cups a day. The berries are also very useful in cough syrup.

LINDEN (Tilia americana)
Common Names: Basswood, American linden, lime tree, spoonwood.
Part Used: Inner bark, leaves, flowers.

Medicinal Properties: Diaphoretic, stomachic, emollient.

Description and Uses: Tea made from parts of the linden, or basswood tree, is an old-fashioned, well-known household remedy. It is useful for colds. The hot tea promotes perspiration and cleanses the system of mucus, especially the kidneys, bladder, and stomach. It is also excellent for female complaints, for poultices on boils, and other painful swellings. It is valuable for coughs, for use as a gargle, for hoarseness, sore throat, epilepsy, and headaches.

MAGNOLIA (Magnolia glauca)
Common Names: Swamp laurel, red laurel, sweet magnolia, red bay, white bay, beaver tree, Indian bark, sweet bay, swamp sassafras, holly bay.
Part Used: Bark.
Medicinal Properties: Astringent, stimulant, febrifuge, tonic, aromatic, antiperiodic, diaphoretic.
Description and Uses: The magnolia tree, which is admired so much for its beautiful and fragrant flowers, has wonderful medicinal properties that are little known to man. The bark is very effective for many ailments. In the first place, it can do the work of quinine, leaving no bad effects after its use. The medical properties of the magnolia will cure the tobacco habit when taken with other hygienic measures. It is good for fever, dyspepsia, dysentery, and erysipelas. It may be used as a douche for leukorrhea. A wash made by simmering one tablespoonful of magnolia bark in a pint of water for ten minutes is fine for many skin diseases. This herb can be taken for a long time without any ill effects.

MAPLE (Acer rubrum)
Common Names: Swamp maple.
Part Used: Inner bark, leaves.
Medicinal Properties: Tonic, sedative.
Description and Uses: The maple tree is one of our

most beautiful shade trees. In my childhood and youth, I admired this tree very much for the syrup and maple sugar that we made from it. We raised plenty of buckwheat and had the whole kernel ground into flour and made into pancakes, upon which we used some butter and plenty of maple syrup. But now we have something better. Look under "Kloss Soybean Pancakes," which are a real health food.

The inner bark of the maple tree and also the leaves are a splendid medicine for both liver and spleen, and are very soothing to these organs. In fact, they are a good medicine for the whole body, acting as a tonic and soother of the nerves.

Take one heaping teaspoonful of the bark or leaves to the cup of boiling water. One to three cups a day may be taken on an empty stomach. Sometimes when there is pain in the liver or spleen, taking a wineglassful every hour or two has a splendid effect.

OAK (Quercus alba)
Common Names: White oak, Tanner's bark.
Part Used: Inner bark, leaves, acorn cups.
Medicinal Properties: Tonic, astringent, antiseptic, anthelmintic.
Description and Uses: The leaves and bark are used: the inner white bark is best and is a very strong astringent. A strong tea made from white oak bark is excellent for vaginal discharge and womb troubles. It will also expel pin-worms. Simmer a tablespoonful in a pint of water for ten minutes. Drink up to three cups a day. It is one of the best remedies for piles or hemorrhoids, hemorrhages, or any trouble in the rectum. It may be used internally or taken as an enema. For enemas and douches, steep a heaping tablespoonful in a quart of boiling water for thirty minutes and strain through a cloth. Use as hot as possible. Stops hemorrhages in the lungs, stomach, and bowels, spitting of blood, and bleeding in the mouth. Increases the flow of urine and helps remove kidney stones. It is helpful for an ulcerated bladder or bloody urine.

Checks excess menstrual flow. The tea is good for use in bathing scabs and sores. In fevers it brings the temperature down.

It is very useful in goiter and hardened neck. For goiter, fold a small towel or some cheesecloth several times to make a compress and moisten with the tea as made for enemas. Tie the compress around the neck, leaving it on all night and covering well with a woolen or flannel cloth. For varicose veins, take the tea internally and bathe the veins externally with a strong tea three or four times a day, diluting the tea a little if there are any open sores. It is also good to moisten a cloth with the tea, wrap it around the legs, and cover well with flannel. This will also reduce the swelling and hard tumors.

A tea made from the bark, with the powder of the acorn cups added, is excellent for bleeding from the mouth, spitting of blood, and to stop vomiting. It resists the force of poisonous medicines and is excellent for ulcerated bladder and bloody urine. The powder of the acorn made into a tea helps to counteract the poison of venomous creatures. The distilled liquid of the buds, before they become leaves, can be used either outwardly or inwardly for inflammations, fevers, and infections. The water from the leaves is especially excellent for the following diseases: leukorrhea, womb troubles, piles, rectal problems, hemorrhages, varicose veins, to normalize the kidneys, liver, and spleen, goiter, tumors, and swellings.

Dose: one ounce of the bark steeped in a pint of water. Use one teaspoonful of the tea three or four times a day for dysentery or diarrhea. Use as a douche for vaginal discharge or as a gargle for sore throat and mucous discharge.

Use the powdered bark on ulcers. It is astringent and antiseptic. It is good in enemas for colon trouble, gonorrhea, gleet (urethritis), leukorrhea and stomach troubles.

PEACH (Amygdalus persica)
Part Used: Bark, leaves, twigs, and kernels.

Medicinal Properties: Relaxant, demulcent, sedative, aromatic, laxative, diuretic, expectorant.

Description and Uses: We go out to the orchard and find the peach tree with its delicious fruit for food. Its leaves are a most healing and specific remedy for dyspepsia, gastritis, and irritation of the stomach lining. Gather plenty of common peach tree leaves and always have them on hand. They are useful to stop vomiting or morning sickness in pregnancy. They are laxative and exert an excellent influence over the nervous system. They are also very useful in coughs, whooping cough, and bronchitis. Excellent for bladder and uterine troubles such as burning urine, inflammation, tenderness and aching in the pelvic region. When the leaves are made into tea and taken hot in small doses (a large swallow every hour or two), it will stop vomiting. The powdered bark or leaves heal sores or wounds. The kernels or buds, bruised and boiled in vinegar until they become thick, are excellent for baldness to grow hair. If necessary they may be used as a substitute for quinine for the treatment of malaria.

Dose: as an infusion, steep one level teaspoonful of the leaves in a cup of water, or one ounce of the leaves to a pint of boiling water. Take two or three cups during the day as needed, taking the first cup before breakfast.

PERUVIAN BARK – See Cinchona.

PINE (Pinus strobus)
Common Names: Deal pine, soft pine, white pine.
Part Used: Inner bark, sprigs.
Medicinal Properties: Expectorant, demulcent.
Description and Uses: White pine is a very old reliable remedy for chest ailments such as bronchitis, coughs, colds, croup, and influenza. It is excellent for use in tonsillitis, laryngitis, and sore throats. It will stop coughing and help to expel phlegm from the throat and lungs. It is even better when combined with wild cherry bark or spikenard.

It has also been found useful in rheumatism, kidney troubles, and scurvy. Combined with uva ursi, marshmallow, and poplar bark, it is excellent for diabetes. The American Indians used the pine tree for food as well as medicine by making a bread from the ground-up bark. This was their remedy for kidney, throat and lung afflictions; especially sore throat and tonsillitis.

Dose: steep one teaspoonful of the inner bark or sprigs with one tablespoonful of wild cherry bark and one tablespoonful of spikenard root in a pint of boiling water for thirty minutes. Take one teaspoonful every hour as needed. Add a little honey for sweetening if desired. A ready-made combination of pine with other herbs is available at many herb shops, with the directions for use on the container.

POPLAR (Populus tremuloides)

Common Names: Quaking aspen, American aspen, quaking asp, quiver leaf, trembling tree, trembling poplar, white poplar, aspen poplar, abele tree.

Part Used: Bark, buds, leaves.

Medicinal Properties: Stomachic, febrifuge, tonic, antiperiodic, balsamic.

Description and Uses: In looking at the tall poplar tree, I see wonderful properties in the buds, bark, and leaves. Poplar is well-known throughout the world as a wonderful tonic. It is better than quinine for all purposes for which quinine is used and has none of the aftereffects as does the continuous administration of quinine. It is very useful for disease of the urinary organs, especially if weak. An excellent aid to digestion and to tone up run-down conditions, either in disease or old age. Very good in all cases of chronic diarrhea. Excellent for acute rheumatism. Good for fever caused by influenza. It is useful in neuralgia, jaundice, liver trouble, diabetes, hay fever, cholera infantum, and will expel worms.

It is splendid when used externally as a wash for cancer, bad ulcers, gangrenous wounds, eczema, strong perspiration, burns, and sores caused by gonorrhea and syphilis. It is more effective than quinine in fever and la grippe (influenza). Place a teaspoonful of the buds, bark, or leaves in a pint of boiling water. Use cold, and take one or two cupfuls a day, one swallow at a time.

The buds from the poplar tree may be boiled in olive oil and made into an ointment, to be used externally for cuts, wounds, burns, and scratches.

PRICKLY ASH (Zanthoxylum americanum)

Common Names: Northern prickly ash, toothache bush, toothache tree, suterberry, suterberry bark, yellow wood, yellow wood berries, pellitory bark, prickly ash berries.

Part Used: Berries, bark.

Medicinal Properties: Tonic, stimulant, diaphoretic, alterative, nervine, deobstruent, and sialagogue.

Description and Uses: The prickly ash is a beautiful little tree, growing from eight to twelve feet tall, full of thorns, and often just covered with berries about the size of a currant. I used to cut off a little of the bark and chew it. It will help sores in the mouth and ease the pain of a toothache. Both the bark and the berries are used. This tree is a most wonderful remedy for many diseases. The berries are generally considered to be more active than the bark and are a most wonderful tonic and stimulant. They are extremely useful in chronic rheumatism and many skin conditions, syphilis, colic, derangement of the liver, scrofula, and chronic female troubles. The berries are also antispasmodic and carminative, acting mostly on the mucous membranes to relieve asthma and colds generally. They are very beneficial in treating paralysis of the tongue and mouth, as they increase the flow of saliva and help to remove obstructions in every part of the body. The berries are very fine in bad cases of cholera and are a splendid blood purifier. The powder is excellent when sprinkled on old wounds and indolent ulcers. Use one teaspoon of the bark or berries in a cup of boiling water. Take a cupful a day, cold, one swallow at a time.

QUASSIA (Picraena excelsa)
Common Names: Quassia wood, quassia bark, bitter bark, bitter quassia, lofty quassia, bitter ash, bitter wood.
Part Used: Wood, bark.
Medicinal Properties: Tonic, febrifuge, anthelmintic.
Description and Uses: The tea is an excellent tonic to tone up a run-down system. It will expel worms and is especially good in dyspepsia and for a weakened digestive tract. It is a wonderful remedy that destroys the appetite for strong drink. In olden days, cups were made of the wood. Water and other liquids were left to stand in them for a short time, thus receiving the bitter property of the wood. Quassia is good in fevers and rheumatism. It is available as a tincture or powder. It is a common component of insecticides.

QUINCE (Cydonia oblongata)
Part Used: Juice squeezed from the fruit.
Medicinal Properties: Mucilaginous, demulcent.
Description and Uses: The quince tree grows to the size of an ordinary apple tree. The fruit has an acid taste and the juice is a good stomach medicine. It is slightly astringent and is quite a good sedative. It will allay gas and vomiting. In children it checks nausea, vomiting, and running off of the bowels. Take two tablespoonfuls of the juice, one-fourth tablespoonful of cinnamon, and one-fourth teaspoonful of powdered ginger. Put in a cup, and fill with boiling water. Take one tablespoonful every hour. More may be taken if needed; children should take less according to their age.

The juice of a quince is really a prevention against sickness and rids the system of poison. The juice makes an excellent gargle. For gargling, it is very effective if a little honey and lemon juice are added. It is also good to apply to sores on the outside. The juice of this fruit, rubbed with the tips of the fingers on the scalp, will keep hair from falling out, and make it grow where the roots of the hair are not entirely dead.

SLIPPERY ELM (Ulmus fulva)
Common Names: Red elm, moose elm, Indian elm, sweet elm, American elm, rock elm, winged elm.

Part Used: Inner bark.

Medicinal Properties: Mucilaginous, demulcent, emollient, nutritive, diuretic, pectoral.

Description and Uses: We all admire the wonderful slippery elm tree. In my childhood we used to go out with a large knife called a drawshave, and shave off the outer rough bark and cut off the inner bark in big strips and carry it home for medicinal use. It contains various medicinal properties that are entirely harmless and of which even small infants can partake to prevent suffering.

Slippery elm is highly nourishing and very soothing to the stomach as a tea. I have used it for many years with wonderful results. It is very effective in diarrhea, bowel, stomach, bladder, and kidney troubles. It is soothing and healing wherever it is used. Slippery elm will stay in an ulcerated and cancerous stomach when nothing else will. It is very nourishing, and in case of famine a person could live for some time on the inner slippery elm bark.

An excellent treatment in female troubles is the following: make a thick paste of powdered slippery elm with pure cold water. Shape into pieces about one inch long and one inch thick. Place in warm water for a few minutes. These are called vaginal suppositories. Insert three into the vagina as far as possible and then insert a sponge with a string attached. Let these remain in place for two days, then remove the sponge and give a douche to remove the slippery elm. This is an excellent treatment for cancers and tumors of the womb, all growths in the female organs, fallen womb (this does not imply that slippery elm by itself will cure cancer), vaginal discharge or inflammation, leukorrhea, and congestion of any part of the vagina or womb.

Slippery elm is one of the most effective ingredients known for a poultice. If the powdered slippery elm bark is mixed with some cornmeal mush and powdered lobelia, it is wonderfully soothing as a poultice. For excellent poultices, mix two parts of powdered slippery elm with one part of any one or all of the following powdered herbs: cornmeal, blood-root, blue flag, comfrey, ragweed, chickweed. Mix well together, add warm water to make a thick paste, and use for abscesses, dirty wounds, inflammations, congestions, or eruptions. The face of the poultice should be smeared with olive oil if it is to be applied to a hairy surface. This poultice is also good for an enlarged prostate, swollen glands of the neck, groin, etc.

Slippery elm will congeal the mucous material troubling the patient and help it pass through the intestines. It cleans, heals, and strengthens.

As a diet, take a teaspoonful of the powdered slippery elm bark and pour upon it a cupful of boiling soybean milk. Sweeten to taste. This is useful in cases of consumption and also in inflammation of the stomach and intestines. This drink makes a good food for children.

To make slippery elm tea, use a heaping tablespoonful to a pint of boiling water. Let steep one hour, then simmer a few minutes. Strain and use. It is well to soak and simmer twice, as the full virtue of the herb does not usually come out the first time.

Slippery elm lozenges are excellent for a sore throat.

SPRUCE (Picea excelsa)

Common Names: Norway pine, Norway spruce, fir tree.

Part Used: Leaves, young shoots.

Medicinal Properties: Expectorant, pectoral, diaphoretic.

Description and Uses: The fir tree or Norway spruce is a well-known tree. Both the leaves and young shoots are used as remedies. A tea made from the leaves is very healing to wounds and ulcers, good for the bladder and for treating gonorrhea and leukorrhea. It is good to use as an enema and also a douche, as well as to take internally; good for stones in the kidney and gravel in the bladder. It is good for lung trouble and will cut phlegm in the throat and lungs, and is very healing. When the breath is short, it helps to open up the air passages.

When the tree is tapped, it yields a pitch that makes a very excellent turpentine that has powerful healing properties.

A tea made of the leaves and the young shoots makes an excellent tea for scurvy and for cleansing the system. It can be steeped or simmered for just a few minutes. This tea is an excellent remedy for those who do not have access to plenty of fruits and greens.

The leaves and branches of this tree have been used in making that well-known spruce beer and have formerly been used in nonalcoholic beer for its wonderful medicinal properties. For a tea, take a heaping teaspoonful to a cup of boiling water, steep for thirty minutes, and drink from one to three cups a day. This tea is excellent used both internally and externally.

TAMARACK (Larix americana)
Common Names: American Larch, black larch, hackmatack.
Part Used: Inner bark.
Medicinal Properties: Alterative, diuretic, laxative.
Description and Uses: The tamarack tree is a tall, slender, straight tree. The sap, a gummy substance, runs out of the bark and as a child I used to chew it as gum. It has a very good flavor, better than other gums on the market. Of course I do not recommend commercial chewing gum as it is injurious to the system.

The inner bark, made into a tea, is good for bleeding of any kind, for the spitting of blood from the lungs or throat, for bleeding hemorrhoids, and to lessen profuse menstruation. The tea is also good medicine for liver trouble, jaundice, and also for colic; very effective for poisonous insect bites; good for the spleen when enlarged and hardened; for earaches, and inflammation of the eyes. Bathe the eyes with the tea, using an eyecup or medicine dropper. Drop some of the lukewarm tea in the ear to relieve earache. This tea is an excellent wash for gangrene or old running sores and ulcers; and will help overcome the itch and kill nits and lice.

A tea made from the ashes of tamarack bark is very healing to burns and scalds and a splendid medicine for a person subject to melancholy.

To make tamarack tea, take one heaping teaspoonful of the granulated bark or leaves to a cup of water and take one-half cup four or five times a day, more or less as needed. To treat constipation, buckthorn bark and calamus root are also used: take a teaspoon of each and mix with a teaspoon of tamarack, using the inner bark. Use a heaping teaspoon of this mixture to the cup of boiling water, steep for thirty minutes, and take as much as needed.

WALNUT (Juglans regia)

Common Names: English walnut, Caucasian walnut, Persian walnut.

Part Used: Leaves, bark, nut.

Medicinal Properties: Astringent, detergent, alterative, and anthelmintic.

Description and Uses: The walnut is a well-known tree. It is too bad that there are not more of them on every farm in the regions where they will grow, for the walnut is an excellent nut and the leaves and bark are an effective medicine for a number of ailments, when taken internally and also applied externally. It will expel all kinds of worms from the intestinal tract, and is an excellent remedy for poisonous snake bites, or other poisonous bites, such as rabid dog bites.

The bark or leaves boiled in honey makes an excellent

throat and stomach remedy, which also is good for lung troubles and sores in the throat and mouth.

Both the leaves and the bark are astringent and are good in diarrhea and excellent for women to take for profuse menstruation, taken both as a tea and used as a douche. Wet the tips of the fingers in the tea and massage the scalp once a day to keep the hair from falling out and to give it a beautiful luster. The tea is also very helpful for running sores. Bathe them with the tea three or four times a day.

Dose: take a heaping teaspoonful of the granulated leaves or bark, steep in a cup of boiling water for thirty minutes, and drink from one to three cups a day.

WHITE ASH (Fraxinus americana)
Common Names: American white ash.
Part Used: Inner bark.
Medicinal Properties: Diuretic, tonic, laxative.
Description and Uses: This is one of the old-fashioned, well-known remedies. Steep one heaping teaspoonful in a cup of boiling water for thirty minutes. Drink one or more cupfuls a day, a half a glass at a time. Useful in dropsy, urinary troubles and constipation. Excellent for reducing.

WHITE OAK – See Oak.

WHITE PINE – See Pine.

WHITE WILLOW (Salix alba)
Common Names: Willow, salacin willow, willow bark, withe, withy.
Part Used: Leaves, bark.
Medicinal Properties: Tonic, antiperiodic, astringent, antiseptic, anodyne, diaphoretic, diuretic, febrifuge.
Description and Uses: The ability of willow bark to reduce fever and alleviate pain has been known for centuries.

It is closely related to the common aspirin. It is useful in all stomach troubles, sour stomach, and heartburn. Excellent in all kinds of fevers, chills, ague, acute rheumatism. The tea made from the leaves or buds is good in gangrene, cancer, and eczema. Use internally and externally. Good for bleeding wounds, nosebleeds, or spitting of blood, as an antiemetic, eyewash, and to increase the flow of urine. Excellent to use in place of quinine and far more effective.

To prepare a decoction, soak one to three teaspoonfuls of bark in a cup of cold water for three or four hours and then bring the water to a boil. Take a mouthful at a time of the unsweetened decoction, to a total of about one cup a day.

WILD BLACK CHERRY (Prunus serotina)

Common Names: Black cherry, black choke, rub cherry, cabana cherry, Virginia prune, choke cherry, rum cherry.

Part Used: Inner bark.

Medicinal Properties: Astringent, tonic, pectoral, sedative, stimulant.

Description and Uses: The cherry tree is a native of Asia and was brought to Italy in the first century B.C. Its wonderful medicinal properties tone up the system, loosen phlegm in the throat and chest, and are very good for colds, influenza, tuberculosis, stomach trouble, dyspepsia, fevers, asthma, and high blood pressure. A common ingredient in cough syrups and cold medicines. Eating large amounts of cherries, a half-pound a day, either fresh or canned, has proven helpful in cases of gout and arthritis. Cherry juice is also good for these same conditions.

The bark of the wild black cherry should not be boiled. Steep one teaspoonful of powdered cherry bark in a cup of hot water. Use one or two cups a day, a swallow at a time; or take one-half to one teaspoon of the fluid extract as needed.

7

SPECIFIC HERBS FOR VARIOUS MEDICAL PROBLEMS

This chapter lists a number of diseases and other conditions and gives the herbs that are most commonly used to treat them. Study the description of each one of these herbs as given in this book and read the directions for their use in Section II, Chapter 3, General Directions for the Preparation and Use of Herbs.

SPECIFIC DISEASES AND COMPLAINTS

ABSCESSES — Carrot (poultice), lobelia, mugwort, slippery elm, charcoal, potato (poultice).

ACHES — Skullcap, motherwort, valerian, catnip, peppermint, angelica.

AGUE — Gentian root, sorrel, tansy, vervain, willow, broom, camomile.

ANEMIA — Comfrey, dandelion, fenugreek, barberry bark, agrimony, centaury, raspberry leaves, quassia chips.

APOPLEXY (STROKE) — Masterwort, black cohosh, hyssop, vervain, blue cohosh, catnip, antispasmodic tincture, skullcap.

APPENDICITIS — Buckthorn bark, vervain, water pepper, lady's slipper. Proper medical attention is also necessary.

ASTHMA — Black cohosh, comfrey, coltsfoot, horehound, hyssop, lobelia, masterwort, milkweed, mullein, myrrh, pleurisy root, prickly ash, saw palmetto berries, skunk cabbage, thyme, vervain, wild cherry, flaxseed, balm of Gilead, red root, red sage, boneset, cubeb berries, elecampane.

BACKACHE — Nettle, pennyroyal, tansy, uva-ursi, buchu, wood betony.

BED SORES — Plantain, balm of Gilead, bayberry bark, bloodroot, witch hazel, golden seal.

BED-WETTING — Plantain, St.John's-wort, buchu, corn silk, cubeb berries, fennel seed, milkweed, wood betony, mullein, willow, hops, fennel.

BILIOUSNESS — Apple tree bark, senna, poke root, camomile, red sage (excellent), wood betony, queen of the meadow, hyssop, agrimony.

BLEEDING — Self-heal, mullein (stops bleeding from the lungs), shepherd's purse (for lungs, stomach, kidneys, and bowels), wild alum root, golden seal, blackberry leaves, comfrey, bayberry, uva-ursi, yellow dock.

BLOOD POISONING AND INFECTIONS — Chickweed, plantain, echinacea, golden seal, myrrh, burdock, bloodroot, water pepper (smartweed) and charcoal (poultice), golden seal.

BOILS AND CARBUNCLES — Balm (poultice), powdered bayberry bark (poultice), burdock, chickweed, comfrey, coral, flaxseed, hops, lobelia, origanum, slippery elm, sorrel, St.John's-wort, turkey corn, white clover, white water lily, wintergreen, wood sage, echinacea, birch (bark or small twigs), plantain, wild cherry (bark or small twigs).

BOWEL TROUBLE — Water pepper, white pond lily, wintergreen, dandelion, wood sanicle, bethroot, chickweed, myrrh, witch hazel, echinacea, bayberry bark, birch, bitter-root, blue violet, caraway seeds (expels gas), catnip (for acid), chickweed, comfrey, coriander, cubeb berries, fenugreek, golden seal, gum arabic, hyssop, magnolia, masterwort, milkweed, mugwort, mullein, origanum, pilewort, rhubarb, rue, sage, sanicle, sassafras, slippery elm, spearmint, strawberry, sumach berries, tansy, vervain, marshmallow.

BREASTS (SORE, SWOLLEN, OR CAKED)
Comfrey, parsley, St. John's-wort and poke root for treating caked breasts.

BRIGHT'S (KIDNEY) DISEASE — Golden seal (combined with peach leaves, queen of the meadow, clover, and corn silk), saw palmetto berries, uva-ursi, wild alum root, yarrow, peach (leaves, blossoms, or twigs), peppermint.

BRONCHITIS — Chickweed, coltsfoot, cubeb berries, golden seal, lungwort, mullein, myrrh, white pine, pleurisy root, sanicle, saw palmetto berries, skunk cabbage, slippery elm, white pond lily, yerba santa, bloodroot, ginger, blue violet, bethroot, red root, red sage, elecampane, horehound, black cohosh.

BRUISES AND CUTS — Bugleweed (for internal bruises), comfrey, hyssop, lobelia, mugwort, giant Solomon's seal, St.John's-wort, bittersweet (combined with camomile as an ointment), pennyroyal, tansy, balm of Gilead, burnet.

BURNS — Aloes, bittersweet, burdock, calamus, chickweed, elder, poplar, onions (bruised), comfrey.
Immerse burned part in very cold water and keep the water cold by changing or adding ice or more cold water. Keep the burned part covered with water until all of the heat is drawn out, and no blisters will form.

CANCER — Blue violet (whole plant, with rock rose and red clover blossoms), chickweed, cleavers, coral, red clover (combined with blue violet, burdock root, yellow dock root, dandelion root, rock rose, and golden seal), rock rose, slippery elm, sorrel, virgin's bower, willow, wood sage, yellow dock, poplar, golden seal, poke root (poultice, also tea), comfrey, blue flag, myrrh, echinacea, aloes, gravel root, bloodroot, dandelion root, African cayenne, agrimony, and wild Oregon grape.

CANKER SORES IN MOUTH — Bayberry bark, bistort (combined with equal parts of red raspberry leaves), golden seal, gold thread, myrrh, pilewort, red raspberry, rock rose, self-heal, sumach berries, white pond lily, wild alum root, birch, burdock, pennyroyal, rosemary, prickly ash, hemlock, wood sanicle, red root.

CARBUNCLES — Carrot (poultice), lobelia (poultice), mugwort, echinacea, burdock, origanum. (See also Boils and Carbuncles.)

CHILLS — Cayenne pepper, bayberry bark tea with pinch of cayenne, myrica, peppermint, willow, peach, sage, catnip, antispasmodic tincture (lobelia).

CHOLERA — Bistort root, cayenne, colombo, elder, fire weed, fleabane, peppermint, prickly ash, wild alum root, wild yam, ginger, water pepper (smartweed), red clover, geranium.

CHOLERA INFANTUM — Birch, poplar, yarrow, wild cherry bark, red raspberry leaves and lady's slipper as an enema, bayberry bark (as an enema and also taken internally), wild alum root.

CHOLERA MORBUS — Peach leaves, bistort, queen of the meadow, raspberry leaves, peppermint, rhubarb, charcoal (take two heaping teaspoonfuls of powdered charcoal in a cup of water every two hours).

COLDS — Bayberry bark with yarrow, catnip, sage, peppermint, wood betony, angelica, blue violet, butternut bark, ginseng, lungwort, nettle, white pine, pleurisy root, prickly ash, rosemary, saffron, summer savory, sweet balm, tansy, valerian, vervain, water pepper, wood sage, yarrow, bloodroot, elder, ginger, gentian, golden seal, hyssop, masterwort, pennyroyal, sarsaparilla, saw palmetto berries, spikenard, wild cherry, horehound.

COLIC — Blue cohosh, caraway seed, carrot seed, catnip, dill, fennel, masterwort, origanum, pennyroyal, peppermint, prickly ash, rosemary, rue, sassafras, spearmint, summer savory, wintergreen, wood betony, flaxseed, valerian, fringe tree, angelica, motherwort.

CONSTIPATION — Balmony, buckthorn bark, cascara sagrada, chickweed, ginger, fennel seed, origanum, psyllium, white ash, elder, blue flag, wild Oregon grape, rhubarb root, butternut bark, licorice, calamus root, aloes.

CONVULSIONS AND SPASMS — Black cohosh, catnip, fit root, rue, skullcap, self-heal, skunk cabbage, valerian, gentian, pennyroyal, mistletoe, antispasmodic tincture, wild yam, lady's slipper, peppermint, fennel seed, sweet balm, sweet weed, hyssop.

CORNS AND CALLOUSES — Bittersweet and camomile combined into an ointment, herbal liniment.

COUGH — Blue violet, comfrey, coltsfoot, ginseng, horehound, hyssop, lungwort, myrrh, origanum, white pine, water pepper (smartweed), black cohosh, bloodroot, borage, flaxseed, marjoram, rosemary, spikenard, balm of Gilead, bethroot, red sage, tansy, wild cherry bark, mullein, golden seal, red clover blossoms, cubeb berries, skunk cabbage.

CRAMPS — Blue cohosh, cayenne (stomach cramps), coral, fennel, motherwort, rue, thyme, twin leaf, wood betony, masterwort, pennyroyal, peppermint, balm.

CROUP — Mullein, white pine, antispasmodic tincture (lobelia).

DANDRUFF — Burdock, nettle, sage.

DEAFNESS — Chickweed, origanum, marjoram, angelica, oil of wintergreen, rosemary, oil of sassafras, oil of hemlock, tincture of myrrh, tincture of lobelia, mullein.

DELIRIUM TREMENS — Motherwort, vervain, wood betony, mistletoe, hops, lobelia, skullcap, lady's slipper, hyssop, quassia chips, black cohosh, valerian, antispasmodic tincture (for quick relief).

DIABETES — Beech, blue cohosh, golden seal, white pine, poplar, queen of the meadow, saw palmetto berries, sumach berries, uva-ursi, wild alum root, wintergreen, yarrow, buchu (first stages of diabetes), dandelion root (especially good), bittersweet, red root, blueberries and blueberry leaves (especially good), raspberry leaves (very good), pleurisy root, white pine combined with equal parts of uva-ursi, marshmallow, and poplar bark.

DIARRHEA (See also BOWEL TROUBLE) — Bayberry bark, birch, bistort root, comfrey, colombo, elder, marshmallow, mullein, nettle, peppermint, pilewort, poplar, red raspberry, rhubarb, St.John's-wort, slippery elm, strawberry, thyme, white pond lily, witch hazel, wild alum root, yarrow, wormwood, ginger, rock rose, hemlock, bethroot, cinnamon, shepherd's purse, plantain, blackberry root, cranesbill, one heaping teaspoonful of powdered charcoal every two hours.

DIPHTHERIA — Golden seal, myrrh, echinacea, lemon juice, red sage, jaborandi, eucalyptus; capsicum (red pepper, make a gargle of it, very effective); lobelia.

DIZZINESS — Peppermint, catnip, rue, wood betony.

DROPSY — Wood betony, hemlock, buchu, blue flag, celandine, juniper berries, holy thistle, lobelia, iris (excellent), bitterroot, black cohosh, blue cohosh, broom, buckthorn, carrot, celery, cleavers, dandelion, elder, hydrangea, milkweed, mullein, nettle, origanum, parsley, queen of the meadow, skunk cabbage, spearmint, tansy, twin leaf, wahoo, white ash, white pond lily, wintergreen, camomile, hyssop, marjoram, masterwort, pennyroyal, plantain, lily of the valley, dwarf elder (excellent).

DYSENTERY — Balm, mullein, bethroot, bayberry bark, birch, bistort, comfrey, colombo, fireweed, fleabane, magnolia, marshmallow, masterwort, nettle, peppermint, pilewort, plantain, pleurisy root, red raspberry, rhubarb, skunk cabbage, slippery elm, squaw vine, St.John's-wort, strawberry, uva ursi, witch hazel, shepherd's purse, ginger (preferably African ginger), hemlock, geranium, white oak bark. (See also DIARRHEA.)

DYSPEPSIA (HEARTBURN) — Beech, buckbean, calamus, cayenne, colombo, gentian root, golden seal, gold thread, horehound, magnolia, origanum, peach leaves, quassia, sage, spearmint, tansy, thyme, wahoo, wild cherry, yarrow, balmony, bloodroot, camomile, Peruvian bark, ginger, charcoal, boneset, motherwort, bitterroot, St.John's-wort.

EARACHE — Hops, origanum, pimpernel, lemon juice (pure), burnet.

EARS, RUNNING — Yellow dock, lemon juice (diluted

one-half with water), oil of origanum, peroxide of hydrogen (put in ear warm), myrrh, echinacea.

ECZEMA — Balmony, beech, cleavers, dandelion, golden seal, nettle, strawberry, strawberry leaves, willow, bloodroot, wild Oregon grape, poke root, white poplar bark, plantain, yellow dock, blue violet, origanum.

EPILEPSY — Black cohosh, elder, mistletoe, Peruvian bark, vervain, valerian, skullcap, lady's slipper, antispasmodic tincture.

ERYSIPELAS — Chickweed, coral, elder, golden seal, lobelia, magnolia, plantain, Solomon's seal, giant Solomon's seal, water pepper (smartweed), wood sanicle, echinacea, slippery elm powder (sprinkled on), cayenne pepper, myrrh, burdock.

FAINTING — Lavender (prevents), cayenne, peppermint, antispasmodic tincture, motherwort.

FELONS — Bittersweet (poultice made of the berries), lobelia, origanum, wintergreen.

FERMENTATION — See HEARTBURN.

FEVER — Catnip, sage, shepherd's purse, sumach berries, sweet balm, tansy, thyme, valerian, vervain, wahoo, wild cherry bark, willow, wintergreen, wood sage, wormwood, yarrow, borage, dandelion, Peruvian bark, apple tree bark (intermittent fever), bitterroot (intermittent fever), buckbean (intermittent fever), camomile, cinchona bark, cleavers, colombo, butternut bark (all fevers), calamus (intermittent fevers), coral, elder, fenugreek, fireweed, fit root, gentian root, hyssop, masterwort, lobelia (excellent), magnolia, mandrake, nettle, parsley, pennyroyal, peppermint, pleurisy root, poplar, quassia, mugwort, cayenne, fringe tree, echinacea, angelica, yarrow (breaks up fever in 24 hours), sarsaparilla, red sage, boneset, lily of the valley, cedron (intermittent fever), black cohosh, willow (bark or leaves).

FLOODING (EXCESSIVE MENSTRUAL FLOW) — Bayberry bark tea, ginger and cinnamon tea, yarrow, shepherd's purse, wood betony, burnet, cayenne pepper, red sage, celandine, bistort.

GALLSTONES — Bitterroot, cascara sagrada, milkweed, camomile, parsley, fringe tree, cleavers, marshmallow, cherry bark, rhubarb, wood betony, goose grass, sweet weed.

GANGRENE — Camomile, comfrey, myrrh, willow, poplar, hemlock, echinacea. Golden seal, smartweed, and pleurisy root are good when combined and used as hot fomentations.

GAS (See also HEARTBURN) — Anise, calamus, caraway seed, catnip, dill, fennel, mint, origanum, peppermint, sage, sarsaparilla, sassafras, spearmint, thyme, wild yam, wintergreen, yarrow, ginger, nutmeg, valerian, angelica, wood betony.

GLEET (URETHRITIS) — Cubeb berries, juniper berries, wild alum root, yarrow, bloodroot, elder, plantain, yellow dock, saw palmetto, wild Oregon grape, red clover, echinacea, prickly ash, golden seal, rock rose.

GOITER — Bayberry bark, white oak bark (internally and externally), echinacea, Irish moss, poke root, seawrack.

GONORRHEA — Bittersweet, black willow, burdock, cleavers, cubeb berries, golden seal, hops, parsley, rock rose, sanicle, squaw vine, sumach berries, uva ursi, witch hazel, wintergreen, poplar, bistort root (combined with plantain), red root, juniper berries.

GOUT — Blue violet, birch, burdock, gentian root, mugwort, rue, sarsaparilla, broom, buckthorn bark, ginger, pennyroyal, plantain, wood betony, balm of Gilead.

GRAVEL (IN BLADDER) — Broom, carrot, hyssop, marshmallow, apple tree bark, hydrangea, nettle, queen of the meadow, ragwort, sorrel, spearmint, valerian, water pepper, hops, masterwort, mugwort, parsley, squaw vine, hemlock, buchu.

GRIPING, IN BOWELS — Anise, caraway seed, catnip, coriander, ginger, pennyroyal, thyme, nutmeg, balm, bay leaves.

GUMS, SORE — Bugleweed, myrrh, golden seal, bistort root, herbal liniment.

HALITOSIS — Rosemary, myrrh, golden seal, echinacea, herbal laxative.

HAY FEVER — Mullein, poplar, skunk cabbage, coltsfoot, black cohosh.

HEADACHE — Blue violet, catnip, coltsfoot, peppermint, rhubarb, rosemary, rue, sweet balm, thyme, vervain, virgin's bower, wood betony, elder, marjoram, calamint, pennyroyal, fringe tree, red root, holy thistle, mountain balm, yerba santa, camomile, tansy.

HEAD TROUBLE (HYDROCEPHALUS) — Sage, rue, rosemary, calamus, broom, catnip, red sage, rosemary, marjoram, wood betony, pennyroyal, skullcap, calamint. Can combine any of these.

HEARTBURN — Balmony, bay leaves, beech, bitterroot, buckbean, cayenne, gentian root, ginseng, golden seal, gold thread, poplar, Peruvian bark, coltsfoot, lobelia, wild cherry bark, bayberry bark, skullcap, nutmeg, balm, bloodroot, marjoram, rosemary, wood betony, wormwood, red root, willow, angelica, burnet (excellent), origanum (excellent to strengthen the stomach and for gas).

HEMORRHAGE — Bayberry bark, comfrey, fleabane (bowels and uterus), golden seal (hemorrhage from the rectum), nettle, pilewort, shepherd's purse, sorrel, St.John's-wort, white oak bark, wild alum root, witch hazel, yarrow. Lemon juice, diluted and taken as cold as possible.

Capsicum (red pepper), taken internally; take one No.00 capsule and immediately drink a glass or two of water as hot as can be drunk freely.

HEMORRHOIDS — See PILES.

HICCOUGHS — Blue cohosh, dill, orange juice, black cohosh, wild carrot seeds, cayenne (in a poultice over the lower chest).

HIGH BLOOD PRESSURE (HYPERTENSION) — Broom, black cohosh, blue cohosh, hyssop, wild cherry bark, valerian, vervain, sanicle, boneset, skullcap, golden seal, myrrh, herbal laxative.

HOARSENESS — Marshmallow, golden seal, lobelia, wild cherry, hyssop, horehound, mullein, coltsfoot, skunk cabbage.

HYDROPHOBIA (RABIES) — Lobelia, skullcap, balm, gentian, white ash, antispasmodic tincture.

HYSTERIA — Skunk cabbage, saffron, skullcap, valerian, mistletoe, peppermint, vervain, catnip, black cohosh, blue cohosh, antispasmodic tincture (quick relief), motherwort, pennyroyal, tansy, rue.

INDIGESTION — See HEARTBURN.

INFLAMMATION — Fenugreek, golden seal, hops, lobelia, marshmallow, mugwort, sarsaparilla, slippery elm, Solomon's seal, sorrel, tansy, white pond lily, witch hazel, water pepper (smartweed) and charcoal poultice, flaxseed oil, hyssop, chickweed, gum arabic, cayenne pepper.

INFLUENZA (See also LA GRIPPE) — Peppermint, white pine, poplar, skullcap, pleurisy root.

INSANITY — Catnip, peppermint, rosemary, rue, vervain, wood betony, holy thistle, skullcap.

INSECT BITES AND STINGS — Black cohosh, lobelia, parsley, plantain, skullcap, balm, bistort root, borage, fennel, gentian, hyssop, marjoram, pennyroyal, wood betony, echinacea, sweet basil, cedron, Kloss liniment.

ITCHING — Buckthorn bark (ointment), origanum, virgin's bower, yellow dock (excellent), borage, marjoram, pennyroyal, plantain, poke root (fine), chickweed.

JAUNDICE — Bayberry bark, balmony, bittersweet, buckbean, cleavers, dandelion, gentian root, horehound, mandrake, peach leaves, poplar, sorrel, St.John's-wort, tansy, wormwood, origanum, bistort root, bloodroot, borage, broom, sorrel, camomile, hyssop, lungwort, marjoram, parsley, pennyroyal, plantain, wood betony, henna leaves, fringe tree, celandine, chicory, fennel.

KIDNEY DISEASE (See Bright's disease)

LA GRIPPE (See also INFLUENZA) — Butternut bark, lungwort, nettle, peppermint, pleurisy root, poplar, saffron, sweet balm, tansy, ginger, golden seal, saw palmetto berries, wild cherry, wood betony, sage, angelica, hyssop.

LEPROSY — Bittersweet, burdock, red clover, yellow dock, pennyroyal, henna.

LEUKORRHEA (WHITES) — Bayberry bark (douche), bistort root, comfrey, cubeb berries, golden seal and myrrh (douche and also take internally), magnolia, pilewort, plantain, ragwort, slippery elm, squaw vine, sumach berries, white oak bark (douche), white pond lily, wild alum root, wintergreen, wormwood, yarrow (increases menstrual flow), blue cohosh, tansy, ragwort (combined with white pond lily), hemlock, buchu, bethroot, cranesbill (douche), wild Oregon grape, juniper berries.

LOCKJAW (TETANUS) — Red pepper, lobelia, antispasmodic tincture, skullcap, fit root, cayenne pepper.

LOSS OF SPEECH — Rosemary, prickly ash, red pepper, golden seal, myrrh, wild cherry, sumach.

LUMBAGO (LAME BACK) — Queen of the meadow, shepherd's purse (excellent), uva ursi, vervain, black cohosh, herbal liniment.

LUNG FEVER — Pleurisy root, bloodroot, coltsfoot, redsage.

MEASLES — Cleavers, pleurisy root, saffron, valerian, yarrow, bistort root, red sage, raspberry leaves.

MENSTRUATION (TO DECREASE FLOW) — Bayberry bark, pilewort, shepherd's purse, sorrel, uva ursi, wild alum root, bistort root, plantain, red raspberry, witch hazel, sanicle, bethroot, burnet, wood betony, red sage, lungwort, celandine, cayenne pepper, yarrow.

MENSTRUATION (TO INCREASE FLOW) — Squaw vine, aloes, angelica, fennel, balm, bittersweet, black cohosh, camomile, catnip, coral, gentian root, ginger, horehound, marjoram, masterwort, mugwort, nettle, origanum, pennyroyal, pleurisy root, ragwort, rue, saffron, St.John's-wort, summer savory, sweet balm, tansy, thyme, valerian, vervain, water pepper (smartweed), yarrow, carrot, coral with blue cohosh, squaw mint, red sage, motherwort.

NAUSEA AND VOMITING — Ginger, lavender, mint, origanum, peach leaves, pennyroyal (but should NOT be taken during pregnancy), peppermint, red raspberry, spearmint, sweet balm, wild yam, anise, giant Solomon's seal, golden seal (will allay nausea during pregnancy).

NERVOUSNESS — Camomile, celery, cinchona bark, dill, fit root, skullcap with golden seal and hops, lobelia, motherwort, origanum, peach leaves, pennyroyal, queen of the meadow, red clover, rosemary, rue, sage, skullcap, skunk cabbage, spearmint, squaw vine, St.John's-wort, thyme, twin leaf, valerian, vervain, wild cherry, wood betony, blue violet, sanicle, buchu, mistletoe, red sage, catnip, peppermint, marshmallow root, mugwort, nettle, poplar bark, Solomon's seal, lady's slipper, antispasmodic tincture (lobelia) for quick results.

NEURALGIA — Bitterroot, blue cohosh, celery, hops, nettle, origanum, peppermint, poplar, queen of the meadow, skullcap, Solomon's seal, giant Solomon's seal, twin leaf, wild yam, wood betony, Peruvian bark.

NIGHTMARES — Bugleweed, thyme, lily of the valley, catnip, peppermint.

NIGHT SWEATS — Coral, sage, strawberry leaves.

NOSEBLEED — Witch hazel, wild alum root, buckthorn, bayberry bark.

OBESITY — Seawrack, white ash, fennel, Irish moss, chickweed, burdock, sassafras.

PAIN — Catnip, fit root, mint, mullein, nettle, skullcap, skunk cabbage, Solomon's seal, giant Solomon's seal, twin leaf, wood betony, camomile, dill.

PALSY — Masterwort, skullcap, elder, wood betony, wood sage.

PARALYSIS — Hydrangea, black cohosh, valerian, vervain, skullcap, ginger, prickly ash (excellent), lady's slipper, cayenne, rosemary.

PHLEGM — Hyssop, nettle, white pine, vervain, wild cherry, borage, pennyroyal, coltsfoot.

PILES (HEMORRHOIDS) — Bittersweet, chickweed, fireweed, golden seal, mullein, myrrh, nettle, plantain, shepherd's purse, Solomon's seal, spearmint, uva ursi, white oak bark, witch hazel, wild alum root, yarrow, bloodroot, pilewort, pimpernel, aloes, burdock, psyllium.

PIMPLES — Spikenard, valerian, gentian, plantain, bistort root.

PLEURISY — Coral, lobelia, pleurisy root, skunk cabbage, flaxseed, cayenne, chickweed, elder, yarrow, boneset.

PNEUMONIA — Marshmallow, vervain, bloodroot, Peruvian bark, sage, red sage, black cohosh, willow, coltsfoot, skunk cabbage, comfrey, elecampane, wild cherry, spikenard, plantain, lungwort, pleurisy root, slippery elm, wild alum root, mustard, flaxseed, hops, hyssop, white pine bark, mullein, yerba santa, yarrow, myrrh, horehound.

POISON IVY — Lobelia, golden seal, myrrh, echinacea,

bloodroot, Solomon's seal. Equal parts of a strong tea made of white oak bark and lime water is very good for poison ivy or poison oak.

Apply a bandage wet with this solution and change as often as it becomes dry.

QUINSY — Hyssop, sage, sanicle, ragwort, sumach berries, agrimony, red sage, raspberry leaves, slippery elm bark, hyssop, cudweed. These are all to be taken internally and also used as a gargle.

RHEUMATISM AND ARTHRITIS (See also LUMBAGO) — Buchu, balm of Gilead, blue flag, wild Oregon grape, cayenne, birch, bitterroot, bittersweet, black cohosh, blue cohosh, buckbean, buckthorn bark, burdock, celery, elder, hydrangea, lobelia, mugwort, nettle, colombo, origanum, peppermint, white pine, pleurisy root, poplar, prickly ash, quassia, queen of the meadow, sarsaparilla, skullcap, skunk cabbage, twin leaf, wild yam, willow, wintergreen, wormwood, yellow dock.

RINGWORM — Golden seal, lobelia, blood root, borage, plantain, sarsaparilla.

RUPTURES — Comfrey, giant Solomon's seal, bistort root.

SCALD HEAD — Sanicle. Make a tea of two ounces of raspberry leaves in one quart of water.

Steep for thirty minutes and add one-half ounce of lobelia powder. Take both morning and evening. Use witch hazel extract to allay itching. Also take a good blood purifier.

SCALDING (BURNING) URINE — White poplar bark, burdock seed, spearmint, cubeb, queen of the meadow, peach leaves or cleavers for cystitis or any inflammatory condition of the urinary organs. If there is bleeding, use shepherd's purse.

SCALDS AND BURNS — Bittersweet, chickweed, elder, onions (bruised).

Submerge the burned part in very cold water, keeping the water cold, and hold the injured part there until it stops burning. If this is done, a blister will not form.

SCARLATINA — Rock rose, twin leaf, bloodroot.

SCARLET FEVER — Cayenne, cleavers, golden seal, pleurisy root, saffron, twinleaf, valerian, red sage.

SCIATICA — Rue, wintergreen, broom, burdock, tansy.

SCROFULA — Bayberry bark, buckbean, burdock, calamus, comfrey, cleavers, coltsfoot, coral, dandelion, elder, gentian root, hyssop, milkweed, nettle, plantain, prickly ash, rhubarb, rock rose, sarsaparilla, seawrack, sorrel, sumach berries, turkey corn, vervain, white pond lily, wintergreen, yellow dock, blue violet, wild Oregon grape, poke root, juniper berries, figwort, echinacea.

ADDENDUM: Scrofula refers to enlarged lymph nodes in the neck due to tuberculosis and is most frequently seen in children. It is now hardly ever seen in the United States.

SCURVY — Buckbean, chickweed, cleavers, coral, dandelion, hydrangea, nettle, origanum, white pine, sanicle, sorrel, marjoram, wood sanicle, lemon juice.

SINUS TROUBLE — Plantain, saw palmetto berries, golden seal, bayberry bark.

SMALLPOX — Yarrow, bistort root, red sage, raspberry leaves; golden seal mixed with vaseline and applied to the lesions will prevent pitting. Lemon juice allays itching. Apply full strength.

SNAKE BITES — Black cohosh, borage, skullcap, bistort root, fennel, gentian root, hyssop, marjoram, pennyroyal, wood betony, echinacea, plantain, sweet basil, cedron.

SORES — Peach, pimpernel, poplar, blue violet, hemlock, echinacea, poke root, aloes, cayenne, bayberry bark, bittersweet, calamus, carrot (poultice), camomile, chickweed, comfrey, elder, flaxseed, golden seal, mullein, myrrh, plantain, sage, sanicle, prickly ash (apply powder), self-heal, skunk cabbage, Solomon's seal, St.John's-wort, sumach berries, valerian, vervain, virgin's bower, white clover, witch hazel, wood sage, yellow dock, bistort root, borage, masterwort, bloodroot.

SORE THROAT — Bayberry bark, bistort root, bloodroot, blue violet, cayenne, fenugreek, ginger, horehound, hops, hyssop, mullein, origanum, white pine, rock rose, sage, sassafras, saw palmetto berries, twin leaf, vervain, white pond lily, wild alum root, wintergreen, wood sage, borage, wood sanicle, echinacea, red root, golden seal, red sage.

SPASMS — Blue cohosh, catnip, cayenne, fit root, masterwort, red clover, rue, sassafras, skunk cabbage, spearmint, twin leaf, wild yam, red root, antispasmodic tincture, fennel, cedron.

SPERMATORRHEA — Sage, buchu, juniper berries, cubeb berries, uva ursi, black willow.

SPINAL MENINGITIS — Black cohosh, golden seal, lobelia.

SPRAINS AND MUSCLE STRAINS — Comfrey, lobelia, origanum, wormwood, bittersweet combined with camomile as an ointment.

STINGS — See INSECT BITES.

ST. VITUS' DANCE — Black cohosh, skullcap, mistletoe (excellent).

SUMMER COMPLAINT (DIARRHEA) — Fireweed, fleabane, shepherd's purse, bayberry bark, white oak bark, colombo.

SWELLINGS — Burdock, comfrey, elder, fenugreek, hops, mugwort, origanum, parsley, tansy, white oak bark, white lily, wintergreen, wood sage, wormwood, yellow dock, camomile, dill.

SYPHILIS — Bitterroot, bittersweet, bloodroot, bugleweed (for syphilitic sores), burdock, elder, golden seal, plantain, prickly ash, rock rose, sumach (berries or leaves), turkey corn, twin leaf, yellow dock, poplar, bayberry bark, barberry, blue violet, sanicle, echinacea, blue flag, red root, poke root, white pine bark, palmetto, wild Oregon grape, red clover, yellow parilla (American sarsaparilla), milkweed, parsley.

TETTERS — Golden seal mixed with borax and vaseline should be used in the first stages.
Borage, plantain, sarsaparilla, sanicle, raspberry leaves, gentian. Kloss's herbal liniment applied externally.

TONSILLITIS — Mullein, white pine, echinacea, red root, sage, golden seal, tansy. (Use the teas strong, gargle every few minutes, and swallow a mouthful).

TOOTHACHE — Hops, origanum (essence), sassafras (oil of), cloves (oil of), summer savory, balm, broom, marjoram, mullein, pennyroyal, plantain, pimpernel, tansy, Kloss's herbal liniment.

TUBERCULOSIS — Comfrey, myrrh, skunk cabbage, wild cherry bark, sanicle, golden seal, bayberry bark, burdock root, coltsfoot, yellow dock, elecampane root, plantain, slippery elm, vervain, celàndine, rosemary, wood betony bethroot, red root, horehound.

TUMORS — Blue violet, chickweed, coltsfoot (for scrofulous tumors of tuberculosis), coral, elder, hops, mugwort, mullein, rock rose, sanicle, skunk cabbage, sorrel, St.John's-wort, tansy, white oak bark, witch hazel, wood sage, yellow dock, flaxseed, sanicle, celandine. Red root taken internally will help destroy tumors.

TYPHOID FEVER — Bitterroot, camomile, golden seal, yarrow, bloodroot, red sage, myrrh.

TYPHUS — Coral, pleurisy root, black root, boneset, borage, camomile.

ULCERS (SKIN) — Bistort root, borage, lungwort, pennyroyal, poplar, blue violet, hemlock, wood sanicle, chickweed, celandine, angelica, cayenne, beech, bugleweed, calamus, carrot (poultice), chickweed, comfrey, fenugreek, golden seal, gold thread, hops, mullein, myrrh, pilewort, prickly ash, psyllium, rock rose, sage, sanicle, sorrel, St.John's-wort, twin leaf, valerian, virgin's bower, water pepper, white clover, white pond lily, wild alum root, wintergreen, wood sage, yarrow; use chickweed tea externally as a wash to heal ulcers and sores; take internally also.

URINARY PROBLEMS — Mugwort, squaw vine, white willow, hemlock, buchu, chicory, juniper berries, angelica, mandrake, blue cohosh, broom, carrot, celery, comfrey, cleavers, corn silk, cubeb berries, dandelion, elder, gentian root, ginseng, fleabane, marshmallow, milkweed, mint, nettle, origanum, parsley, peach leaves, poplar bark, queen of the meadow, ragwort, sarsaparilla, spearmint, St.John's-wort, sweet balm, white ash, wild yam, yarrow, burdock, hops, marjoram, masterwort, tansy, fennel, uva ursi.

UTERUS (PROLAPSED) — Witch hazel, black cohosh, white oak bark (used in douche), bayberry bark (douche), slippery elm (douche). Tampons saturated in a strong tea made of bayberry bark or white oak bark, combined with slippery elm, make a very fine medicinal support for prolapsed uterus. Witch hazel bark may also be used.

VARICOSE VEINS — White oak bark, witch hazel, bayberry bark, wild alum root, burnet.

VOMITING, PREVENTION — Sweet basil, colombo, peach leaves, white poplar bark, clover, spearmint. Use equal parts of white poplar bark and clover to stop vomiting during pregnancy.
Give peppermint and peach leaves in small doses.

WARTS — Buckthorn bark, mullein, celandine.

WHOOPING COUGH — Black cohosh, blue violet, coltsfoot, lobelia, peach leaves, red clover, saw palmetto berries, skunk cabbage, thyme, vervain, red root, red clover, blue cohosh, bloodroot, slippery elm, elecampane. Drink the tea generously–it is excellent. Antispasmodic tincture; take according to directions.

WORMS — Birch, bitterroot, buckbean, buckthorn bark, butternut bark, carrot, camomile, horehound, hops, nettle, quassia, rue, sage, self-heal, senna, sorrel, tansy, vervain (take three days), white oak bark, wormwood, bistort root, catnip, hyssop, motherwort, peach, poplar, wood betony, aloes.

WOUNDS — Burdock, carrot (poultice), camomile, chickweed, comfrey, fenugreek, plantain, prickly ash, sage, self-heal, Solomon's seal, St.John's-wort, white pond lily, wild alum root, yarrow, bistort root, pilewort, pimpernel, poplar, wood sanicle, echinacea, balm of Gilead, aloes, beech. Wood sage, self-heal, chickweed, golden seal, myrrh and slippery elm can be effectively used as poultices and washes.

DISEASES AFFECTING SPECIFIC
BODY ORGANS

ADENOIDS — Bayberry bark, bloodroot, golden seal, myrrh, echinacea, red root.

BLADDER (URINARY) — Celandine, aloes, juniper berries, comfrey, apple tree bark, balm, beech, broom, carrot, camomile, cleavers, corn silk, cubeb berries, fleabane, golden seal, hydrangea, hyssop, nettle, peach leaves, birch, buchu and uva ursi combined, pimpernel, queen of the meadow, sassafras, slippery elm, spearmint, sweet balm, uva ursi, valerian, vervain, water pepper, white pond lily, wild alum root (pus in bladder), wintergreen, wood sage, yarrow, hemlock, bethroot.

CHEST TROUBLE — See LUNGS.

COLON TROUBLE — Colombo, fireweed, fleabane, peppermint, vervain, aloes, slippery elm bark, bayberry bark, white oak bark, golden seal, myrrh.

EYES (INFLAMMATION) — Rosemary, borage (inflamed or sore eyes), camomile (cataract), chickweed, elder, fennel, golden seal, hyssop, marshmallow, rock rose, sarsaparilla, sassafras, slippery elm, squaw vine, witch hazel, wintergreen, yellow dock, plantain, golden seal and burnt alum, tansy, white willow, angelica.

FEMALE TROUBLE — Black cohosh, milkweed, motherwort, mugwort, parsley, prickly ash, queen of the meadow, ragwort, rosemary, slippery elm, Solomon's seal, giant Solomon's seal, squaw vine, sweet balm, vervain, yarrow, comfrey, Peruvian bark, dandelion root, gentian root, bethroot, red sage.

GALLBLADDER — Golden seal combined with equal

parts of red clover, yellow dock, dandelion, and parsley. Milkweed is excellent for gallbladder and bile troubles.

GENITALS (BURNING, ITCHING) — In cases of itching, raspberry leaves, marshmallow, slippery elm, or pleurisy root should be taken internally. Peach leaves should be used for swelling.

Chickweed may be used internally and also externally as a wash for burning or itching.

GLANDULAR SWELLING — Bittersweet, mullein, parsley, seawrack, yellow dock, myrica, poke root, echinacea, slippery elm (both internally and as a poultice), queen of the meadow.

HAIR — Nettle, rosemary (prevents hair from falling out), sage, peach, burdock.

HEART — Angelica, blue cohosh (for palpitation), borage (strengthens heart), cayenne (stimulant), coriander, golden seal, peppermint, sorrel, valerian, vervain, wintergreen, wood betony, bloodroot, motherwort, sorrel, mistletoe, holy thistle, tansy. Combination: golden seal, skullcap, cayenne, lily of the valley.

INTESTINES — Fenugreek, golden seal, mint, nettle, pennyroyal, psyllium, slippery elm, giant Solomon's seal, strawberry, wild alum root, cascara sagrada.

KIDNEYS — Cayenne, chicory, water pepper, white oak bark, white pond lily, wood sage, birch, black cohosh, bloodroot, buckbean, masterwort, parsley, hemlock, cayenne, wood sanicle, bethroot, wild Oregon grape, fringe tree, poke root, juniper berries, balm, beech, bitterroot, bittersweet, broom, carrot, camomile, comfrey, cleavers, corn silk, dandelion, elder, golden seal, hydrangea, hyssop, marshmallow, celandine, holy thistle, milkweed, mustard (plaster), nettle, white pine, pleurisy root, poplar, queen of the meadow, sage, sanicle, sassafras, seawrack, sorrel, spearmint, sweet balm, tansy, uva ursi, buchu, aloes.

LIVER — Bitterroot, black cohosh, bloodroot, buckbean, fennel, parsley, plantain, wood betony, fringe tree, celandine, aloes, chicory, holy thistle, angelica, beech, bittersweet, butternut bark, carrot, cascara sagrada, celery, cleavers, dandelion, elder, golden seal, lobelia, magnolia, mandrake, milkweed, motherwort, poplar, prickly ash, rhubarb, sage, self-heal, wahoo, white oak bark, wild yam, wormwood, balm, blue flag, wild Oregon grape, red root, poke root, gentian root, red sage, hops, uva ursi.

LUNGS — Bayberry bark, chickweed, comfrey, coltsfoot, ginseng, lobelia, lungwort, marshmallow, mullein, mustard, myrrh, nettle, pimpernel, white pine, sanicle, shepherd's purse, skunk cabbage, slippery elm, thyme, wahoo, witch hazel, yarrow, yerba santa, pennyroyal, wood sanicle, bethroot, holy thistle, angelica, red sage, black cohosh, hops, sassafras, giant Solomon's seal, vervain, wild cherry, spikenard, elecampane, horehound, hyssop.

MUCOUS MEMBRANES (DISEASES AFFECTING) — Bitterroot, coltsfoot, golden seal, gum arabic, hyssop, myrica, red raspberry, white pond lily, wild alum root, yarrow, fireweed.

NASAL TROUBLE — Black willow (combined with palmetto berries or skullcap), witch hazel (bleeding nose), wild alum root (bleeding nose), white willow, bloodroot, fringe tree, buchu.

OVARIES — Saw palmetto berries, pennyroyal, black cohosh, blue cohosh, bayberry bark, pleurisy root (for inflammation of ovaries), burdock, peach leaves.

PANCREAS — Bittersweet, dandelion, golden seal, uva ursi, wahoo, cayenne, blueberry leaves, huckleberry leaves.

PROSTATE GLAND — Corn silk, golden seal, saw palmetto berries, white pond lily, buchu, garlic.

SKIN DISEASES — Beech, bittersweet, blue violet, buckthorn bark, burdock, chickweed, cleavers, coral, dandelion, elder, golden seal, magnolia, rock rose, saffron, sarsaparilla, sassafras, sorrel, turkey corn, vervain, white clover, wintergreen, bloodroot, pennyroyal, plantain, blue flag, wild Oregon grape, poke root, prince's pine, hyssop, red root, red clover, spikenard.

SPLEEN — Bittersweet, dandelion, golden seal, uva ursi, wahoo, white oak bark, balm, broom, fennel, gentian root, hyssop, marjoram, parsley, wood betony, cayenne, red root, aloes, chicory, angelica.

STOMACH (INDIGESTION AND GAS) — Angelica, strawberry, thyme, valerian, vervain, witch hazel, wild cherry, willow, wintergreen, wood betony, camomile, marjoram, echinacea, bethroot, chickweed, aloes, chicory, bayberry bark, balmony, blue violet, buckbean, calamus, caraway seed, catnip, cayenne, cinchona bark, comfrey, colombo, cubeb, fennel, ginseng, golden seal, golden thread, sage, sassafras, slippery elm, giant Solomon's seal, spearmint, St.John's-wort, gum arabic, hyssop, milkweed, mint, mugwort, nettle, origanum (especially for sour stomach), peach leaves, pimpernel, plantain, rue, anise, bay leaves, cedron.

TESTICLES (INFLAMMATION AND SWELLING) — Chickweed, mullein, saw palmetto berries to be taken when testicles are swollen and painful. The following herbs are to be used in a mixture as a poultice or taken internally in the usual manner: burdock, 2 ounces; clivers (cleavers), 1 ounce; sanicle, 1 ounce; bittersweet root, 1 ounce.

THYROID — Bayberry bark, white oak bark, skullcap, black cohosh.

WOMB (UTERUS) TROUBLES — Slippery elm, bayberry bark (douche), black cohosh, blue cohosh, fit root and fennel, gum arabic (in inflammation of uterus), mandrake, peach leaves, rue, squaw vine, St.John's-wort, witch hazel, fenugreek, bethroot, wild Oregon grape, shepherd's purse (to stop excessive flow), yarrow (increases menstruation), smartweed, uva ursi. For douches, use wild alum root or white oak bark.

GENERAL MEDICAL USES OF HERBS

ANTIEMETIC (PREVENTS OR STOPS VOMITING) Sweet basil, colombo, red raspberry leaves, lobelia in small doses, peppermint and peach leaves in small doses, white poplar bark, clover, mint, spearmint, giant Solomon's seal. Use equal parts of white poplar bark and clover to stop vomiting in pregnancy.

APPETITE, HERBS TO IMPROVE — Agrimony, beech, calamus, camomile, colombo, gentian root, ginseng, golden seal, origanum, strawberry, wood sage, wormwood, balmony, marjoram.

ASTRINGENTS — Bistort root (strongest astringent known), fireweed, white oak bark, wild alum root, bayberry bark.

BEVERAGES — Red clover blossoms, sage, mint, sassafras, strawberry leaves, peppermint, spearmint, fennel, red raspberry leaves, hyssop, chickweed, catnip, wintergreen, sarsaparilla, wild cherry bark or small twigs, birch bark or small twigs, chicory, dandelion, yellow dock, camomile, hops, calamus root (sweet flag), meadow sweet, juniper berries, alfalfa, green celery leaves, horsemint, rue.

BILE, TO INCREASE — Bitterroot, hops, cascara sagrada, fringe tree, celandine (will cause bile to leave the gallbladder).

BLOOD PURIFIERS — Bittersweet, blue cohosh, burdock, chickweed, dandelion, elder, fireweed, gentian root, hyssop, nettle, prickly ash, red clover, sanicle, sassafras, sorrel, spikenard, St.John's-wort, turkey corn, white clover, yellow dock, borage, cleavers, echinacea, blue flag, wild Oregon grape, fringe tree, holy thistle, elecampane, sarsaparilla.

BREASTS, TO DRY UP MILK — Sage, wild alum root (the strong tea rubbed over breasts), camphor applied to breasts.

CHILDBIRTH, TO HELP EASE — Black cohosh, blue cohosh (brings on labor pains when time), shepherd's purse, spikenard, or squaw vine (taken some time before, they shorten the length of labor), red raspberry leaves–a teacupful (including the juice from one orange), three cups daily through the last month will make childbirth easier. Combine with squaw vine. Angelica to expel the afterbirth.

CIRCULATION, TO INCREASE — Cayenne, gentian, golden seal, hyssop, witch hazel, holy thistle.
Combination: golden seal, skullcap, cayenne, bayberry bark.

DOUCHE (VAGINAL) — Fit root and fennel, gum arabic, marshmallow, slippery elm, uva ursi, white oak bark, white pond lily, wild alum root, fenugreek, bayberry bark.

EMETIC (PRODUCES VOMITING) — Bayberry bark, buckbean, large doses of lobelia, mustard, myrica, white willow, ragwort, boneset, bitterroot.

ENEMA — Catnip, chickweed, bayberry bark, white oak bark, shepherd's purse, wild alum root, echinacea, strawberry leaves, raspberry leaves.

GARGLE — Bayberry bark, bistort root, hyssop, myrrh, pilewort, rock rose, sage, golden seal, Kloss's liniment diluted.

LAXATIVE — Golden seal, horehound, hyssop, mandrake, mullein, peach leaves, psyllium, rhubarb, sage, senna, wahoo, elder, blue flag, wild Oregon grape, fringe, aloes, Kloss's herbal laxative.

LIQUOR HABIT (ALCOHOLISM) — Lady's slipper (American valerian) and lobelia—equal parts; one ounce of skullcap and one-half ounce of valerian (lady's slipper) given every half hour in hot water until results are obtained, then continue taking until taste for liquor is gone. Quassia chips, magnolia bark, ivy (five-leaf).

PERSPIRATION, TO INDUCE — Bayberry bark, elderberry leaves, coral, sage, holy thistle, horehound, hyssop, marjoram, pennyroyal, saffron, thyme, vervain.

POULTICES — Balm, flaxseed, gum arabic, hyssop, marshmallow, mustard, slippery elm, virgin's bower, wintergreen, chickweed, poke root, cayenne pepper, flaxseed meal, smartweed and charcoal, red sage, burdock, lobelia, comfrey.

PREVENTION OF DISEASE — Juniper berries (prevents contagious diseases), holy thistle, angelica, gentian root (wonderful), garlic, dandelion and dandelion greens, blueberries and leaves, lemon juice. Take the juice of four lemons daily, diluted one-half with water.

QUININE SUBSTITUTES — Fit root, golden seal, magnolia, white poplar bark, yarrow, willow (excellent), dogwood blossoms, Peruvian bark, skullcap, gentian root, peach, sage, vervain, wahoo, wood betony, willow bark and red pepper (act quickly: they are tonic and stimulating without any unhealthy reaction), boneset, capsicum (red pepper), turnips (grated skin and all), and given in tablespoonful doses whenever a dose of quinine is indicated.

ADDENDUM: It is best to use quinine in cases of malaria.

RELAXANTS — Lobelia, boneset, queen of the meadow, pleurisy root, antispasmodic tincture.

SEXUAL DESIRE, TO INCREASE (aphrodisiacs) — Ginseng, plantain, English walnut, fenugreek, jasmine, saffron, savory, saw palmetto.

SEXUAL DESIRE, TO LESSEN — Black willow, hops, sage, skullcap, star grass, wild Oregon grape.

SLEEP, TO INDUCE — Hops, motherwort, mullein, vervain, skullcap, peppermint. Equal parts of skullcap, nerve root, hops, catnip, and black cohosh.

STIMULANTS — Cayenne, elder, prickly ash, peppermint, ginger, cloves, red sage, raspberry, nettle, pennyroyal, rue, shepherd's purse, valerian.

TOBACCO HABIT — Calamus, magnolia, myrtle leaves and seeds, skullcap, vervain, peppermint, catnip, valerian, motherwort, quassia chips, angelica, black cohosh, blue cohosh, sweet flag. Use burdock or echinacea for cleansing the bloodstream.

Section III
Treating Diseases
with Herbs

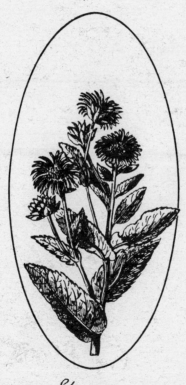

Elecampane

III

TREATING DISEASES WITH HERBS

In this section are listed a number of diseases along with their causes, symptoms, and treatment with herbs and other natural methods, which I have used for many years in association with competent physicians.

No one should try to do the work of a physician, of course. When you are sick, call a competent physician and have a correct diagnosis made of your illness so that the proper herbs and other natural methods of treatment can be selected.

Addendum: The following herbs should not be used in foods, beverages, or drugs, according to a list compiled by the FDA in October 1983: bittersweet, bloodroot, broomtops, calamus, lily of the valley, lobelia, mandrake, mistletoe, St. John's wort, wahoo bark, and wormwood. *Please heed the cautions that are included in the information about each of these herbs.*

For additional information on herbs and their use, see Section II, Chapters 1 through 7.

ACID DYSPEPSIA

Causes: Meats, fish, fowl, tea, coffee, tobacco, alcohol, pepper, mustard, spices, vinegar, excessive use of salt, baking powder, soda, jellies, sweet desserts, candy, preserves, pancakes, hot breads, pastries, fried foods, irregular eating, eating late at night, excess starch, improperly cooked foods, starchy or poorly baked bread, foods too hot or too cold, and foods cooked in aluminum utensils.

Symptoms: Loss of appetite, headaches, sleeplessness, acid urine, acid or strong perspiration, acid taste in the mouth, sour stomach, lassitude, occasional vomiting, a burning, hot feeling in the chest or abdomen, gas on the stomach.

Treatment: Soybean products are excellent as a remedy

for an acid condition. A diet of soybean milk, buttermilk, or orange juice for a few days or a week is excellent. Avoid constipation. Use zwieback, soybean, or whole grain breads. The drier the food that is eaten, the sooner the acid condition can be overcome. Chew! Chew! Chew until your food becomes liquefied and thoroughly saturated with saliva, which is alkaline in reaction. By so doing the normal digestive process can begin in your mouth. Do not drink with meals.

Do not eat between meals or for several hours before going to bed!

After you have been on this diet for a few days to a week, eat one good vegetable meal every day, preferably at noon. Be careful of combinations of food. Avoid eating fruits and vegetables at the same meal, since fruits digest more quickly than vegetables, and when the two are combined digestion is delayed. Do not use any of the foods listed under CAUSES in the first paragraph of this section, because when these are used the acid condition will recur.

ALL OF THESE SYMPTOMS ARE THE RESULT OF YEARS OF WRONG LIVING. YOU MUST NOT EXPECT THEM TO DISAPPEAR IMMEDIATELY. It will require persistence, but persistence can win and you will be greatly rewarded.

The following foods are rich in sodium and magnesium, and should be eaten in abundance:

oranges	apples
beets	cherries
carrots	strawberries
celery	radishes
cucumbers	figs
okra	string beans

Burnet, sanicle, wood betony, calamus, and peppermint are very beneficial herbs. Golden seal powder, taken one-fourth teaspoon in a glass of hot or cold water an hour before meals, is also very healing. Because of the unpleasant taste, you will very likely prefer taking golden seal in capsule form.

ALCOHOLISM – See LIQUOR HABIT

APPENDICITIS

Causes: Constipation may to some extent promote appendicitis; as does eating a diet composed largely of devitalized foods such as white flour products, cane sugar and cane sugar products, greasy and fried foods, tea, coffee, chocolate, and wrong combinations of food. These must be strictly avoided in appendicitis, as must alcoholic drinks, tobacco, and all stimulating food and drink.

The appendix becomes inflamed when its opening into the intestine is blocked, and it cannot empty its contents properly. If the swelling and inflammation continue without proper treatment, the appendix may rupture, producing a very severe infection in the abdomen that may under certain conditions prove fatal.

Symptoms: Nausea and vomiting, pain and distress around the navel and in the right lower abdomen, constipation or loose stools, rapid pulse, and usually a rise in temperature to 100° to 102°F. The pain is usually made worse by pressing on the abdomen or by movement. Drawing the knees up may ease the pain.

Treatment: Cleanse the colon thoroughly with an enema, preferably an herbal enema. Use as much water as possible, as warm as can be tolerated comfortably. This treatment is of great value, and while it will often relieve the pain immediately, it will seldom cure the appendicitis. If using an herbal enema, use either spearmint, catnip, white oak bark, bayberry bark, or wild alum root. When herbs are not available, use plain water. If the pain continues, a very warm enema of catnip alone will often help to relieve the discomfort.

At night, apply a poultice prepared as follows: use a large

handful of granulated or crushed mullein leaves; add a table-spoonful of granulated or powdered lobelia, and sprinkle with ginger. Mix the herbs together in boiling water, making the mixture thick enough to spread as a paste by adding powdered slippery elm or cornmeal. Apply the poultice warm and leave on until cool, then repeat.

When suffering an attack of appendicitis, go on a liquid diet, drinking alkaline broths, fruit juices, and several glasses of slippery elm tea every day. When the attack is over, follow the nourishing diet recommended in Section V, Chapter 11, Normal Diet.

Caution: If you think you are suffering from an *acute* attack of appendicitis, do not apply heat over the abdomen and do not use enemas; you should seek competent medical help *immediately*. Any significant delay may result in dangerous complications.

ARTHRITIS – See LUMBAGO and RHEUMATISM

ASTHMA

Causes: Most, but not all, patients with asthma are found to be allergic to certain substances (antigens), that provoke an acute attack. These substances range from various foods, drugs, and chemicals to pollens, and many other substances. The respiratory passages become filled with mucus, making breathing very difficult. It is not infrequent in asthma sufferers to find that there is some associated problem in the stomach, intestines, or kidneys. Eating certain foods will sometimes bring on an attack.

Symptoms: Most frequently there is shortness of breath, wheezing, and coughing. This becomes so bad at times that the patient fears he may choke to death. The severest attacks frequently occur during the night or early morning. The patient feels that he must fight for air, and may have to get up and go to an open window, or some place where there is a great deal of fresh air. In severe cases, the patient may become almost black in the face or the complexion may become livid because of a lack of oxygen.

Treatment: If the substance that brings on the asthmatic attack is known, it should be avoided at all costs. If the patient with asthma is a smoker, he should give up this habit immediately. An emetic is beneficial when the attack follows shortly after a meal. I have found the following emetic to be very effective: pour one pint of boiling water over one teaspoonful of lobelia; allow to steep a few minutes, and drink several cups lukewarm. If vomiting does not occur freely, place your finger far back in the throat until vomiting occurs. If lobelia is not available, drink lukewarm water with a little salt in it, one cup after another until vomiting occurs. The addition of a little mustard will be found beneficial in cleansing the stomach and lungs, a tablespoonful to a glass of water. When the stomach has been cleansed in one of these ways, there is usually immediate relief. Following this, drink a cup of hot spearmint or peppermint tea or hot lemonade (unsweetened) to settle the stomach.

Give hot fomentations over the stomach, liver, and spleen. You may also give them over the lungs. Then place the patient in a tub of hot water, just above body temperature, and have him remain in the tub for forty-five minutes to an hour or longer. Do not let the water cool off, but keep adding more hot water. Finish the bath by sponging with cool water or by taking a cool shower. Cold morning baths are very valuable in the treatment of asthma, applying the cold water particularly to the neck and shoulders.

It is a good practice to use some tonic herbs. A mixture that I have found excellent is the following: equal parts of lobelia, wild cherry bark, skullcap, gentian, valerian, calamus, and cubeb berries. Mix thoroughly and use a heaping teaspoonful to a cup of boiling water. Drink a cupful of this tea three or four times a day an hour before meals, and a cupful hot upon retiring. If you do not have all of these herbs, use the two, three, or more that you do have. If you are constipated, use the herbal laxative as given in Section II, Chapter 3, taking it at night.

Any one of the following herbs may be used as a tea in the same way as those given above: hyssop, vervain, skunk cabbage, coltsfoot, mullein, horehound, poplar, black cohosh, yerba santa, milkweed, jaborandi, boneset, chickweed, lungwort, masterwort, pleurisy root, thyme, blue cohosh, calamus, and cubeb berries. Select any one, two, or more and mix in equal parts. Take as given above. For children, the amount should be less according to age, or make the tea weaker and give it more frequently. I have had good results when using only one herb indicated for asthma, so read their descriptions and take the one or ones that you feel are best suited to your case.

Antispasmodic tincture and the herbal cough preparation are valuable for treating asthma. Formulas for both are found in Section II, Chapter 3.

Diet: Diet is a very important factor in helping asthma cases. A simple, nourishing, nonstimulating diet is always helpful. It is better to have the heavier meal in the middle of the day and a light meal in the evening. A fruit diet for a few days is highly recommended, after which eat only sparingly of nourishing foods, with few mixtures at a meal. Either zwieback or whole wheat flakes with soybean milk are excellent. French toast (see index) may also be used with soybean milk. Vegetables may be eaten, the leafy ones being especially good. Potatoes, steamed with their jackets on, or baked and mashed, may be eaten; also natural brown rice cooked in very little water, as well as three-minute oatmeal eaten with a little honey or soybean butter.

Remember, the bowels must be kept open. Take baths daily, or more often if desired, and get plenty of outdoor exercise. Practice deep breathing. Have good ventilation in your sleeping room. The water treatments and also the enemas, if they are necessary, should be kept up for some time. Follow the above treatment faithfully and you will obtain splendid results.

BED SORES

Causes: Pressure on the skin from lying too long in one position. The position of a bedridden patient should be changed frequently. If good care is taken of such patients, and they are bathed and turned frequently, they will rarely get bed sores.

Treatment: Hot and cold applications with thorough rubbing will produce good circulation and prevent bed sores, or will greatly relieve them. Make a tea of witch hazel and bathe the sores at least three or four times a day. Kloss's liniment, as given in this book, is also excellent to heal sores of any kind. If there is any proud flesh, sprinkle it with powdered burnt alum. The best wash for bed sores is made of one teaspoonful each of golden seal, myrrh, and boric acid added to a pint of boiling water. After washing the sore, it should be sprinkled with equal parts of powdered golden seal and myrrh. This will help to neutralize the poison and heal the infection, and is very healing. Cover the sore with a bandage saturated with olive oil. Expose the sore to the open air occasionally.

BED WETTING (ENURESIS)

Causes: About ten percent of young children are bothered by bed wetting at night. This is more common in boys than in girls. It is usually a functional or emotional problem and may be associated with sleep walking. Weak and undernourished children are most likely to have this habit. Other causes may be kidney or bladder trouble, eating or drinking late at night just before going to bed, or various problems with the intestines, such as constipation, excess gas, or worms.

Treatment: Do not let the child eat or drink for several hours before going to bed. No stimulating foods or drinks, such as tea, coffee, soft drinks, white bread, or cane sugar products should be allowed. No liquids or foods should be allowed after four or five p.m. If possible, the child should sleep on his side or stomach rather than on his back. It sometimes helps to elevate the foot of the bed a little. Cold morning baths with massage, if possible, and plenty of outdoor exercise, will be a great help. A special effort must be made to discover at about what time the child wets the bed. Usually it is about an hour and a half after retiring and again at about 3:00 in the morning. The child should be awakened and taken to the bathroom a little before this time until the habit is broken. Sometimes when the kidneys or bladder are very much irritated, fomentations over the bladder and along the entire length of the spine will relieve the situation.

In addition, make a tea of plantain and St. John's wort, equal parts mixed together. Use a small teaspoonful to a cup of boiling water. Steep. Give the child one to two cups a day in doses of one-fourth cup at a time. The tea may be sweetened with a little honey so that the child will not object to taking it. Either one of the above herbs is effective alone, but it is well to use both.

See to it that the child is not constipated. Good elimination is very necessary. Warm herb enemas are helpful to relieve this situation when it is present.

It is of absolutely no use to scold the child, as this will only make him nervous and make it harder for him to conquer the habit. Special efforts should be made to help him overcome this distressing habit that he himself dislikes but cannot prevent unless his parents help him.

BLADDER INFLAMMATION (CYSTITIS)

Causes: The immediate cause of most cases of cystitis is some type of bacteria. The bacteria that is the usual cause is the one that is normally found in the large bowel. Cystitis may also be caused by injury, blows or falls, infectious diseases, or the passage of catheters into the bladder. Exposure to cold after perspiring, wrong eating habits, constipation, piles, and extreme nervousness may also be contributing causes. Cystitis may be found in men suffering from venereal diseases.

Symptoms: Cystitis is found much more frequently in females than males. The most frequent symptoms are a burning pain on urination, frequency of urination, the passage of cloudy urine that may be tinged with blood, and a feeling of urgency to empty the bladder. There may be a slight or even high fever, little or no appetite, great thirst, and a distressed countenance.

Treatment: The very first thing to do is to take a high enema of catnip tea; you will find this very soothing. Make the catnip into a tea, using a tablespoon to a quart of water. Take the enema as hot as can be borne, 105° to 110°F. Then take some laxative herbs; equal parts of senna, buckthorn bark, spearmint, cubeb berries, and marshmallow are an excellent combination. After mixing these together, make the tea by using a teaspoon to a cup of boiling water. Drink one to four cups per day, more or less, to suit your case, but keep the bowels loose.

A most effective remedy is to inject an herb tea into the bladder: THIS MUST BE DONE BY A GRADUATE NURSE, OR SOMEONE WHO IS COMPETENT TO TEACH YOU.

Take one heaping teaspoon of golden seal, one of cubeb berries, and one of marshmallow. Mix these together and dissolve them in a quart of boiling water. Steep for twenty minutes, stirring well. After it has settled, strain the tea carefully, so that it will not have any sediment in it. Use a small sterile soft rubber catheter and a sterile enema can. (Sterile, disposable equipment for catheterization is now readily obtainable.) Put the herb tea, a little more than lukewarm, in the enema can and attach the catheter to the rubber tip of the enema tube; lubricate the catheter and gently insert it into the bladder. Permit the tea to flow into the bladder slowly until there is a feeling of fullness. One or two ounces will usually give this feeling, but continue until several ounces are used. Retain the liquid as long as possible. This process should be repeated two or three times a day and you will have good results. An injection of slippery elm water (see index) into the bladder in this way is also excellent, as it is very soothing and healing.

There are two herbal teas that are particularly good for inflammation of the bladder. One is flaxseed tea; use one teaspoonful of the herb to a cup of boiling water and drink three cups a day. The other is an equal mixture of buchu and uva ursi. Make a tea the same way as for flaxseed and drink one to four cups a day. These herbs may also be used in capsule form, but if you take the capsules, you must be sure to drink a large amount of water.

Give fomentations over the bladder and along the entire length of the spine. Hot sitz baths are extremely beneficial. In severe cases, the sitz bath must be repeated two or three times a day until relief is obtained.

Diet: The diet should be light and nourishing. All irritating and stimulating foods are strictly forbidden. Avoid foods high in protein. Mashed potatoes, prepared according to the recipe in Section V, Chapter 2, are very good, as they are unlike the ordinary mashed potatoes because of the addition of soybean milk, which is highly alkaline, and because the potatoes are not peeled before cooking. It must be the whole potato, for when you remove the peeling, the mineral salts are lost. Also use potassium broth as given in this book. (See the index.) It is very good. In addition, soybean cottage cheese, soybean milk with zwieback, all leafy vegetables, carrots, okra, cauliflower, and eggplant are very good.

A fruit diet is the best means of cleansing the system. Fruits are always good as they are rich in alkaline salts and help to overcome acidity.

Drink two or three quarts of water daily, so that the urine will be bland and nonirritating. This is very important. The same treatment is excellent for any kind of bladder trouble.

The bladder should be emptied as soon as the urge to urinate is felt, and also after sexual intercourse.

BLOOD POISONING AND INFECTION

Causes: Uncleanliness, various infections, improper dressing of sores.

Symptoms: The disease begins with a decided chill and a feeling of depression. Shivering sensations, followed by profuse perspiration, are frequent. The pulse rate becomes very rapid and the area around the wound looks red and angry. The breathing grows rapid and there is an anxious expression on the countenance. The temperature becomes elevated.

Treatment: Echinacea is a very good herb to correct impure blood conditions, especially when there is a tendency to develop gangrene. It is useful when given internally in acute appendicitis to prevent gangrene and peritonitis, and is helpful in scarlet fever, malaria, septicemia following child-birth, tonsillitis, diphtheria, and typhoid.

Take a high enema. Take as many cups of echinacea tea a day as possible, using a teaspoonful to the cup; or if taken in powdered form in capsules, take two No.00 capsules every two hours.

Take nothing but fruit juices for a number of days, especially grapefruit, orange, lemon, and pineapple. Do not mix the juices. Take them one at a time but drink plenty of them. Keep the temperature even and have an abundance of fresh air.

When the patient feels chilly, give a cup of hot water in which a little cayenne pepper has been dissolved. This can be given often. One heaping teaspoonful of charcoal powder put in a cup with enough hot water added to make a paste, diluted, and drunk at once, is very good. Charcoal can also be used to advantage as a poultice. (See Section IX, Chapter 4, The Value of Charcoal.)

Wash the wound thoroughly with boric acid solution, and if the discharge is thin and unhealthly looking, sprinkle equal parts of powdered myrrh and golden seal directly on the sore. (See herbs listed under Blood Poisoning in the index.)

BOILS AND CARBUNCLES

Causes: Poor habits of cleanliness, infections on the skin, inactivity of the skin, bad blood from putrefaction in the system. The fact that one has boils or carbuncles shows that the body contains poisons and waste matter and is in a low state of resistance. Some of the minute glands die; sometimes the root of a hair dies; then a little pimple appears, which if treated immediately, would soon disappear. The red spot or pimple is followed by tenderness and great pain. Boils seldom come singly. Frequently, one is followed by several others.

Treatment: When the carbuncle or boil is at the root of a hair, it is best to pull out the hair and apply a little liniment, for which the formula is given in Section II, Chapter 3. If treated early, and if the liniment is applied repeatedly, the boil should soon disappear. In case of a pimple, it should be opened, the pus squeezed out, and liniment applied. Pimples around the face and head, however, should never be squeezed. It is very necessary that the system be cleansed from waste matter. The bowels must be kept open. Take some of the laxative herbs. Echinacea is excellent for cleansing the blood; take two capsules twice a day. A cleansing diet for a week or more with proper elimination is a very effective means of ridding the system of boils and carbuncles. A hot bath followed by a vigorous salt glow is a very successful measure for preventing the spread of boils or carbuncles. Cold baths are excellent to increase the circulation and stimulate the system. The general health must be built up.

Oranges are practically a specific when a person is afflicted with boils or carbuncles. They assist in restoring the body to a healthy condition so that the cause of the boils and carbuncles can be removed. Eat them freely, a dozen or more a day, either alone or combined with grapefruit. Also use plenty of fresh vegetables, especially the leafy ones, such as turnip greens, spinach, etc. Eat canned or fresh tomatoes without seasoning. The fresh tomatoes are preferable. It is better to make a separate meal of them than to combine them with other foods.

Hot and cold fomentations applied to the boils for half an hour three times a day are very helpful. Leave the hot fomentation on for about three minutes and the cold one on for about thirty seconds. Alternating hot and cold water treatments can be used if the boils are in an accessible part of the body, such as the arms or legs.

It is important to never squeeze or incise a pimple, boil, or carbuncle unless the area has been completely cleansed with alcohol or some other suitable solution, the hands and fingernails thoroughly cleaned, and any needle, knife, or other instrument that you will be using has been sterilized by boiling in water for ten minutes. This is very important, as squeezing helps to force the infection into the blood which carries it to other parts of the body.

BREASTS (CAKED OR INFLAMED)

Causes: Infections of the breast are frequently associated with nursing and milk production. Bacteria may enter the breast through small abrasions, cracks or lacerations near the nipple.

Symptoms: A hard, painful swelling occurs in the breast, accompanied by a throbbing, burning pain, restlessness, and fever. A lump may be felt beneath the skin, which is very tender and warm to the touch. The skin over the area often has a pinkish-red color.

Treatment: Often just bathing an inflamed breast with alder tea will relieve the inflammation and pain. The following treatment is excellent when the breast is inflamed, swollen, or caked, or when the nipples are sore. Use dry hot and cold applications to ease the soreness and inflammation. These should be given continuously until relieved. Then apply a solution made as follows: mix well together one pint of linseed oil, four ounces of spearmint and four ounces of spirit of camphor. Soak a cloth in this solution, place it on the breast, and make sure it covers all of the affected part. Apply as often as required.

When the breast is swollen, a poultice of slippery elm with a little lobelia added will give great relief. (See Section II, Chapter 3.) Also a poultice made of grated poke root and cornmeal, applied warm, is very good.

Drink three or four cups of tea a day made of equal parts of ginger, golden seal, and black cohosh.

If the lump does not disappear or if the redness, heat, and soreness continue after this treatment has been used, seek out competent medical help.

BRIGHT'S DISEASE (NEPHRITIS)

Causes: Bright's disease is a broad descriptive term commonly used for kidney infection. It frequently follows streptococcal infections of the throat and skin. It is sometimes associated with other diseases, such as typhoid, influenza, diphtheria, pneumonia, smallpox, or scarlet fever. Alcoholic drinks, tea, coffee, and spices may cause some injury to the kidneys. Patent medicines may be a cause. Food cooked in aluminum utensils is injurious and should never be eaten, especially when one is suffering from Bright's disease, either acute or chronic.

Symptoms: One of the most common symptoms is loss of appetite. At other times there is a great desire for food; then, when it is set before the patient, he refuses to eat. In some cases, the skin becomes dry and there is fever, shortness of breath, and palpitation of the heart. There may be swelling of the ankles and under the eyes, which is a sign that the heart is affected. Pain in the kidneys may occur and there may be blood in the urine. The patient is usually pale, especially after the condition has advanced to some extent. At first there may be scantiness of urine, but later the amount of urine greatly increases and contains protein, which your family physician will be able to find when he tests your urine. Often there is frequent urination at night, accompanied by a burning sensation. Sometimes these symptoms begin very suddenly, but at other times they appear slowly. There may be fever, chills, headache, dizziness, nausea, and vomiting, and the patient becomes very weak. This disease occurs frequently in children from three to seven years of age and should receive early adequate treatment to prevent permanent kidney damage.

Treatment: Regular and adequate elimination is necessary and may be obtained by the use of enemas containing white oak bark, bayberry bark, or wild alum root bark. In the absence of these herbs, use very warm tap water made slightly sudsy with ivory soap. It is important to keep the skin clean and a daily bath, sufficiently warm to bring a glow to the skin, should be taken. While the patient is in the tub, he may be given two or three cups of pleurisy root or sage tea. This treatment will open the pores in the skin and encourage perspiration. It is good to stay in the bath at least one-half hour. Finish off with a short cold shower or a short cold towel rub and dry thoroughly. Be sure to keep away from drafts so that no chilling occurs. A salt glow will greatly stimulate the activity of the skin. An excellent thing to do after the bath is to wrap the patient in a blanket, put him to bed, and continue giving the pleurisy root tea or sage tea to encourage perspiration. Applying fomentations to the spine, and then sponging the spine with cold water after each one and rubbing the skin thoroughly dry before applying another, are excellent methods to allay pain. Also give the same treatment over the stomach, liver, and spleen.

A tea of broom top and marshmallow leaves (equal parts) is very good. Be sure the patient gets plenty of rest and try to eliminate all causes for restlessness or worry. The room should be well ventilated, warm and free from drafts. Salt and water intake should be reduced at first to a minimum.

The patient should frequently change positions in bed so that bed sores do not develop.

Diet: The diet should be light and nourishing. All stimulating and heavy foods should be strictly forbidden. Salt should be restricted, as should foods high in protein. Sprouted soybeans and lentils may be eaten.

The soybean recipes given in Section VI, Chapter 2, and also cauliflower, asparagus, eggplant, and vegetable broths are good. The free use of fruit juices or a fruit juice diet for a few days, before starting to partake of other foods, is excellent. Soybean milk, with whole wheat flakes dissolved in it, is extremely nourishing and very easily digested. Avoid the use of salt as much as possible, and do not mix fruits and vegetables at the same meal.

BRONCHITIS, ACUTE

Causes: Changeable weather, catching cold, exposure, wet feet, chilling when not sufficiently clothed, insufficient ventilation in the house, especially in the bedrooms. Bronchitis would be uncommon if people ate the right food, kept their systems free from mucus and poisonous waste material, and dressed properly. Stomach trouble and constipation are frequently associated with bronchitis.

Bronchitis is an infection by a virus or bacteria that affects the mucous membrane lining of the bronchial tubes, causing a large amount of mucus to form, which is called phlegm. It may start as a cold or as influenza and then, because of inadequate treatment, extend down the air passages into the lungs.

Symptoms: Chills and fever, tightness and stuffiness in the chest, difficulty breathing. Sometimes there is a severe cough and the attack comes on like croup. In most cases it is the larger bronchial tubes that are affected. The cough is often worse when the patient lies down and there is usually a bad coughing spell the first thing on waking in the morning. At first there may be but little mucus, but after several days it increases and turns to yellow pus, sometimes becoming frothy. Children sometimes have convulsions and become unconscious.

Treatment: The same treatment as for chronic bronchitis, following. Everyone should have on hand the antispasmodic tincture and cough medicine made according to the formulas given in Section II, Chapter 3 for use in acute and chronic bronchitis and asthma.

BRONCHITIS, CHRONIC

Causes: Acute bronchitis may become chronic if it is not properly treated and relieved. When a cold is allowed to continue, the infection may extend down into the lungs and become chronic. Occasionally, if it is not cured, it may encourage the development of tuberculosis or some other serious chronic lung disease. Some forms of stomach trouble may be a cause of bronchitis and even pneumonia. This is particularly true of those persons who bring up acid and other stomach contents into the mouth while asleep, and then aspirate it into their lungs.

One of the major causes of chronic bronchitis is cigarette smoking. Air pollution may also be a factor, particularly in those who smoke cigarettes.

Symptoms: Almost continual coughing; coughing up quantities of mucus and phlegm; shortness of breath and wheezing. These symptoms may become very severe and disabling.

Treatment: If the person afflicted with this disease is a smoker, the most important thing to do is STOP SMOKING, and if at all possible stay out of smoke-filled rooms.

Take equal parts of wild cherry, mullein, coltsfoot, yarrow, horehound, and buckthorn. Mix these together, using one teaspoonful to a cup of boiling water. Take a cupful four times a day. It may be taken more often in smaller doses if preferred. If you do not have all of these herbs, read the description of the different ones in Section II, Chapter 5 and then select the one best suited to your case.

All acid-forming foods must be eliminated from the diet and scrupulously avoided. Do not drink with your meals, as taking liquid with meals causes fermentation, acid, and gas;

it delays digestion as the liquid must be absorbed first. Eat alkaline foods. (See the preceding paragraphs on Acid Dyspepsia in this section.) Fruit juices of all kinds, especially pineapple, lemon, orange, and grapefruit are best, as they help to loosen and cut the phlegm.

A full hot bath, steam bath, or vapor bath, followed by a short cold shower, is beneficial. In the absence of a shower, finish with a cold towel rub of short duration. Hot fomentations to the chest and spine, finishing with cold, will do much to relieve the congestion. Hot footbaths with a tablespoonful of mustard added to the water often gives great relief. A hot fomentation applied around the neck, followed by a cold compress, is also beneficial. The cold compress must be thoroughly covered with a woolen cloth to heat it up. If for any reason it should get cold, it must be removed and the neck rubbed thoroughly dry, leaving a dry woolen cloth on.

The air in the patient's room should not be too dry. Place a dish of water on the stove or radiator to produce moisture in the air. The room should be kept at an even temperature, but good ventilation is necessary.

If breathing is difficult and the cough is severe, one of the most effective things to do in order to clear the throat and facilitate breathing is to take an emetic using warm water. Make a weak tea of cubeb berries, using one heaping teaspoonful to a pint of hot water. A pinch of red pepper added is excellent to loosen the phlegm so that it can be expelled. After doing this, take a drink of the hot tea to wash out the stomach. Good results will be obtained. A very little lobelia (one-fourth teaspoonful) added will relax the throat, stomach, and bronchial tubes at once. Be sure the bowels are kept open. If there is any problem with this, take laxative herbs or high enemas.

Everyone should keep herbs on hand for colds and influenza and not let them develop into chronic bronchial trouble. Chickweed, coltsfoot, cubeb berries, golden seal, lungwort, mullein, myrrh, white pine, pleurisy root, sanicle, saw palmetto berries, skunk cabbage, slippery elm, white pond lily, yerba santa, bloodroot, ginger, blue violet, bethroot, red root, red sage, and lobelia can be used singly or in any combination you desire. Everyone should have on hand the antispasmodic tincture and cough medicine made according to the formulas given in Section II, Chapter 3.

BURNS AND SCALDS

Treatment: Immerse the burned part in cold water and keep the water cold by adding more ice or cold water. Keep the part covered with water until the heat is all drawn out and there will not be any blisters. If the clothing should catch fire, a blanket or some large piece of cloth (wet if possible) should be quickly wrapped around the person to smother the fire. The one who is on fire should *never* start to run or walk, but must throw himself immediately on the ground and roll, or grab a blanket and roll up in it. The clothes should be quickly removed. Do not even wait to undress but cut the clothes off as soon as possible. The patient should be taken to a quiet place where the burn may be dressed. The first thing to be considered is the nature of the scald or burn, where it is, and to what degree the skin is burned. Dip a cloth in kerosene and cover the burn. This will quickly allay the pain. If there are any blisters, prick them on the edge with a sterile, clean needle and press out the water. The writer has healed large burns with very little pain by the kerosene method. A hot water burn should be treated in the same way.

Large burns may be bathed with the following lotion: take one teaspoonful of golden seal, one of myrrh, and one of boric acid and add them to a pint of boiling water. Let this mixture stand for one-half hour, then pour off the clear liquid and apply with absorbent cotton. This solution is very soothing and healing and is an excellent remedy for deep burns. Herbal salve and liniment (see Section II, Chapter 3) are also very excellent for this. If the burn is deep, it will heal more quickly if just the mixture of powdered myrrh, golden seal, and boric acid is sprinkled on the sore, thus keeping the burn dry so that it will heal more readily. Cover with gauze. If there is any proud flesh, sprinkle it with burnt alum.

The following tea taken internally will stimulate the circulation and greatly aid the healing of burns: take one teaspoonful each of powdered valerian, skullcap, and peppermint. Mix these together and use one teaspoonful to a cup of boiling water. It is very quieting and soothing to the nerves.

IF THE BURN IS EXTENSIVE OR DEEP, CALL YOUR FAMILY PHYSICIAN OR GO TO THE NEAREST HOSPITAL EMERGENCY ROOM AS SOON AS POSSIBLE.

CANCER

Causes: Although cancer in some parts of the body is increasing at an alarming rate, in other areas, such as the stomach and uterus, the incidence of cancer is decreasing. Certain types can be prevented to a great degree, and it is estimated that well over one-half of all cancers are due to the unhealthy living and eating habits followed by the majority of Americans.

Through chronic autointoxication, constipation, and the inactivity of the organs of elimination – lungs, liver, kidneys, skin, and bowels – the system becomes poisoned and the poisons accumulate around the weakest organs or where the body has been injured by a blow, fall, or bruise. Poisoning of the body is caused by the use of improper foods, tea, coffee, soft drinks, liquor, tobacco in all forms, meats of all kinds, especially pork, cane sugar and cane sugar products, white flour products, white rice, and all denatured foods, which cause waste matter in the system. Cancer would be rare if devitalized foods and meats were not eaten and all unhealthy living habits were eliminated. The life-giving properties and minerals are removed from much of the food that is eaten. These properties keep the bloodstream pure, and cancer will not develop readily where there is a pure bloodstream.

Symptoms: Skin cancers are most frequently the result

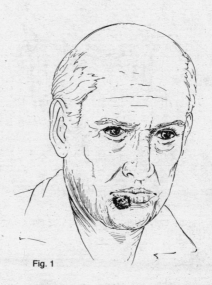

Fig. 1

of exposure to the sun over a long period of time. These cancers often begin on the face close to the nose, sometimes in the middle of the cheek, behind or below the ear, and sometimes on other parts of the face or neck. The skin becomes rough and eventually forms an open sore, which slowly grows larger and larger. Lip cancer (Fig. 1) is usually caused from smoking a pipe, cigars, or cigarettes. Sometimes cancer begins inside the mouth.

Cancer may appear in any part of the body. It may start in the stomach. The victim thinks it is merely indigestion, but as the cancer grows and invades the surrounding tissues it causes abdominal pain, loss of weight, and poor appetite.

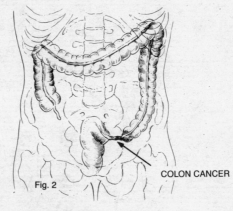

COLON CANCER

Fig. 2

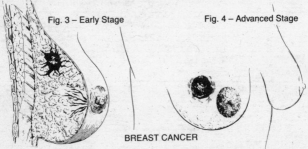

Fig. 3 – Early Stage

Fig. 4 – Advanced Stage

BREAST CANCER

Eating may cause an increase in the stomach pain, followed shortly by nausea or vomiting. Often a brown-colored matter is vomited. Constipation, sleeplessness, and a feverish condition are usual. There is a general wasting away and finally death. Very frequently cancer begins in the colon (Fig. 2) or rectum and may cause bleeding from the bowel or great distress at stool. Sometimes the liver is cancerous, causing pain in that region and general debility. Cancer of the female organs is quite common, and manifests itself in the form of a tumor on the uterus, as a sore at the mouth of the uterus, or as a growth in the ovaries. Cancer of the breast is very common in women and there may be an associated cancer of the female organs when cancer of the breast is present. (Figs. 3 and 4) Cancer of the lung is the most common cancer in men and is rapidly approaching that same position for women also. Its most common cause is cigarette smoking.

Treatment: No type of cancer is to be taken lightly. If it is not treated properly and completely removed, it will continue to spread and eventually will probably prove fatal. The first step is to cleanse the bloodstream by thoroughly relieving constipation and making all the organs of elimination active – skin, lungs, liver, kidneys, and bowels – and keeping them active. For constipation, take the herbal laxative given in Section II, Chapter 3. It is very good. Use high enemas to cleanse the colon of any bad condition there. It is necessary to take a fruit diet of oranges, grapefruit, lemons, apples, cranberries, unsweetened blueberries, red raspberries, cherries, peaches, pears, ripe strawberries, avocados, pineapples, and tomatoes. All fruit should be well ripened on the tree or vine to be fully beneficial.

Tomatoes should be eaten separately, not with other foods. Make a meal of them. For the first ten days (or a longer or shorter period depending upon the condition of the patient), it is advisable to take nothing but unsweetened fruit juices, preferably orange, grapefruit, pineapple, lemon, or grape. Do not mix the juices but take different ones at different times.

Vegetable juices are very useful also – celery, cucumber, parsley, lettuce, and carrot. Carrot juice is especially valuable in cancer. These juices may be mixed.

Drink six glasses of fruit juice and six glasses of herbal tea a day. If you can take more, so much the better. If the herbs are taken in capsules, take No. 00 size capsules according to the correct dosage for that herb, and be sure the capsules are full. Follow this with a glass of hot water, as hot as can be taken comfortably. Take the herbs one hour before taking any fruit juice.

If the patient is thin or has been losing weight, after a few days of fruit diet, give an alkaline nourishing diet – vegetable soups (recipes given in Section VI, Chapter 2); mashed potatoes, prepared as described in this book; natural brown rice; soybean cheese; carrots; greens of all kinds; red cabbage (especially valuable); the green leaves of cabbage; parsley; eggplant (especially valuable); okra; tender corn, on the cob or canned; tender peas (fresh or canned); naturally cured ripe olives; celery; green lima beans; onions; garlic; cauliflower; baked Irish potatoes; lentils; cucumber; garden-grown lettuce; radishes; watercress; spinach; squash; kale; asparagus; young beets; dandelion greens; endive; collards; Swiss chard; Chinese cabbage; soybeans or wheat, sprouted; salsify; wild rice; yellow cornmeal; watermelon; and tomatoes. Watermelon should be eaten alone and not with any other foods. Likewise, tomatoes should be eaten alone. Make a separate meal of them. Tomatoes are high in vitamin content. Use fresh ripe tomatoes or the best canned ones. Fresh vine-ripened tomatoes are best. Eaten with whole wheat zwieback, they make an excellent meal.

Never cook food in aluminum cooking utensils. Never eat fruit and vegetables at the same meal, nor drink fruit and vegetable juices at the same time.

Get plenty of fresh air and exercise, outdoors in the sunshine if possible, to cleanse the lungs and increase the circulation. If the patient is unable to be outdoors, he must be in a sunshiny room, which is well ventilated at all times. He should take deep breathing exercises and all the other exercise he is able to perform in the house.

Give frequent sweat baths to keep the skin active, followed by salt glows so that the skin will eliminate the poisons. While giving sweat baths, keep the head cool by placing a cold towel wrung out of very cold water around the neck, changing often to keep it cold. Put an ice bag over the heart if the patient has any heart trouble. If the patient is strong enough, give a cold towel rub every morning. This increases the circulation. Apply alternate hot and cold applications to the liver, stomach, spleen, and spine.

Thorough massage is very helpful in the treatment of

cancer. It assists in eliminating the poisons from the body by increasing the circulation.

As mentioned earlier, when I was a child, I gathered red clover blossoms for the postmaster in our town, who used them to make a tea for cancer. I do not remember the particulars of his case, but I do remember he lived to be an old man. Use plenty of red clover blossom tea. Drink it instead of water. The tea may be prepared by using a handful of dried blossoms to a quart of cold water. Let it come to a boil and simmer for fifteen minutes. Keep it covered until cool enough to drink; then strain and drink as many glasses a day as you possibly can. See also the list of herbs suitable for treating cancer given in Section II, Chapter 7.

One of the principal aims of this book is the prevention of disease. One of the great causes of cancer is the food we eat and the way in which it is prepared. Statistics show that many of the cancers today are caused by improper foods and improper eating habits. A faulty diet irritates the stomach and causes an ulcer, which if not cured may develop into cancer without the victim ever realizing what is taking place.

There are foods in which cancer germs cannot develop – food that is very nourishing and palatable – and there are nonpoisonous herbs that can heal cancerous sores both inside and outside the body.

Violet leaves (or you may use the whole plant), have been known to cure cancer when the diet and other improper living habits were corrected. Make a tea of the leaves by using one-half ounce of leaves to a pint of boiling water. Steep one-half hour and drink a cupful every two hours. Dip a piece of cloth into some of this tea and apply warm over the affected part. Leave on until dry. A poultice can be made of chopped fresh violet leaves, steeped in boiling water for thirty minutes, with some linseed meal added to make the poultice. As an enema, use one-half ounce of violet leaves to the pint of water; strain and use morning and night.

Agrimony and ground ivy are also excellent. They will help to dry up and heal skin cancers.

Herbs for Cancer: Red clover blossoms, burdock root, yellow dock root, blue violet (the whole plant), golden seal root, gum myrrh, echinacea, aloes, blue flag, gravel root, bloodroot, dandelion root, African cayenne, chickweed, rock rose, agrimony, Oregon grape and equal parts of echinacea and chaparral. Most of these herbs are available in either the powdered or capsule from. In addition, an old Chinese herb in use for over 5,000 years, called ho shou wu or fo-ti, has been used to shrink cancer.

Many years ago, before I attempted to treat cancer and had taken it for granted that there was no cure, I made up my mind that I would find out the cause of cancer; so I looked up the records to find out in which countries of the earth cancer was most prevalent. When I learned this, I looked to find out what food the peoples of these countries ate. I found that in the civilized nations of the earth where a large amount of meat and rich, luxurious foods were consumed, cancer was more prevalent. In the developing nations where they ate plain, natural foods, cancer was very rare. In some parts of the world where cancer was rare, after the people learned of the diet used by the "civilized peoples" and started using it, cancer increased.

People used to think that meat was the great cause of cancer, but in my research I discovered that some people who ate no meat at all still developed cancer. I also found that people who did not eat meat, and with whose habits of diet I was well acquainted also had cancer. They were eating refined food and bad combinations of food of such a nature that much waste matter accumulated in the system. This caused the different organs to become diseased and many times cancer resulted.

After learning this, I felt quite sure that I was on the right road to finding the cause of cancer, and since then I have known it. Refined, processed foods have been robbed of their minerals and vitamins, which are the life-giving properties, the very parts which God put in the different foods to keep the blood pure and to sustain the nervous system.

After deciding that the food people ate and the things they drank were primarily the cause of cancer, I started to search for a cure. While taking a course in one of the best dietetics schools, I also learned the water cure and took a medical electrical course. I also made a study of the body and foods, and the effects of food upon the various organs of the body. I recalled how, during my youth when in my parents' home, I learned something of the value of herbs from my parents and from the Indians, who were numerous in those days in northern Wisconsin.

As stated earlier, I gathered herbs for my parents and the herb doctors, thus learning the value of herbs which I have never forgotten. I very distinctly remember gathering red clover blossoms, witch hazel bark, white pine bark, white willow bark, white poplar bark, bloodroot, mandrake root, hemlock bark, golden seal root, sarsaparilla, and many other herbs which grew all around us in abundance.

After learning the water cure and taking a course in medical electricity, I wanted to know more about herbs; so I took a medical herb course. I also obtained from different parts of the world the best books I could find and subscribed to the best magazines dealing with the medicinal value of herbs.

By experience I learned how herbs could be used to cure bad sores and ulcers. I determined to try them on cancer, and I have seen the most malignant cancer sores heal on various parts of the body externally. The herbs have the same healing qualities, too, when taken internally.

I have been asked many times what my cancer cure is. Here it is in a nutshell: correct food, herbs, water, fresh air, massage, sunshine, exercise, and rest.

If herbs are used that can heal the most malignant cancerous ulcer externally, and herbs are used internally that may kill the malignancy of internal cancers, then there must by an elimination of waste matter to clean the entire system and bloodstream if you want the patient to live. Now, how is the waste matter to be eliminated and the bloodstream purified?

First, the five eliminating organs must be made active; the lungs, skin, liver, kidneys, and bowels. Then there must be enough fluid taken into the body so that this waste material can be eliminated. This is done by the copious drinking of herb teas, fruit juices, vegetable juices, and pure water; also hot baths to open the pores, massage, rest, fresh air, and the remainder of the prescribed treatment.

Not long ago a woman came to me who had cancer involving the liver, lungs, and stomach. She lived only a few weeks after I saw her. A postmortem was held, and we found that her liver was almost entirely gone. Parts of both lungs were hardened, and the throat and stomach had growths in them. She had not been able to retain anything in her stomach for some time. Portions of her intestines were very much shrunken. Upon inquiring into what had been her diet, we found that it had been white bread, jellies, jams, soda crackers, and denatured foods.

Many times I have caused hard swellings in the breast, bowels, rectum, and vagina to disappear with herbs and applications of heat. In different parts of the earth, people are searching for the cure for cancer and other so-called incurable diseases. The treatment for them is found in this book.

Cancer is a treacherous disease. When there is any suspicion of cancer, take a cleansing diet — fruit and vegetable juices, taken separately. Cancer cannot live in a system where all the mineral elements, which God put there in the beginning, are present.

If cancer is suspected, clean out the system, and get a new supply of pure blood. There are nonpoisonous herbs that will purify the blood and kill malignant growths internally or externally, leaving no bad after-effects. Cancer will not live in a system when the bloodstream is pure.

While it may be all right to treat symptoms, the cause of a disease must be ascertained and removed before there can be a permanent cure.

Since I have been asked many times about my experiences with cancer cases, I will give a few.

Many years ago I was asked to see a man who was in a charity hospital. His trouble had been pronounced cancer. In fact, he had no outward sign of cancer, just a little swelling on the underside of his jaw, which was not painful; but he complained of pain in the region of the navel. There was no outside swelling on or near the navel, but a tumor could be felt there. Something gave way in this region that caused his death. A postmortem was held and it was found that the cancer had eaten through the bowels. It had not only spread through all the bowels, but had also affected all his organs. From the crown of his head to the soles of his feet, the tissues of his body were full of cancerous growths.

Another man — quite fleshy — who had been sick for some time and whom I had nursed for nearly a year, died suddenly. The attending physician, who was a prominent surgeon, said to me, "We will have a postmortem on this man." We found this man's bowels to be full of cancerous growths. His liver was very much enlarged and full of tumors, large and small. His heart was much enlarged and upon opening it, we found a large amount of fat in each part. There were no growths in the stomach, but it was full of mucus and the walls were a very dark color. This man was a big user of pie, ice cream, iced tea and coffee, white bread, peeled potatoes, denatured foods, liquor, tobacco, and other harmful things. Many times when I talked to him about his eating and drinking he would reply, "I'm going to have what I want while I live."

Another man had a cancer on his cheek. It was in the form of a tumor about the size of a fist and was extremely painful. The cancer had eaten completely through the cheek and spread on the inside of the cheek to his gums on both upper and lower jaws and had started to eat his tongue. Pus ran out of his mouth and he was kept alive by inserting a tube in the other side of his mouth, through which he took liquid nourishment. This sore was so painful that it could not be touched with a little cotton without excruciating pain. After about seven weeks of treatment as I have outlined, this cancer healed so that this man could sit at the table and eat with his family. The last I heard from him he was doing some work. To heal this cancer, the herbs which I have enumerated in this book were used.

In another patient the cancer had spread from the gums to the throat and it then progressed to the stomach. Pus was exuding freely on the outside and also from the throat. The patient was kept alive by tube feeding and by treatment with the herbs and other natural remedies. In seven weeks this man was able to sit with his family again, and to eat at the table. The last I heard from him he was once again able to do some light work.

Another woman who had cancer of the breast, had had one breast removed and had been overtreated with radium and x-rays. She was burned from it so that the flesh came off her ribs and she could not eat or drink anything, even water. I did not try to do anything for her except to make her as comfortable as possible.

A man who had cancer of the rectum had his folks come for me. I injected some of the herbs given in this book, and the terrible pain stopped about the fourth day. In about seven days a lot of slush came from the rectum, including a big chunk that looked like a crab. In seven or eight weeks after I began to treat him, he said he felt as well as he ever did in his life, and began to do some light work.

A woman who also had cancer of the rectum, about the size of an egg and causing her constant pain, came to see me. After I had treated this woman for five weeks, the tumor was gone and she had no more symptoms. Her health was very much improved generally. She continued taking the herbs and some of the treatment to be sure her bloodstream was purified. I heard from this woman some years later, and her health was good.

Another woman had developed a painful, swollen breast, which was surgically removed. A short time later she developed a large tumor in her bowels. This also was removed. Then she developed another tumor larger than the first one.

When the surgeon attempted to remove it, he found that the cancer had spread through the entire abdomen. He simply closed up the incision without removing anything, stating that she could not live more than three to ten days. She was taken home to die and her nurse was instructed to give her plenty of medicine to relieve her pain.

Her husband was advised to get in touch with me. He came for me and took me to see his wife. When I arrived at their home and examined her, I found that nothing would go through her bowels. She had a tube in one side of her colon, through which the waste matter came out. In the other side of her abdomen, there was an opening through which the urine passed. There was another opening through which pus oozed all the time. She had to lie flat on her back and could retain nothing on her stomach, not even water.

Her husband and family wanted me to try to help her. I gave them no hope whatever, but I said I would try. It indeed took some courage to undertake to help a person in that condition.

We did not give her any more hypodermics to quiet her, but tried to soothe her pains with fomentations, liniment, massage, etc. We gave her herbal enemas, which cleaned out the impaction and swelling from the colon until she had a natural bowel movement through the rectum. Then I removed the tube from her colon and healed the opening. I worked hard to heal the side where the urine passed; but this was harder to heal, as a little urine oozed away all the time. It finally healed, however. Just as soon as her side was healed, we gave her hot tub baths, so she would sweat freely.

At first she was so weak that it took four persons to put her in the tub and take her out again. There was improvement from the first day we put her in the bath. She perspired freely. We gave her a hot sweat bath every day until she got well, followed by a salt glow, cold towel rub, and a massage. She also had fomentations every day over the stomach, liver, spleen, spine, and over the entire abdomen, after which her abdomen and back were thoroughly saturated with the liniment (recipe for which is given in Section II, Chapter 3). Her abdomen was thoroughly massaged several times a day for quite a while to assist in removing the poisons and cancerous growths.

This treatment was followed for about four months. In the meantime she went to Florida in a touring car, stayed there for a while, and came home on the bus. She stood the trip by bus fine, and after returning, went every day to visit some of her many friends. Soon she began to do her own housework and has done it ever since, besides raising beautiful flowers and helping materially in the family vegetable garden.

She took the herbs and diet as given in this book and also made many meals of fresh, vine-ripened tomatoes for some time. In addition, she ate freely of leafy greens.

This was six years ago and today she is the picture of health. My wife and I were invited to her home some time ago and what a fine dinner she had prepared! It was delicious and all of the dishes were healthful dishes. We enjoyed this dinner immensely for two reasons: seeing this woman enjoying life in the nice new home that her husband had built for her and partaking with them of the fine dinner she herself had prepared.

Right here I must say that part of the credit for the recovery of this outstanding case I give to my wife and youngest daughter, Naomi, who were the faithful nurses on this case. The following is a letter from this patient.

I write this for the benefit of others. During the summer of 1933, I was taken seriously ill, and was taken to a large institution in the vicinity of Washington, D.C. They found that I had cancer of the breast, so they removed the entire breast. A little later it was discovered I had a large tumor in my abdomen. They then operated and removed it, and then another tumor developed in the bowels which was larger than the first one, so much so that it completely shut off any movement from passing through the bowels to the rectum.

They then made an opening in the colon and put a tube in to eliminate the waste matter. My suffering was so intense that they kept me under heavy opiates all the time. I was failing fast and they told me there was no chance for any recovery. I was taken home in an ambulance, and my family was told I could not live more than three to ten days. My husband purchased a burial plot, and about that time we learned of a man by the name of Jethro Kloss that could cure cancer, so we looked him up and my husband brought him to our house. He made no promises, as the case was very hopeless: nothing would go through my bowels, I could keep nothing on my stomach, and was paralyzed with opiates. But he said that he would try to help me, but would not make any promises.

He treated me with natural remedies, herbs, proper diet, water treatments, massage, sunshine, fresh air, and rest. I was treated by him for four months, when I made a trip to Florida with Mr. Kloss in an auto and stayed there under his care for one month. I then left Miami and went to visit relatives elsewhere in Florida, returning home to Washington from there by bus. This was five years ago and I am a well woman today, doing my own housework, working in my garden, etc.

I write this so that others suffering from the dread disease of cancer may know that there is help for them.

Mrs. John Rhine

Another case was that of a woman who had large breasts. One was very much enlarged and inflamed, and there were sharp, cutting pains shooting in all directions and into her arm. She had been advised to have her breast removed at once, as that seemed to be the only help.

She came to see me in that condition, and in about three days I had the excruciating pains allayed. I continued the treatment for about four weeks.

After that, I instructed her what to do, and she took the herbs for some time. About three years later I saw her, and she said she never felt any further trouble in her breast and that her health was good.

To allay the inflammation in the breast, I applied hot and cold applications alternately twice a day, and thoroughly saturated the breast with the liniment recipe given in this book. As soon as the inflammation was all gone, we thoroughly massaged the breast twice a day and gave her heavy sweat baths daily, followed by salt glows and cold towel rubs to assist in cleansing her system and building up her general health. She took the diet and herbs as given in this book.

Now I feel sure that a good many who read this are going to come to me for help, and right here I want to say that I am not practicing, nor do I want any practice. The only way I can help anyone is through their family physician or some other practitioner.

My ambition is to give my findings to the practitioners so the people may receive the benefit of them. I have written the American Medical Association in Chicago, Illinois, and they have asked me to come to Chicago and give it to their clinic. I wrote the following letter to the National Cancer Research Institute in Washington, D.C.

> 712 18th St., N.W.
> Washington, D.C.,
> March 27, 1939

DOCTORS OF THE NATIONAL CANCER
RESEARCH INSTITUTE
WASHINGTON, D.C.

Dear Gentlemen:

Knowing that you are vitally interested in the work to which our government has called you and in which it has shown a deep interest by the large appropriation it has allowed, and realizing that the people generally are looking and watching for the National Cancer Research Institute to accomplish great things for the benefit of the many, many rapidly increasing sufferers from cancer, I am constrained to write you and tell you that I absolutely have a cancer cure that will cure any cancer which has not gone too far.

I know the cause, prevention, and cure of cancer, also of heart diseases, pneumonia, asthma, infantile paralysis, gonorrhea, syphilis, and tuberculosis. I use no poisonous drugs. What I use would harm no one, no matter what his trouble, but would benefit him. I have spent a great deal of money, much labor, and deep research in finding out these things.

I am getting along in years and do not myself want any practice. I wish to give what I have discovered to practitioners who have a license to practice. This is what I would like to do for the benefit of the Cancer Research Institute that the people of the world may have the benefit of what I have found to be a real cure.

Will you permit one or more of your research doctors who know of a cancer patient who has not been treated by radium or x-ray to let me treat this patient under their special observation by the methods which I have found successful? Thus they will see everything done for this patient and will know that a cure really can be effected by the means which I use. You may provide the patient and the patient may be kept anywhere where there are necessary facilities for treatment.

Not a few prominent citizens of this city who know of my work are urging that I write you thus. They feel sure that you will be pleased to give me this opportunity, for we all know that the government has appointed you to make every effort to find a remedy for cancer. I feel concerned that I have not done more to make public my findings. I must make them public and I would like to do it through you.

If the above terms do not meet with your approval, please advise me.

Most respectfully yours,
JETHRO KLOSS

The Cancer Research Institute doctor who answered my letter said they were not in a position to accept my offer, but they suggested that I go to some hospital that takes cancer patients or to some regular practitioner.

They asked me to write out my treatment. To do this means a great deal. Other physicians have asked me again and again to put my findings on paper, not only on cancer but on other diseases as well. One army surgeon asked if I were going to take all this knowledge with me into the grave. Because I am willing to help any physician or group of physicians in helping humanity, I an now presenting the treatments that I have found to be highly successful.

No animal experimentation is required. Nothing poisonous is used. What I use would benefit anyone.

I have been asked many times by physicians and others how I know that certain cases were cancer. My reply was that I know only what their physician said it was, and what the laboratory test showed.

In advanced cases of cancer and in other serious cases, it is necessary to have a nurse who is very thorough and persevering in her work and who understands the value of the treatment, diet, water, massage, herbs, sunshine, fresh air, exercise, and rest.

It is very hard to write out all my findings and practical experiences, but I trust I have said enough and made it plain enough so that somebody will be benefited by them.

Addendum: The preceding section on cancer was written by Jethro Kloss in the 1930s and much has been learned regarding cancer since that time.

In the 1930s stomach cancer was the most common cancer in men and the second most common cancer in women. But for some reason, the incidence of stomach cancer has been decreasing rapidly during the past several decades, so that now it is one of the less commonly encountered cancers. Cancer of the uterus, which was the most common cancer in females in the 1930s, has also been decreasing at approximately the same rate as stomach cancer. The incidence of most other cancers has stayed relatively stable during the past several decades, with one very notable exception and that is cancer of the lung. This is by far the most common cancer in men. For women, in some states it now surpasses the incidence of breast cancer. Thus, cancer in the lung is probably now the most common cancer in women, with breast and colon cancer taking the second and third places. In men, cancer of the lung is by far the most frequent, with colon and prostate cancer taking second and third places respectively. Overall, in the United States during 1988, there will be an estimated 140,000 deaths from cancer of the lung, nearly all of which can be attributed to smoking. This is nearly one-third of all deaths from cancer. Not only is smoking responsible for most cases of cancer of the lung, larynx, oral cavity, and esophagus, but it is also a contributing factor in cancer of the pancreas, kidney, and bladder, and perhaps in the uterus and stomach. Those who chew tobacco or smoke pipes or cigars also have a higher incidence of cancer in the mouth.

Smoking is also strongly linked to chronic pulmonary conditions, such as bronchitis and emphysema, and to peptic ulcers and coronary heart disease. On the average, only about nine percent of patients with lung cancer survive five or more years after the diagnosis is made. Diseases associated with smoking cost the United States taxpayer approximately $22 billion a year in medical care, $43 billion in lost productivity and cause about 350,000 deaths per year. According to the 1982 U.S. Surgeon General's Report, cigarette smoking is "the chief, single avoidable cause of death in our society and the most important public health issue of our time."

Some recent reports show that smoke that is given off from the cigarette between puffs and inhaled by nonsmokers contains substances that induce cancer. In some countries it has been found that nonsmoking wives of cigarette-smoking husbands have an increased risk for the development of lung cancer. These findings should put one on guard to avoid inhaling tobacco smoke whenever possible.

In adults, cancer is the second most common cause of death next to heart disease.

The following is quoted from a letter written by a medical

scientist to the *New York Times*. "Two radioactive isotopes, polonium-210 and lead-210, are highly concentrated in particles in cigarette smoke. The major source of polonium is the phosphate fertilizer used in growing tobacco. In a person smoking one and one-half packs of cigarettes per day, the annual radiation dose is equivalent to that of 300 x-ray films of the chest." (*DOW THEORY LETTERS 848*, November, 1982, page 5.)

One location where cancer can be prevented or cured if treated promptly is skin cancer. Approximately 400,000 cases of skin cancer occur every year in the United States and most of these are caused by frequent overexposure to sunlight. Direct exposure to the sun should be avoided if possible between about 10 a.m. and 3 p.m. when the ultraviolet rays are strongest.

If it is necessary to be in the sun during this time, protective clothing should be worn. Also there are a number of sunscreen preparations that will protect the skin from ultraviolet rays if used properly.

CANCER'S SEVEN WARNING SIGNALS

1. Change in bowel or bladder habits.
2. A sore that does not heal.
3. Unusual bleeding or discharge.
4. Thickening or lump in the breast or elsewhere.
5. Indigestion or difficulty in swallowing.
6. Obvious change in a wart or mole.
7. Nagging cough or hoarseness.

CATARRH (COMMON COLD)

Causes: There are many poor health habits that lower our resistance and thereby permit infection with the common cold virus. Among these are eating foods robbed of their life-giving properties, poor circulation, lowered vitality, lack of sunshine, fresh air and exercise, eating wrong combinations of foods, poor elimination as a result of eating too much soft food, and drinking insufficient fluids, particularly water.

Symptoms: The mucous membrane lining the inside of the nose becomes swollen and makes breathing difficult. The mucous cells in this lining membrane secrete an abundant, thick mucus. Sneezing is common. There are dryness and soreness of the throat, mouth breathing, snoring at night, frontal headaches, and impairment of hearing. The turbinate bones in the nose enlarge to such an extent at times that they completely obstruct one or both sides. This may be accompanied by nosebleed, and a dull aching pain between the eyes.

Treatment: The mucous membranes of the nose must be kept clean, for when mucus collects around the turbinate bones, it becomes putrid and causes trouble.

The first thing to do is to wash the nose out thoroughly. A safe and effective way of doing this is as follows: take a pint of soft, lukewarm water and add one teaspoonful of salt. Bend over a wash bowl, pour your hand full of this water, and sniff it up the nose. Keep repeating this until the water comes out of the mouth. Then blow the nose, holding one passage shut and then the other. Repeat this process until the nasal passage is entirely clean and no more mucus in expelled. To hold one side of the nose shut while blowing through the other has a tendency to suck the mucus out of the sinus cavities of the cheek and forehead.

After the nose passages are clean, gargle well with the salt solution to clean the throat.

Make a solution of one teaspoonful of powdered golden seal to a pint of boiling water. Let it steep for a few minutes and then pour the liquid carefully off. Add one-half teaspoonful of boric acid and sniff this up the nose in the same way as the salt water. Then gargle with this solution.

This is not only cleansing, but also soothing and healing. It is a very effective remedy when done along with other things that build up the body's strength, such as getting adequate rest, drinking abundant fluids (especially fruit juice), proper eating, outdoor exercise, proper elimination, and deep breathing.

If the nose is stopped up so that the water cannot be drawn through, practice for a few minutes what is called the "jumping-jack" exercise (see Fig. 5). I have seen a nose that would not open up otherwise do so when this exercise was done.

Attention must be given to the diet, which should be simple but nourishing. A fruit diet for a few days will do much to cleanse the system of mucus. Pineapple juice in particular is beneficial, but all fruit juices are good for this condition. A total of eight to twelve glasses of some form of liquid should be taken during the day; however, milk should be limited as it tends to produce mucus. When eating other foods, they should be taken dry and chewed thoroughly.

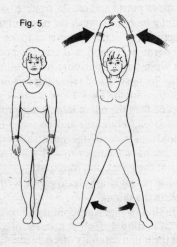

Fig. 5

The bowels must be kept open. Take one high herb enema a day for a while. This will not hurt you and will do much to cleanse the colon of mucus: bayberry bark would be suitable.

Take tonic cleansing herbs, such as black cohosh, calamus, and valerian, according to the directions in Section II, Chapter 4. Golden seal should be taken, a teaspoonful to a pint of boiling water. Let it steep, and take two or three swallows several times during the day, or take one No.00 capsule three times a day, drinking plenty of water with each dose.

Any one of the following herbs is good for this condition: lungwort, coltsfoot, jaborandi, skunk cabbage, buckthorn, wild cherry bark. Look them up in Section II, Chapter 5 and take those that are best suited to your needs.

The faithful taking of exercise, plenty of fresh air, and following other good health habits will often prevent catarrh from progressing into something more serious such as bronchitis, pneumonia, or tuberculosis. Using the salt solution for the nose and also gargling with it will help prevent the cold from going down into the lungs.

CHOLERA

Cholera is more frequent in hot climates than elsewhere. It is always present in certain sections of India and occasionally an epidemic of cholera spreads around the world.

Causes: Cholera is caused by drinking water or eating food that is contaminated with the microbe vibrio cholerae. This organism grows in the small intestine and produces a toxin that causes severe diarrhea.

Symptoms: Cholera usually begins abruptly with severe watery diarrhea.

There is usually no fever, severe abdominal cramping, or blood in the stools. If the diarrhea continues, however, muscle cramps, prostration, and kidney failure may develop.

Treatment: Treatment should be directed mainly at replacing all of the liquids and important chemical elements lost from the bowels because of the diarrhea.

With cholera, as well as with other forms of diarrhea, the patient should be kept quiet and in bed. Frequent doses of antispasmodic tincture (the formula for which is given in Section II, Chapter 3) may be taken with benefit. Take eight to fifteen drops in one-half glass of water, according to age, followed by more water if desired.

Give hot fomentations over the bowels and also to the full length of the spine.

Often there is vomiting of mucus accompanied by great pain. If this is the case, give weak peppermint tea or spearmint tea lukewarm, and drink a pint to a quart, or as much as you can possibly take. Then place the finger far down the throat until you vomit. After you have thoroughly cleansed the stomach out in this manner, drink a cupful of hot peppermint tea made strong. This will settle the stomach and relieve the distressed feeling. If the pain or vomiting of mucus returns, this can be repeated.

A weak person or an invalid might not be able to do this, in which case, give a cup or two of very hot peppermint, catnip, or camomile tea. This will relieve the stomach.

Two hours after the peppermint tea has been taken, it would be well to take a cup of golden seal, gentian, or bayberry tea. This will greatly strengthen the stomach and kill the poisons in it.

Cholera usually begins with a watery diarrhea, which may be checked at once by the use of a high enema, as hot as can be borne. Use an enema made of the following: two tablespoonfuls each of bayberry bark, white oak bark, sumach, or wild cherry. Use the granulated herbs and steep this mixture in four quarts of boiling water for thirty minutes, strain, and use.

The stools and all discharges should be disinfected or burned, as this disease is contagious. No one should touch articles used by the patient until they have been disinfected.

The best diet to use in cholera is oatmeal water, slippery elm water, which is highly nourishing, or soybean milk. (See the index for recipes.) If the diarrhea continues after these measures have been used, it may be necessary to have fluid replacement given intravenously.

CIRCULATION — TO INCREASE

Treatment: Take deep breathing exercises each morning

and evening and during the day. In the morning, a cold towel rub, followed by a thorough rubbing with a dry, coarse towel, is beneficial. Get plenty of outdoor exercise, breathing deeply while exercising. For constipation, which is one cause of poor circulation, go on an eliminating diet and use herbal laxatives as given in this book.

The following herbs are good to increase the circulation: gentian root, skullcap, colombo, rue, valerian, vervain, peppermint, catnip, spearmint. (See Section II, Chapters 3, 5, and 7 for directions).

Take African red pepper in No.1 size gelatin capsules, one capsule one hour before each meal, drinking a full glass of water or more with each capsule. This can be taken any time during the day or with other herbs. It is fine to increase the circulation; however, cayenne, as well as most other herbs, should not be taken continuously over a long period of time.

COLIC (INFANTS)

Causes: Eating too rapidly, excessive air swallowing, indigestion, improper food, constipation.

Symptoms: Sudden loud crying spells, pulling knees up on the stomach, red face, distended stomach, clenched fists.

Treatment: Warm catnip tea given in a bottle, and also a catnip tea enema will be beneficial. Spells of crying come on at regular intervals, and if a very warm bath is given an hour before the expected attack, the attack can sometimes be prevented. Have catnip tea on hand to use in an emergency.

A hot footbath or hot fomentation over the abdomen may give relief. Breast feeding is ideal; however, if the baby is fed from a bottle, dissolve wheat flakes by pouring boiling water over them, put them through a sieve, and add soybean milk to make the desired consistency. Potassium broth and oatmeal gruel (see index) are also very good for nourishment.

COLITIS

Causes: There are many causes of colitis, most of which are known, but some are unknown. Many cases of colitis are caused by infectious organisms, while others may be caused by faulty diet, constipation, improper mixtures of food that irritate the stomach and bowels, too much cane sugar and too many cane sugar products, grease, white flour, eating too hastily, too much liquid and very soft foods, taking of excessive cathartics, stress, and food cooked in aluminum utensils.

Symptoms: Running off of the bowels or constipation. Mucus passes in the feces and discharges are stringy. There is a feeling of weakness through the abdomen, at times headache, often great pain and dizziness, emaciation, weakness, and pains in various parts of the body. In severe cases of colitis, there may be severe abdominal cramps, bleeding from the rectum, and fever.

Treatment: The following treatment is very beneficial. Take a high enema made of one tablespoonful of bayberry bark to every quart of water. Yellow dock root and burdock root are also good and are very healing. Cover and let simmer for a few minutes; then steep for fifteen or twenty minutes.

After the herbs settle, pour off the tea and take it as hot as you can stand (from 100° to 108°F. — or in some cases even hotter).

Wild alum root, golden seal, or myrrh are also excellent herbs to use as an enema. Use a heaping teaspoonful of golden seal and a heaping teaspoonful of myrrh to four quarts of boiling water. Steep and let the mixture settle.

A liquid diet for a short time is advisable. When eating solid food, thoroughly chew and liquify it with saliva, drinking no liquids with meals. All roughage and foods containing skins and seeds should be avoided until the condition is better. Puree the vegetables until the condition clears up. Soybean milk, zwieback, and wheat flakes are an excellent diet for this condition.

Herbs to be taken internally: Use a teaspoonful of golden seal and one-fourth teaspoonful of myrrh to a pint of boiling water. Let it steep and take a tablespoonful of this mixture six or eight times a day. If the case is severe, take a tablespoonful every hour; or take from one-fourth to one teaspoonful, as per directions for taking herbs, one hour before each meal and upon retiring.

In places where sumach grows, a tea may be made from the bark, leaves, or berries. For an enema, take a handful of any of these in four quarts of water and steep for an hour.

CONSTIPATION

Causes: Nearly the entire human race is afflicted with constipation. Waste matter is left entirely too long in the body. Wrong diet is the main cause. Eating refined, devitalized foods that do not contain enough fiber or bulk; lack of muscular tone in the bowels; improper mastication of food; meat diet; too many varieties of food at one meal; eating food that is too concentrated; using coffee, tea, and liquor of all kinds; irregular habits of attending to the calls of nature; sedentary life and lack of exercise are other contributing factors to this almost universal ailment.

Constipation, diverticulosis, and cancer of the colon are all prevalent diseases in North America and European countries where the diet contains large amounts of refined foods and is low in bulk. In Africa, where the diet contains large amounts of bulk, these diseases of the colon are rarely found. The life-giving properties that would aid digestion are removed from the foods we eat or are spoiled by improper cooking and wrong combinations.

Excessive use of drugs and patent medicines is a frequent cause of constipation, tumors, etc.

Symptoms: Coated tongue, foul breath, backache, headache, mental dullness, depression, insomnia, loss of appetite, and various pains.

Treatment: Regulate the diet. Take high enemas of red raspberry leaves, wild cherry bark or leaves, or bayberry bark, using one heaping teaspoonful to a quart of water. This is a very good disinfectant and stimulant to bring back the normal peristaltic action of the colon. Take an enema every evening until the bowels are moving normally by themselves.

Eat your food as dry as possible. When food is eaten dry and thoroughly saturated with saliva, it is a wonderful help to lubricate the bowels. It will make the system alkaline and will greatly increase the rapidity of digestion.

Do your drinking one hour before or two or three hours after eating. Drinking with meals is very harmful. No liquid of any kind should be taken with the meals. Eat freely of fresh and stewed fruits, apples, figs, peaches, oranges, bananas, and blueberries, selecting the fruits that agree best with you. But don't forget, it is best not to eat fruits and vegetables at the same meal.

Get plenty of outdoor exercise with deep breathing, brisk walking, golf, horseback riding, rowing, bicycling, tennis, or swimming. Practice deep breathing while walking, and in the morning before getting up, lie on your back, knees flexed, and pant, breathing in short rapid gasps. Roll on your right side, stomach, and left side, and continue panting. This exercise massages the bowels.

The number of bowel movements per day varies greatly from person to person. It may be normal for an individual to have one bowel movement per day, while in others, two or three times a day may be normal. Food should digest readily and the waste matter be eliminated from the body without undue delay. If it stays too long in the colon, peristaltic action may be decreased. Look in the index for the recipes for bran water and oatmeal water. These two products, which may be used in many food stuffs and in baking, are an effective means of making the bowels active. Oat bran is also very effective in correcting this problem.

Plenty of baths and massage to the abdomen are also excellent aids in overcoming constipation. A happy mental attitude is very helpful.

The following is an excellent formula for a laxative: mix thoroughly one tablespoon each of mandrake, buckthorn bark, rhubarb root, fennel seed, and calamus root, and one teaspoonful of aloes. This is a real body cleanser. Mandrake is one of the finest herbs to cleanse the liver. If powdered, take one-fourth teaspoonful in a half glass of cold water followed by a glass of hot water. This can be taken after meals or upon retiring. Take more or less than the one-fourth teaspoonful according to your individual needs.

Another laxative herb formula that is very good is this: mix thoroughly one ounce mandrake root, one ounce cascara sagrada bark, one ounce buckthorn bark, one ounce fennel seed, one ounce calamus root, and one-fourth ounce aloes. Putting this mixture through a fine sieve is a good way to mix it thoroughly. The above herbs are available in powdered form. Take one-fourth teaspoonful or one No.00 capsule with one glass or more of hot water upon retiring. Increase or decrease the amount taken so as to keep the bowels moving normally.

Moderate exercise after meals is very helpful. Never lie down or go to sleep immediately after meals. Practice deep breathing just before and right after eating. The oxygen that is gained is one of the greatest factors in helping digest your food and in making good red blood. It is impossible to get the full benefit of your food without exercise.

Plenty of liquids are imperative in the treatment of constipation. Try to drink six to eight glasses of water or fruit juice a day, and be sure the diet contains an abundance of fiber and bulk-forming foods.

CONVULSIONS, SEIZURES, OR SPASMS

Causes: Infants and children are most frequently affected and in most of the cases the cause is not known. Sometimes the seizure will occur with the beginning of a fever. This may indicate the beginning of a severe illness, such as meningitis or encephalitis, or it may indicate the onset of one of the infectious diseases, such as measles or whooping cough. Other less frequent causes include rickets, teething, indigestion, worms, brain congestion, and eating some articles of food, such as candy, ice cream, cake, pies, meat and gravy, and heavy indigestible foods. Undernourished, nervous children with emotional problems are apt to be troubled with seizures. Children of this type should be given plenty of fresh air, sunlight, nourishing food, and emotional support in the home.

Symptoms: The child straightens out and becomes stiff. Many times the back is arched and there may be twitching or spasms of the extremities. Breathing seems to stop and the eyes are fixed and staring or turned upwards. The head is drawn back. Several severe attacks in succession are dangerous, and the child may never awaken. It is reassuring, however, to know that death seldom results from convulsions, unless the child is very weak. The convulsion may come on suddenly and without warning. If the child is old enough to talk, he may be able to tell when a convulsion is coming on, or if the child is very young, there may be a behavioral change. There may be difficulty in breathing, with frothing at the mouth. Often the extremities are cold and the child usually becomes unconscious. The seizure may last from a few seconds to nearly an hour.

If a child is disturbed during the night and grits his teeth and rubs his nose, it may be a sign of worms. If these signs are not very prominent and yet the child is not well, it would not be amiss to give the worm treatment (see Worms, following in this Section), as this would be very beneficial to the system and does no harm.

Treatment: The first thing to do is to loosen the clothing and give plenty of fresh air. Place a tongue blade wrapped with cloth between the teeth to prevent the child from biting the tongue. Put the child in a full bath at 100 F. and increase the heat by adding hot water. Wring a towel out of cold water and put around the neck and on the head. If the gums are hot and swollen, give cold water and rub them with a cloth that has been held on ice. Keep the child in the bath from ten to twenty minutes, as may seem best. Dry thoroughly, wrap in a warm blanket, put into bed, keep quiet, and give plenty of fresh air. If the child goes to sleep, let it sleep as long as it will.

If the child is constipated, give immediately a warm enema of catnip tea, made by putting a heaping teaspoonful of catnip in a quart of boiling water. Let it steep for fifteen minutes, strain, cool to a tepid temperature, and use. Keep the bowels rather loose. If catnip is not at hand, give a warm water enema, giving as much as the child can hold.

Always have antispasmodic tincture on hand. The recipe is given in Section II, Chapter 3. The dose for children is 5 to 8 drops in a tablespoonful of water, according to age. Follow by drinking more water. The herbs may be sweetened with a little malt honey, honey, or malt sugar to make them more palatable.

For nourishment, give potassium broth (see index), fruit juices of all kinds, and oatmeal gruel, to which some soybean milk has been added. After serving a liquid diet for two or three days, give vegetable puree, mashed potatoes, and baked potatoes. A light nourishing diet is best for some time, as often a too-rich diet is to blame for the convulsions.

If there are no further convulsions after the child has had the first one; if all solid food is withheld for a few days and the child is given plenty of catnip tea and warm catnip enemas; and if the bowels are kept regular and the worm treatment is given; there may not be a recurrence.

The same treatment applies to adults. Often, if the convulsion is very severe, the antispasmodic tincture will stop it at once. The dose for adults is fifteen drops to one teaspoonful in a glass of warm water. This may be repeated as often as necessary.

If seizures continue, a serious underlying disorder may be present and appropriate medical help should be obtained.

COUGHS AND COLDS

Causes: A cough is caused by inflammation of the throat

and bronchial tubes. This inflammation causes mucus to form, which the system tries to expel by coughing. The vitality of the system has been lowered by improper diet, loss of sleep, lack of exercise and fresh air, and improper elimination. If the stomach and entire body were kept in good condition, there would be but few colds. Improper clothing and bedding at night are often causes of colds. The poisons and waste matter in the body make one more susceptible. If the system were kept in good health and the powers of resistance good, coughs and colds would be rare.

Treatment: A cold can be treated and overcome in just one day. When the first symptoms of a cold, influenza, or cough appear, it is an indication that there is waste matter and mucus in the system. Take a pint of soft warm water and add a teaspoonful of salt. Sniff this up the nose and then blow it out. Repeat this until the nose is entirely free of mucus. Then gargle and rinse the mouth out thoroughly. After the nose is clean, take one of the good herbs such as golden seal, peppermint, hyssop, yarrow, or black cohosh, sniff it up through the nose, and then gargle, swallowing some of it. This helps to prevent the cold from developing into bronchitis, asthma, pneumonia, or maybe even tuberculosis. Whenever there is a cold, the first precaution is to keep the nose and mouth clean. This will keep the infection from going down into the lungs and causing further trouble.

When the head is stuffed up and there is tightness in the chest, as well as an irritable, drowsy, stupid feeling, we sometimes hear people say, "My head is all stuffed up," but the fact is that they are aware of it only in their head. The whole system is involved. Anything we can do to relieve this condition in the system will help break up the cold.

Colds would not be so prevalent if the body were not filled with mucus and waste products, so one should immediately rid the body of these poisons. There is no better way to do this than to cleanse the entire colon by high enemas, continuing them until they reach the upper end of the colon and get it clean.

Keep quiet and stay in bed if possible. Take only fruit juices for nourishment. If you do not have fruit juices, drink water (hot or cold) with lemon juice, then later potassium broth (see index), which is nourishing and alkaline. This treatment will break up the cold.

If the cough continues, an excellent help is to take one teaspoonful each of colt's foot, black cohosh, and cubeb berries, mix thoroughly and steep in a pint of boiling water. Take a glassful every hour according to age. Also see the herbal syrups given in Section II, Chapter 3.

Occasionally there may be a feeling of severe nausea. If this is the case, take an emetic. This can be done with just lukewarm water or water with a little salt added. Drink all the water possible and run the finger down the throat to promote vomiting. This will wash the stomach out. Repeat this until the stomach is clean and then take a hot herb tea. Several cups of hot tea should be taken immediately, followed by two or three cups a few hours later. The following herbs are excellent: Sage, red sage, hyssop, yarrow, black cohosh, peppermint, and camomile. The use of one rounded teaspoonful of composition powder in a glass of water every hour for five or six hours is also excellent.

CROUP

Causes: Croup is caused by an inflammation of the larynx or "voice box." Overeating may cause symptoms that resemble croup. This is caused by overloading the system with food, which makes it very easy to catch cold. The fermentation in the stomach causes phlegm, which in turn causes coughing and choking spells. These same symptoms may also be caused by worms.

Symptoms: Croup is most often seen in children under five years of age. Although a high fever may be present, the temperature may be normal or only slightly elevated. The child's face is flushed and the eyes may be bloodshot. The attacks are usually much worse at night. The child is awakened by a hard spasmodic barking cough and the attacks last anywhere from fifteen minutes to several hours. These attacks may occur several times during the night. The child seems unable to get his breath and it may seem that he is strangling. It is particularly difficult for the child to take in a breath, and a whistling sound may be heard. There is usually no difficulty in breathing out. In struggling to breath, the child often sits up.

Treatment: The most important part of the treatment for croup is to have the child breath warm, moist air. This can be done by forming a croup tent, by draping a sheet and blanket over the crib and directing the moist vapor from a croup kettle into the tent. Constant attention must be given so the child is not burned by the condensation of the hot steam. Make a tea of equal parts of cubeb berries, horehound, and lobelia. Put it in the croup kettle, letting it steam so that the child will inhale the vapor. This will many times give immediate relief. If this is done before the child goes to sleep and is continued during sleep, it will sometimes prevent him from having an attack during the night. When the child is very ill, he must be kept in bed in a warm well-ventilated room, away from drafts.

During the day if the child is peevish, an attack can be modified or prevented by a warm bath or hot footbath. Vick's Vaporub rubbed on the chest, throat, and back is helpful. It can be obtained almost anywhere. The child must be watched at night and kept warm and well covered. Give a catnip tea enema and then keep the bowels open with laxative herbs given in proportion to the age. Take a teaspoon of senna pods or granulated senna, coltsfoot, horehound, white cherry bark, cubeb berries, or black cohosh and mix these well together. Take one teaspoonful to a cup of boiling water, let steep one-half hour, then give the child a tablespoonful every hour until the bowels move naturally. (If you do not have all of these herbs, use senna with cubeb berries.) This mixture will cut the phlegm and relieve spasm in the throat.

Give a prolonged hot bath, but be sure that the child does

not go out and catch more cold afterwards. Give a thorough rubbing with oil of some kind, such as olive oil or cocoa fat, as a good preventive against catching more cold.

Hot and cold applications to the chest and neck often bring speedy relief. Antispasmodic tincture (given in Section II, Chapter 3), can be applied to the throat as a liniment and will give relief. This can be taken internally: three or four drops to a teaspoonful of water for infants, and increasing the dose for older children. Give every fifteen minutes if necessary.

Diet: The child's diet should be regulated. Give a fruit diet for a few days consisting of baked apples, pineapple juice, grape juice, or orange juice. There is nothing that is more nourishing or better than soybean milk, either with toast or whole wheat flakes. This is very easily digested. If cow's milk is used at all, boil a little oatmeal in it and strain. For young infants about five or six months old, dissolve four tablespoonfuls of whole wheat flakes in a little hot water and add either soybean milk or cow's milk. This will keep the child from losing weight and strength. Potassium broth is excellent. It is nourishing and will cleanse the entire system.

DELIRIUM TREMENS

Causes: Habitual intoxication with alcohol.

Symptoms: Loss of appetite, nausea, vomiting, feeble and rapid pulse, wild expression on the face, delusions, fright because of horrible fancies, such as snakes. It is sometimes hard to control the patient who is full of such fears. When the patient is very violent, it takes two strong persons to take care of him. In such a case, the patient must be shut in where he cannot do himself or anyone else harm. Sometimes patients have convulsions, talk incessantly, and are not able to sleep. These symptoms usually begin two to three days after the end of a drinking bout. Nearly all cases have associated stomach disorders and poor elimination.

Treatment: Place the patient in a lukewarm bath and keep him there as long as possible — two or three hours or more.

While he is still in the bath, give him hot drinks of soothing, quieting herb tea, such as tea made from the following: valerian, gentian, catnip, peppermint, spearmint, calamus root, sweet balm, skullcap. Do not make the tea too strong. Use a small teaspoonful of herbs to a cup of water. Keep the head cool with towels wrung out of cold water. Put these around the neck and on the head. Give either a shower or sponge bath, short and cold, several times during the bath. Just before finishing, give a good brisk salt glow. Put the patient in the warm water afterwards, letting him become thoroughly warmed and then give the final cold shower or rub. Dry thoroughly, rubbing vigorously with a rough Turkish towel and put him to bed.

To destroy the taste for liquor, give quassia chips, skullcap, and cayenne. Take a teaspoonful of hops to a cup of boiling water with a little lobelia added, steep, strain, and give this hot. It will prove very quieting and produce sleep. Give more than one cup if necessary.

Take a teaspoonful of golden seal steeped in a pint of boiling water, strain, and give two or three swallows four or five times during the day. This will be very beneficial to the stomach.

Give a light nourishing diet. The stomach is usually in such poor condition that it cannot retain much food at a time and digest it. It is best to give a liquid diet for a while, such as oatmeal water, potassium broth, soybean milk, and fruit juices.

Take the patient out in the open air for exercise and have him practice deep breathing. For violent cases of this kind, when they are treated at home, tie the hands and feet with wide bandages made of towels or sheets. There is also a restraint called a "straightjacket" that may be used. Kind, gentle treatment and soothing words will help a great deal to hasten a speedy cure. You will absolutely have success if this treatment is strictly followed.

Select one or more of the following herbs and take as directed: antispasmodic tincture (for quick relief), valerian, black cohosh, quassia chips, hyssop, lady's slipper, skullcap, lobelia, mistletoe, wood betony, vervain, motherwort, hops.

If there is a problem with elimination, give a high herbal enema or use an herbal laxative as given in Section II, Chapter 3.

DIABETES

Causes: Diabetes is essentially a disease of degeneration of some part of the digestive tract, nearly always the pancreas. When the pancreas fails to function normally and does not produce enough insulin, you have diabetes. Call on your family physician for an examination and diagnosis. In diabetes mellitus, when starchy foods are broken down to sugar in the body, the pancreas is unable to rid the system of the excess sugar.

Most people know that diabetes has something to do with the function of a large gland called the pancreas, which lies just behind the stomach. However, from study and research into the cause of diabetes, it has been found that failure of the pancreas to function normally is not the only cause for this condition. Another, but less common, cause of diabetes in some persons is obesity caused by eating an unbalanced diet, consisting largely of sugars, fats, and starches, prepared so as to delight the eye and palate, but which are to a great extent denatured (refined). The greater part of the food, as eaten by the majority of people from day to day, is denatured in one way or another.

Resulting from a large consumption of meat, sugar, white flour products, etc., diabetes has become a common disease in the United States. Diabetes will continue to increase as long as people partake of artificial sweets, white flour products, tea, coffee, tobacco, liquor, Coca Cola, soft drinks, and all denatured food and harmful drinks.

Many of the food preparations that are used daily are prepared with baking powder and soda. Soda decreases the activity of the pancreatic juices. These juices are used in the body to digest protein, fat, and carbohydrates. The pancreas is one of the most important organs of digestion.

Symptoms: Constant hunger, frequent urination, great thirst, progressive weakness, loss of flesh, inordinate appetite, mental depression, dyspepsia, and a dry red tongue. The patient is irritable, restless, and morose. Not all these symptoms are present in every case.

Treatment: There is no known remedy for diabetes. Generally, there is some colon trouble; therefore, using either powdered burdock root, yellow dock root, or bayberry bark, a high enema should be taken to help cleanse and heal the colon. Pour four quarts of boiling water over one tablespoonful of the powdered herb, stir thoroughly and use when cool enough. Daily hot baths followed by cold towel rubs are very beneficial. For best results, take the enema before the bath. Lying in a tub of hot water for one-half hour to two hours will greatly help to eliminate the sugar and waste matter from the system. Excellent results are obtained in diabetes by having the water as hot as the patient can comfortably stand, and have him drink a hot tea while in the tub, made either from red raspberry leaves, blueberry leaves, dandelion root, or pleurisy root. Raise the patient up when he feels too warm or if there is slight palpitation of the heart, and sponge off with cool water. If you have a shower bath, have the patient stand and shower off with cool water, getting right back into the hot water. Repeat a number of times, then finish with a cool shower and vigorous towel rub.

A salt glow is very beneficial. I recommend this highly, as it will increase the circulation and remove the old dead skin from the body so that the pores are open and the skin is more active. Much of the poison in the system will escape through the skin. A general massage after the bath is very restful and beneficial, as it also helps the circulation. When massaging, always stroke towards the heart.

Fomentations should be applied to the spine, stomach, liver, spleen, and pancreas daily. Do not fail to take a cold bath upon arising, thoroughly rubbing the body with a cold wet towel, and then vigorously with a dry towel.

The bowels should be kept loose with one to three good

eliminations every day. Do not take harsh cathartics. Use an herbal laxative compound as given in Section II, Chapter 3, or other laxative herbs.

Diet: The general health must be improved if the patient expects to keep the diabetes under control. Correct the diet, which is one cause of diabetes. The food question is an important item to be considered in the treatment of this disease. There are many herbs which have medicinal properties that can be used and will greatly aid the vegetables and fruits in supplying the needed alkaline elements for the body. All foods that can be enjoyed in their natural state are best adapted for normal nutrition.

Meat of all kinds must be excluded from the diet. Milk and eggs should be reduced to a minimum. Stimulating foods are strictly forbidden, as well as such foods as oysters, chickens, clams, crabs, etc. Avoid all starches and sugars, except natural sweets such as juices of ripe fruit.

Bran, oatmeal, and slippery elm water are very beneficial in diabetes. A very wholesome dish, that is high in life-giving properties and is also an alkaline food, is the soybean. Prepare by using soybeans that have been sprouted a half inch or more, boil until tender, and then place in a baking dish and bake a little. Flavor with vegetable extract, onions, garlic, or tomatoes to suit the taste.

The following list of foods is very good in diabetes: Greens of all kinds, Chinese cabbage, red cabbage, cauliflower, watercress, cucumbers, okra, brussel sprouts, asparagus, onions (baked or boiled), sprouted lentils, peas (tender and young), ripe olives, lettuce, beets and tops (tender, young), string beans, carrots, carrot juice, celery, spinach, eggplant, radishes, endive, parsnips, sprouted lima beans, green corn (very tender), soybean milk, soybean cottage cheese, whole wheat, zwieback, buttermilk, cream, baked Irish potatoes, coconut milk, peanuts, almonds, walnuts, pecans, and Brazil nuts. Do not eat roasted peanuts or peanut butter made from roasted peanuts. Raw peanuts and butter made from them is good. Avocados are excellent in diabetes. When thoroughly ripe, they are almost a specific.

Use all kinds of fresh fruits that are ripened in the sun, such as strawberries, oranges, apricots, currants, blueberries, peaches, pears, pineapples, apples, lemons, red raspberries, huckleberries, grapefruit, cherries, and limes.

Fruits should never be sweetened with sugar. Cane sugar, raw or natural brown sugar, and all sugar syrups are harmful. The natural sugar contained in grapes and other fruits is beneficial. A small amount of malt sugar may be used.

Never eat fruits and vegetables at the same meal. Eat as many raw fruits and vegetables as possible. Those requiring cooking should not be cooked more than just enough to make them palatable. It is best to steam or bake vegetables, but when boiled, boil them in as little water as possible so there will not be any to throw away.

Your tender beet tops and young tender beets are very desirable. The full-grown beets or old beets contain an excessive amount of sugar and should not be eaten by diabetics.

Deep breathing and as much vigorous outdoor exercise as the condition of the patient will permit must be taken.

Blueberry leaves, red root, and dandelion root tea are especially beneficial in diabetes.

The following list of herbs is helpful and beneficial in diabetes. Study them separately and use one or a combination of several that best suit your needs. Beech, blue cohosh, golden seal, white pine, poplar, queen of the meadow, saw palmetto berries, sumach berries, uva ursi, wild alum root, wintergreen, yarrow, buchu (in first stages of diabetes), dandelion root (especially good), white pine combined with uva ursi, equal parts of marshmallow and poplar bark, raspberry leaves (very good), and pleurisy root. If the kidneys or nerves are affected, use one of the following herbs: cornsilk, cubeb berries, fennel, skullcap, wild cherry bark, and nerve root.

Addendum: Many new and important discoveries have been made in regards to the cause and treatment of diabetes since the preceding section was first written by Jethro Kloss in the 1930s. While diabetes mellitus has many different causes, they all share an intolerance to glucose (sugar) as a major feature. It has been estimated that up to five percent of the American population will at some time be affected with diabetes. While eating a special diet remains the mainstay of the proper treatment of diabetes, some patients with more severe diabetes will require additional help in the form of insulin injections, or medicine given orally, to control the amount of glucose in the blood and urine. It is very important for obese persons to lose weight. Because of the severe complications that commonly occur in diabetics, it is extremely important that this disease be kept under proper control. These complications occur earlier and with greater frequency and severity if diabetes is not controlled properly. Some of these complications are: an increased incidence of coronary artery disease and strokes, gangrene and infection in the feet due to poor circulation, cataracts, kidney disease and high blood pressure, various neurological diseases, poor digestion, and various skin diseases. Because of the prevalence and seriousness of this disease and the need for constant monitoring and control of the sugar in the blood and urine, qualified medical advice is recommended.

DIPHTHERIA

Because of mass immunization in the United States, this dreaded disease in not nearly as common now as it once was. It is most common in children about two to six years of age. It is a contagious disease affecting the throat and upper air passages. The first thing to do is to call your family doctor, as this is a life-threatening disease.

Causes: Diphtheria is an acute infectious disease caused by specific bacteria. It is spread by intimate contact with someone who has the disease. Some people who have no symptoms may also be carriers of this disease and spread it to others. Many cases of acute sore throat and acute tonsillitis are mistaken for diphtheria and vice versa. A "sore throat," when persistent and improperly treated, is sometimes later found to be diphtheria. Impure blood, unhygienic measures, contaminated milk and foods, and excessive starchy diet may be contributing factors.

Symptoms: Chills, fever, sore throat, headache, difficulty swallowing, foul breath, and sometimes nausea, vomiting, and diarrhea are the primary symptoms. There may be associated headache, weakness, listlessness, and rapid heart. Children usually complain first of being tired and sleepy. The tonsils appear inflamed, dark red, unevenly swollen and covered with white patches that look like parchment. The glands of the neck swell in most cases. The tenacious membrane in the throat and on the tonsils spreads very rapidly unless checked. The membrane may appear yellow or greenish, but it does not always look the same. In severe cases, it is gangrenous. In a very short time, if nothing is done, this membrane will spread to cover the back of the throat and the entire cavity of the mouth. When it spreads down into the air passages it causes difficulty in breathing, and the patient has a frightened look. If there are no white patches or exudation, the disease is probably not diphtheria.

Treatment: The most important points to remember in the treatment of diphtheria are isolation of the patient, strict bed rest, and the early use of diphtheria antitoxin.

If you have a sore throat of any kind, whether there is any danger or not of its being diphtheria, the treatment given below may be used with benefit. Do not wait until the actual symptoms have developed.

Steep one teaspoonful of powdered golden seal and one teaspoonful of powdered myrrh with a pinch of cayenne in a pint of boiling water for one-half hour. Gargle and swab the throat thoroughly with this solution. It will kill the poisons that are there. Do this until you have the throat clean. A hot fomentation to the throat, followed by a cold compress, will give great relief.

Thoroughly saturate the neck and spine with the liniment given in Section II, Chapter 3. Take ten or twelve drops of antispasmodic tincture in a glass of water five or six times a day, or every ten or fifteen minutes if the case is severe. A hot tub bath or sitz bath is a very valuable measure.

The patient must be in a well-ventilated room, but must be kept warm until the most serious stage of the disease is over.

Diphtheria is a very serious disease, particularly in its more severe forms. Without proper treatment, up to ninety percent of patients may die with severe diphtheria. If proper medical treatment is not available, no time should be lost in giving the treatment as outlined in this book. This treatment should be continuous until the patient has recovered.

If there is any problem with constipation, herbal enemas or laxatives should be given to keep the bowels moving freely. Use either bayberry bark or red raspberry leaf tea.

If an emetic is needed, I have used bayberry bark and lobelia with splendid results. Bayberry bark and lobelia clean off the mucous membranes. After you have vomited once, it must be repeated until the stomach and throat are entirely clean. Treat children the same way, using only about one-half the amount of the tea that you would use for adults. Bayberry not only cleans the mucous membranes, but it also is stimulating, so that the poisonous exudation can be thrown off. It is also healing and antiseptic. It is also good to add a little capsicum or ginger to the bayberry, as these are both excellent stimulants.

Sleepiness is not a good sign. Always give the emetic and stimulating herbs with the enema before you allow either a child or an adult to sleep, if you wish to save them. After the throat and colon have been thoroughly cleansed and the patient has been given at least three cups of prickly ash bark tea, if there is wheezing or choking during sleep, wake the patient up and give a dose of red raspberry tea and bayberry. Also give fresh or unsweetened pineapple juice.

Red clover, yellow dock, sweet flag, prickly ash berries, golden seal, myrrh, and jaborandi are also excellent to take internally. Use only liquids such as fruit juices until the patient is well cleaned out, the exudation has stopped, and the throat is clean.

When the patient begins to recuperate, the following diet may be used: baked apples, potassium broth, soybean milk, fresh fruits and vegetables (properly cooked).

DROPSY

Causes: Dropsy (edema) is an accumulation of fluid in the cellular tissues or in any of the cavities of the body, such as the chest or abdomen, and it may be due to disease of the heart, lungs, liver, or kidneys. Anything that will cause the blood to become poisoned or the red corpuscles to die may result in dropsy. In most cases, it is caused by a crippled heart. Sometimes the liver and gallbladder are so diseased and inflamed that they will not function normally and a dropsical condition will arise, causing the abdominal cavity to fill with fluid. It may be that the kidneys are the cause, as is the case in Bright's disease when the kidneys do not function properly, and dropsy results. Tumors in the abdomen may irritate the lining membrane (peritoneum), causing it to produce a large amount of fluid that results in a large, swollen abdomen.

Treatment: Generally a complete change should be made in the diet, leaving off all alcoholic drinks, cocoa, chocolate, tea, coffee, Coca Cola, and other such drinks. No flesh foods, pies, cakes, or rich pastries should be indulged in. All foods should be eaten as dry as possible, thereby causing the patient to chew his food thoroughly. No fluids should be taken with the meals, but water can be taken one hour after meals. Do not use any salt. Fruits or tomatoes should occupy a large part of the diet. One vegetable meal a day (preferably at noon), should compose the diet of all patients. It is best to avoid eating fruits and vegetables at the same meal. Sprouted lentils and sprouted soybeans are very good, as well as all of the soybean preparations mentioned in this book. Eat freely of vegetables, such as eggplant, young beets, parsley, celery, okra, kale, asparagus, collards, mustard, lettuce, spinach, parsnips, onions, cucumbers, watercress, pumpkin, potatoes, peas, yellow corn, Swiss chard, cauliflower, endive, fresh beans, and peas.

Fresh grapes should be eaten freely in season. Thoroughly ripe bananas may be eaten often. Nuts or nut preparations can help to take the place of meat. Coconut is also good. If a patient cannot take the whole coconut, the coconut milk is excellent. Whole wheat zwieback should be eaten instead of fresh bread. Never eat bread made with soda or baking powder.

Drink plenty of water and fruit juices to flush the kidneys and bladder. A hot bath daily (preferably at night) to produce perspiration will help rid the body of impurities. Cold morning baths and washing the limbs and abdomen two or three times a day with cold water are also very beneficial.

Drinking plenty of herb tea made of red raspberry or pleurisy root will produce perspiration. If the herbs are in powdered form, take a half- teaspoonful in one cup of boiling water. Let it steep thirty minutes and drink; or the powder may be taken in capsules four to six times a day. An excellent herb combination for this purpose is one-half teaspoonful each of wild yam and black cohosh, with a pinch of cayenne pepper, to a cup of water. Keep the bowels active so that they move one to three times a day by using the herbal laxatives as given in Section II, Chapter 3. A tea made of the following may be taken freely with benefit, as much as four to six cups a day: wild carrot (blossoms or seeds, ground), dandelion root, yarrow, burdock root, queen of the meadow, dwarf elder, and broom. You may use equal parts of these herbs, adding one teaspoonful of the mixture to a cup of boiling water, and steeping for twenty or thirty minutes.

Burdock and broom make a good combination. They are also prepared in the same way. Dwarf elder is especially good since it cleanses the kidneys.

The following remedy has been known to cure dropsy many times: take grapevine root and burn to ashes. Use one dessert-spoonful of these ashes in a glass of water three or four times a day, always drinking plenty of water with it. The inner bark of the vine is good too, prepared in the same way.

Frequent bathing in the ocean is very helpful for dropsy.

If one cannot do this, take one pound of Epsom salts and one pound of table salt and add these to your bath.

Wild carrot, which grows so abundantly in many of the states of the United States, has been known to cure dropsy, together with the proper diet, after leaving off the harmful drinks, food, and habits.

Since dropsy is actually not a disease in itself, but merely a reflection of some trouble in another organ, such as the heart or kidneys, the cause for the dropsy should be determined and proper treatment directed to this cause.

DYSENTERY (DIARRHEA) OR SUMMER COMPLAINT

Causes: Inflammation of the rectum and large intestine, insufficient foods, improper diet, drinking too much liquid with meals, overeating, wrong combinations of foods, stimulating foods, liquor, tea, coffee, drinking impure water, unhygienic surroundings, eating fruits or vegetables that have begun to decompose, eating foods that have been standing in pantries that are not well ventilated, and eating improperly refrigerated, contaminated foods. Irritable bowels, habitual constipation, and taking certain types of medicine, such as laxatives, may also be the cause.

Mild Symptoms: Frequent, small, and painful passages from the bowels, or the passage of mucus streaked with blood. A constant desire to evacuate the bowels. Great straining. More or less fever, loss of appetite, sleeplessness, and restless at night. Sometimes the abdomen is distended.

Severe Symptoms: Increasing fever, great thirst, red tongue, the abdomen may appear sunken in some cases, straining ceases, and the bowels become relaxed and may protrude. Passage of urine is infrequent and is accompanied by a burning sensation. The pulse becomes slow, breathing is rapid, and generally the patient looks pale and emaciated. Do not let this condition continue. Give the following treatment in either mild or severe cases and good results will be obtained.

Treatment: The patient should be put to bed. Take equal amounts of slippery elm, lady's slipper, gentian, wild yam, bayberry bark, and skullcap. Mix thoroughly. Use a heaping teaspoonful to a cup of boiling water; steep one-half hour; drink a half cupful every half hour until relieved; then take three or four cups a day. The addition of calamus root will prevent griping, fermentation, and gas. These herbs can usually be obtained in either powder or capsule form, which makes their administration quite easy.

Another excellent combination of herbs is equal parts of red raspberry and witch hazel leaves. If the kidneys are affected, add peach leaves. Mix thoroughly together. Use a heaping teaspoonful to a quart of boiling water and drink four or five cups a day as hot as possible.

The diet must be light. Use potassium broth, soybean milk, or oatmeal milk, and drink at least a pint a day of slippery elm water and barley water. Whole wheat flakes can be completely dissolved in soybean milk: a diet of this is most nourishing and highly alkaline. It contains all the elements the system requires. For solid foods, see Section V, Chapter 11. Chew your food thoroughly, until it is a cream, before swallowing.

Give hot fomentations to the abdomen and spine, continuing for half an hour. If the case is severe, repeat three or four times a day. These are indispensable.

The herbal liniment, as given in Section II, Chapter 3, when thoroughly applied to the abdomen and spine after the fomentations, is excellent.

Give a high enema, using either white oak bark, bayberry bark, or wild alum root tea. All of these act as an astringent. Give the enema as hot as the patient can tolerate without burning. This will usually be between 102° and 108° F. It may be hard to retain the tea at this temperature, but it will give great relief.

DYSPEPSIA (SOUR STOMACH)

Causes: Nonnourishing and devitaminized food, such as white flour and cane sugar products and polished rice, eating too many soft foods, drinking with meals, hasty eating, eating or drinking shortly before retiring, irregular meals, highly seasoned foods, improper mastication, iced tea, coffee, all iced drinks, overeating. People who lead a sedentary life need plenty of outdoor exercise and deep breathing, and should obtain a proper amount of rest.

Symptoms: Heartburn, headache, pain in the chest, heaviness in the stomach, irregularity of bowels, cold feet, weak pulse, general prostration in chronic cases, irritability, nausea, bloating, and gas. In long-standing cases, there may be a hacking cough, intermittent fever at times, or palpitation of the heart.

Treatment: The herbs listed below will prove soothing and add tone to the system. Any one, two, or three of them may be used together and will be of great advantage in treating dyspepsia.

tansy	gentian root	thyme
wild cherry	boneset	summer savory
origanum	buckbean	yarrow
magnolia	horehound	golden seal
sweet flag	quassia	white oak
masterwort	spearmint	peach leaves
golden thread	wahoo	myrrh

The taking of soda and magnesium is very injurious. The antispasmodic tincture, also discussed in Section II, Chapter 3, given in a dose of eight to ten drops in a glass of water, will give relief. Golden seal, taken one-quarter of a teaspoonful to a glass of water an hour before meals, will help the digestion greatly; or a teaspoonful of it can be steeped in a pint of boiling water. Drink one-half cupful an hour before meals. A cup of skullcap or gentian tea taken every three hours will prove most beneficial, since many cases of dyspepsia are primarily caused by nervous troubles.

When overeating is the cause, a mild emetic to empty the stomach will often bring immediate relief. This can be done by drinking as much warm water with a little salt in it as the stomach can hold. Put the finger down the throat after drinking the water and you will be surprised at the matter that comes up. You will not have to strain if plenty of water is taken.

Diet: The old idea of starving dyspepsia is a wrong one. Ordinarily dyspeptics should eat more than the usual amount of food, but it should be light, nourishing, and easy to digest, so as to give plenty of nourishment and not burden the stomach. Quick elimination is essential. The following foods are recommended: whole wheat zwieback, mashed potatoes (as given in Section V, Chapter 2), soybean cottage cheese, asparagus, tender corn, cauliflower, eggplant, a good grade of string beans, tender canned peas (if the fresh cannot be obtained), spinach, lettuce (the curly head or leaf lettuce is better than the iceburg lettuce). Vegetables are best baked. Season a little with soybean butter. Crisp whole wheat or bran crackers are good. If raw vegetables, such as spinach, lettuce, and celery do not agree with you, do not eat them; for in this kind of diet, you obtain all of the vitamins that are needed. Bran muffins, soybean muffins, and potassium broth are excellent for a weak stomach. Masticate your food thoroughly. Never eat in a hurry, but eat regularly with no late meals. If you are hungry before retiring, drink fruit juice, hot soybean milk, or soybean coffee. Don't forget, however, that it is best not to eat or drink anything for several hours before retiring. Be happy, relax at mealtime, and avoid nervous tension.

EAR TROUBLE

Causes: Earaches are usually caused by colds, tonsillitis, or influenza; but sometimes by other less common diseases such as measles, erysipelas, smallpox, diphtheria, scarlet fever, or typhoid fever.

Symptoms: When the ear becomes red or swollen on the inside, it is a sign of inflammation. There may be a sensation of fullness or ringing in the ears. When an infant or young child pulls at his ears, he may have an earache.

Treatment: Whatever the cause, earache can be relieved by the application of heat over the ear and around the neck. A hot footbath with a tablespoonful of mustard in it often gives relief. Bake a large onion until it becomes soft and tie it over the ear; this will often give great relief when the pain is severe. A lobelia or slippery elm poultice is very effective in allaying the inflammation and pain. An injection of oil of lobelia or origanum, or a tea made of these herbs injected warm with a medicine dropper, will often afford relief. If the ear has abscessed and the abscess has broken, use warm peroxide to wash the ear out. Peroxide will loosen all the putrified matter and bring it out of the ear. This should be repeated until the ear is clean. Do this before injecting any medication or applying poultices. A saturated solution of boric acid may be used for an ear wash. Never introduce objects, such as toothpicks, match sticks, etc., into the ear.

ECZEMA

Causes: The exact cause of eczema is unknown; however, allergy seems to play a large part in most instances. Foods that cause eczema most frequently are eggs, wheat cereals, milk, and certain fruits, especially citrus fruits. Lack of sunshine, fresh air, and constipation may be contributing causes.

Symptoms: Eczema may occur at any age, but is most frequently seen in infants. It is most common and severe on the face, but also occurs on other parts of the body. It causes severe itching, burning, and stinging of the skin. Sometimes it begins in the form of small pimples that develop into larger blisters filled with water. Usually the skin dries up and forms little scales that itch intensely. There are two kinds of eczema, dry and moist (weeping) eczema. Both forms are usually worse during the winter months. The following treatment is beneficial for either type of eczema.

Treatment: Select alkaline foods (see Section V, Chapter 1, Fruits, and Chapter 11, Healthful Diets). The bowels must be made to move regularly, one to three times a day. Do not use soap and water for cleansing the skin; instead, use a weak boric acid solution. Using a salt solution of one teaspoonful to a quart of water is also helpful.

Take equal parts of burdock root, yellow dock, yarrow, and marshmallow; using a heaping teaspoonful of this mixture of granulated herbs to a cup of boiling water, steep, strain, and drink one-half cupful four or five times a day. Also bathe the affected parts freely with this same tea. Healing herbal salve, as given in Section II, Chapter 3, applied freely will relieve the itching and heal the skin.

Use whichever of the following herbs is best suited to your case: golden seal, willow, poplar, yellow dock, blue violet, strawberry leaves, origanum, cleavers, plantain.

When eczema occurs in infants, gentle restraint of the hands must be used to prevent scratching of the lesions, which may result in infection. When an infant has eczema, he should not be vaccinated for smallpox, nor should he associate with other infants or children who have been recently vaccinated.

EPILEPSY (FALLING SICKNESS)

Causes: The main cause is eating a wrong diet, which in turn has caused stoppage of the bowels and affected the sympathetic nerves, which in turn affects the cerebrospinal nerves. This condition calls all the blood away from the head, which at times almost stops the heart and causes the face to become very pale, or purple, and the body limp. It is often caused from trouble in the bowels and intestines, or can be caused by falls, blows, fractures, and other injuries. Many epilepsy cases have worms.

Addendum: The foregoing paragraph lists many of the

causes that were felt to be responsible for epilepsy in the early part of the twentieth century. It is now felt that epilepsy may be either hereditary, in which case it usually is first manifested during childhood and persists throughout life, or is due to injury, tumors, or infections in the brain.

Symptoms: The patient uusually becomes unconscious and this may or may not be associated with a convulsion. There is sometimes gnashing and grinding of the teeth or foaming at the mouth. The eyes usually roll upward and become fixed. The patient usually falls forward. Before an attack there may be a peculiar sensation (aura) felt throughout the body, dizziness, twitching of the muscles, or sudden perspiration. When the patient feels any of these unnatural sensations, he should lie down immediately.

Treatment: The patient must develop a program that fits his needs and must strictly follow this schedule every day.

Have some antispasmodic tincture on hand and give from eight to fifteen drops in one-half glass of water. If the patient cannot drink, put a few drops on the tongue. This will check the convulsion at once.

When the attack first comes on, or even if possible during the attack, have the patient lie down. Have plenty of fresh air in the room. In severe seizures, when there is danger of biting the tongue, place a tongue blade or piece of wood wrapped with cloth between the teeth to prevent injury. When possible, give the antispasmodic tincture before the attack.

To make an excellent tea for use in epilepsy, mix equal parts of the following herbs: black cohosh, valerian, lady's slipper, and skullcap. Steep a heaping teaspoonful of this mixture in a cup of boiling water for thirty minutes. Have the patient drink two or three cups of this tea just as warm as possible, when he feels the attack coming on. This tea should also be continued after the attack.

If the patient complains of pain in the bowels, apply the herbal liniment, as given in Section II, Chapter 3, to the abdomen. Rub it in freely and thoroughly.

Many times I have treated bad cases by giving them either

the foregoing herbs or some from the list in the second paragraph following, combined with a simple, nourishing diet, and plenty of fresh air; and often there has been a decrease in the severity of the attacks or occasionally they have stopped altogether.

When using the herb teas and baths, you must stop eating the things that have caused epilepsy. If you do not, those same things that brought on the attacks in the first place will bring them on again. Discontinue the use of tea, coffee, tobacco, alcoholic liquors, and all stimulating and constipating foods. It would be a great help if all the bread that is eaten was made into zwieback before using. Do not drink with meals; masticate your food thoroughly. The cleansing and nourishing diets discussed in Section V, Chapter 11, would be excellent taken in connection with the herbs given. If, in addition to following the above treatments, enemas are taken and the bowels are kept thoroughly cleansed, the patient will have a good chance of overcoming the attacks.

Take the following herbs either singly or in any combination you desire, study them, and use those best suited to your case. Take a cupful of the tea an hour before each meal and one upon retiring: black cohosh, elder, mistletoe, Peruvian bark, vervain, valerian, lady's slipper, skullcap; and use the antispasmodic tincture.

ERYSIPELAS

Causes: Erysipelas is a disease caused by a disordered condition of the system that allows it to become infected with the streptococcus organism.

Symptoms: Erysipelas appears as an inflammation of the skin in splotches of deep red and copper color, causing an itching and burning sensation. It is most common on the face, but may spread to other parts of the body. It appears as a very red, hot, swollen area on the skin with a sharp margin. It sometimes starts from a slight wound or abrasion of the skin, although at times it seems to arise spontaneously. The involved area may contain blisters. It spreads rapidly, covering the face and neck in a short time. Even in only moderately severe cases, the face is swollen, the eyes are swollen shut, the lips and ears thickened, and the patient is feverish.

When it begins from a wound or scratch, the spot becomes slightly reddened before spreading. Occasionally, the first symptoms begin with a chill or fever, and in a few hours a slight redness appears over the bridge of the nose and on the cheeks. In about twenty-four hours, blisters begin to appear in the red areas. An attack of this disease generally leaves the patient particularly susceptible to the disease for a long time.

Treatment: Erysipelas is very contagious and strict isolation with special nursing care should be used. Do not wash the sores with soap and water. Use a saturated solution of boric acid exclusively. Make a solution of the following herbs: one-half teaspoonful golden seal, one teaspoonful lobelia, one teaspoonful burdock, one-half teaspoonful of yellow dock root, one tablespoonful of boric acid, and one-fourth teaspoonful of myrrh. Dissolve in a quart of boiling water. Dip a piece of cotton in this and lightly touch all of the affected parts. A piece of gauze may be moistened with this solution and left on the sores with good effect, as it is very cleansing and healing. It will greatly ease the pain. Do not wipe the skin.

Chickweed tea, made as follows, is excellent used in the same way. Use one heaping tablespoonful of the granulated herb to a pint of boiling water.

A poultice of raw cranberries, applied cold, will allay the intense burning in erysipelas; also lemon juice, diluted half-and-half with boiled water.

Take internally a tea of pleurisy root, burdock root, sage, or ginger. These herbs affect the skin and keep it moist, also aiding in keeping the pores open. It is good to take a heaping tablespoonful of pleurisy root, a tablespoonful of sage, and one teaspoonful of ginger steeped in a pint of boiling water. Drink one-half cup of this tea every two hours.

Herbal salve, as given in Section II, Chapter 3, will give splendid results when applied to the affected parts.

Another excellent wash is the following: mix equal parts of gum myrrh, echinacea, witch hazel, and golden seal, all granulated. After thoroughly mixing, use one tablespoonful to a pint of boiling water; steep one-half hour and strain. Apply gently with cotton.

A very good, but simple remedy is as follows: cover the affected parts well with grated raw potatoes, about one-fourth inch thick. When the potatoes become dry, remove them and replace with fresh raw potatoes. Keep the bowels open with herbal laxatives or enemas.

FELONS

A felon is a painful abscess, usually found on the end of a finger, thumb, or toe, near the nail.

Causes: A felon is usually caused by some type of blow or injury that becomes infected.

Symptoms: Pain, redness, and swelling. There is usually also some fever.

Treatment: Warm some kerosene and immerse the affected part in it four or five times a day, keeping it in the kerosene from ten to fifteen minutes (or longer) each time. This alone will cure a felon or check one that has just started. This treatment is also good for painful ringworm on the end of the finger. An excellent poultice for this is made of equal parts of slippery elm, lady's slipper, and lobelia herb. Granulated herbs can be used if the powdered herbs are not obtainable.

To relieve the pain when the felon is on the end of a finger, cut a small hole in the end of a lemon and stick the finger in it. If the felon is located on some other part, slice the lemon and bandage a thick slice of it over the felon. This gives excellent results and will often cure a felon.

Addendum: In some cases when the germs causing the infection are very resistant and the individual's general health is poor, these slower acting natural remedies may not be successful and antibiotics may become necessary.

FEMALE TROUBLE

There is so much needless suffering and disease among women that could be prevented if they would use remedies that are simple, harmless, and inexpensive. (See also Menstruation and Pregnancy, following.)

Charcoal poultices with smartweed will do much to relieve womb inflammation. A high enema should be taken, and if there is colon trouble, use herb enemas, such as burdock root, yellow dock root, bayberry bark, or witch hazel. The foregoing herbs are excellent for enemas, douches, or both. If there is any soreness or piles in the rectum, inject a little healing herbal tea as given in this section under Hemorrhoids or Piles. Do this with a small syringe and warm the solution before using. When there is laceration, ulceration, or tumors, make a strong tea of one of the following: white oak bark, witch hazel bark, golden seal, myrrh, or wild alum root. Use a heaping teaspoonful of the herb to a pint of boiling water. Use this in a douche. These teas are very disinfectant and healing.

An exceptionally fine solution is a rounded teaspoonful each of golden seal and myrrh steeped in a quart of boiling water and used as a douche.

Some precautions to observe when your monthly period first arrives are well worth their seeming inconvenience. Stay off your feet as much as possible and keep your hands out of cold water. During the entire time, keep your limbs and feet warm. In the winter and during cold weather, do not go to bed with cold feet. Take a hot footbath on retiring or use a hot water bottle or an electric pad or blanket. A gallon jug of hot water at the foot of the bed is excellent.

Fomentations are a great household weapon, as they will relieve much suffering and pain. They are very beneficial when applied to the lower spine and abdomen of a woman suffering with menstrual cramps.

FEVER

Causes: A fever is nature's way of warning us that something is wrong with our body. It is usually due to an infection somewhere in the body, but many other diseases, including tumors, may cause a fever.

Treatment: If there is nausea and waste matter is present in the stomach, it may be necessary to take an emetic to cleanse the stomach.

Should the temperature be too high and the patient too ill for this, give a cup of golden seal and myrrh. This will help take care of the poisons in the stomach. To make a pint of this tea, steep a heaping teaspoon of golden seal and one-half teaspoon of myrrh in a pint of boiling water for twenty minutes. After taking the first cupful, take a teaspoon every hour thereafter. More can be taken with benefit.

Cool water enemas will bring down the temperature rapidly. Have the water slightly below body temperature. If the enema contains herbs, it is even more effective. Soap may be used, but it is not necessary and may be irritating to the colon. If it is used, the water should be slightly sudsy. It is the removal of the poisons from the system that brings the temperature down. Remove the clothing and then place the patient between cotton blankets. Sponge with tepid water, beginning with the face and sponging downward over the entire body. Sponge well around the head and especially around the back of the neck. Sponge the feet thoroughly, leaving the soles moist. Do this every five minutes if the fever is very high. Also give sips of cold water every five minutes. If the patient becomes chilly, stop the sponging, cover the patient well, and place hot water bottles or hot fomentations over the stomach. This will usually stop the chill. If it does not, apply a hot fomentation to the spine, or give a hot footbath and a hot drink. This should stop the chill at once.

I have again and again broken up very severe cases of fever with this treatment. The bowels must be kept open with laxative herbs. If the temperature is only slightly elevated, sometimes lemon juice alone will break the fever. Take the lemon juice diluted in water without any sweetening.

I well remember my father and mother breaking up severe cases of fever with herb teas and fruit juices. They used red raspberry leaves, willow bark, and other herbs.

Slippery elm tea is excellent in all cases of fever, since it is a powerful cleanser and is soothing to the stomach and intestinal tract.

Any one of the following herbs is useful in fevers. Make them into a tea and drink copiously until the fever breaks: yarrow, red sage, catnip, peppermint, wild cherry bark, valerian, black cohosh, tansy, camomile, elder, boneset, willow (bark or leaves), pleurisy root, marigold, nettle, and lobelia.

Red raspberry leaf tea is excellent for the reduction of fever in children.

Diet: In all cases of fever and severely prostrating diseases, a few days of liquid diet will lessen their severity and give the stomach a much needed rest. The first point to be emphasized is to drink plenty of water, as this dilutes and carries away the toxins through the kidneys. Remember that water is the greatest solvent known.

Special benefit will be derived from using orange juice. Fruit drinks of any kind are beneficial when taken without cane sugar. The use of cane sugar will increase the fever and tend to acidify the blood. Weak lemonade, given freely, is very good. Sweeten drinks with malt honey, malt sugar, or honey, if at all. Use fresh fruits whenever possible. When the fever subsides, special care must be taken to eat light, nourishing, easily digested food. The following foods are nourishing, and can be used during convalescence: soybean milk, potassium broth, zwieback, baked Irish potatoes, natural brown rice, and bananas (very ripe).

Soybean milk is alkaline, very nourishing, and easy to digest. Dissolve whole wheat flakes in hot soybean milk. This is very strengthening. Well-ripened bananas made into a puree are excellent, especially for underweight patients.

The following foods are to be strictly avoided during a fever: meats of all kinds, meat broths, fish, fowl, oysters, pickles, condiments, cheese, mushrooms, and eggs. These foods should be avoided because of the high amount of protein they contain, and when the intake of protein is greater than the requirements of the body, putrefaction results. As a matter of fact, the continual use of these foods always brings on disease in one form or another. Use salt as sparingly as possible, or eliminate it entirely. This will not only allow you to taste the wonderful natural flavors in the food, but it will also help to lower your blood pressure if it is too high.

Two quarts of orange juice and an equal amount of oatmeal water is a daily ration for typhoid or any other fever. More can be taken with good results, but do not take orange juice at the same time that oatmeal water is taken: take them at least one hour apart.

GALLSTONES

Cause: The exact cause for the formation of gallstones is unknown.

It is, however, known that certain groups of people tend to develop gallstones much more frequently than others. Heavy eaters who live on a high calorie, high fat diet, are much more apt to develop gallstones. They are more commonly found in middle-aged females, especially those who are over-weight. They are exceedingly common in some tribes of American Indians, but are rarely seen in certain races, such as the Japanese. People with gallstones should be on a low-fat diet, and should not eat greasy or fried foods, mayonnaise, eggs, highly seasoned foods, high protein foods, cheese, salad dressing, pork products, and rich pastries. There are certain foods that some people tolerate very poorly, and when this is found to be the case, these foods should be omitted from the diet. Examples of such foods are beans, onions, cucumbers, cabbage, turnips, radishes, sauerkraut, and highly spiced foods. There may be associated constipation

and liver trouble. If the liver is overloaded it will not be able
to perform its work of eliminating the poisonous waste matter
that comes to it. A fruit diet for a week or ten days is a
wonderful medicine for the liver, especially if a high enema
is taken every day with enough laxative herbs so that the
bowels move at least one to three times a day. If you would
do this when gallstones are suspected, it would help prevent
their formation.

Even if you have had your gallbladder removed, you can
still develop gallstones, since they not infrequently form in
the bile ducts; either in the small bile ducts within the liver
or in the large bile duct that leads from the liver to the small
intestine.

Symptoms: In advanced cases there is pain in the region
of the liver, which is located under the right lower ribs. The
pain may extend to the right shoulder blade and violent pains
may occur in the abdomen. There is often jaundice because
of obstruction of the bile duct. There may be chills, fever,
nausea, or vomiting. These symptoms are not always present,
but they are brought on many times by dietary indiscretion.

Treatment: If the pain is not too severe, give an enema,
preferably of catnip tea. Apply hot fomentations of lobelia
and hops over the region of the liver; but if the patient is
having too much pain and you do not have these herbs, use
plain hot water fomentations until you are able to obtain the
herbs. Give a hot footbath and a cup of hot tea just as soon
as possible, made of equal parts of the following herbs:
hyssop, gentian root, skullcap, and buckthorn bark. Mix
thoroughly and use a heaping teaspoon to a cup of boiling
water. Take a cup of this tea every hour the first day, then take
one cup four times a day an hour before each meal and one
upon retiring. This will liquefy the bile, and improve the liver.

Continue with the fomentations. One-half hour after taking
the tea, take four ounces of olive oil and four ounces of lemon
juice or grapefruit juice beaten thoroughly together. After
taking the lemon juice and olive oil, lie on your right side,
with the hips elevated by placing two pillows beneath them.

Fomentations of lobelia and hops will not only soothe the pain but will dilate the bile duct so the lemon juice and oil may pass. A thorough massage under the right ribs, rubbing towards the center of the body, will greatly facilitate the passage of the gallstones after the fomentations have been applied and the oil has been given. Remember, if the herbs are not available, use hot water fomentations.

When suffering from gallstones, you should go on a fruit juice diet, using oranges and grapefruit. Unsweetened pineapple juice is also especially recommended for gallstones. Be sure your diet contains plenty of alkaline foods. Potassium broth (see index) is one of the best things that can be taken. It is highly nourishing and alkaline. This same diet is also good for gravel in the bladder, stones in the kidneys, and liver trouble.

Be sure to take the lemon juice and olive oil for three days. You may also take them separately as follows: two tablespoons of lemon juice, followed by two tablespoons of olive oil, or vice versa, on an empty stomach.

The following herbs are very valuable in cases of gallstones. Take one rounded teaspoon of either powdered wood betony or milkweed mixed in one-half glass of cold water; follow this by drinking a glass of hot water. Do this one hour before each meal and also upon retiring.

Dr. Lee, one of New York City's great physicians, said that if people would stop eating acid-forming foods and eat alkaline foods, any case of gallstones could be cured. Dr. Clark, of Chicago, once said to me that any case of gallstones, appendicitis, tonsillitis, piles, or hemorrhoids could be cured without the knife. It has been my experience for years that God has a remedy for every ill of man, and operations are rarely needed.

GANGRENE

Causes: Gangrene, either internal or external, is caused by a lack of oxygen and blood to a part of the body so that decay and death of tissue sets in. This is seen most frequently in elderly persons and diabetics with poor blood supply to the extremities due to hardening of the arteries (arteriosclerosis). Blocking or narrowing of the arteries stops or decreases the normal flow of blood, and therefore the amount of oxygen supplied to the tissues is diminished, and gangrene may set in. Gangrene may also occur following a severe injury to the tissues in which all of the dead tissue is not removed. In these instances the gangrene is caused by a class of bacteria called clostridia that thrive in dead tissue and produce a poison that permits the gangrene to spread rapidly through the surrounding tissues. This form of gangrene can be rapidly fatal if it is not treated properly as soon as it is discovered.

Burns, injuries caused by acid, or frostbite, are often followed by gangrene. Severe bruises or sores, such as boils or carbuncles, that are not properly cared for, may become gangrenous.

Symptoms: There are two kinds of gangrene, moist and dry. There is always inflammation before the moist gangrene sets in. The part affected is painful and becomes bluish or black. Soon the tissues become completely dead; thereafter, there may be no feeling in the part at all. Dry gangrene usually begins as a small spot in any location, but most often where the circulation is poor. Frequently the toes or fingers are affected and turn yellow or black. At first the area of skin becomes cold and painful, particularly during muscular activity. This is seen especially in the toes, feet, and legs. Gangrene of the feet occurs frequently in diabetics, because of the poor blood supply due to hardening of the arteries.

Treatment: Follow the diet given under purifying the blood. A person who has pure blood and a good circulation will not develop gangrene. I have used the following treatment with excellent success in very bad cases of gangrene.

Take one-fourth pound of powdered charcoal and one ounce of water pepper or smartweed; put these in a pan and pour one pint of boiling water over them; let them steep for twenty minutes. Then mix two tablespoons of whole wheat flour and enough dry charcoal with this solution to make a poultice. Spread this on a piece of gauze that is a little larger than the involved area. Apply this to the affected part. Lay another piece of gauze over it and bandage it on.

If the part is painful, add a tablespoon of lobelia when steeping the herbs. You may need a little flaxseed meal or cornmeal to make the poultice stick together.

When there is pus and ulceration, first warm some hydrogen peroxide and use it to bathe the affected part thoroughly, repeatedly applying and wiping it off with a piece of cotton, until the area is absolutely clean. Do this *before* applying the poultice.

Another excellent poultice may be made as follows: two tablespoons of ground flaxseed (or flaxseed meal), one teaspoon of golden seal, and one-half teaspoon of myrrh. Add enough hot water to make a paste. The paste must not be too stiff, but must be soft enough to penetrate. Apply the same as any other poultice. Renew this every six hours, cleaning each time with peroxide if pus forms.

To take internally, mix equal parts of skullcap, valerian, yellow dock, and buckthorn bark. Use a heaping teaspoonful to a cup of boiling water. Let steep for one-half hour. Take a cupful one hour before each meal and a cupful hot upon retiring. If constipated, take an herbal laxative. The bowels must be kept open.

In case of gas gangrene, which is caused by the toxin produced by a bacteria, proper medical attention should be sought as soon as possible. This type of gangrene usually follows severe trauma, frequently gunshot wounds.

Caution: It should be remembered that heat should never be applied to the affected area if gangrene due to a lack of adequate circulation is present or impending,

GAS IN THE STOMACH OR BOWELS

Causes: Gas in the stomach and bowels is the result of improper digestion. Most of the gas in the intestinal tract is composed of nitrogen, carbon dioxide, and methane. The amount of hydrogen and carbon dioxide in the intestines largely depends upon the diet, since these gases are mostly produced by bacteria in the colon acting on unabsorbed carbohydrates and proteins in the diet. Approximately 600 cc of gas is passed each day, and about two-thirds of this is produced in the intestines. Air that is swallowed during routine everyday activities contributes only a small amount to the total gas content of the intestinal tract. Certain conditions, such as strictures or spasm in the small intestine or colon, may cause some obstruction to the bowel, thereby producing "gas pains."

Large amounts of gas in the intestinal tract may be produced by eating certain foods, by improper absorption of some foods, particularly carbohydrates, or by an overgrowth of gas-producing bacteria. Eating wrong combinations of food will cause gas to form in the stomach and bowels.

Drinking with meals causes a sour stomach and fermentation, as does hasty eating and poor mastication.

Treatment: Peppermint and spearmint tea are excellent for reducing gas in the stomach. Equal parts of calamus root, valerian, and granulated or powdered peppermint or spearmint should be taken: mix these together using a teaspoon to a cup of boiling water; steep, strain, and drink one-half cupful an hour before meals, and another half cupful after meals.

The above herbs can be used in powdered form, as well as in capsules, if desired.

To strengthen the stomach and cleanse it so that this condition will be overcome, take one-fourth teaspoon of powdered golden seal in one-half glass of warm water an hour before each meal. You may also take it as follows if you prefer: one heaping teaspoon of golden seal and one-fourth teaspoon of myrrh to a pint of boiling water, steep, and take a swallow just a few minutes before eating.

Rinse the mouth and throat thoroughly with this every morning, swallowing a little.

If you find that certain foods such as beans, sauerkraut, apples, etc., form excessive gas, eat these foods sparingly or omit them entirely from your diet.

It has also been found that as a person grows older, different foods may react differently in the body, whereby foods that could previously be eaten without any trouble may, as the person reaches middle and older age, begin to produce considerable gas. If this occurs, the diet must be adjusted accordingly.

GOITER

The term goiter refers to an enlargement of the thyroid gland, a rather large gland that is located in the neck on either side of the "Adam's apple."

Causes: The most common cause of goiter is a lack of iodine in the diet. In North America goiter has been practically eliminated by the introduction of iodized salt in 1924. There are, however, areas in the world where goiter is still common due to a lack of iodine. In Asia alone, there are over 400 million iodine-deficient people; this is due to growing crops, which are staple foods in the Asian diet, in iodine-deficient soil.

A less common form of goiter also exists for which the cause is not known. In this form of thyroid disease, the gland becomes overactive (hyperthyroidism) and the patient complains of nervousness, rapid heart beat, increased appetite, weight loss, excessive perspiration, weakness, and diarrhea. This form of thyroid disease is much more common in females than males. There are certain vegetables that contain substances called goitrogens. When excessively large amounts of these foods are eaten, the body's normal use of iodine is interfered with and a goiter in the thyroid gland may be the result. These vegetables are: broccoli, cauliflower, brussels sprouts, turnips, raw cabbage, kale, rutabagas, and horseradish.

Treatment: Build up the stomach by eating a plain nourishing alkaline diet. A good stomach remedy is composed of
the following: a heaping tablespoon each of golden seal and
bayberry and one teaspoon of myrrh. Mix these thoroughly
and take one-half teaspoon in a cup of water an hour before
each meal and one upon retiring. Use also as a mouthwash
and gargle thoroughly with it. Kelp is an excellent source of
iodine.

If there is no diarrhea the bowels must be kept loose. Use
high herb enemas to cleanse the colon thoroughly. Also take
an herbal laxative.

Bathe the neck thoroughly with the liniment recommended
in Section II, Chapter 3.

A bayberry poultice used at bedtime and kept on all night
is excellent. It must be well covered with a woolen cloth to
keep it warm. See poultices in Section II, Chapter 3.

Sweat baths and massage to increase the circulation and
build up the nervous system are very helpful. Take herbs for
nerves.

If these simple natural remedies do not relieve the symptoms given above, and the pulse remains rapid, the blood
pressure high, the skin warm and moist, the eyes prominent,
and the thyroid enlarged, the aid of a physician should be
sought.

GONORRHEA

Cause: Gonorrhea, like syphilis, is a venereal disease
nearly always transmitted by sexual contact. It is caused by
an organism, neisseria gonorrhoeae, that produces urethritis
in males and females. This bacteria may also infect the throat,
eyes, rectum, vagina, and joints. Following the introduction
of antibiotics, the number of cases of gonorrhea declined
dramatically until the "sexual revolution" took place in the
1960s and 1970s. Since then there has been a marked resurgence of this disease as well as all the other venereal diseases.
Gonorrhea is much more common than syphilis and is now

the most common reportable infectious disease in the United States, with between one and two million new cases reported annually. The control of this disease is difficult because while approximately fifty percent of females and ten percent of males who have gonorrhea do not have symptoms, they are still capable of infecting others.

Symptoms: Symptoms usually begin from two to seven days following exposure. The genitals become inflamed and there is a yellowish urethral discharge with a painful, stinging sensation during urination. The complications of gonorrhea that occur in males, such as strictures of the urethra and prostatitis, were once fairly common but are rarely seen today.

The most serious complication in females is infection of the fallopian tubes (salpingitis), which may lead to sterility. The chances of this occurring increase with each attack of gonorrhea, so that after three or four attacks the incidence of sterility approaches seventy-five percent.

Approximately 15 percent of women with gonorrhea develop salpingitis. Without treatment, the symptoms may persist for two to three months and the complication rate becomes much higher.

Treatment: The treatment used most commonly today for gonorrhea is the administration of an appropriate antibiotic. This is curative in a short time in nearly one hundred percent of patients and dramatically reduces the complications in both males and females.

If antibiotics are unavailable, or if it is felt best that they should not be used, the following treatment program may be followed. The length of the illness may be greatly shortened if the infected person can go to bed at once. A cleansing fruit juice diet, as given in Section V, Chapter 11, should be started immediately. Take absolutely nothing into the stomach that is the least irritating.

Take two high enemas a day, preferably herb enemas. An excellent douche for women is equal parts of red raspberry leaves and witch hazel leaves. Good results will be obtained if a douche of this tea is given after every urination. Steep a heaping tablespoon of the mixed leaves in a quart of boiling water for twenty minutes. Use warm. This solution is also a fine wash for the genitals in both men and women.

If there are sores and ulcers, make a solution consisting of one-fourth teaspoon of powdered aloes, one teaspoon of golden seal, and one teaspoon of powdered myrrh. Steep these in a pint of boiling water for half an hour. Bathe the sores thoroughly with this; then sprinkle them with equal parts of powdered golden seal and myrrh. Herbal salve, as recommended in Section II, Chapter 3, is also fine to apply to either the sores or ulcers.

Drink at least one pint of slippery elm tea a day. It can be mixed with fruit juices or taken plain. Drink at least eight glasses of water a day.

If the patient stays in bed, be sure the room is well ventilated at all times. A hot sitz bath two or three times a day will give relief from pain. For pain in the legs or any part of the body, apply hot fomentations or rub thoroughly with the herbal liniment recommended in Section II, Chapter 3.

Black willow, saw palmetto berries, and skullcap are especially beneficial in acute gonorrhea. Steep a heaping teaspoon in a cup of boiling water for one-half hour. Take two tablespoons six times a day.

You may also use other herbs as given under the section on Syphilis, following.

GOUT

Gout, which has also been called the "disease of kings" and "rheumatism of the rich," was first described at least 2500 years ago by Hippocrates. Many great people of the past, including John Calvin, Charles Darwin, Benjamin Franklin, and Martin Luther, suffered from gout. Gout is not a very common disease, although there are certain groups of people, such as the Philippinos living in the United States, in whom there is a very high incidence. It usually affects adult males; only five to ten percent occurring in women. Patients with gout comprise approximately five percent of all patients having arthritis.

Causes: While the cause of most cases is not known for sure, approximately ten to twenty percent of patients with gout have an inherited form of the disease. All patients with gout have increased urates in the blood. These are deposited in crystalline form in the joints and may produce severe arthritis. Many patients with gout also have kidney stones.

Symptoms: The peak age for the onset of symptoms in men is between forty and fifty, while in women gout is rarely seen before the menopause.

A classical description of an acute attack of gout was given in 1863 by Sydenham: "The victim goes to bed and sleeps in good health. About two o'clock in the morning he is awakened by a severe pain in the great toe; more rarely in the heel, ankle, or instep. This pain is like that of a dislocation, and yet the parts feel as if cold water were poured over them. Then follow chills and shivers, and a little fever. The pain, which was at first moderate, becomes more intense. With its intensity the chills and shivers increase. After a time this comes to its height, accommodating itself to the bones and ligaments of the tarsus and metatarsus. Now it is a violent stretching and tearing of the ligament, now it is a gnawing pain, and now a pressure and tightening. So exquisite and lively meanwhile is the feeling of the part affected that it cannot bear the weight of the bed clothes nor the jar of a person walking in the room. The night is passed in torture, sleeplessness, turning of the part affected, and perpetual change of posture; the tossing about of the body being worse as the fit comes on. Hence the vain effort, by change of posture, both in the body and the limb affected, to obtain an abatement of the pain."

More than half the patients with gouty arthritis experience their first attack of pain in the great toe. Other common sites are the ankle, knee, wrist, fingers, and elbow. The pain usually occurs suddenly and frequently begins at night. The affected joint becomes red, hot, and exceedingly painful. Overindulgence in an abundance of rich foods and alcohol frequently brings on an attack, which may last anywhere from a few hours to weeks. Between attacks the patient usually has no symptoms, but subsequent attacks occur at unpredictable intervals. In a small percentage of patients (about five percent), after the first attack no further attacks occur. As the episodes of gout become more frequent and severe, the joints become more deformed and painful.

As previously mentioned, many patients with gout develop kidney stones, and as these stones slowly pass down the ureter, the slender tube leading from the kidney to the urinary bladder, the symptoms of renal colic appear, consisting of severe abdominal or flank pain, nausea and vomiting, and perhaps reddish discoloration of the urine.

Treatment: The diet is of great importance. During an acute attack of gout, the diet should be high in carbohydrates and low in fat and protein. Meat should be eliminated and peas, beans, and lentils should be limited. The calories must be strictly limited so that the patient does not gain weight, and if the patient is obese he must be placed on a diet to lose weight. Alcohol must be eliminated. A large fluid intake is very helpful.

Take equal parts of granulated skullcap, yarrow, and valerian, and mix thoroughly together. Use a heaping teaspoon to a cup of boiling water.

Steep, and drink a cupful an hour before meals and one upon retiring. Take laxative herbs to keep the bowels open; this is important. The liniment, as recommended in Section II, Chapter 3, if applied freely and thoroughly rubbed in, will greatly allay the pain. The herbs given in the section on Rheumatism and Arthritis, following, may also be taken for gout with good effect. Study each herb separately, and take the one or combination that suits your case best.

Any one of the following herbs will be found beneficial and may be taken singly or in any combination you desire. Use a teaspoon to the cup of boiling water, steep for twenty minutes, and take four cups a day, an hour before each meal and at bedtime: blue violet, burdock, gentian root, mugwort, rue, birch, broom, sarsaparilla, buckthorn, ginger, penny-royal, plantain, wood betony, and balm of Gilead.

For an acute attack of gout, colchicine is the standard medicine and has been used successfully for hundreds of years. Colchicine is obtained from the meadow saffron (Colchicum autumnale). This plant is poisonous and should be used only under medical supervision.

HAIR AND SCALP

Any disease that impairs the vitality of the body has an effect upon the hair. When the circulation is diminished by a general nervous condition, the scalp cannot be properly nourished. Diseases of the scalp and loss of hair are expressions of bodily ailments. A poisoned or impure bloodstream carries little or no nourishment to the hair. The color, luster, dryness or oiliness, and brittle condition of the hair are all due to the condition of the system. The real treatment for diseases of the hair and scalp lies not in the many tonics that are used, but in the attention to the foods that are eaten, many of which cause diseases of the body, thereby affecting the hair and scalp. The blood that nourishes the hair must be purified by using wholesome, nourishing foods, that will build a healthy body.

Loss of hair may be caused by catarrh, nervous diseases, fevers, worry, mental disorders, skin diseases, injurious tonics, eczema, and anesthetics. Curling and crimping with metal curlers and hot irons dries the hair and breaks it.

Since an analysis of the hair shows it to be composed of iron, oxygen, hydrogen, nitrogen, carbon, and sulphur, the blood must be supplied with these minerals so that nourishment will be carried to the scalp. Raw foods contain the highest percentage of minerals obtainable. Many of the best foods are prepared in such a way that most of the minerals are drained off in the water. Proper nourishment and good health will do more to make beautiful hair than any external treatment it is possible to give.

A thorough brushing of the hair every day keeps it free from lint and makes it silky and lustrous. To manipulate the scalp lightly with the tips of the fingers, always using a rotary movement, is good. It should be done very thoroughly.

The leaves and bark of the willow tree, made into a tea, will cure dandruff. A tea made of marshmallow leaves and thoroughly applied to the scalp will do much to prevent falling hair.

Any of the following herbs are useful to nourish and brighten the hair and make it grow: nettle, pepper grass, sage, henna leaves, or burdock.

Steep a tablespoon in a pint of boiling water for one half hour and add a level tablespoon of boric acid. Massage the scalp with this solution. It may also be used before a shampoo or between shampoos.

HAY FEVER

Causes: We hear all kinds of theories about the cause of hay fever, but the general belief is that it comes from the pollen of various plants, especially trees, grass, and weeds. It is most frequent in the spring and fall, but may be present all year round. I have known men to get hay fever every summer while cutting and loading hay. Ragweed and grass pollen are reported to be the most frequent causes of hay fever in the United States. This may all be true as far as I know, but it is also true that it would be a rare thing for anyone to have hay fever who had good digestive organs and whose nasal membranes were in a healthy condition. Wrong eating habits may have much to do with it.

Symptoms: Hay fever usually comes on suddenly, and at about the same time every year with many people. There is a stinging, tickling or prickling sensation in the nose, with a watery discharge, sneezing, itching and watering of the eyes, and swelling of the mucous membranes in the nose and mouth. There may be coughing or difficulty breathing, with a feeling of being smothered, much the same as in asthma. These conditions may continue until colder weather arrives.

Treatment: If the offending item causing the hay fever can be discovered, it should be strictly avoided. People are frequently allergic to the hair of their pets, particularly cats or horses, and if this is true, the hay fever symptoms will continue as long as contact is made with these animals.

Warm saltwater may be used for both the throat and the nose. Dissolve one heaping teaspoonful of salt in a pint of warm water and use as a gargle. Blow the nose entirely clear of mucus, then sniff the salt water into the nose.

In addition to this, make a solution using a rounded teaspoonful of golden seal and a heaping teaspoonful of borax in a pint of boiling soft water. Shake well. Let stand an hour or two, shaking occasionally; it is then ready for use. Pour some into the hand and sniff it into the nose, one side at a time. Repeat this a number of times until the nose is entirely clean. This is very healing and soothing to the membranes and should be repeated four or five times a day.

I have had good success in treating hay fever by using ragweed and goldenrod. Use one teaspoon of each herb and also one teaspoon each of skunk cabbage and calamus root. Mix thoroughly and take a teaspoon in a glass of warm water an hour before each meal and upon retiring.

Another treatment is to put one tablespoon of ephedra in one pint of boiling water. Let steep one-half hour, strain through a cloth, then sniff up the nostrils, drawing it into the throat. Repeat this several times until relieved, using the same treatment three or four times a day. This treatment is also excellent for other nasal troubles.

It may be helpful to take one heaping teaspoon of powdered bayberry bark and pour over it one pint of boiling water. Steep for twenty minutes. Let settle and then sniff into the nostrils four to six times a day. This is also good when one-half glass is taken internally three or more times a day.

HEADACHES

There are three common kinds of headaches.

1. *Sick Headache.* This type of headache occurs if undigested food stays in the stomach, during times of increased stress, if there is a disordered liver, or when there is mental or physical overwork. In women, disorders of menstruation may cause a sick headache.

Treatment: Relief is sometimes obtained by taking a hot footbath with a tablespoon of mustard in it, or use just plain water as hot as can be borne. Keep the feet and legs in the hot water nearly up to the knees. Place a cold washcloth on the forehead and one on the back of the neck. Drink a cup of hot peppermint, spearmint, valerian, black cohosh, or skullcap tea. If you do not have these herbs, drink a cupful of hot water, adding the juice of a lemon, but no sweetening.

2. *Bilious Headache.* Caused from indigestion, disordered liver, overeating, wrong food combinations, and insufficient exercise. People who overeat of rich heavy foods and take little or no exercise at all are the frequent suffers of this type of headache. Unless the diet is changed and a regular exercise program established, this may develop into a chronic type of headache.

Symptoms: Dull pain in the forehead, throbbing temples.

Treatment: Avoid all harmful articles of diet. High enemas initially, to cleanse the colon, may be helpful in bilious headaches. Often the stomach is overloaded when the headache comes on. If this is the case, use an emetic. (See Section II, Chapter 3.) Take the treatment as given for sick headache.

3. *Nervous (Tension) Headache.* Nervous people and those whose work is sedentary usually suffer from this form of headache. Mental strain and worry will cause a nervous headache. Bright lights or noises of any kind usually make the headache worse.

Treatment: Lie down and rest where it is quiet, and where there is plenty of fresh air. Take a cupful or two of hot peppermint, catnip, red sage, or spearmint tea. Upon retiring, take a cupful of hot hops tea, or if it is possible to retire when the headache comes on, take it then; it will soothe the nerves and produce sleep. Red sage is one of the best herbs for headache.

The herbal liniment that is recommended in Section II, Chapter 3, when thoroughly applied to the forehead, temples, and back of the neck, will many times give prompt relief.

If the headache continues, use an enema of catnip, blue cohosh, or black cohosh tea. The enema should be very warm and retained as long as possible, using a pint or more of liquid.

HEART TROUBLE

There are many causes of heart trouble. Frequently there are wrong eating habits that cause obesity, thereby placing an extra strain on the heart. Too much salt in the diet also causes a strain on the heart by elevating the blood pressure. Palpitation of the heart is often due to gas and fermentation in the stomach. Some years ago an elderly woman who had complained for years of heart trouble came to see me. I advised her to take a sweat bath and thorough salt glow with vigorous rubbing of the body, and also cold morning baths. I also advised her to correct her diet.

Before a week had passed that woman had forgotten all about her "heart trouble". I knew this woman for years and she never had a recurrence of the attacks, as far as I know.

Not long ago, shortly after a dinner that I attended, a woman complained to me of severe heart trouble. I told her that there was nothing wrong with her heart. She simply had gas in her stomach that was pressing against her heart. I told her to lie face down, roll on her left side and then her right, then drink a cup of hot water, and her "heart trouble" was gone.

Much so-called heart trouble is not due to actual damage to the heart muscle or valves, but rather the heart has been weakened by impure blood caused by a wrong diet, lack of exercise, and poor circulation. Thus, the blood that should be circulating near the surface of the body, nourishing the skin, muscles, etc., is diverted to the inside and overburdens the digestive organs and heart.

Some forms of heart trouble may be made worse by tea, coffee, tobacco, and alcohol. Excess body weight and too much salt in the diet cause an extra strain on the heart by raising the blood pressure. Sometimes heart trouble is caused by eating too much food made of white flour and cane sugar products. When a large amount of food is eaten that has been robbed of its life-giving properties, and since the real health-giving properties that have been refined out of the foods are those properties that strengthen our bodies and heart, the heart grows weaker and weaker.

Most heart trouble can be overcome. My heart was so weak many years ago that in my weakened condition I could scarcely walk across the floor.

I am now almost seventy-six years of age and only a short time ago I ran five miles. There was not the slightest sign of a flutter or palpitation in my heart. Those who witnessed this said it was too good to believe when they felt my pulse and listened to my heart. I only mention this to show what right habits of living and correct food will do for a weakened body.

Diet in heart trouble. See Section V, Chapter 11, for cleansing and nourishing diets, which are good for any kind of heart trouble. Salt in the diet must be severely restricted and a good reducing diet must be followed to get rid of any excess weight.

Herbs. A number of herbs are a great help in any kind of heart trouble. Tansy is very good for palpitation of the heart. Make it into a tea by using one heaping teaspoonful to a cup of boiling water and take three or four cups a day; or it may be taken in half cup doses an hour before meals and upon retiring.

When the heartbeat is irregular or there is weakness of the heart, the following tea may be used with excellent results. Take one teaspoon each of black cohosh, skullcap, valerian, lobelia, and a pinch of cayenne. Mix thoroughly and use a heaping teaspoonful to a cup of boiling water. Steep one-half hour. Drink four cups a day, one an hour before each meal and one upon retiring; or you may take a swallow every two hours or a half cupful as needed. This is very beneficial.

Look up the following herbs, read the description of each herb, and use the one that best suits your condition. Any one may be combined with others. Lily of the valley is excellent in palpitation and for quieting the heart. Angelica, blue cohosh, borage, cayenne, golden seal, wood betony, hawthorn, valerian, vervain.

For any kind of heart failure, physical and mental rest is a necessity.

In case of severe heart trouble, call your physician.

HEMORRHAGES

Causes: Whenever a blood vessel, either artery or vein, large or small, is severed or cut, or ruptures from any other cause, hemorrhage (bleeding) will start at once. The bleeding may be in the lungs, stomach, bowels, brain, skin or any other part of the body. If an artery is cut, the blood spurts and flows fast and is usually bright red in color. If a vein is cut, the blood will be dark and the flow will be slower and more constant. When the wound is small, the blood usually clots rapidly and the bleeding stops, provided that the proper blood components, especially the platelets, are present in sufficient amounts.

Hemorrhage from the stomach. Quiet and rest are required. Put an application of ice over the stomach for a short time and have the patient swallow small bits of ice. Shepherd's purse, made into a tea, is very reliable in hemorrhage. One cupful has been known to stop a hemorrhage. Witch hazel leaves, wild alum root, bistort root, red raspberry, and sumach are also good. Make any one into a tea by steeping a teaspoon in a cup of boiling water thirty minutes, strain, and drink. Ulcers, tumors, and inflammation (gastritis), are the most common causes of bleeding from the stomach.

Hemorrhage from the lungs. Give a hot footbath and have the patient refrain from coughing as much as possible. A tea made of hemlock spruce with a pinch of cayenne added has been known to stop bleeding from the lungs almost immediately. Also use the same herbs as for stomach hemorrhage. Cancer of the lung is a frequent cause of coughing up blood.

Hemorrhage from the uterus. Have the patient lie down and elevate the foot of the bed. Give a hot douche made of bayberry bark or bistort root. Use either in powdered or granulated form. Steep one tablespoon in a quart of boiling water for a few minutes. Use a spiral douche if available; if not, use a regular douche tip.

A tea made from red raspberry leaves, white oak bark, witch hazel bark, or wild alum root is also good. If used in the granulated form, use two tablespoons to a quart of boiling water; steep for twenty minutes; let settle, strain, and drink as hot as possible.

Bleeding between the menstrual periods or after the menopause may indicate a serious problem, and if it continues a physician should be consulted.

Hemorrhage from the bowels. Keep the patient lying down. Give an enema of warm wild alum root tea. White oak bark or red raspberry tea may be used. Inject two or three ounces of the tea through the enema tip and have the patient retain this as long as possible. Repeat. Shepherd's purse, raspberry leaves, bistort root, witch hazel, bayberry, or sumach, may be taken as a tea. Use either one of the herbs by itself, or make a mixture of any two or three and take according to the directions given in Section II, Chapter 3.

Hemorrhage from the nose. Make a tea of golden seal, using one teaspoon to a pint of boiling water. Steep a few minutes, let settle, and when cold pour a little into the palm of the hand and sniff it up the nostrils. Sometimes cold or pressure applied to the back of the neck helps to prevent the free flow of blood to the head. Use the golden seal tea a number of times during the day. If this is done thoroughly, the hemorrhage will rarely recur. Tea made from a combination of wild alum root, blackberry leaves, witch hazel leaves, and white oak bark is also very useful to check nosebleeds, as these herbs are astringent.

Pinching the nostrils together tightly for three to five minutes, while breathing through the mouth, will stop most ordinary nosebleeds.

Caution: Continued bleeding, even if only in small amounts, from any place in the body, may indicate a serious problem such as cancer, and the exact cause for the bleeding should be found as soon as possible.

HEMORRHOIDS OR PILES

Hemorrhoids are dilated veins around the anus and rectum, They may be either internal (not visible from the outside) or external. Approximately half the population of the United States over fifty years of age has hemorrhoids.

Causes: Wrong eating habits may be a cause of hemorrhoids. Eating a diet that contains a large amount of refined foods that are low in bulk (fiber), tends to cause small, hard stools, resulting in straining and constipation; this causes the pressure inside the colon to increase.

Taking ordinary commercial laxatives that are on the market may also be a cause, as many of them irritate the membranous lining of the colon.

Symptoms: Swollen veins are present around the anus or inside the rectum. These swollen blood vessels frequently become irritated and bleed.

Sometimes the bleeding is quite severe and may even result in anemia and weakness. If a blood clot forms in a hemorrhoid, it becomes swollen, blue, tense, and extremely painful. At times the veins inside the rectum are so swollen that when the stool passes they are forced to the outside. In this case, some oil should be used and they should be replaced inside. Often there is extreme itching.

Treatment: First take a high hot enema at a temperature of from 102° to 108°F. Use white oak bark, bayberry bark, or white alum root tea. This will cleanse the entire length of the colon.

Make a strong tea of witch hazel bark and one teaspoon of

catnip, one-half teaspoon of bloodroot and one teaspoon of yellow dock root. If you do not have the other herbs, you may use just the witch hazel bark and catnip. Use a tablespoon of witch hazel bark and a teaspoon of catnip to a cup of boiling water. Steep twenty minutes. If the hemorrhoids are external, dip a small piece of cotton in this tea and bathe the affected parts. If the hemorrhoids are internal, use a soft rubber enema tip and inject two tablespoons at a time into the rectum. This will give good relief in a short time.

When taking the herb enemas you will find that it is less painful, and the piles will go back inside easier, if you take the knee-chest position; this will cause the intestines to drop forward.

Another herb tea injection that is very effective is powdered white oak bark or alum root tea. Use a teaspoon of either to a cup of boiling water, steep twenty minutes, strain, bathe the affected parts, and inject a little into the rectum. This will give relief. This alone will sometimes cure the hemorrhoids, if the enemas and diet are taken as recommended.

I have cured bad cases with kerosene alone. Apply to the affected parts either inside or out. If inside, inject a little. Clean, pure kerosene gives instant relief. Lemon juice is also excellent when used in the same way.

Take the following tea internally: use equal parts of mullein, yarrow, wild alum root, and pilewort. Mix thoroughly and use one teaspoon to a pint of boiling water. Boil and then let steep one-half hour. Take half a cup three or four times a day. The following is a very excellent remedy for healing when used as a suppository:

2 ounces powdered hemlock bark
1 ounce golden seal
1 ounce powdered wheat flour
1 ounce boric acid
1 ounce bayberry bark

Mix with glycerine until it is stiff enough to form suppositories. Insert one into the rectum at night and leave it in place.

Diet: All heavy and stimulating foods should be avoided, as should tobacco, tea, coffee, vinegar, alcoholic drinks, and meats of all kinds.

The diet should be simple and light. Potassium broth (see index) is very excellent. So is soybean milk, soybean zwieback, thoroughly ripe bananas, and vegetable broths of any kind. Staying on a fruit diet for a few days is very helpful.

In using all these treatments, good judgment must be exercised. There are perhaps other things that could be eaten, but a simple alkaline diet will hasten a cure.

A hot sitz bath, as hot as can be borne, should be taken. Sit in this bath for fifteen minutes or longer until the body is thoroughly heated. Have another tub ready containing cold water, and sit in this for a minute or two. Return to the hot water and repeat. If you use a bathtub, have the water well over the hips. Place the other tub alongside the bathtub, and tilt it by using wood or some other solid article under one side. Continue this treatment for one hour. (See also Section VIII, Chapters 3 and 5.)

HICCOUGHS

Causes: Irritation of the phrenic nerve, resulting in contraction and spasm of the diaphragm. Excessive food or drink in the stomach.

Treatment: A woman was once brought to me who was nearly dead from hiccoughs. I gave her the juice of half an orange and the hiccoughs stopped immediately. The juice of an orange will usually stop hiccoughs.

Eating regular blackboard chalk, taking a swallow or two of very hot or very cold water, or taking onion juice in teaspoonful doses, have all been used to stop hiccoughs. Another helpful thing to do is to make a tea of wild carrot seed, using a heaping teaspoon to a cup of boiling water; let steep one-half hour. Invariably a half cupful will stop hiccoughs. The blossoms are also good, used in the same way.

A poultice made from one-half teaspoon of cayenne pepper to a pint of vinegar, thickened with cornmeal, whole wheat flour, or linseed meal, and applied over the diaphragm, is excellent. One-fourth teaspoon of antispasmodic tincture, taken in a half glass of water every fifteen minutes until relief is obtained, is also very good.

A tea made of blue cohosh or black cohosh, taken either separately or mixed in equal parts, is also good.

HIGH BLOOD PRESSURE (HYPERTENSION)

Causes: There are many causes of high blood pressure. The blood pressure in normal individuals rises about one point each year until the seventh decade and then it usually levels off. Early in life, women usually have slightly lower blood pressures than men, but after the fourth decade this is reversed. A wide range of normal pressures exists, but the average pressure for a young adult is considered to be 120/80 mm Hg.

Overeating, which usually results in obesity, contributes to high blood pressure, as does eating the wrong diet, particularly a diet that is high in salt. High blood pressure would be less common if the liver and kidneys were not burdened with an overabundance of irritating foods. Some forms of high blood pressure are inherited, in fact in some groups of people this may be the cause in as many as seventy or eighty percent of the cases.

Symptoms: Patients with high blood pressure frequently complain of headaches, particularly in the morning, difficulty breathing, dizziness, flushed complexion, and blurred vision. They may first be seen with symptoms of heart failure or a stroke. In fact, one of the most frequent causes of a stroke (cerebrovascular accident) or heart attack (myocardial infarction) is hypertension.

Treatment: Please see also the section on Impure Blood (How to Cleanse), following. High herbal enemas should be given, for there is always putrid waste matter in the colon. Put one teaspoon of golden seal in a pint of boiling water, and take a swallow of this at least six times a day. Take plenty of red clover tea, as this will purify the blood; it is good to drink this in place of water. The following herbs are useful for high blood pressure: wild cherry bark, vervain, rue, broom, black cohosh, boneset, peppermint, blue cohosh, red pepper, valerian, hyssop, sanicle, and skullcap.

Diet and Rest: White flour products, cane sugar products, meat, tea, coffee, pepper, vinegar, mustard, pickles, alcohol, and all other stimulating foods and drinks are very harmful and should be omitted from the diet. Tobacco should also be eliminated, as it is one of the main causes of heart attacks. A fruit diet for a few days is one of the best things you can take. Then use a simple nourishing diet, get plenty of outdoor exercise, and practice deep breathing. Most people with high blood pressure do not get enough rest. They worry about business affairs, have too many social duties, too much stress, and keep too late hours. We mention these things because too much excitement and being overtired will always cause the blood pressure to rise. Rest is imperative. A warm bath at night and plenty of sleep in a well-ventilated room will do a great deal to lower the blood pressure. If troubled with sleeplessness, take an' herb tea that induces sleep. These teas are harmless and will leave no bad aftereffects. If you follow the above treatment and instructions, your blood pressure will surely come down.

The following treatment will greatly aid recovery: hot and cold applications to the spine, liver, spleen, and stomach; cold towel rubs in the morning upon arising; warm baths at night and salt glows; hot and cold showers. A general massage is excellent, as it will help work the waste matter out of the system, equalize the circulation, and greatly relieve the heart and nerves.

The blood pressure reflects the contractile powers of the heart and the resistance of the blood vessels. The blood pressure increases slowly during life so that the normal pressure at age thirty is approximately 125 and at age sixty it is about 140 mm/Hg. Persons who are weak physically have a slightly lower pressure. The blood pressure rises to some degree during exercise, depending upon the amount of exercise you are accustomed to taking. The more regularly you exercise, the less the blood pressure will rise.

If the blood pressure is too high or too low, there may be something wrong with the circulation of the blood; therefore a course of treatment must be followed to improve the circulation. When this is done it helps the blood pressure to become more normal. Two very important things which you can do to lower your blood pressure are (1) restrict the amount of salt in your diet and (2) make sure you are not overweight.

If after using the above simple measures your blood pressure does not come down to within the normal range, medical help should be sought because of the great frequency of strokes and heart attacks (coronary artery occlusion) in people who have high blood pressure.

HYDROPHOBIA (RABIES)

Causes: Rabies is caused by a virus that is present in many warm-blooded animals, and is transmitted to humans by the bite of an infected animal. Prior to the 1950s most cases of rabies in the United States were caused by the bites of rabid dogs or cats. Because of an intensive rabies control program, however, the number of cases of rabies has been reduced dramatically and the majority of cases now result from the bites of bats, foxes, skunks, and raccoons.

Symptoms: The length of time between the animal bite and when symptoms of rabies appear is extremely variable, but it is usually between three and eight weeks. During this period of time the person feels well except for the effects at the location of the animal bite. The closer to the head the person is bitten, the sooner the symptoms will appear. The early symptoms consist of tiredness, headache, fever, and loss of appetite. There may be persistent pain and swelling at the site of the bite. A feeling of anxiety, irritability, and nervousness is common, as is a lack of sleep. More severe symptoms involving the nervous system follow, including paralysis, stiffness of the neck, hallucinations, convulsions, agitation, and other hyperactive movements, which may come on by themselves or which may be brought on by noise, touch, or other kinds of stimulation. Attempts at drinking water are followed by severe pain due to spasm, which causes choking and gagging. If nothing is done, the patient goes into a coma, stops breathing, and soon dies.

Treatment: As soon as possible after the bite, the wound should be rinsed with water, then washed thoroughly with soap and water for five minutes and rinsed again. The locally injured tissue should be removed. If bitten by a healthy-appearing dog or cat, the animal should be confined for ten days, and if it does not develop rabies during this time, no further treatment is necessary. But if the animal develops rabies, or if it cannot be confined and observed for this length of time, which is usually the case with wild animals such as skunks, raccoons, foxes, etc., rabies vaccine must be given as soon as possible.

Until adequate medical assistance is available, the following measures can be used. Immediately after being bitten, tie a tight bandage above the wound and apply warm water and vinegar. The rabies virus usually remains localized in the tissues near the bite for quite some time before it finally travels up the nerves to the brain. After the wound has been washed thoroughly with warm water and vinegar or soap, it should be permitted to dry. Then apply a few drops of hydrochloric acid if available. This will neutralize and destroy the poison in the saliva from the animal's mouth. After this, apply a poultice made of granulated slippery elm with a teaspoon each of powdered golden seal, myrrh, and lobelia. Make the poultice large enough to cover the entire wound and change it every four hours. A poultice of burdock is also good. (See poultices in Section II, Chapter 3.)

For an internal tonic, take a compound of the following: one teaspoon each of golden seal, gentian, myrrh, lobelia, and one-eighth teaspoon of cayenne. Steep in one quart of boiling water for one-half hour. Take a swallow every hour.

It is best to take the herbs as a mixture, as just given, but, in case you cannot get them all, use any of them that you can obtain. I recommend this compound very highly. This treatment has been very successful in mad dog bite, snake bite, or insect bites, when the treatment was strictly followed. (Snake bites and insect bites never cause rabies.)

If the patient becomes nauseated or weak, give the following herbs: skullcap, black cohosh, valerian, gentian, and angelica. Use equal parts and mix thoroughly together, adding a little cayenne. If you do not have all these herbs, use the ones you have. Take according to directions for use of nonpoisonous herbs.

A tea made of plantain leaves is very effective and cleansing for a wash. A poultice made of the plantain leaves is also very good.

All poisonous insect bites and snake bites should be lanced. If this is not possible, the bite should be sucked by someone who does not have a sore of any nature in the mouth. Remember that insect bites and snake bites never result in rabies, since rabies only occurs in warm-blooded animals.

Rabies is an extremely ancient disease, and is mentioned as long ago as 2300 B.C. in old Egyptian writings. Before Pasteur introduced rabies vaccine in 1885, the bites of animals with rabies were treated with local cautery (burning).

The following paragraphs on hydrophobia are included mainly for historical interest, and are quoted from *The Model Botanic Guide to Health,* pp. 189-192.

Dog and Snake Bites and Hydrophobia

This terrible, always to be dreaded, affliction exists in both the human and animal species; it is produced by a specific virus, and is taken up by the absorbents, and carried through the medium of the saliva into the circulation, when after a certain period, the wound becomes red and inflamed, accompanied by pain and spasms.

They (the victims) have always a dread of liquids, particularly of water, even the sight of it causing spasms.

There is a frothy saliva ejected, and often a desire for biting anyone near them is manifested; and if not speedily attended to, alarming convulsions are experienced. Most people know that hydrophobia is madness caused by the bite of a mad dog or other rabid animal, while laboring under the disease.

M. Buisson read an interesting paper on the subject before the French Academy of Arts and Sciences, as a discovery and remedy for hydrophobia, in which he gives the particulars of his own case. He was called to attend a woman who was suffering from hydrophobia, and some of the poisonous saliva coming in contact with an ulcerated sore on one of his fingers, he contracted the disease himself. He says: "The ninth day after the accident I suddenly felt a pain in my throat and a still greater pain in my eyes. My body seemed to have become so light that I fancied I could leap an immense height; and the skin of my ulcerated hand became so acute in feeling that I thought I could have counted every hair on my head with it, without seeing. The saliva was constantly rising in my mouth, and not only the shining objects but the very contact of the atmosphere became painful to me. I felt a desire to run about and bite every animate and inanimate object but my fellow creatures. In time I experienced a great difficulty of breathing, and the sight of water was more distressing to me than the pain in my throat. The effects returned at intervals of five minutes after each other, and it appeared to me that it originated in the diseased finger, and then extended as high as the shoulder blade."

M. Buisson's account is thus concluded in a London Medical journal: "Concluding from these various symptoms that he was suffering with hydrophobia, he resolved to make an end of himself by suffocating himself in a vapour bath. With this view he raised the heat to 140°F. but was delighted, no less than surprised, to find that all his pains disappeared. He went out of the bath completely cured, ate a hearty dinner, and drank more freely than was usual with him. He adds that he has treated more than fourscore persons who have been bitten by mad dogs in a similar manner, and they all recovered, with the exception of a child seven years old, who died in a vapour bath he was administering."

Dr. Buisson mentions several other curious facts: "An American had been bitten by a snake away from home. Wishing to die with his family, he ran all the way home, and, going to bed, perspired profusely, and the wound healed as a simple cut."

Mr. Hubbard of Illinois, in a letter, says: "Eighteen years ago, my brother and myself were bitten by a mad dog; a sheep was also bitten at the same time; we were then ten or twelve years old. A friend suggested the following, which he said would cure the bite of a rattlesnake: Take the bark from the root of common ash, and boil it into a strong decoction, and of this drink freely. Whilst my father was preparing the above, the sheep spoken of began to be afflicted with hydrophobia; when it had become so fatigued from its distracted state as to be no longer able to stand, my father drenched it with a quantity of the ash bark tea, hoping to ascertain whether he could depend on it as a cure for his sons; four hours after the drenching had been given, to the astonishment of all, the animal got up and went quietly with the flock to graze.

"My brother and myself continued to take the medicine for eight or ten days, a teacupful three times a day. No effects of the dread poison were ever discovered on either of us. It has been used successfully in snake bites. To our knowledge the author has used the seeds or keys of ash for more than twenty years, and they are an old English remedy, but we have no hesitation in saying that the bark of the roots is much better."

A Saxon forester named Gastell, at the age of 82, unwilling to take to the grave with him a secret of so much importance, has made public in the *LEIPSIC JOURNAL* the means which he used for fifty years, and he affirms he has rescued many human beings and cattle from the fearful death of hydrophobia. His remedy is: wash the wound immediately with warm water and vinegar; let it dry, and then pour upon the wound a few drops of hydrochloric acid, and that will neutralize and destroy the poison of the saliva.

Treatment: These are remedies we also recommend; the vapor or hot water bath is an invaluable auxiliary in the treatment of hydrophobia. While in the vapor bath, give the following to all above ten years of age: half a teaspoon of tincture of lobelia with a teaspoon of antispasmodic tincture. Wash the wound with acid tincture of lobelia, oil tincture, or tincture of gum myrrh; keep the part constantly wet with it. At night apply a poultice of bloodroot and lobelia powder, equal parts, mixed with yeast.

HYSTERIA

Causes: Those who have hysterical attacks are very nervous as a rule. There is a long list of causes, but to mention a few will suffice. Anxiety, sudden fear, indigestion, extreme nervousness, temper tantrums, and menstruation in young girls. In some cases it is simply perverseness and nothing else. The cause should, of course, be ascertained in order to deal with it successfully.

Symptoms: An attack of hysteria never comes on when a person is asleep, since it usually indicates a desire for sympathy, or is brought on to frighten and disturb others. It always occurs when others are around. The beginning is usually a sob or a sigh, then there may be a twitching of the limbs or perhaps violent convulsions, the person throwing himself about. After the attack, there is usually a free discharge of urine.

Treatment: Always be firm with a person like this. They should not have excitement or sympathy, but be kind. Do not make fun of them after the attack, but take as little notice as possible.

Any one of the following herbs is useful: black cohosh, blue cohosh, valerian, vervain, skullcap, or catnip. Use a heaping teaspoonful to a cup of boiling water, steep thirty minutes and take a cupful four or five times a day. It is good to take a cupful hot upon retiring. Valerian, skullcap and catnip are available from your herbalist in capsule form.

For quick relief, take one-fourth teaspoon of antispasmodic tincture (see Section II, Chapter 3) every fifteen minutes.

IMPURE BLOOD (HOW TO CLEANSE)

Causes: A wrong diet, constipation, overeating, eating a combination of food at the same meal that causes fermentation, or devitalized foods. The very elements that would keep the blood pure are removed from many foods by the way they are prepared; for example, the heart and the outside of the wheat, the eyes and peelings of potatoes, the outside of rice, and the heart of corn, which is taken out of the meal. These are wonderful alkaline medicines and do a great deal toward keeping the blood pure.

Some other causes of impure blood are improper breathing, sleeping in rooms that are not properly ventilated, and lack of exercise. Often the muscles are poisoned and feel tired because of the accumulated waste matter from insufficient exercise.

Drinking impure water and other harmful drinks, such as tea, coffee, liquor, and all kinds of soft drinks, are other causes. These confuse the mind and cause wrong thoughts and ideas. The brain is made up of about 90 percent water and when we drink these unwholesome drinks, many of which are stimulating, the blood is made impure and the mind is very much affected.

Worry, fear, anger, unhappiness, and hate generally hinder the circulation of blood, and thus the impurities are not carried off as they should be. A stagnant condition of the skin is another cause of impure blood. Many times the blood that should be circulating near the surface of the body is in the deeper structures, overloading the various organs and causing congestion and various diseases.

Symptoms: The symptoms cover a large list of diseases

and complaints: pimples, boils, discolorations of the skin, jaundice, headaches, drowsiness, wrinkles, premature aging, insanity, nervousness, getting angry easily, continually frowning when we should be smiling, thinking evil thoughts when we should think evil of no man, seeing darkness where there is light, gray hair, loss of hair, loss of eyesight, loss of hearing, stiff joints, and pain in various parts of the body. All of these symptoms will be helped to a greater or lesser degree when the bloodstream is purified.

Treatment: To make the blood pure, the first thing to do is to eliminate all harmful articles of food and drink such as tea, coffee, all alcoholic drinks, soft drinks, all white flour products, all cane sugar products, and the liberal use of free fat or grease. The bowels must be kept open by proper diet and the use of herbal laxatives when needed. Take high herbal enemas to clean out the colon and make it active and strong. Drink plenty of fresh, pure water. Take regular outdoor exercise with deep breathing and get plenty of sleep in a well-ventilated room.

Echinacea and red clover are good blood purifiers. Both can be purchased in convenient capsule form.

Keep the skin active by cold morning baths and vigorous rubbing with a coarse Turkish towel. Take a hot bath or shower every day. Wash the body thoroughly with some good soap. A thorough salt glow is good after a hot bath. This will stimulate the skin, make it active, and open the pores.

A massage from head to foot is beneficial. Give it thoroughly on the neck and upper part of the spine and especially on the feet.

Go on a fruit diet for one week. In the absence of an abundance of fruit, eat vegetables prepared as discussed in Section V, Chapter 2, and Section VI, Chapter 1. For example, eat the green part of leafy vegetables and carrots — either raw, grated, or baked until tender — carrot juice, and potatoes. Reader, if you want to see wonderful results, live on the food that God originally gave to man. There is an abundance of it. Just live on fruit for a while and follow the sanitary habits previously mentioned. Make use of the herbs that God let grow for the healing of the nations and you will say with many whom the writer has heard say, "Truly the day of miracles has not passed." The fruit of the tree is for man's food, and the leaves for his medicine. (Ezekiel 47:12)

INFANT FEEDING

The natural food for infants is mother's milk, which is by far the best. Mother's milk is richer in iron than cow's milk. If the mother is on a good diet, eating a wide variety of fruits and vegetables, including daily citrus fruit, the baby will receive all the necessary vitamins, minerals, protein, fat, and carbohydrate. Unless the mother is in a weakened condition, or is suffering from disease, she should nurse her child, and nine times out of ten would be able to do so by using the right diet. Diet recommendations for nursing mothers are given in the article on Pregnancy, which follows later in this section.

Regularity in infant feeding is essential. The child should not stay at the breast more than thirty minutes, and if the milk supply is plentiful ten to fifteen minutes is usually adequate. All infants should be weaned by the end of the first year. Weaning should be gradual. Give a bottle once a day with the breast feeding, increasing the number of bottles each day until the child is entirely weaned.

Cane sugar in any form should never be given to infants under any circumstances. Many times cane sugar is the cause of fever and other ailments. Malt sugar, malt honey, or honey should always be used in place of cane sugar.

Diarrhea in infants can be stopped by the use of thin rice or barley water. For an older child, use oatmeal gruel. This should be given until the looseness is checked.

Soybean milk is a good food for infants and children and can be given from the first day. In using soybean milk, you eliminate the danger of contaminated milk and also disease is not encountered. Note the analysis of soybean milk as compared with other kinds of milk, in the chart in Section V,

Chapter 8. The flavor of soybean milk can be improved by the addition of a little powdered oatmeal, powdered wheat malt, or barley malt.

For infants, soybean milk should be diluted by using one-fourth water to three-fourths soybean milk. Discretion must be used in diluting soybean milk as in other infant's food, depending upon the needs of the infant. When the infant has a weak stomach, or is not strong constitutionally, dilute the milk more. The milk can be given full strength at the age of five or six months. When the baby is six months old, dilute four tablespoonfuls of whole wheat flakes in boiling water until completely dissolved, put through a fine sieve, and add to the baby's bottle. This will give added nourishment in an excellent form. A smaller amount of wheat flakes may be added earlier with benefit.

Begin feeding wholesome simple foods in puree form, such as greens, vegetables, fruit juices, and gruels, when the first teeth appear. Orange juice and tomato juice may be given from the beginning, starting with a half teaspoonful at about the age of one month.

When a child is given meat, white flour products, cane sugar products, candies, etc., he loses his taste and desire for wholesome natural foods. The eating of these detrimental things by children is responsible for many illnesses.

Never allow children to eat between meals. Irregularities in eating ruin the digestive organs by keeping them overworked, causing indigestion and nervousness.

If the baby is being fed cow's milk, vitamin C and D may be lacking. A simple way to make sure the infant is getting sufficient vitamins is to use a multivitamin concentrate which contains vitamins A, C, D, and sometimes B complex. But overdosage with vitamins, particularly vitamin D, should be avoided.

INFANTILE PARALYSIS (POLIOMYELITIS)

Causes: Infantile paralysis is caused by a virus and is

transmitted by human contact. This virus enters the body through the mouth and passes into the intestines. From there it may be absorbed into the lymph nodes and the nervous system. Poliomyelitis is a worldwide disease, but it has largely been eliminated in the United States and western Europe since the advent of effective vaccines in the 1950s.

Symptoms: There is nothing characteristic of poliomyelitis in the early symptoms. These symptoms consist of a low-grade fever, a feeling of tiredness, aching muscles, running nose, and sometimes headache. There may be nausea and diarrhea. The more serious symptoms soon follow; these are weakness, stiff aching muscles, severe headache, gastrointestinal complaints, restlessness, stiff neck, and eventually weakness and paralysis of muscles. Read about my experiences in treating and curing cases of infantile paralysis in Section I, Chapter 1.

Treatment: Prevention. With proper vaccination, this dread paralyzing disease has been all but eliminated in the United States and other developed countries of the world. The immunization program should begin in infancy at about two months of age. It is no longer recommended that adults living in the United States receive routine immunization against poliomyelitis.

See Section V, Chapter 11 on diets. If the elimination diet is used, followed by a nourishing diet, proper water treatments given, and a similar course followed as given in Section I, Chapter 1, this terrible disease can be cured.

The following herbs are used with excellent results. See their descriptions in Section II, Chapter 5: prickly ash berries, wild cherry bark, English or American valerian root, poplar bark, dandelion root, skullcap, golden seal, black cohosh, catnip, red clover, yellow dock. Select one or several that are best suited to the case, and mix equal parts to make an herbal tea.

An excellent compound is made of the following: one tablespoon each of valerian, catnip, and calamus root. Mix together, then steep a teaspoon in a cup of boiling water. Give one-fourth cupful every two hours. Considerable amounts of this tea may be taken as it is harmless. For a small child, give the tea in tablespoon doses, several times a day, sweetened with a little honey or malt sugar.

Antispasmodic tincture given in doses of eight to fifteen drops in one-fourth glass of water (hot) is also very good. Adjust dose according to age.

INFLUENZA (LA GRIPPE)

Causes: Influenza is caused by three types of influenza virus — types A, B, and C. Type A causes the most severe disease. Influenza may occur worldwide involving millions of cases, or it may appear sporadically in a single community. Exposure to cold or dampness, or when the body is weakened by disease, or by following poor health habits, makes one more susceptible to the influenza virus.

Symptoms: There is usually a chilly feeling, various muscular aches and pains, backache, poor appetite, ringing in the ears, dizziness, cough, sometimes a sore throat, stuffiness, and hoarseness. Headache is frequent. The fever may be more severe in the evening. Influenza starts rapidly and lasts for seven to ten days. The real danger of influenza is that if it is not checked by proper treatment, complications may set in. Pneumonia is one of the most frequent complications, and it may prove fatal unless treated vigorously. Patients who already have heart or lung disease or are pregnant are particularly prone to develop viral pneumonia with influenza. After an attack of influenza, the system should be built up with good nourishing foods.

Treatment: If treatment is started when the symptoms first appear, influenza may be overcome in twenty-four hours.

Stop eating and go to bed. Use the following internally: one tablespoon yarrow, one teaspoon pleurisy root and a small pinch of cayenne. Steep in a pint of boiling water for twenty minutes and take a cupful every hour. Drinking this tea will cause profuse perspiration, and when the bed clothes become wet they should be changed. If there is fever, bathe the entire body with tepid water thoroughly, having the towel very wet and exposing only one portion of the body at a time.

Alternate the herbs with fruit juices; orange and grapefruit preferably. Lemon juice is also excellent to reduce the fever. Do not use sugar in any of the juices. Orange juice is very strengthening. If you follow the treatment outlined, being sure to keep the bowels moving normally with some laxative herbs, you will find your influenza practically gone the next day.

If the disease progresses, take the herbs given above and also the orange juice and other fruit juices. Take sweat baths and some tonic herbs such as wild cherry bark, skullcap, valerian, lady's slipper, or feverfew (Chrysanthemum parthenium). Plenty of fresh air in the patient's room is essential.

Dr. Zalabak gave me this formula many years ago, saying that it would cure a cold in twenty-four hours: equal parts of cinnamon, sage, and bay leaves. Use a heaping teaspoon of this mixture to a cup of boiling water, steep, and drink as much as desired.

A very effective remedy that works like a charm is made by using equal parts of the following herbs: agrimony, vervain, boneset, and culver's root. Use a heaping teaspoon of this mixture to a cup of boiling water. Take a cupful every hour.

More herbs that are good for influenza are: peppermint, white pine, poplar, butternut bark, lungwort, nettle, pleurisy root, saffron, sweet balm, tansy, ginger, golden seal, saw palmetto berries, wood betony, angelica, hyssop, boneset, vervain, Culver's root, agrimony, and feverfew. Use singly or in combination. Read their description in Section II, Chapter 5 and use those best suited to your condition.

Influenza is usually much more difficult to cure than a common cold. The symptoms may be helped, but they may not completely disappear with the above treatments. If so, do not become discouraged, but stay in bed, drinking lots of liquids, particularly fruit juices. This disease is usually self-limited and will gradually disappear within seven to ten days, although the cough may last longer than this, sometimes for weeks or even months.

INSOMNIA

Causes: Common causes are overeating, indigestion, eating late at night just before retiring, stress, tension, worry, fear of something that might happen, etc. Cold feet, poor circulation, nervousness, and poor ventilation in the bedroom are also causes. A constant loss of sleep, whatever the cause, is always injurious to health.

Treatment: A full warm bath or a hot footbath taken with a cup of hot tea, as given in the next paragraph, will often bring sleep immediately. If the person is very tired, nervous, and worn out, a fomentation to the spine, liver, and stomach will help produce sleep. The extremities should be kept warm, and a hot water bottle or electric heating pad should be used if necessary. Some people are put to sleep by having their hair brushed, or sometimes by having their feet gently rubbed.

The following herbs are very effective in producing sleep: lady's slipper, valerian, catnip, skullcap, and especially hops. Use a teaspoon of any one of the above, steep in a cup of boiling water twenty minutes and drink hot. These herbs will not only produce sleep, but they have many other good qualities: they tone up the stomach and nerves, without ever leaving any bad aftereffects. Instead, they act as a tonic to the entire system. Aspirin or bromides taken for this purpose may seem to help for a time, but as their effect is to deaden the nerves, every dose taken makes the condition decidedly worse, and finally they lose their effectiveness altogether.

If you do not have herbs on hand, either hot sour lemonade or hot grapefruit juice may be tried. A cup of warm soybean milk is also sometimes helpful.

ITCH

Causes: There are various kinds of itch: seven year's itch, barber's itch, bricklayer's itch, and others. The itch that went by the name of "seven year's itch" for a great many years, is caused by a very small insect called the "itch mite." These small mites bore beneath the skin where it is thin, warm, and moist, usually between the fingers, wrist, forearm, etc. When they get on children, they attack especially the feet and buttocks. The itching is greater at night when the body is warm. The irritation and scratching cause pimples and scabs to form. This type of itch is also commonly known as scabies. It is most frequent in people who do not bathe frequently. Close physical contact with an infected person is all that is needed to acquire scabies.

Treatment: Before each application of the following salve, thoroughly wash the affected parts with tar soap. All clothing must be washed in boiling water. When the clothes cannot be washed or boiled, press them with a hot iron to destroy any insects that may be on them. Take one tablespoon of each of the following: burdock root, yellow dock root, and yarrow. Steep them in a pint of boiling water for a half hour. Strain through a cloth into a cooking pan (not aluminum), and add one pound of cocoa fat or Crisco. Boil this slowly, stirring frequently until it has boiled down to the consistency of a salve. This is an excellent salve for itch or eczema of any kind. If you do not wish to make the salve, bathe the affected parts with the tea as directed above. Herbal salve, as given in Section II, Chapter 3, is very useful in itch and eczema. It is healing and soothing.

If students are found to be infected with the scabies mite, they should be kept at home until cured. Frequent washing of the body is necessary. There are now many lotions available for the treatment of scabies that are very effective. These lotions should be applied to the entire body below the neck and washed off the following day. One or two additional treatments at weekly intervals may be necessary to rid the body of all the mites.

JAUNDICE

Causes: Jaundice is caused by obstructive diseases of the liver or bile ducts that result in an increased absorption of bile into the blood. This makes the skin and whites of the eyes turn yellow. There are many diseases that may cause jaundice. Some examples are cancer, gallstones, infections, cirrhosis of the liver, various drugs and toxins, blood transfusions, and some virus and bacterial diseases that involve the liver. Jaundice may occasionally result from a rapid destruction of red blood cells in the body.

Bile is produced by the cells in the liver. It leaves the liver through the bile ducts and enters the small intestine just beyond the stomach. Some of the bile passing from the liver to the intestine is sidetracked into the gallbladder, where it is stored and concentrated before reaching the intestine. About one or two ounces of bile is normally stored in the gallbladder. Eating fatty foods, particularly cream and egg yokes, causes the gallbladder to contract and expel its content of bile into the intestine.

Bile has several important functions. Its main function concerns the digestion and absorption, in the intestine, of the fat in our food. Bile also serves as a method for getting rid of certain waste products. It helps to neutralize the gastric juice and alkalinizes our food; thus enabling the body to absorb it. A lack of bile entering the intestines contributes to constipation.

Symptoms: Yellow skin; whites of the eyes turn yellow; bitter taste in the mouth; constipation, dark urine, slight fever, headache, dizziness, and itching of the skin.

Treatment: Take one-fourth teaspoon of golden seal in a glass of water one hour before meals, three times a day. At first, take nothing but fruit juices, especially lemon and grapefruit. These will help to alkalinize the system and wash out the poisonous toxins. Potassium broth may then be given, as it is very nourishing and will keep the patient's strength up if nothing else is given except the fruit juices. The patient should drink a glass of lemon juice every hour as long as there is fever, and continue drinking it freely after the fever has gone down. During the acute stage, fomentations to the liver and stomach will help ease the pain.

In infectious jaundice there is usually itching of the skin. Washing with very hot boric acid water will allay this. Also see the herb washes given under the treatment for itch, preceding.

The following herbs are excellent for overcoming jaundice: dandelion, agrimony, yarrow, and self-heal. Make an herb tea according to directions given in Section II, Chapter 3. Self-heal and dandelion are especially beneficial. Self-heal alone is very good. Also use the herbal laxative. The bowels must be kept open.

Another good remedy is to take a handful of peach pits and grind or crush them. Make a tea by putting the ground pits into two cups of water and let simmer slowly for thirty minutes. Strain and take one-fourth cupful of this tea upon arising every morning, and the same dose before each meal and at bedtime. If the pits cannot be obtained, use a handful of the bruised leaves or twigs, with enough cold water to cover them. Simmer the twigs a little longer than you would the leaves. Take the same as directed for tea made from the pits.

Unsweetened lemonade may be taken with benefit in place of water. The same treatment as that given for gallstones is also good for jaundice.

If the jaundice does not clear with the above treatment, it may indicate that a more serious disease is present, and you should seek the help of a physician so that the cause for the jaundice can be found.

KIDNEY STONES

Causes: Some of the causes for kidney stones are wrong dietary habits, drinking an insufficient amount of liquids, infection and obstruction in the urinary tract, certain diseases involving the intestinal tract, and other diseases such as gout, etc. Many patients develop kidney stones without any apparent cause. For some reason, people living in the southeastern United States are much more likely to develop kidney stones than those living in other parts of the country.

Symptoms: Severe pain in the back, lower abdomen, or groin is the most common symptom. If this pain is not relieved, nausea and vomiting will develop. The urine may turn a dark orange or reddish color. If the stones are in the urinary bladder there may be a great desire to urinate, but without success. If urination stops, a catheter must be used. The amount of discomfort ranges from a mild intermittent ache to severe unrelenting pain.

Treatment: In order to prevent the formation of kidney stones, a very high fluid intake of two to four quarts a day is necessary. This will keep the urine dilute and prevent the formation of stones. Kidney stones are frequently composed of calcium oxalate, and it may help to prevent this type of stone from forming by eating a diet that is low in oxalates and dairy products. Vegetables high in oxalates are spinach, parsley, beets, beet greens, Swiss chard, asparagus, okra, collards, celery, leeks, and sweet potatoes. Many fruits are also relatively high in oxalates, particularly berries; but the highest of all is rhubarb. Several nuts are high in oxalates, particularly almonds, cashews, peanuts and peanut butter. Ovaltine and cocoa should be eliminated from the diet as should tea, coffee, and all dark cola drinks. If there is any infection in the urinary tract, this should be controlled, as it tends to promote the formation of stones.

Once a stone that has formed in the kidney begins to pass down the ureter — the slender tube leading from the kidney to the urinary bladder — the pain becomes intense. When this happens, apply hot fomentations across the back in the region of the kidneys. A poultice made of hops with a little lobelia added and applied just below the waist line on the back will help relieve the pain. Make this as hot as can be borne. Herbal liniment, as given in Section II, Chapter 3, should be freely and thoroughly applied and rubbed in well. This will also help to relieve the pain.

Give a hot bath starting with a temperature of 100° and increasing to 112°F. Keep the head and neck cool with cold applications. If the patient becomes very weak, have him stand and sponge off with cool water, getting immediately back into the hot water. This should be continued for at least thirty minutes. Give a hot enema before the bath, using catnip tea if possible. This will give great relief. It soothes the kidneys and warms up the bladder. Use a tablespoon of catnip herb to every quart of water. Use a one or two-quart enema for adults. Children use less in proportion to their age.

Also drink a tea of the following: equal parts of wild carrot seeds, valerian, and peppermint. Mix these together and use a teaspoon to a cup of boiling water; steep for one-half hour. Take one-half cupful every hour until relieved. Queen of the meadow, peach leaves, or cleavers may also be used with good results.

In case of hemorrhage from the kidneys or bladder, use shepherd's purse. This will help stop the bleeding. Use a heaping teaspoon to a cup of boiling water, steep thirty minutes, strain, and drink half a cupful five or six times a day, and more if needed.

For tumors or inflammation of the bladder, use a teaspoon of golden seal, one-half teaspoon of myrrh, and one-half teaspoon of boric acid, in a pint of water. Inject through a soft catheter into the bladder. This should be done by a graduate nurse or someone with experience. I DO NOT RECOMMEND THAT PATIENTS DO THIS FOR THEMSELVES UNLESS THEY HAVE BEEN SHOWN BY A PHYSICIAN OR GRADUATE NURSE HOW TO DO IT.

Follow the diet as given for treating gallstones. This diet should be used in all kidney and bladder troubles.

LEPROSY

Another name for leprosy is Hansen's disease. This disease is caused by a bacillus and affects mainly the skin and peripheral nerves. It is a very old disease, and it is estimated that at the present time between ten and twenty million people worldwide are infected; about 60 percent of the cases are in Asia. In India alone, there are about 3.5 million lepers. Leprosy is found mostly in tropical regions. In the United States it is most prevalent in Louisiana, Florida, Texas, California, and Hawaii. Only 244 cases were reported in the United States in 1981; however, many cases are now being brought into the United States from foreign countries. Puerto Rico also has a high incidence of leprosy.

The exact way that leprosy is spread from one person to another is not known for sure. It is thought to be spread through the respiratory tract much more frequently than by coming in direct contact with the skin of a person who has leprosy. The longer the time of contact, the greater will be the chance of contracting leprosy. The infective rate of leprosy is not high, however, and only about 5 to 10 percent of close family members will contract the disease — about the same as for active tuberculosis.

Symptoms: One or several large, flat, whitish areas appear on the skin. The margins are usually rather red and the centers of the white plaques do not contain hair and are quite dry. The patches are usually numb when touched or pricked, and the surrounding nerves may be enlarged. These lesions may occur anywhere on the body surface or within the mouth. Leprosy progresses slowly, with eventual loss of fingers, toes, nose, and sometimes other portions of the body. The diagnosis is best made by taking a small piece of the involved skin and examining it under a microscope.

Treatment: Fresh air and a nourishing diet are absolutely necessary. Fish and meats of all kinds are strictly forbidden. Eat plenty of fresh fruits and vegetables.

Take a heaping teaspoon of golden seal and one-half teaspoon of myrrh. Steep them in a pint of boiling water. Take one cupful of this solution one-half hour before each meal and upon retiring.

An excellent herb combination to use in leprosy is one heaping teaspoon of red clover blossoms, one teaspoon of yellow dock root, one teaspoon of calamus, one teaspoon of burdock, and one-half teaspoon of mandrake. Mix these together and use a heaping teaspoon to a cup of boiling water. Take four cups a day, an hour before each meal and one upon retiring.

The following herbs are also good. Look up their descriptions in Section II, Chapter 5, and take those best suited to your case: bittersweet, dandelion, and myrrh.

LIQUOR HABIT

Taking alcohol into the system always produces an unnatural condition. Habitual users of alcohol often have stomach ulcers, since alcohol injures the mucous membrane lining. Many who drink alcohol freely develop cirrhosis of the liver, which is eventually fatal.

The continual use of alcohol makes a total wreck of the person, and may lead to insanity. The heart becomes weak and the blood vessels are affected. It ruins the nervous system and weakens the mental powers. It makes one coarse and unrefined. Alcohol is certainly a snake in the grass. It is stimulating to the senses and makes a person feel happy and strong for a short while, but misery and weakness soon follow. Alcohol numbs the nerves to such an extent that a person feels warm when he is actually cold. It makes him quite active while he is under its hellish influence, but there is great collapse as the effect wears off. It surely mocks a man and makes a fool of him. Solomon, the wisest man that ever lived, said that "wine is a mocker, strong drink is raging; and whoever is deceived thereby is not wise." Proverbs 20:1.

While in Minnesota many years ago, the foreman of the

red marble works, who was not a drinking man, had stomach trouble and the doctor prescribed brandy in tablespoon doses. In order to quiet his misery, he kept taking more and more brandy until he became a wreck and was afflicted with what is known as the "snakes." It took two men to control him, for when he imagined he saw the snakes coming he would try to get away from them and go through any door or window near at hand, using all the power that was in his body to get away. Often he looked for a gun to kill the snakes. Two men brought this man to me when I had a sanitarium. The first thing I did was to give him a warm bath. These two men placed him in the tub. When he could not be kept in the bath tub any longer, we would put him under a shower. I went in the shower with him, keeping him under it as long as possible and using cold water. Then we had him drink all the quieting herbs we could make him drink or force down him. He slept for two hours the first night. When he woke up he said, "Oh! how good I feel." The men who brought him to me told me that previous to the treatment he had absolutely not slept for three weeks or more. They said that he would doze off, and then wake up all excited and try to get out of the way of the snakes.

The next day we went through quite a program. We gave him several warm baths, which he was made to stay in for quite long periods. He was given hot and cold fomentations to the spine and over the stomach, liver, and spleen; and then cold fomentations to the spine and over the stomach, liver, spleen, and pancreas. He was given nourishing food that was easy to digest. The second night he slept for six hours. The third day we went through the course of treatment again, and that night he slept all night. In three days he had improved so much that he could be left alone. In three weeks, this man who had been a wreck physically and very weak, went back to work and took his former position.

The happy part of it all was that this man, who was separated from his family because of drinking, was restored to them, and there was great rejoicing. The beauty of it was that he quit drinking and could not be hired to touch alcohol under any circumstances. Many a family that has been torn apart through the curse of alcohol has been brought together again, through the loving service and simple remedies that God has given to man. We could cite many such cases, but space does not permit.

In order to help anyone overcome the drinking habit, he must be willing to quit. When he decides to give it up, it is very easy and simple to help him stop.

Treatment: A fruit diet is very effective, followed by a light nourishing diet. Heavy sweat baths should be given every day. Take some of the laxative herbs to keep the bowels loose.

Give hot baths, with thorough rubbing, while in the tub. This helps eliminate the waste matter from the system. A massage every day is very valuable. Give the patient a vigorous cold towel rub every morning upon arising, followed by brisk rubbing with a rough Turkish towel.

To help destroy the taste for liquor, quassia chips are very beneficial. Use one teaspoon to a cup of boiling water. Steep for one-half hour and keep covered. Take a swallow every two hours. In very bad cases, the patient should have a constant attendant, so he will not be able to get more liquor.

Never taper off! QUIT and NEVER taste the stuff again. That is the way I did. I was a very heavy drinker when I made up my mind one day that I would give up this damnable stuff, which was ruining my health and my life. I never tasted it again, and that was about forty years ago. I was also a heavy tobacco user, both chewing and smoking. That was also given up and I have never used tobacco again either.

LOW BLOOD PRESSURE (HYPOTENSION)

The diagnosis of low blood pressure must be made with care. In adults, the blood pressure is usually considered low if it is below 110/70. But many healthy adults consistently have a systolic pressure (the highest number) of 90 to 100 mm/Hg.

Causes: Lack of proper nourishment, rest, and exercise; lack of vitality and loss of blood. Certain neurological and muscular diseases.

Treatment: Increase the circulation by means of deep breathing, hot baths, and cold morning baths, thoroughly rubbing with a coarse towel when drying. Any one of the following herbs, mixed with a very little red pepper, will greatly increase the vitality: hyssop, golden seal, vervain, prickly ash, blue cohosh, gentian, wood betony, burnet, and skullcap. Take any of the tonic herbs listed in Section II, Chapter 4.

Diet: Eat plenty of nourishing food; potassium broth and mashed potatoes (see Section V, Chapter 2), baked potatoes (skin and all), soybean milk, soy cottage cheese, plenty of leafy vegetables, and vegetables of all kinds. Do not eat any devitaminized or stimulating foods. If you are troubled with indigestion, drink peppermint or spearmint tea. You will not likely have indigestion if you eat proper food, and eat it dry. Drinking water and other liquids with meals causes fermentation and slows digestion. If you thoroughly cleanse your system, and follow the above instructions, your blood pressure will soon become normal.

Regular exercise out-of-doors is very necessary.

Echinacea is an excellent tonic for the blood and is available in capsule form; take one capsule three times a day.

LUMBAGO — See also RHEUMATISM and ARTHRITIS

Lumbago is a form of rheumatism that may be brought on by becoming very warm, and then suddenly cooling off or getting in a draft. Sometimes lumbago is caused by rupture of a spinal disc, which causes pressure on the spinal nerves. A back injury or strain will sometimes bring on an attack.

Symptoms: Pain and tenderness in the muscles, sometimes affecting one and then another muscle. At times the pain comes on suddenly, and it feels as though there was a kink in the back. Adults are the most frequent victims, but children are also sometimes affected.

Treatment: In all cases of lumbago, rest is very important. Hot fomentations followed by a thorough massage of the painful area, using herb liniment, is very helpful, and will greatly relieve the pain. The patient should be kept warm. Use the same herbs as listed for the treatment of rheumatism.

Those who suffer from lumbago should not use tea, coffee, liquor, tobacco, or any stimulating or unwholesome food. If constipated, an herbal laxative or enema may be needed.

LUNGS, INFLAMMATION OF

Inflammation of the lungs is usually referred to as pneumonia.

Causes: The direct cause of pneumonia is usually infection with some form of bacteria, virus, or fungus. Exposure to cold and dampness, with lowered resistance, is a contributing factor.

Treatment: Proper treatment, given at the first signs of a cold or chilliness, will likely prevent a severe attack and will in all probability prevent any attack. For a cold and sore throat, the nose and throat should be kept clean by sniffing salt water up the nose and then blowing the nose, holding one side shut while blowing through the other. Use one teaspoon of salt to a pint of water. Do this several times a day. Gargle and rinse out the mouth with salt water. Take a rounded teaspoon of golden seal and one-fourth teaspoon of myrrh, steep in one pint of boiling water and use in the same way as above. Be sure to gargle deeply and thoroughly with this, as it will clean all the germs and impurities out of the mouth and throat.

If this is repeated often enough, the cold or flu will not go down into the lungs. Take internally one tablespoon of this same solution of golden seal and myrrh six times a day.

If the lungs are not already seriously affected, take the above treatment, giving hot footbaths at the same time. The bowels must be kept open by taking proper enemas or herbal laxatives. Drink large quantities of water. Give the patient hot fomentations to the chest and back of the lungs, with a short cold rub between each hot fomentation.

Only liquids should be given for the first few days. The best ones to use are lemonade without sugar, grapefruit juice, orange juice, pineapple juice (unsweetened); other fruit juices may also be used. When there is a high fever, this diet should be followed until the fever returns to near normal. When it is advisable to administer more nourishment, give strained vegetable broth. Soybean milk with whole wheat flakes or whole wheat zwieback is also very good.

The herbs that are lung tonics are comfrey, cudweed, elecampane, horehound, ground ivy, and ginger. A small amount of cayenne added to any of these herbs when making the tea is beneficial. Take as directed in Section II, Chapter 3.

Any one of the following herbs may also be taken. Look up the descriptions of these herbs in Section II, Chapter 5, and take the ones which are best suited for your case: plantain, lungwort, pleurisy root, slippery elm, wild alum root, coltsfoot, mustard, vervain, flaxseed, hops, hyssop, white pine, spikenard, wahoo, mullein, herba santa, yarrow, skunk cabbage, horehound, myrrh.

MEASLES (RUBEOLA)

Causes: Few persons escape having measles during childhood, but adults may also catch this very common disease. Measles is caused by a virus, and is one of the most contagious diseases. One attack of measles usually produces a permanent immunity against a second attack. Measles is caused by coming in contact with another person who has measles, while they are in the active stage of the disease. The measles virus is present in the greatest concentration in discharges from the patient's nose, mouth, and throat.

Symptoms: The symptoms begin to appear about ten

days following exposure, and at first they resemble a common cold with fever, runny nose, cough, and sore throat. After three or four days the rash breaks out, usually on the head or face, and after a few days it has spread over the entire body. It appears as blotchy, red areas with normal skin in between. Reddish white spots may be present inside the mouth before the rash appears. When the rash has fully developed, the fever drops to normal.

Complications such as pneumonia and ear infections are common and must be guarded against.

Treatment: The patient must be kept isolated for at least five days following the appearance of the rash, and should be put to bed for as long as the fever persists or there is any sign of cough or lung infection. The eyes should be protected from bright light by darkening the room, wearing dark glasses, or turning the bed so it is not facing toward a window. A tea made as follows should be given: one teaspoon of pleurisy root and one-fourth teaspoon of ginger steeped in a pint of boiling water. You may sweeten the tea a little for children by using honey or malt sugar. For a nervous person, add a teaspoon of lady's slipper or catnip to the above. Two tablespoons of the tea should be given every hour, more or less according to age. Catnip or peppermint tea given separately is also excellent.

The patient must be kept in a dimly lit room of even temperature and with good ventilation. Drink plenty of water and take hot footbaths.

In the event the patient's eyes become sore, make a solution of one-fourth teaspoon of golden seal steeped in a pint of boiling water (soft or distilled), for thirty minutes; then add enough boric acid to make a saturated solution. Strain through a cloth and bathe the eyes two or three times a day or oftener.

The same diet recommended for fevers is excellent after the fever has broken. A simple, nourishing diet is essential, such as soybean milk with wheat flakes and whole wheat crackers. If cow's milk is used in the absence of soybean milk, boil a little oatmeal in it or use half cow's milk and half oatmeal and barley water. Very ripe bananas with soybean milk and whole wheat toast are good. Potassium broth (see index) is nourishing, cleansing, and tasty, and would be fine. Ripe fruits of all kinds may be used.

Any of the following herbs are also good for treating measles: catnip, peppermint, camomile, vervain, yarrow, or lady's slipper. Steep a teaspoon in a cup of boiling water, covered. Give one-fourth cupful every two hours.

If coughing is a problem, the air in the room should be kept moist by using a kettle of boiling water or a vaporizer.

MENSTRUATION

Causes of Tardy or Suppressed Menstruation: Most young girls start to menstruate at about the age of thirteen or fourteen years. The menstrual periods during this time may normally be scanty and irregular and may not become well established until the age of fifteen or sixteen. Occasionally a young woman may not begin menstruating until sixteen or seventeen years of age. If the menstrual cycle has been well established and then ceases, the most common cause is some form of stress or emotional disturbance. When these problems are resolved satisfactorily, the menstrual cycle will return to normal. Occasionally undernourishment, or a lack of fresh air, sunshine, and proper exercise, results in absent or diminished menstruation. Nervousness, caused by tension in the home or at school, may also affect the normal menstrual cycle.

Treatment: The following herbs can be taken with confidence that there will be no harmful aftereffects and that they will help to reestablish normal menstrual periods. Select one, after looking up their descriptions in Section II, Chapter 5, and take according to directions in Section II, Chapter 3: tansy, black cohosh, wild yam, mugwort, camomile, and gentian. Take a hot bath before retiring. Hot sitz baths are beneficial. The legs and feet must be covered and kept warm at all times. The same treatment applies to all women troubled with suppressed or scanty menstruation.

Causes of Profuse Menstruation: There are many causes, including hormone imbalance, diseases of the womb, metabolic diseases, improper diet resulting in iron deficiency, and general debility.

Treatment: Eat plain, simple food. All stimulating foods, drinks, and narcotics are harmful and should be discontinued. Keep off the feet as much as possible when menstruating. The body, including the legs and feet, must be kept well covered and warm. A warm douche of white oak bark, wild alum root or bayberry bark is very helpful; taken, of course, after the menses have ceased. Use a heaping tablespoon of one of these herbs to a quart of boiling water, steep covered, and use as a douche four or five times a day if needed. Also take bayberry, white oak bark, or wild alum root internally.

If the bleeding is extremely profuse, make or purchase tampons of absorbent material, immerse them in a tea made from equal parts of wild alum root and white oak bark with a little lobelia added. Tie a piece of strong string around the middle, if one is not already present, leaving it long enough so that the end remains outside of the vagina. The tampon should be inserted far enough into the vagina so that it presses snugly against the womb. Remove the tampon every twelve hours and wash the vagina out with an herb douche.

Painful Menstruation: Painful menstruation is quite common in girls around the age of fifteen or sixteen. Perhaps as many as fifty percent of girls in this age group suffer from this problem at one time or another. In most cases, this can be considered a normal phenomenon that needs to be explained and dealt with sympathetically. Painful menstruation that develops later in life frequently has a more serious underlying cause. In a rather large percentage of adolescent girls, college students, and even older single women, one or two days of each month must be spent in bed because of the severe abdominal cramps and pain.

Treatment: The girl should be reassured that she is not

abnormal in any way and that the pain can usually be relieved by simple measures. She should also be made aware that this will not interfere with normal sexual function nor have any effect on childbearing.

Keep the body warm at all times, using a hot water bottle or heating pad at night, if necessary. Keep off the feet as much as possible, especially the first day.

A douche made as follows will give relief: one tablespoon of lady's slipper and one-half teaspoon of lobelia, steeped in one quart of water. Use warm. For internal use, make a tea using equal parts of black cohosh, pennyroyal, and bayberry, adding a little lobelia: take one-half cup every three hours. If you do not have all these herbs, use as many as you have. A hot sitz bath or hot fomentations to the lower spine and abdomen often afford great relief. Repeat these as often as necessary.

During the winter, never permit the feet to get cold or wet. It is also best to keep the hands out of cold water when possible. As far as possible, the patient should be urged to carry on all of her normal activities.

If, in spite of the above treatment, absent, irregular, or profuse menstruation persists, or if bleeding between menstrual cycles or following the menopause occurs, see your family doctor.

MUMPS

Causes: Mumps is caused by a virus. It usually occurs in children between the ages of three and sixteen, but is sometimes seen in adults also. But when it does occur in adults, the complications can be quite serious. Mumps is not as contagious as measles, and one attack usually affords lifetime protection.

Symptoms: At first there is a slight fever and chilliness, loss of appetite, and headache. This is followed shortly by swelling of the glands located just below the ear, near the angle of the jaw. The glands on one or both sides of the face may enlarge and become very painful. Occasionally the glands grow so large that it becomes difficult for the patient to open his mouth. The swelling begins to go down after two or three days, and it is usually completely gone in 10 to 14 days.

Treatment: The child should be kept isolated and in bed if possible, until two or three days after the swelling has disappeared.

A light, nourishing diet such as fruit juices, potassium broth, soybean milk, and zwieback should be given. Acid foods may increase the pain, and if this happens they should not be used. If there is a fever, a hot bath may be taken twice a day for about twenty minutes. If there is a high fever, sponging with tepid water will help lower the temperature. Herbal liniment (see Section II, Chapter 3) is most excellent to lessen the pain of the affected part. It should be applied freely.

A poultice made of the following will give relief. Use a small handful of mullein, add one tablespoon of lobelia. Mix together, and pour enough boiling water on them to make a poultice. A little flaxseed meal or cornmeal may be mixed with these to make them stick together. Apply hot between pieces of gauze, and cover with a woolen cloth to keep the poultice warm. Remove it when it cools and replace with another similar poultice. Nearly any form of heat will help to relieve the pain.

For internal treatment, take equal parts of ginger and skullcap and mix them together; steep a small teaspoon of this mixture in one cup of boiling water. Have the patient take a swallow of this every hour. You may sweeten it with a little honey or malt sugar.

If there should be trouble with constipation, keep the bowels open with an enema of catnip tea.

NAUSEA AND VOMITING

If the nausea is due to undigested food or fermentation in

the stomach, take an emetic and clean out the stomach. (See emetics in Section II, Chapter 3.)

A cup of hot peppermint or spearmint tea, taken after the stomach is cleansed, will strengthen and settle it.

A hot fomentation applied over the stomach or a hot water bottle with a moist towel under it will often prove beneficial.

The following herbs are excellent for nausea and vomiting: spearmint, peppermint, catnip, sweet balm.

To stop severe vomiting, use origanum, peppermint, spearmint, or peach leaves. Sweet balm settles the stomach. Use one teaspoon of the herbs to a cup of boiling water and steep. Lobelia is also good. Use a teaspoon to a pint of boiling water and steep. Take a teaspoon of this tea every fifteen minutes until relief is obtained.

Antispasmodic tincture given in small doses is very good; use ten drops in a glass of warm water.

NERVOUSNESS

Causes: A large variety of circumstances and conditions may cause nervousness. The stomach and intestinal tract are very closely connected with the nervous system. Many times a woman becomes extremely nervous because of overwork, worry, care of children, improper food, lack of sleep, and in many instances it is true that a woman's work is never done. Many times the husband finds fault and makes unpleasant remarks, which make her more nervous and which would be unnecessary if he understood the situation and lent a helping hand. Excessive novel reading, sedentary or dissipating habits, and lack of exercise and fresh air are also causes.

Waste matter in the system gets into the blood and affects the nervous system, especially the nerves of the brain, causing irritability and headaches. We must never forget that the food we eat affects all the nervous system, because what we eat and drink is what feeds and nourishes the nerves.

Treatment: Hot and cold fomentations, to the spine, stomach, liver, and spleen, are very beneficial for nervous people. A prolonged warm bath of an hour's duration or longer if agreeable, finishing with a cool bath or spray and vigorous rubbing, is excellent. Gentle massage after a bath, or for that matter at any time, will help greatly.

A nervous person must also get the system cleaned out. Use high enemas and herb laxatives. The bowels must move freely to maintain good health. Plenty of rest in a well-ventilated room is essential. Skullcap is one of the best herbs for nerves. Red sage is excellent for nervous headaches. Take a cup of the tea, strong, as often as necessary.

The following herbs are excellent for strengthening the nerves, or for any nervous disorder: horehound, lady's slipper, motherwort, mugwort, marshmallow, poplar bark, catnip, spearmint, camomile, ginger, peach leaves, vervain, blue and black cohosh. Prepare and take according to the directions for use of herbs.

NEURALGIA

Causes: Neuralgia is due to irritation of a nerve from a variety of causes. Exposure to dampness and cold with resultant infection, dental decay, lack of proper diet, eye strain, and infections around the nose are some of the causes.

Symptoms: Pain is usually felt in the part of the body supplied by the irritated nerve. There may or may not be accompanying muscle weakness, paralysis, or areas of decreased sensation on the skin. One side of the face may be affected or there may be pain in the temples and neck.

Treatment: Hot and cold compresses to the painful area are very effective. The cold portion of the treatment must be kept very short. A hot fomentation wrung out of a tea made of mullein and lobelia and applied to the affected parts, will do much to relieve the pain. Herbal liniment (see Section II, Chapter 3), applied freely and rubbed in thoroughly, will relieve the pain in a short time.

Placing the opposite hand and arm in very hot water for twenty minutes will frequently give relief.

Choose the following herbs best suited to your case and

follow the directions given in Section II, Chapter 3: valerian, origanum, skullcap, queen of the meadow, nettle, poplar bark, peppermint, Solomon's seal, hops, lady's slipper, twin leaf, motherwort, and wood betony.

Daily massage to the area is very helpful. Rest in bed and a nourishing diet, including adequate vitamin E, are essential.

NIGHTMARES

Anyone who eats a heavy evening meal or midnight supper is likely to have nightmares. They are caused by overloading the stomach just before bedtime, and are made worse by sleeping on the back. No food should be taken for four or five hours before bedtime, as it normally takes about this long for the stomach to empty. Anyone who has frequent nightmares should sleep on his right side or stomach.

Children troubled with bad dreams, sometimes termed night terrors, frequently have trouble digesting their food properly. If they are bothered by constipation, they should be given catnip enemas and catnip tea to drink. They must also have a well-balanced diet.

NIGHT SWEATS

Anyone suffering from night sweats will be greatly benefitted by taking a hot saltwater sponge bath before retiring. Use two tablespoons of salt to a quart of water. A hot bath followed by a salt glow is also good. Wild alum root or white oak bark tea is excellent when used in the same way. Use a tablespoon of the herb to a quart of boiling water; steep twenty minutes.

Make a tea of golden seal by steeping one teaspoon in a pint of boiling water, and drink two cups upon retiring. This will do much to prevent night sweats. Sage, coral, or strawberry leaves may be used in the same way with good effect. The bowels must be kept open and the colon clean by using herbal laxatives or enemas, if necessary.

NOSEBLEED

Causes: Injury to the nose, excessive heat, occasionally high altitude, acute congestion in the head, and abnormality of the blood.

Treatment: The application of very cold water or ice over the nose and on the back of the neck will sometimes stop the bleeding. Pressure on the back of the neck hinders the free flow of blood to the head. Pinching the nostrils tightly for three to five minutes while breathing through the mouth, will usually stop the nosebleed.

Take a heaping teaspoon of golden seal and steep in a pint of soft or distilled water that is boiling; add enough boric acid to make a saturated solution. Put in all the boric acid that will dissolve in the water; if some is left undissolved it will do no harm. Shake it thoroughly and let it stand until it settles, and then it is ready for use. After this solution is cold, sniff some up the nose. Do this several times a day until the bleeding stops.

Wild alum root, white oak bark, or bayberry bark are also very good. Use one heaping teaspoon to a cup of boiling water; steep thirty minutes, then strain or let settle. Then sniff up the nose. Gargle with it also, as no harm is done if you swallow some.

The above things are all good remedies for nosebleed, as well as for colds in the head, and sinus trouble.

Another most effective herb for running nose or nosebleed is ephedra valgaris. Use one heaping teaspoon to a cup of boiling water, and steep for thirty minutes. Let settle or strain all the sediment out. Sniff up the nose and repeat until relief is obtained. Another herb that can be used in the same way is golden seal, in powdered form.

In making any of the above solutions, use the best water obtainable, preferably soft or distilled water.

OBESITY

Causes: Obesity can be overcome to a great extent by proper living and eating. It is made worse by wrong habits of eating, excessive starch, fatty foods, and sugar in the diet; and also a lack of exercise. The basic reason for most cases of obesity is simply taking into the body more calories than are used in daily living. A small number of cases are due to a disturbance in the function of the thyroid or pituitary glands.

Symptoms: Excessive fat, shortness of breath, palpitation of the heart upon slight exertion.

Treatment: Reduce the calories in the diet, and eat only nourishing and nonfattening foods. Start exercising moderately, slowly increasing in vigor, and always in the open air if possible. In order to lose weight you must use up more calories than you take in. Oxygen burns up fat and waste matter in the system; therefore, deep breathing and exercise are essential. Chickweed is especially helpful to those suffering from obesity, as it thoroughly cleanses the system and will reduce fat. Steep a heaping teaspoon to a cup of boiling water. Drink at least four cups a day, one an hour before each meal and one on retiring. If there are other troubles, clear them up with the herbs indicated. Seawrack, burdock, and nettle can also be used with good results.

Great care must be exercised when using commercially prepared weight reduction formulas that are being widely promoted at the present time. Several deaths have been caused by using these preparations.

PALSY

Causes: Palsy is a nervous or physical condition caused by fatigue or nerve injury. The use of tea, coffee, or liquor as well as eating stimulating foods, white flour, and cane sugar are both contributing factors, as they lack the properties that sustain and strengthen the nerves. Collapse, in one form or another, is frequently the result of living on a diet composed mainly of such foods.

Symptoms: Trembling and shaking of the limbs, arms, hands, and sometimes the head: a peculiar manner of walking.

Treatment: Tea, coffee, liquor, and all stimulating foods must not be used if a person wants to be helped. Use the elimination diet given in Section V, Chapter 11. If the nerves have been permanently damaged, a lasting cure is impossible.

Hot and cold applications to the affected parts, followed by vigorous massage, is very beneficial, as it increases the circulation. A warm bath and salt glow can also be given with good results. The pores of the skin must be kept open and a good circulation started. Keep the bowels open with laxative herbs or enemas.

The following herbal medicine is also good. Steep one tablespoon of prickly ash bark or berries, a pinch of cayenne, and one teaspoon of lobelia in a pint of boiling water. Take a tablespoon every two hours.

Take internally any one of the following herbs. Look up their descriptions and use the one or ones best suited to your case: masterwort, skullcap, vervain, lady's slipper, and black cohosh.

Addendum: Since "palsy" is a general term that refers to any type of paralysis, weakness, or uncontrolled movement, and there are many different forms of palsy, some additional remarks about this condition are necessary. The two most common forms of palsy are Bell's palsy and cerebral palsy.

Bell's palsy comes on suddenly and results in paralysis of the muscles on one side of the face. This results in a drooping of the mouth, and an inability to close the eye or wrinkle the forehead, all on the affected side. There is no loss of sensation and little pain. The cause is not known, although it occasionally occurs with shingles. Most cases recover completely in 4 to 8 weeks, but about 10 to 20 percent remain partly or completely paralyzed.

The eye on the affected side must be protected until it can close by itself; heat and gentle massage to the muscles on the paralyzed side will help to maintain their position and tone.

Sometimes Bell's palsy is confused with a stroke, but when a stroke occurs the paralysis involves the muscles in the lower part of the face and rarely affects the eyes or forehead.

A far more common and much more tragic form of palsy is that which develops in the infant at or shortly after childbirth. This type of palsy is called cerebral palsy.

There are several causes of cerebral palsy, and they may occur before, during, or after childbirth. In many cases a specific cause can never be determined; however, they all have in common some degree of damage to the brain. Sometimes the amount of damage is slight and the symptoms can hardly be noticed; while at other times there is severe damage and the afflicted child must spend his entire life as a helpless cripple.

Some of the possible causes of cerebral palsy are: a difficult labor that results in a lack of oxygen or actual injury to the brain; a severe childhood illness such as encephalitis, high fever, pneumonia, meningitis, or head injury. Before birth there may be injury to the brain from a disease contracted by the mother during early pregnancy, especially rubella (German measles), from an inadequate diet, or from the use of drugs or alcohol.

The symptoms of this tragic disease may not be apparent at birth, but as the infant continues to grow a lack of muscle tone and coordination soon become evident. In many cases the diagnosis is not made until the child is between one and two years of age.

The bodily changes range from mild, hardly detectable muscle spasm to severe spasticity and weakness, There may or may not be mental changes and they are not related directly to the degree of muscle impairment. There is a lack of balance; difficulty walking; a clumsy unsteady gait; awkward, jerking movements of the muscles, especially in the arms and legs; muscle spasm, mostly in the legs where it tends to make the legs cross and the toes point inward; and sometimes there are convulsions, impaired speech and varying degrees of mental retardation.

The treatment is difficult and prolonged and requires considerable patience. It is directed towards speech therapy, muscle training and reeducation, and special vocational guidance. The symptoms do not progress as the person grows older; in fact many of those with cerebral palsy can live a fairly normal life.

PANCREAS (INFLAMED)

Causes: The main cause of inflammation of the pancreas is the use of alcoholic beverages. Gallstones that cause a blockage of the pancreatic duct are another fairly common cause. Denatured foods, and combinations of food that cause fermentation in the stomach, such as fruits and vegetables used together, white flour products, cane sugar, and unpolished rice, may be contributing factors and should not be used in the diet. When the pancreas becomes inflamed and hardened, it does not produce enough enzymes to properly digest the food in the intestines. Inflammation of the pancreas may lead to other serious diseases such as diabetes.

Symptoms: Gas and disturbance in the bowels and colon. Severe pain in the upper abdomen sometimes going through to the back. Nausea, vomiting, fever, and chills may also be present.

Treatment: Give hot fomentations to the spine, stomach, liver, and pancreas. In severe cases, follow the treatment and diet as given under diabetes. Use slippery elm enemas. Cut the slippery elm bark into pieces the size of a match. Put a large handful of these in four quarts of cold water, put on the stove, and allow to simmer for ten to fifteen minutes, stirring frequently. Keep covered tightly and allow to set for thirty minutes. This will draw the wonderfully healing jelly out of the bark. Strain it and use warm.

Drink the slippery elm tea made in the same way. Steep a heaping teaspoon of lobelia in a cup of boiling water for a half an hour and add a tablespoon of this lobelia tea to every cup of slippery elm tea that you drink. Take a cup one hour before each meal and one upon retiring. Alternate one of the following herbs, made into tea, with the slippery elm as given above: bitterroot, vervain, wahoo, buchu, dandelion, yarrow, and blueberry.

PARALYSIS (STROKE)

Causes: Strokes (cerebrovascular accidents) are the third most frequent cause of death in the United States. They are the result of a decreased blood supply to a portion of the brain, usually caused by plaques forming in the arteries and blocking off the normal circulation of blood to the brain, or by rupture of a blood vessel in the brain.

Symptoms: The entire body or only a portion of the body may be paralyzed. Often in cases of paralysis half of the body will be paralyzed so that the patient is entirely helpless, unable to talk, and there is no sign of life, even when pricked with a needle. I have treated and cured such cases, as related in the beginning of this book.

Treatment: The following treatment can be used with benefit no matter what part or parts of the body are affected. I have restored feeling in a single day to the affected part by using hot and cold fomentations, massage, liniments, and herbs when the attack first came on. A stimulating liniment used on the part affected is always beneficial. Liniment, as recommended in Section II, Chapter 3, should be thoroughly rubbed in, and the part well saturated. Use the treatment described under my experiences in Section I, Chapter 1, and use the same herbs as given for infantile paralysis. Give a cleansing and nourishing diet. Massage and exercise, as tolerated, are also beneficial. When giving hot fomentations, be sure you do not burn the skin, since the patient may have no pain sensation in the area affected by the stroke.

PLEURISY

Pleurisy occurs when the very thin, delicate lining around the outside of the lungs, called the pleura, becomes infected. Sometimes this causes fluid to collect in the space surrounding the lungs. There is a variety of causes of pleurisy, among which are tuberculosis, pneumonia and other infections, cancer, and blood clots that lodge in the arteries to the lungs. These clots usually come from the blood vessels in the legs or pelvis. Fluid in the pleural spaces around the lungs can also result from heart failure or kidney disease. Cancer frequently causes bloody fluid to collect around the lungs.

Symptoms: Pleurisy frequently begins with fever, chills, and a sharp chest pain, which is made much worse by breathing. A cough is frequently present. Large amounts of fluid cause shortness of breath. The pain in the chest is increased by coughing, breathing, lying on the affected side or pressure. In chronic pleurisy, the symptoms are slight pain, rapid pulse, dry hacking cough, shortness of breath, and increasing debility.

Treatment: Strict bed rest and a highly nutritious diet are important. Apply hot fomentations to both the chest and back. Have the fomentation large enough to cover the lungs. Keep this up for an hour or two, then let the patient rest and repeat the treatment. Keep this up until the pain has ceased. Change the fomentations often, as cold or chilliness will increase the pain. The hot fomentations will help disburse the water from the lungs.

Give a hot herb tea made from equal parts of pleurisy root, yarrow, buckthorn bark, and valerian. Steep a heaping teaspoon in a cup of boiling water for twenty minutes and drink a half cupful every two hours. If the tea is not laxative enough, add more buckthorn bark. If the pain is severe and does not subside quickly, mix together equal parts of lady's slipper, skullcap, and calamus root. Steep a heaping teaspoon in a cup of boiling water for twenty minutes, and take a large swallow every hour.

A specific cure for pleurisy can be made by steeping one tablespoon of yarrow, one tablespoon of pleurisy root, and a pinch of cayenne in a quart of boiling water. Take a large warm swallow every hour. This has been known to cure many cases of pleurisy. Pleurisy root alone is very effective when taken freely.

A slippery elm poultice is also very good. Use three heaping tablespoons of granulated slippery elm, one tablespoon of lobelia and one-half teaspoon of cayenne. (See directions for poultices in Section II, Chapter 3.) If both lungs are affected, a larger quantity will have to be used to make the poultice large enough to cover both lungs. Place the poultices on the chest and the back over the lungs. If you do not have slippery elm, use flaxseed or cornmeal with the lobelia and cayenne.

The diet should be restricted to oatmeal water, fruits, vegetables, and grains. Positively no meat, milk, or stimulating foods such as condiments or intoxicating drinks of any kind should be given.

If these directions are faithfully followed, and the treatment thoroughly given, the pain should soon cease and any fluid that has collected will be absorbed.

PNEUMONIA — See LUNGS, INFLAMMATION OF

POISON IVY

Poison ivy and poison oak are caused by exposure to these poisonous plants. In sensitive persons, this causes a red area that may be slightly swollen and covered with small blisters. Exposed areas such as the hands, arms, and face are most frequently involved. The itching may be intense.

Treatment: The following herbs are good for poison ivy or poison oak: lobelia, golden seal, myrrh, echinacea, bloodroot and Solomon's seal. A strong tea made of equal parts of white oak bark and lime water is very good for poison ivy or poison oak. Apply a bandage wet with this solution and change it as often as it becomes dry. Apply Antiphlogistine (a trademark formerly used for a poultice made of glycerin, kaolin, and aromatics) cold and renew every twelve hours for poison ivy or poison oak. Spread on one-half inch thick and cover the surrounding healthy skin to prevent it from spreading. The juice that comes from squeezing the leaves of aloe vera can also be applied directly to the rash to help stop the itching.

PREGNANCY

The first sign of pregnancy is stopping of the monthly menstrual periods. Occasionally the periods continue, but this is rare and it is usually not a normal period. An early symptom is morning sickness. Some women do not suffer from this at all, but in others it is very severe and disabling. In about six or eight weeks the breasts begin to enlarge and the nipples become prominent with a dark ring around them. Movements of the child are felt between four and five months.

Regular but not strenuous exercise must be taken during the entire nine months to keep the muscles in good condition, as childbirth is chiefly a muscular action. The habit that a large majority of women have of lying or sitting most of the time, is a most injurious one both to the child and mother, as it causes the muscles to become weak and the health to generally run down. To have a beautiful baby, take plenty of gentle exercise. Brisk walking in the open air is one of the best exercises. When sleeping or resting, lie in different positions on either side, then on the stomach, then on the back.

I have seen many instances where women were obliged to do their own housework, as well as work in the garden, right up to the time of confinement and they had an almost painless delivery. Care should be taken, however, not to exercise to the point of exhaustion.

All bad habits must be abandoned and all unnecessary

medications discontinued. Due to the fact that nowadays so many women smoke and drink, it cannot be overemphasized that this will have an extremely damaging effect on the child, mentally, morally, and physically. The mother should have plenty of rest, fresh air, and moderate exercise. A simple nourishing, nonstimulating diet is necessary if you would have a happy, healthy, normal child. Meats of all kinds should be eaten very sparingly, if at all.

Inflammation of the kidneys is a frequent occurrence during pregnancy, and is greatly encouraged by the use of meat. The diet should consist largely of fresh fruits and vegetables. It is an erroneous idea that the infant will be marked if the craving for some particular article of food is not satisfied.

Special attention must be given to the bowels. They should move every day. Use laxative herbs if necessary to keep them regular, but it is preferable to keep the bowels regular as far as possible with the diet. Figs, bran cereals, whole grain bread, raisins, and prunes are good for this.

Breast feeding is the best method for healthy mothers who have full-term babies. There are three main advantages: nutritional, psychological, and immunological. There is also an economical advantage, and no time is needed for the preparation of formulas. Breast feeding is clean, and contamination of any kind is infrequent. Breast feeding also offers some degree of protection against pregnancy, but it should not be relied on as a completely safe means of contraception during this time.

The nutrient content of breast milk is especially suited for infants. It produces a small curd in the infant's stomach that can easily be digested. The total protein content is much lower than cow's milk, so less nitrogen has to be removed by the infant's immature kidneys and liver. The amount and type of protein in human milk are ideal for the infant's growth and it is unlikely to cause any type of allergic reaction. The relatively large amount of cholesterol in human milk is needed for proper development of the nervous system and for the manufacture of steroid hormones and bile acids. Human milk contains slightly more carbohydrate than cow's milk.

Breast milk contains immunoglobulins, lactoferrin, and bifidus factor that protect the infant from many diseases such as tetanus, whooping cough, diphtheria, shigella, salmonella, infantile paralysis, and other bacterial and viral diseases.

There is also a great psychological benefit for both mother and child. The child develops a sense of trust and closeness to the mother, and the mother is offered an excellent opportunity to develop a stable, affectionate relationship with her child.

In order to get the most benefit from breast milk, it should be the main source of food for the infant for the first 4 to 6 months of life, despite the fact that many are advocating feeding solids as early as 1 to 2 months of age. This gives the child the best protection against disease, since the infant's own immunological defense system is not developed totally before 9 to 12 months of age. It also reduces the risk of introducing foreign proteins, which may cause an allergic reaction in the infant.

If it is not possible to satisfy the infant totally using only the mother's milk, some type of formula may have to be added as a supplement. The mother should continue nursing as long as possible, however, since the infant will receive benefit from any human milk it can get. Fresh cow's milk should never be used before the age of 12 months.

When the diet of the mother is nutritionally adequate, the breast milk will meet all the growth requirements of the infant except for vitamin D, iron, and fluoride. A vitamin supplement of 400 I.U. a day of vitamin D should be started at birth. Vitamin D is necessary for the absorption of calcium and phosphorus, which are the two minerals most important in the formation of bones.

In order to prevent an iron deficiency anemia in the infant, an iron supplement should be started at 4 to 6 months of age, since at about this time the infant's store of iron is used up. Never give more than 15 mg of iron a day.

Dress: The wearing of tight clothing by the mother-to-be is extremely detrimental to the child and such garments should not be worn. The dress should be loose and suitable for the different seasons. When the abdomen becomes greatly enlarged, it will be found beneficial and comfortable to wear a wide band to support the abdomen, but do not have it tight. Tight clothing should not be worn around the breasts.

Baths: Frequent sitz baths will relieve many of the local ailments that women suffer during this period. They should be taken at least two or three times a week. During the last few weeks of pregnancy they should be taken daily. A full bath should be taken daily to keep the skin and circulation in good condition.

Mental Attitude: If you want a cheerful, happy child with a sunny disposition, that is just how you will have to be during your pregnancy. Special effort should be made by the mother to avoid as much unpleasantness as possible. A fit of anger, great fright, or novel reading have a very bad effect on the child. The surroundings should be made as pleasant as possible, and it is positively the husband's duty to bring this about, as far as lies in his power. By proper living, care, and treatment, pain can be almost entirely banished at childbirth.

There are special herbs that will help to make childbirth less painful and save a great deal of suffering. Spearmint tea is good to take for morning sickness. Red raspberry leaves made into a tea help to relieve nausea and vomiting, is an aid to labor, and is efficacious in promoting uterine contractions. If red raspberry tea were taken continuously during pregnancy in place of ordinary tea, and a cupful taken every hour during labor, hemorrhages would seldom occur and the use of instruments would rarely be required.

Spikenard is an old Indian remedy to promote easy and painless childbirth. Indian women were noted for their painless childbirths.

I have stopped a very profuse hemorrhage after childbirth with a hot douche of around 120°F., using a tea made of wild alum root and white oak bark. The hot water coagulates the blood and stops the flow. In the absence of these herbs, a solution may be made of alum crystals, which can be obtained in nearly every drugstore.

Diet: Tea, coffee, rich and heavy foods, fish, oysters, condiments of all kinds, and all stimulating foods and drinks should be strictly avoided in the diet of a nursing mother. Very little, if any, meat should be eaten as meat contains many bacteria that cause poisons in the intestines, and the infant as well as the mother may become poisoned by it.

To avoid constipation, eat as much bulk-containing food as possible, for example: lettuce, carrots, spinach, beets, prunes, figs, apples, apricots, zwieback, shredded wheat biscuits, wheat flakes, bran cereals, ripe olives, grapes, and berries of all kinds. Fruit juices of all kinds, especially orange juice, are also excellent.

Two of the most important things when nursing a child are to keep the bowels regular and to keep calm at all times.

Foods to Increase the Milk: Potassium broth (Section VI, Chapter 5) and mashed potatoes are both very strengthening and nutritious and will increase the milk, as will whole grain cereals, especially oatmeal and oatmeal water.

Always drink six to eight glasses of water a day. Insufficient water will always cause insufficient milk. Dill herb tea will help to increase the milk also.

To Decrease the Flow of Milk: The drinking of sage tea will dry up the milk. Do not take much liquid and eat dry foods.

During the entire nine months it is very helpful to thoroughly massage the entire area of the stomach and abdomen with cocoa butter or some good oil every evening before retiring. This will help prevent the marks on the skin that are caused by stretching of the abdomen during pregnancy, as it lubricates the skin and helps make it more elastic.

PROSTATE GLAND (INFLAMMATION)

The prostate gland may become infected by many organisms, including the one that causes gonorrhea. Infections elsewhere in the body may also be carried to the prostate gland through the bloodstream. Sometimes the prostate may become inflamed simply by enlargement of the gland, or by excessive sexual activity. Truck drivers and heavy equipment operators are very prone to develop inflammation of the prostate.

Symptoms: There is usually frequency, urgency, and burning on urination, pain in the rectum, and slowness of urination with incomplete emptying of the bladder. Fever may be present.

Treatment: Hot sitz baths at a temperature of 105° to 115°F. may be taken with great benefit from two to four times a day. The entire pelvis should be covered with the hot water and the bath should last for at least twenty minutes. It may be necessary to put a cold pack on the forehead and back of the neck during the bath. All stimulating foods and drinks, particularly all alcoholic drinks, are strictly forbidden. A man suffering from this disease must eat a diet consisting mainly of fruits, vegetables, and grains. Several of the recipes in this book are good such as soybean milk, zwieback, potassium broth, etc. (See Section VI, Chapter 2.)

If the infection is acute, and fever is present, antibiotics may have to be given.

A high enema, as hot as can be borne, of either catnip or valerian gives great relief when there is much pain.

A slippery elm poultice is extremely beneficial when applied between the legs in the fork of the thighs.

Drink a tea made of equal parts of gravel root and either cleavers or peach leaves, using a teaspoon to a cup of boiling water. Drink one to four cups a day, more or less as needed. A tea made in the same way, composed of equal parts of buchu and uva ursi is also good; or these herbs may be used in capsule form; directions on the bottle.

As an injection in any bladder trouble, take a teaspoon of golden seal, one-half teaspoon of myrrh, and one-half teaspoon of boric acid; pour on one quart of boiling water and steep for thirty minutes. This is a wonderful herbal solution to heal bladder trouble when the cause is removed. It is very powerful to remove poisonous mucus or inflammation from the bladder. Inject the solution into the bladder through a sterile catheter and let the fluid flow in freely. Everyone should learn to use a catheter correctly, but PROPER DIRECTIONS FROM A NURSE OR PHYSICIAN ARE ESSENTIAL!

PROSTATE GLAND (ENLARGEMENT)

Causes: Enlargement of the prostate gland is very common. It is usually seen in men over the age of fifty. The cause of the enlargement is not definitely known, although it may be related to hormone production.

Arrow Points to Narrowed Urethra

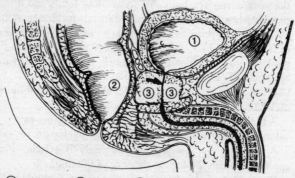

① Bladder   ② Colon   ③ Enlarged Prostate Gland
                          Constricting The Urethra

Symptoms: The first thing that is noticed is a slowing down of the urine stream. This is followed by increased frequency of urination. If infection is also present there is an urgency to urinate and a burning sensation while urinating. There is occasionally blood in the urine, fever, cloudy urine, lower abdominal pain and distention, loss of appetite, and weakness. A hard lump is present in the fork of the thighs or rectum which becomes very painful when pressed.

Treatment: In mild forms, no treatment may be required. Hot sitz baths taken two to four times a day are helpful. Follow the treatment given for inflammation of the prostate.

Alcoholic beverages must be completely eliminated. The patient should keep warm at all times. If symptoms are not relieved, and urination becomes increasingly difficult, a physician specializing in diseases of the urinary tract should be consulted.

PYORRHEA

Causes: Pyorrhea is infection of the gums and the most important cause is poor dental hygiene. Toxins in the system caused from wrong diet and poor elimination also contribute.

Symptoms: Bleeding and swelling of the gums. In bad cases the gums recede and the teeth become loose.

Treatment: Correct the diet by using alkaline foods. Go on a fruit diet for a time, as this is always good in overcoming an acid condition in the body. Take one teaspoon of golden seal, one teaspoon of myrrh, and steep in a pint of boiling water. Rinse out the mouth with this solution and gargle with it freely. Also brush the gums thoroughly with this solution at least three or four times a day. You will be pleased with what this one measure will do to overcome pyorrhea.

Herbal liniment (see Section II, Chapter 3) is also very effective. Apply it to the gums with a small swab or rinse out the mouth with it. The golden seal and myrrh can be used as a powder on the toothbrush instead of making the tea. If the disease is far advanced and there is danger of losing the teeth, help should be sought from a dentist.

RHEUMATISM AND ARTHRITIS
See also LUMBAGO

There are many kinds of arthritis. *Osteoarthritis* is the most common type and is often seen in older patients. It is caused by the everyday wear and tear on the joints over a period of many years. Sometimes it develops in a joint following an injury. *Rheumatoid arthritis,* which can be a very crippling disease, is most common in young and middle-aged women. *Gouty arthritis* is most frequent in middle-aged men, and is hardly ever seen in women. The exact cause of most forms of arthritis is not known; however, wrong dietary habits, which fill the system with uric acid and other poisons, seem to play a part in some types of arthritis, especially gout. Exposure to wet and cold may increase the pain and suffering.

Symptoms: The joints become stiff and sore. Sometimes they may enlarge and become very deformed. The skin over the joints may become hot and very tender to the touch or to any type of motion. Not infrequently, the joints become so stiff that they cannot be moved. In some forms of arthritis the pain is intermittent, while in others it is quite constant. The muscles may become smaller and almost useless. In some cases the joints farthest from the trunk are involved; for example, the wrists and hands; while at other times the spine and larger joints are most severely involved.

Treatment: All unwholesome, devitaminized food must be strictly avoided. Tea, coffee, liquor, white flour products, cane sugar products, soda biscuits, fried potatoes, meat, pork, and bacon especially. When fed on the foregoing foods, the blood cells will not be able to rid the system of impurities. See cleansing and nourishing foods in Section V, Chapter 11. All food should be eaten as dry as possible, and well masticated so that it is thoroughly mixed with saliva to help digestion. This will alkalinize the system as much as any other one thing you can do. Wonderful results may be obtained from a prolonged fruit diet. After taking the fruit diet for two or three weeks, use potassium broth, French toast, and mashed potatoes (recipes given in Section VI). Drink slippery elm tea; it is very nourishing, cleansing, and strengthening. Solid food must be taken sparingly at first, after the fruit diet.

Take a good sweat bath every day and drink two or three cups of pleurisy tea. Use a teaspoon of pleurisy root to a cup of boiling water and let steep for twenty minutes. Drink this while in the tub. Thorough massage after the bath is very beneficial. If there is *inflammation* of the joints, do not massage those parts.

Mix equal parts of the following herbs: black cohosh, gentian root, angelica, columbo, skullcap, valerian, rue, and buckthorn bark. Use a heaping teaspoon to a cup of boiling water; steep and drink three or more cups per day, as the case may require. Drink a half-cupful at a time.

An excellent poultice for swollen joints is made as follows: two tablespoons of mullein, three tablespoons of granulated slippery elm bark, one tablespoon of lobelia, and one small teaspoon of cayenne; mix thoroughly together, then mix with enough boiling water to make a stiff paste. Spread a layer of paste about one-fourth of an inch thick on a cloth. Cover the swollen joints with this poultice and it will bring great relief.

Another excellent way to relieve the pain is to mix equal parts of oil of origanum and oil of lobelia, then add a few drops of oil of capsicum or extract of capsicum (red pepper). This can be applied full strength or mixed with coconut oil. Massage thoroughly with this, as long as there is no inflammation of the joint.

The following herbs are also very beneficial in rheumatism and arthritis: bitterroot, buckthorn bark, burdock, saw palmetto berries, black cohosh, wintergreen, yellow dock, sassafras, skullcap, and bearsfoot. Look up their descriptions and take those best suited to your case. Use singly or in combination.

RICKETS

Causes: Children would not have rickets if they were properly fed and were exposed to adequate sunshine. The use of devitaminized foods and refined products such as white flour, polished rice, and cane sugar, predisposes to rickets. The specific cause for the development of rickets is a lack of vitamin D. Rickets is found almost exclusively in infants, and is more common in artificially fed babies than in breast-fed babies. It is more frequent in infants growing up in those parts of the world where there are long periods of time without sunshine, and it is also more common in the black-skinned races.

Symptoms: The abdomen becomes enlarged and protruding. There is a delay in the normal appearance of the teeth. The skull has a square shape and may be quite soft. The muscles in general become weak and constipation develops because of this. The bones in the spine, as well as the extremities, tend to bend and become deformed, resulting in knock-knees and bowlegs. There may be fretfulness and restlessness at night. The lungs may become affected and even enlargement of the heart may result.

Treatment: The treatment for rickets consists primarily in the administration of an adequate amount of vitamin D. This can readily be given in the form of cod liver oil. Children suffering from rickets should be exposed to plenty of fresh air and sunshine. Frequent warm baths with friction to increase the circulation may help.

The diet is of great importance. The diet for infants given in this section under Pregnancy is very good. If cow's milk is used, vitamin D has already been added. For older children, give all the fresh vegetables, simply prepared, fruits of all kinds, mashed potatoes, soybean cottage cheese and potassium broth. It is best not to let children combine fruits and vegetables at the same meal or to drink with meals, as this hinders digestion.

Steep a heaping teaspoon of skullcap in a cup of boiling

water; strain, and give a tablespoon six or seven times a day. Catnip tea is also excellent in all children's diseases and may be taken freely. Sweeten the tea a little with honey or malt sugar.

Because of the tendency to constipation, the bowels must be kept open. Enemas using only plain warm water or catnip tea may be used. Senna tea taken internally is also good. If possible, the bowels should be kept open with fresh fruits and vegetables, so that enemas are not necessary. Give plenty of fruit juices of all kinds between meals.

RINGWORM (TINEA)

There are many kinds of ringworm, and each one is caused by a fungus. Ringworm can occur on various parts of the body, but it is most common on the head, trunk, groin, feet, finger, and toenails. When ringworm occurs on the scalp, the hair falls out, leaving a small, round, scaly area. When it involves other parts of the body, it looks like a pale round area surrounded by a zone of redness that is slightly elevated and may contain small blisters. Any form of ringworm is very contagious, and proper care should be taken so that the disease is not spread to others.

Treatment: Ringworm of the scalp may be difficult to cure. The hair should be shampooed with a good quality of soap or tar soap. Every morning and evening moisten the spots with the following solution: one teaspoon of golden seal and one-half teaspoon of myrrh, steeped in a pint of boiling water. Daily application of wet dressings with boric acid is good.

For internal use, adults should take a level teaspoon of golden seal in a cup of water twice a day; make it weaker for children, according to age. Hops, boneset, and plantain may also be taken internally with good results. Bloodroot tea, made strong and applied externally, is excellent. Whitfield's ointment, available at nearly any drug store, may be used in cases of severe itching. For ringworm of the body, special ointments that will kill the fungus are readily available at nearly any pharmacy.

SINUS TROUBLE

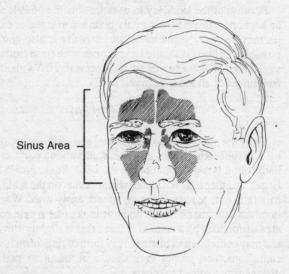

Sinus Area —

Causes: The sinuses are air-filled spaces within the bones of the face and skull. They are lined by mucous membrane and connect with the nasal cavity through small channels. The sinuses may become infected whenever an infection is present in the nose and throat, such as occurs in the common cold, influenza, etc. The normal drainage channels from the sinuses become blocked by the infection, and this may also cause the sinuses to become infected. People who do a lot of swimming, diving, snorkeling, or scuba diving are also prone to develop sinus trouble. Any poor health habits such as eating an unhealthy diet, lack of proper exercise, uncleanliness, lack of fresh air, or an inadequate fluid intake may prolong sinus trouble.

Symptoms: Pain over the sinuses, sometimes becoming very severe, aching eyes, discharge from the nose or down the throat, low-grade fever, headache, running eyes and nose. The symptoms may be very similar to those seen in hay fever, which, however, is usually due to an allergic condition. In fact, the two diseases frequently occur at the same time.

Treatment: Remove the causes. Regulate the bowels so as to have one to three good eliminations a day. Thoroughly cleanse the colon with a high enema. You may have to take a high enema every day for several weeks to help rid the system of mucus and poisons.

Remain on a fruit juice diet for four or five days, drinking all the juice you can of oranges, grapefruit, lemons, pineapples, and grapes (all unsweetened). Do not mix the juices; drink one at a time, alternating them. Then go on a vegetable diet, using all kinds of greens, red cabbage, and eggplant, which are especially useful as they are very rich in potassium; but use all kinds of vegetables. Continue the fruit juices, but drink them between meals.

At times cold applications over the sinuses will give great relief; and at other times alternate hot and cold applications will help. Use whichever gives you the most relief. Have a pan of both hot and cold water available. Bathe the whole face with hot water, as hot as you can stand; then briefly apply the cold water.

Herbal liniment (recipe in Section II, Chapter 3) thoroughly applied and well rubbed in over the sinuses often gives relief. Inhale it also. But the only cure is to thoroughly cleanse the body of all poisons; then there will be no sinus trouble.

To cleanse and heal the nose, make a tea of bayberry bark or golden seal. Use a teaspoon to a cup of boiling water; let it simmer for thirty minutes; strain when cool or just warm; sniff it up the nose, getting it up both sides, one side at a time; this will cleanse and heal at the same time.

SKIN DISEASES

Many skin diseases are caused by impure blood or infection. If you have boils, carbuncles, blackheads, pimples, or a skin infection of any kind, a prolonged fruit diet would be very helpful. Stop using meats of all kinds and do not eat between meals. Use no cane sugar, white flour, or white flour products. Take plenty of exercise in the fresh air. Eat plenty of fresh fruits and vegetables and well-cooked grains.

Cold towel rubs are very helpful, rubbing vigorously to increase the circulation.

Make a strong tea of red clover blossoms, using three or four tablespoons of the granulated herb to a quart of water. Steep covered for one-half hour in boiling water. Drink this tea freely in place of water. Chickweed tea may be used in the same way, the taste being similar to spinach and not at all disagreeable. If you follow this treatment, using either of the herbs as directed, the skin condition will greatly improve.

The following herbs are also beneficial in skin diseases: burdock root, yellow dock root, hyssop, sanicle, blue violet, golden seal, plantain, echinacea, beech, bittersweet, buckthorn bark, elder, bloodroot, dandelion, sassafras, sarsaparilla, and spikenard. These can be taken singly or you may combine two or more of them in equal parts. Take four cups a day, one an hour before each meal and one on retiring.

The following is a very effective external remedy when made into a tea and applied a number of times a day to the affected parts: equal parts of golden seal, echinacea, yellow dock root, burdock root, and witch hazel bark mixed thoroughly. Use a heaping tablespoon of this mixture to a pint of boiling water; steep one-half hour; pour off the liquid or strain, and add a level tablespoon of boric acid: this will keep the fluid from souring.

Citrus fruits are especially beneficial in all skin troubles.

SMALLPOX

Smallpox is a very contagious disease caused by a virus. The sores tend to leave permanent scars when they heal. This disease is contagious from the time the first symptoms appear until all of the sores have healed completely. In the United States, smallpox is no longer the common dreaded disease it once was. In fact, while smallpox was once one of the world's most dreaded diseases, it was officially declared eradicated in 1977 by the World Health Organization, thanks to worldwide cooperation and vaccination.

Symptoms: After exposure to smallpox, the symptoms usually appear in about ten or twelve days. These symptoms consist of fever, headache, weakness, vomiting, and constipation. In a few days the sores begin to appear, usually on the face and around the wrists. Later the entire body is involved, with more of the pustules located on the arms, legs, and face, than on the back, chest, or abdomen. The sores gradually heal over a period of four to six weeks, and when the crust comes off a scar very often remains. Smallpox has a fairly high fatality rate, particularly in small infants.

Treatment: Because of the highly contagious character of this disease, the patient must be kept in isolation, and all persons and articles that come in contact with the patient need to be disinfected. The isolation needs to be continued until all the sores have healed and the crusts have come off.

The patient must be kept clean and the room darkened. Good ventilation and an even temperature of not over 70°F. are best. During the fever stage, give plenty of lemonade without sugar. When the skin is hot and dry, take equal parts of pleurisy root and ginger; steep a teaspoon in a cup of boiling water for twenty minutes and give a cupful every hour or until there is free perspiration. Equal parts of yarrow and valerian taken in the same way will also produce perspiration. Red sage, made into a tea or taken in the powdered form in capsules, is very good.

If there is severe itching of the skin, bathe with a tea made of burdock root, golden seal root, or yellow dock root. When the pustules are well advanced and begin to rupture, the skin can be kept clean with boric acid compresses. Bathing the pustules with golden seal tea is a help against permanent scarring. Cleansing with hydrogen peroxide is also helpful.

The diet should be very light. Soybean milk, oatmeal water, or bran and barley water are good. Vegetable broth is very nourishing. Fruit juices are excellent.

When there is exposure to smallpox or any danger of contracting it, cleanse your system with high enemas. Take the herbal laxative given in this book or any good herb laxative; go on a fruit juice diet for a number of days; then take vegetable broth, or vegetable puree (made from leafy vegetables combined with thick potato peelings, with some oatmeal or natural brown rice added; and after cooking, strain, and use).

Hot baths taken before contracting smallpox or after contracting it will make the skin active and shorten the course of the disease.

SORE EYES

Causes: Eye troubles may be caused from a deficient diet. The eating of unhealthful foods and drinks such as tea, coffee, condiments, alcohol, as well as the use of tobacco, weakens the nerves and hinders the free circulation of blood to the eyes.

Unhealthful foods and drinks cause impure blood, and when the circulation carries impure blood to the eyes it weakens them. The all-important thing is to eat food that will give you a pure bloodstream. Inflammation of the eyes from any cause will greatly benefit by the following treatment.

Treatment: For eye trouble it will be necessary to correct the diet and leave off all harmful foods and drinks. Get plenty of sleep in a well-ventilated room. Cleanse the system thoroughly with blood-purifying herbs such as echinacea, fruit and fruit juices, and cleansing vegetables such as cucumbers, carrots, celery, and leafy greens.

Take the juice of a lemon every morning one hour before breakfast in a cup of hot water. Steep one teaspoon of red raspberry leaves and one teaspoon of witch hazel leaves in a cup of boiling water, and strain through a cloth. When using the powder, use one-half teaspoonful in a cup of water. Saturate a soft cloth with this tea and apply it as a wet pack to the eyes or bathe the eyes with it often, using an eyecup. Fennel tea is excellent when taken internally. It will benefit the eyes as it strengthens them. When used in an eyecup, dilute one-third with water.

Charcoal or slippery elm poultices, applied cold to the eyes, will relieve inflammation.

An excellent eyewash for everyday use as well as when there is particular difficulty is the following: one teaspoon of golden seal and one level teaspoon of boric acid dissolved in a pint of boiling water; shake well and let settle. You may pour off the liquid, or use just as is.

Hot and cold applications to the eyes with a heavy wash cloth will relieve itching and soreness. Aloe vera gel applied to the eyelids relieves itching and burning eyes.

SORE MOUTH

In infants and children, when there is a general redness and soreness in the mouth, it should be carefully sponged with the following solution: one teaspoon of powdered golden seal and one-half teaspoon of powdered myrrh steeped in a pint of boiling water, adding one tablespoon of boric acid. When this has settled, pour off the clear liquid. For adults, use this as a mouthwash and gargle several times a day, holding some in the mouth for a few minutes.

White oak bark, wild alum root, and red raspberry leaf tea, used as a gargle and mouthwash, are also very beneficial.

SPINAL MENINGITIS

Symptoms: High fever, vomiting, headache, prostration, pain in the back, legs, and neck, and convulsions, are the most frequent symptoms. Drowsiness, irritability, vomiting, loss of appetite, constipation, diarrhea, and sometimes a rash may also be present. This disease usually occurs in children under the age of ten. Any movement of the patient causes much pain, and a position with the head and neck bent backward and held rigid is frequently assumed.

Treatment: The earlier in the disease that treatment is begun, the better will be the results. The disease is much more severe and more frequently fatal in infants less than a year of age. The older the child, the fewer the complications, which include paralysis and various degrees of brain damage. Since the introduction of antibiotics the mortality rate has dropped dramatically.

Good nursing care is essential. The patient must be kept quiet and in bed. No visitors should be allowed, and while the room should be somewhat darkened, it must be well ventilated at all times. Fomentations may be given to the spine and abdomen. This will help to increase the circulation. Thorough massage will also be beneficial.

Make sure the bowels stay open, using herbal laxatives as necessary.

Any one of the following herbs is helpful. Make a mixture of two or three of the following: skullcap, catnip, blue and black cohosh, golden seal, prickly ash bark, queen of the meadow. Use one teaspoon of the mixture to a cup of boiling water. Take at least four cups per day, one an hour before each meal and one upon retiring.

The diet must be nonstimulating and light. A fruit diet at first is advisable. Bran, oatmeal, and barley water are excellent. Use vegetable broth freely, as given in Section VI, Chapter 6. It is very nourishing, alkaline, and cleansing.

SPLEEN, INFLAMMATION OF

Causes: Inflammation or enlargement of the spleen may be associated with enlargement of the liver or other organs.

It may be found with serious forms of blood disease, cancer, some infectious diseases, malaria, and various other diseases.

Symptoms: There is usually some degree of pain in the left side just under the ribs. This pain may extend up to the shoulder. There may be a chill followed by fever. The skin may become hot and dry. Constipation may be present. In some cases the urine is scanty and very dark in color. The person is very thirsty.

Treatment: A light, nourishing diet must be provided. A fruit diet for a few days is excellent. Hot fomentations applied to the left side over the spleen, followed by a short cold application, will do much to relieve the inflammation and pain. This treatment should be repeated two or three times a day until the pain is relieved and then given once a day.

Herbal liniment (see Section II, Chapter 3) should be rubbed in well over the spleen. This will do a great deal to relieve the pain. Use the same herbs and in the same way as given under Pancreas (Inflamed), preceding. This treatment applies to either acute or chronic enlargement of the spleen. If the spleen continues to enlarge, your family doctor should be consulted.

The bowels should be kept open with laxative herbs, or by giving an enema of slippery elm tea.

SPRAINS AND STRAINS OF JOINTS AND MUSCLES

Sprains generally occur in the ankles, wrists, fingers, knees, or back.

Causes: The cause is usually some type of injury such as a sudden or unexpected movement, missing a step in going downstairs, stumbling, falling, etc. When ligaments are torn there is extreme pain and swelling around the joint.

Treatment: If the sprain is a very bad one, see a physician as soon as possible in order to prevent any possible permanent deformity of the joint.

If the injury is in the hand, wrist, elbow, or ankle, place the injured part in very hot water. Every few minutes remove it from the hot water and place it in ice water for about a minute, then back into the hot water. This can be kept up for an hour or longer. I have kept it up for two hours with gratifying results and repeated it two or three times a day. After this, *gently* massage the injured part for fifteen or twenty minutes. If it should be the ankle or foot, massage the entire foot and leg well up over the knee. If the injury is in the hand, massage the entire hand and arm to above the elbow. If using hot water makes the pain worse, use only ice water or an ice bag for 24 to 48 hours and then start using the alternate hot and cold.

Keep the injured part at rest. If the ligaments are badly torn, a fairly tight bandage (Ace bandage) may help to ease the pain and give stability to the joint. If this treatment is repeated for a few days the results will be most gratifying. Massage the area gently at least twice a day. If swelling and fever set in before you have an opportunity to treat the injury, use hot fomentations followed by short cold applications. Usually a total of three fomentations are applied. This will reduce the swelling and inflammation. Then use the alternate hot and cold water, as described earlier. If you do this, the soreness and swelling will soon leave. After the inflammation and soreness have abated, you can massage directly over the spot; although at first you may have to massage around it.

If the sprain or strain is in the back or shoulder, first treat the area with hot fomentations, then short applications of cold, and end with massage.

Make an herb tea of equal parts of gentian, skullcap, valerian, buckthorn bark, and a pinch of red pepper. Mix thoroughly together, using a heaping teaspoonful of the herbs to a cup of boiling water. Take a tablespoonful every hour. More may be taken if needed.

Herbal liniment, as given in Section II, Chapter 3, will take most of the soreness out of a bad sprain in a single day. Everyone should make this liniment for himself and always keep some on hand. Apply the liniment freely and massage gently before the inflammation sets in. Keep this up for 15 to

20 minutes at a time, using it three or four times a day. The liniment will also take the soreness out of black and blue spots. Massage the spot gently as you apply the liniment. A bad bruise on any part of the body, or a pain in the back, may be treated the same as a sprain or torn ligament. Treat with hot fomentations and short cold applications; then apply the liniment thoroughly. I have taken a bad kink out of the back in a single day with this treatment. Keep up the applications, giving them thoroughly.

STOMACH INFLAMMATION (GASTRITIS) — See also GAS IN THE STOMACH OR BOWELS

Causes: One of the most common causes of gastritis is the drinking of alcohol. Another frequent cause is aspirin or other antiinflammatory medicines that people often take for arthritis. People with ulcers also frequently have gastritis. The ingestion of strong acid or alkali products causes severe gastritis. It is usually associated with either a suicide attempt or accidental ingestion by a child. Excessive use of spices, mustard, condiments, and all stimulating foods, also favor the development of gastritis.

Symptoms: The most frequent symptoms are pain in the upper abdomen, nausea with or without vomiting, loss of appetite, weight loss, gas, burning sensation in the chest or upper abdomen. These are the most frequent symptoms.

Treatment: Discontinue all irritating medicines, particularly aspirin. Drink no alcoholic beverages. Eat a bland, nourishing diet with no stimulating or irritating foods or condiments.

Take oatmeal, bran, or barley water. Oatmeal water with soybean milk is an excellent nourishing drink when mixed half-and-half. To get the stomach into shape to retain food, steep a teaspoonful of golden seal in a pint of boiling water. Take six or more large swallows a day.

Hot and cold applications to the stomach, liver, and spine are helpful.

The following herbs are excellent in stomach trouble. Look up their descriptions and use the one or ones best suited to your condition. They may either be taken singly, or two or more may be combined. Sage, wood betony, poplar bark, bitterroot, cayenne, slippery elm (excellent) columbo, pleurisy root, hyssop, plantain, wild yams, sweet flag, yarrow, strawberry leaves, wild alum root, rue, violet leaves.

Red raspberry tea is very soothing to the stomach. Excellent results will be obtained by drinking chickweed tea or red clover tea in place of water, six or eight glasses a day. Slippery elm tea should be used in all stomach troubles. It heals, strengthens, and nourishes.

An excellent stomach remedy is to mix equal parts of golden seal, echinacea, burnet, wood betony, myrrh, and spearmint (use powdered herbs). After thoroughly mixing these together, take one-half teaspoonful in a glass of hot water an hour before meals and one upon retiring.

STOMACH TROUBLE

Stomach troubles arise from eating and drinking harmful foods, wrong combinations of foods, eating fruits and vegetables together, milk and cane sugar together, pies, cakes, white flour products, greasy and fried foods, taking too much fluid with meals, and poor mastication. No matter what or how much you eat, if it is not properly masticated it will not digest properly. Drinking with meals will dilute the digestive juices so that they cannot do their work properly. Ice cold drinks are especially harmful, because they chill the stomach as well as dilute the digestive juices.

The best thing to do for any kind of stomach trouble is to go on a fruit diet for at least a week or more. Give the stomach a chance to rest so that the normal gastric juices may become strong enough to digest the food.

When on the fasting or fruit diet, do not drink anything but pure water and the prescribed herbs. Upon arising, drink one-fourth teaspoonful of golden seal or take one No.00

capsule in a glass of very warm water, before taking anything else into the stomach. This is one of the best remedies. Continue doing this after you have completed taking the fruit diet. If this is taken regularly, good results will follow.

SYPHILIS

The following quotation is from Edward N. Bran, Jr., M.D., Editorial, *Journal of the American Medical Association,* October 22-29, 1982, p. 2032, Vol. 248, No. 16.

Physicians and Sexually Transmitted Disease: A Call to Action

Syphilis, the most common and dreaded venereal disease in the early 1900s, was thought to be conquered at last with the advent of penicillin in the early 1950s. This was not to be, however, and along with a resurgence of syphilis, other sexually transmitted diseases (STD) have also appeared and have now reached epidemic proportions.

The epidemiologic features of STD have changed and the number of diseases categorized as sexually transmitted has climbed drastically. Estimates of the annual statistics are staggering: 200,000 to 500,000 new cases of genital herpes; 200,000 cases of hepatitis B, a significant proportion of which are sexually transmitted; 3 million cases of trichomoniasis; more than 1 million episodes of pelvic inflammatory disease that lead to 80,000 to 100,000 forced sterilizations among our young women; 2.5 million cases of nongonococcal urethritis and related Chlamydial infections; 80,000 new cases of syphilis; and 2 million new cases of gonorrhea. The human tragedy is terrible, and the conservatively estimated 2 billion dollar cost to all of us is an enormous burden.

Cause: Syphilis is caused by an organism called treponema pallidum, a "screw-shaped" protozoan that will die after only a few minutes exposure to cold or drying. In recent years, due in large part to the so-called "sexual revolution" of the 1960s and 1970s, the number of cases of venereal disease, including gonorrhea and syphilis, has been rapidly increasing. Syphilis is nearly always transmitted by direct sexual contact; however, it can be transmitted by kissing an individual with an active lesion around the mouth. It may very rarely be contracted by such things as contaminated needles, clothing, toilet seats, etc. A baby may be born with syphilis if the mother is infected; particularly if she acquired the infection during the course of her pregnancy.

Symptoms: The primary sore of syphilis, called a chancre, appears on the genitals about two to four weeks following sexual contact. It is an ulcerated yet painless sore, and there is no pus or other discharge from it. The lymph nodes in the groins become enlarged. Without any treatment, the sore usually disappears in a few weeks, leaving a permanent scar. The infection spreads throughout the body and, if nothing is done, a few months later a skin eruption appears that persists for several weeks. It is usually painless and does not itch. The hair may drop out. There may be pain in the bones and joints, swelling of the lymph nodes, sore eyes, ear aches, and enlargement of the liver and spleen. Following these symptoms, the patient may appear to be well for a few years, but later develops a special form of severe arthritis particularly involving the knees, infection in the aorta and heart, and involvement of the brain and many of the internal organs. Ulcerations may appear on any part of the body. These ulcers are very difficult to heal and are great destroyers of tissue. It is not unusual for several ulcers to start at the same time.

Treatment: This disease is constitutional; that is, it affects the entire body. The treatment must be continued several months after all the symptoms have disappeared in order to be effective. It is imperative to lead an active life in the open air as much as possible. Eat simple nourishing foods for years, to build up a constitution that has been weakened by the poison of syphilis.

Syphilis can be treated successfully with natural remedies that leave no bad aftereffects.

Meats of all kinds, especially pork, also tea, coffee, oysters, shellfish, tobacco, all condiments, stimulating foods, and drinks must not be used. These foods tend to irritate and heat the blood, and they fill the system with waste material and poisonous toxins.

Mix thoroughly together two tablespoons each of the following herbs: Oregon grape, uva ursi, burdock root, blue flag root, red clover blossoms, prickly ash berries, buckthorn bark, and one teaspoonful of bloodroot. Steep a heaping teaspoonful in a cup of boiling water for one-half hour. Drink at least four cups a day, one an hour before each meal and one upon retiring. This combination may also be taken in capsules; take two No.00 capsules four times a day. Continue taking these herbs for at least one year.

Bathe the sores with a solution of golden seal and myrrh, using a teaspoonful of each to a pint of boiling water. When the eruptions first appear, bathe them thoroughly with this tea. Since these sores are contagious, make sure you are careful to protect yourself and to dispose of all contaminated material properly. Heavy sweats and salt glows will help to eliminate the poisons. Take high enemas every day, using either bayberry bark, burdock root, yellow dock, or echinacea.

Any of the following herbs can also be used with good results: red clover blossoms, holy thistle, archangel, Oregon grape, parsley, uva-ursi, witch hazel, burdock root, bitterroot, red raspberry, yellow dock root, elder, bittersweet, turkey corn, wintergreen, cleavers, poplar, witch hazel, golden seal, prickly ash, rock rose, spikenard, twin leaf, wild elm root. Look up the descriptions and use those best suited to your case, in the event you also have some other disease.

If the treatment outlined above is started immediately when the symptoms first appear, you need not suffer greatly at all. The worst cases of syphilis have yielded to the above compound of herbs, when the rest of the treatment, diet, and hygiene, were strictly adhered to.

Addendum: Nearly all cases of syphilis are now treated rapidly and successfully with antibiotics, which became widely available in the 1940s and 1950s. The treatment given in this book may still be used, but is quite costly and time-consuming compared with treatment by antibiotics. For early cases of syphilis, which have been present for less than a year, one injection of penicillin is usually adequate for a complete cure; if the disease has been present for over one year, three or four weekly injections are usually adequate.

TOBACCO HABIT

Cigarette smoking is the main cause of lung cancer. This is now the most common cancer in men in the United States, and in some states is now the most common cancer in women also. Smoking cigarettes also predisposes to cancer of the esophagus and the bladder, is one of the main contributors to heart attacks, and is implicated in some stomach diseases, such as ulcers.

Chewing tobacco is a common cause of cancer in the mouth, while pipe smoking is responsible for the development of cancer on the lips. Smoking and chewing tobacco weakens and debilitates the digestive organs. The loss of saliva that is caused by chewing tobacco is one of the ways by which the system sustains loss and injury through the use of tobacco.

Many girls smoke to keep thin, but it is destructive to the system. The same can be said of many of the advertised reducing pills and medicines. Everyone knows that the first attempt at smoking usually makes one deathly ill and pale and causes nausea and vomiting.

I had the same experiences when first starting to use tobacco. It made me deathly sick, so sick I could hardly stand on my feet. But gradually the system becomes accustomed to it and builds up a resistance so that the evil effects are not so noticeable; however, even though they are hidden, they are still there. All the time I was using tobacco I was confident it was injuring my stomach and digestion, and while giving it up, I was extremely nervous and lonesome in the midst of pleasant surroundings. It took a long time until this feeling wore off. Had I known then what I know now, I could have overcome the habit in a few weeks; instead, it took me half a year to accomplish it.

The poisons in tobacco very readily find their way into the bloodstream, and anything that affects the blood affects every organ and tissue of the body. It greatly harms the blood corpuscles, has a very damaging effect on the nervous system, causing poor circulation. Smoking is not only the main cause of cancer of the lungs, it also causes other serious lung diseases such as emphysema and bronchitis.

Persons suffering from tuberculosis, palpitation of the heart, irregular pulse, cancer, inactivity of the skin, or paralysis of the nervous system who use tobacco in any form, will find that these ills may in many cases be traced directly to the use of tobacco.

Too much emphasis cannot be placed upon the fact that people who use tobacco in any form will finally find their bodies in a weakened and diseased condition. Medical workers see the truth of the above statements lived out before their eyes every day.

Treatment: The following treatment will be found extremely successful in curing anyone of the habit.

Go on a diet of fruit juices and vegetable broths for a period of eight to fifteen days. Vegetable broth is very nourishing and is therefore helpful in keeping up the strength.

Take plenty of hot baths, warm enough so that you perspire freely; at least one a day. Finish with a cold towel rub or spray. Remain in the tub thirty minutes to an hour, or longer if possible, and keep continuously adding hot water. Put cold cloths on the head and throat if you feel weak or faint. Copious drinking of water while in the tub helps one to perspire more. Poisons are given off through the skin by means of perspiration. Rub vigorously while drying off, in order to increase the circulation. Those who take Turkish baths should have one every day, with thorough rubbing.

Red clover tea is very effective in cleansing the system. Use the blossoms, one teaspoonful to a cup of boiling water. Steep, and drink from five to twelve cups a day.

Magnolia tea is specifically used for curing the tobacco habit. Also, myrtle leaves and seeds. Make the tea as you do when using other herbs.

Drinking slippery elm tea is excellent while curing the tobacco habit.

The following herbs are also good: skullcap, vervain, peppermint, catnip, nerve root, quassia chips, motherwort, angelica, burdock root (for cleansing the blood), black cohosh, blue cohosh, echinacea.

TONSILLITIS

Causes: A disordered stomach from eating the wrong diet may lower the natural resistance of the body; however, the specific organism responsible for tonsillitis is usually a virus, and occasionally a bacteria. Wrong habits of eating and living lower the natural resistance, and permit these organisms to gain a foothold in the body and cause various diseases, including tonsillitis.

I know of cases where I had been sitting at the table with people whose throat was all right the day before, but they ate a large amount of rich food, and the next day they developed a case of fever with tonsillitis. They blamed the food, but it was not the food, but the abnormal amount of it that they had eaten. The stomach and intestines could not handle it, so it became a poison in the system and inflamed the entire digestive tract. This permitted the virus to gain a foothold in the tonsils and they became swollen and sore. Most throat and adenoid troubles, sinusitis, bronchitis, and various coughs, can be traced directly to a bad condition in the stomach.

Symptoms: The throat becomes very sore and swollen and sometimes nearly closed, so that it is almost impossible to swallow. There is usually fever and sometimes chills. The throat and mouth may become dry. Lots of poisonous mucus accumulates. The tonsils are swollen and red in color, sometimes with ulcers or whitish spots on the surface. Often the glands of the neck are swollen and tender.

Treatment: Crush some ice and wrap it in a towel; put it around the neck, pinning securely in the back with safety pins, or use an ice bag if available. When this becomes too painful, take it off and apply a hot fomentation, keeping it on for three to five minutes. Then put the ice on again for a short time. Keep this up for an hour or more, then gargle the throat with a solution made of one teaspoonful each of golden seal and myrrh to a pint of boiling water. Let steep one-half hour. Gargle thoroughly with this solution every half-hour, swallowing a little. If the tonsils are swollen so large that the tea does not reach the back of the tonsils when gargling, swab the tonsils with it. Lemon juice may be used in the same way with splendid results.

A hot bath and a good salt glow in the evening before retiring are beneficial.

Take some hot tea made of red raspberry or sage, one teaspoonful to the cup of boiling water. Slippery elm is an excellent remedy for sore throat and stomach trouble. This may be taken freely during the day, a cupful at a time. Take five or six times a day. See Section II, Chapter 6, under slippery elm, for how to prepare this tea. Slippery elm lozenges are available at many pharmacies; take as directed on the box.

Diet: The diet should be very light for the first few days. A fruit diet is excellent. If fruit is not available, make a vegetable soup (see index). It may be used as a hot or cold drink, and is very nourishing.

Give hot soybean milk over whole wheat flakes. This may also be taken by a small child or infant. When used for infants, it should be put through a fine sieve and given in a bottle.

Soybean milk does not form curds like cow's milk.

Use plenty of fruit juices during the attack of tonsillitis. Pineapple and citrus fruit juices are especially valuable.

Another excellent gargle can be made by steeping one teaspoonful each of wild cherry bark and sumach and a small teaspoonful of powdered lobelia, in a pint of boiling water for one-half hour. Gargle or swab the tonsils with it often, and swallow a little. Do this every hour until the condition is better, and then as often as needed. A tea may also be made from red sage, wood betony, or bistort, for an excellent gargle in tonsillitis.

TUBERCULOSIS (CONSUMPTION)

Causes: Tuberculosis may affect not only the lungs, but other parts of the body as well, especially the bones and kidneys, but also sometimes the intestines, spleen, and liver. Since the turn of the century, the number of cases of tuberculosis in the United States has decreased dramatically, due to an improved standard of living and a better understanding of the disease. Despite this decrease, however, tuberculosis is still seen quite frequently, and during 1980 there were approximately twenty-eight thousand new cases of tuberculosis reported. This disease is caused by a bacteria, and is contracted by the inhalation of small droplets that are dispersed by persons who have active tuberculosis. These small droplets, containing the tuberculosis germs, are given off by coughing, talking, or sneezing, and because they are so small, they remain suspended in the air for a long time. These droplets may be inhaled by an unsuspecting person, and finally come to rest in the lungs, where they produce tuberculosis. Intemperance in eating, drinking, and dressing, exposure to cold, loss of sleep, impure air, lack of proper exercise, not breathing deeply enough to open up all the lung cells, leading a sedentary life, overwork, lack of properly prepared nourishing food, and an unbalanced diet all pave the way for the tuberculosis germ to gain a foothold. Persons with feeble constitutions are often infected with tuberculosis.

Contaminated milk, use of tobacco in any form, liquor of all kinds, tea, coffee, and all harmful drinks are also contributing causes.

Symptoms: The symptoms may be slow in developing. There is usually a cough, and many times the sputum that is coughed up contains blood. The cough may gradually become more severe. There is frequently an associated fever, profuse sweating at night, fatigue, weakness, loss of appetite, and weight loss. Chest pain may be present when there is an associated pleurisy. Sometimes the lymph nodes in one or both sides of the neck are enlarged (scrofula). These may get very large and rupture if not treated properly. Years ago this form of tuberculosis (scrofula) was frequently caused by drinking milk that was contaminated with the tuberculosis bacteria; however, it is now very rare to contract tuberculosis in this manner, since pasteurization of milk kills the germs that cause tuberculosis.

Treatment: A moderate temperature in the sickroom should be maintained at all times, never having it excessively warm. There should always be good ventilation. The patient should avoid becoming chilled, and the room should be sunny, airy, and dry. Get plenty of outdoor exercise, and stay outdoors as much as possible. If the patient is not too weak, clean the stomach out thoroughly with an emetic. It will be surprising how much mucus will be brought up that otherwise would have been brought up in paroxyms of coughing.

Steep one teaspoonful of powdered golden seal, one teaspoonful of cubeb berries, and one-fourth teaspoonful of lobelia in a pint of boiling water for one-half hour. Take a swallow every hour. Mix two tablespoonfuls of powdered bugleweed with a pinch of cayenne and use a level teaspoonful of this mixture to a cup of boiling water. Take a swallow of this every two hours. A cupful of this tea is also useful to check bleeding from the lungs. Powdered bayberry bark or shepherd's purse is also very good to check hemorrhage from the lungs. Use half a teaspoonful to a cup of boiling water; let steep, strain, and drink it cold.

Drink at least one quart of slippery elm tea daily, drinking one cup an hour before each meal and one at bedtime. This will strengthen, heal, and nourish. If the digestion is not good, take one-fourth teaspoonful of powdered golden seal in a glass of water an hour before each meal.

A nourishing diet is essential. Soybean milk can be taken

freely. Soybean milk with whole wheat flakes is very nourishing. Other good foods to use in the diet are very ripe bananas, oatmeal with malt honey, whole wheat or soybean bread, zwieback, potassium broth (see index), tender fresh peas, steamed figs, dates, graham crackers, all kinds of vegetables (seasoned with soybean milk or soybean butter), natural brown rice, and baked Irish pototoes.

When there is fever, follow the treatment in Fevers, preceding, in this Section.

Deep breathing and plenty of fresh air are absolutely necessary, taken in connection with gentle exercise. Sun baths are excellent. Expose the entire body. Take sweat baths to open the pores, and while in the tub drink two or three cups of tea made from pleurisy root.

All sputum and discharges from a patient suffering with tuberculosis should be burned or buried.

The following herbs may also be used to advantage in tuberculosis; look up their descriptions and use those best suited to your condition: wild cherry, flaxseed, sanicle, mullein, vervain, hyssop, skunk cabbage, coltsfoot, lungwort, and marshmallow root.

In treating this disease, one must take into consideration its extent and the length of time the patient has suffered with it. If we find that tubercles have formed, we must find a preparation of a solvent nature to soften and break up the cheesy particles of the tubercles so they can be eliminated. An agent must be used that will clean away the pus and accumulation, and at the same time be of a healing nature. Such herbs as powdered comfrey, marshmallow, chickweed, and slippery elm are beneficial. Mix together equal parts of the foregoing herbs, and use four ounces of this mixture to four quarts of water. Let boil down to two quarts, strain, and take a half-cupful of this solvent every two hours either hot or cold. This will ease the irritation or inflammation, as well as dissolve and break up the cheesy substances.

In addition to healing properties, there must be something having astringent and healing properties, which will cause the cavities to heal and become sound again. For this, use one ounce each of powdered black horehound, hyssop, lobelia, and one-half ounce of ginger to four quarts of water. Boil this down to two quarts and take a half-cup every two hours. Give these two preparations alternately. Give a dose of the first solvent, followed in one hour by a dose of the second healing preparation.

Short, hot fomentations alternating with short cold applications should be applied to the front and back of the chest. Also give these along the full length of the spine, and over the stomach, liver, and spleen. These will prove very beneficial.

Warm baths followed by a thorough salt glow and massage are helpful. Judgment must be used in giving these, of course; give them according to the strength of the patient.

Take the cough medicines as given under Coughs and Colds, preceding, in this Section. Give freely; and always take some after a coughing spell.

The patient must always be kept warm with warm clothing, especially the feet, legs, and arms.

The foregoing treatment has been used successfully in many cases of tuberculosis, but it takes a long time, and the final outcome is uncertain. Science has recently developed specific medications that will cure this disease. So if you think there is a chance that you might have tuberculosis, out of consideration for your family and others that you associate with, as well as for your own good, you should consult a physician.

TUMORS

The word tumor simply means a "swelling." There are many kinds of tumors. They are named according to the tissues involved, such as glandular, muscular, fibrous, fatty, etc., and there are also cancerous tumors.

Any one of these tumors may enlarge rapidly and become ulcerated.

Tumors may be caused by impure blood, impurities of the system, unbalanced diet, constipation, or a generally run-down condition. The cause of many tumors is not known.

Sage poultices have been known to remove external tumors. Slippery elm poultices are also excellent. See poultices in Section II, Chapter 3.

Take any one of the following teas internally for tumors, or a combination of any two or three: bayberry, slippery elm, mugwort, white pond lily, chickweed, sage, or wild yam. These are all good.

When suffering from tumors, use the same treatment as for cancer. (Please read the paragraphs on Cancer, preceding, in this section).

TYPHOID FEVER

Typhoid fever is a communicable disease. It is contracted by the ingestion of water or food that has been contaminated by the feces or urine of patients with active typhoid fever or by someone who carries the typhoid germ but has no symptoms — an asymptomatic carrier. The specific organism that causes typhoid fever is a member of the salmonella family. This type of bacteria is also frequently the cause of food poisoning. Approximately five hundred cases of typhoid fever are reported every year in the United States, and many times it is contracted by overseas travelers. A small percentage of those who contract the disease become asymptomatic carriers; that is, they do not have any symptoms of typhoid fever and yet they spread the disease. At one time, contaminated milk was a great source of typhoid fever in the United States, but this is no longer true. There are still fairly frequent reports of milk contaminated with salmonella, causing local epidemics of food poisoning, the most recent one being in the Chicago area in the spring of 1985, when several thousand people were infected and thousands of gallons of milk had to be destroyed.

Symptoms: There is a gradual onset of fever, which

becomes higher until it reaches to between 103° and 105°F. Fatigue, loss of appetite, chills, headache, muscle pain, and tenderness in the abdomen also develop. After about a week, severe diarrhea, which may be bloody, begins. Red spots form on the skin over the chest and abdomen, and the spleen may become large and tender. These symptoms get progressively worse for about three or four weeks, and then recovery begins. If no treatment is given, the patient may continue to grow weaker, with severe loss of fluid, an enlarging abdomen, and a rapid pulse. Approximately ten to fifteen percent of patients die if no treatment is given. The usual cause of death is severe intestinal hemorrhage or perforation.

Treatment: Pure air and good ventilation are essential in every case. If the patient has a high temperature, see the diet for fever in the preceding article in this section on Fevers.

A sponge bath of a temperature agreeable to the patient should be given morning and evening, or much more often if the patient has a high temperature. Give a high herb enema every day, using white oak bark, red raspberry leaves, or wild alum root. After giving the high enemas, inject two ounces of the enema tea into the rectum with a small syringe and retain. It will help to heal the ulcers in the rectum. The high enema and the injected solution will greatly relieve the patient and hasten recovery.

Pleurisy root tea is excellent when the skin is dry and hot. Give wild cherry bark tea when there is diarrhea. Cold cloths placed over the right groin will often stop bleeding from the bowels. Injections of cold witch hazel tea are also helpful in this condition. (See Hemorrhages, preceding, in this Section.)

Often those who suffer from typhoid fever have ulcers in the stomach and rectum. If such is the case, steep a heaping teaspoonful of golden seal and one of wild alum root in a pint of boiling water and take a swallow every hour.

Have the patient drink all the water he possibly can. Orange juice and oatmeal water taken at separate intervals are good nourishment. A vegetable broth made from several vegetables such as carrot, celery, a little onion, and spinach will be nourishing: strain it, and give as a liquid broth.

Antibiotics are used successfully in typhoid fever and have helped to reduce the mortality rate to one percent in the United States.

It is important for those traveling in areas of the world where typhoid fever is common to avoid drinking unboiled water or eating raw vegetables or unpeeled fruit.

ULCERS, SKIN

Ulcers may form where the skin has been cut or broken and has failed to heal properly. When the tissue has been destroyed by a burn, cut, or wound of any kind, bacteria may enter and produce an infection with the formation of pus. An ulcer that forms on the skin surface that has been exposed to the sun for a long period of time may be cancerous, and medical attention should be sought if it does not heal. Ulcers may also be caused by poor circulation, or excessive pressure on an area of skin over a period of time. The latter is frequently seen in bedridden patients who do not receive proper nursing care.

Treatment: A light diet is necessary, and the food must be well digested. The bowels must move at least once a day. Use laxative herbs and high enemas as necessary. Steep one teaspoonful of golden seal and one-half teaspoonful of myrrh in a pint of boiling water. This solution cannot be excelled for washing the ulcers, and also for applying to the dressings covering the ulcers. Also take a tablespoonful of this six times a day internally.

Mix together two teaspoonfuls of powdered golden seal and one teaspoonful of myrrh, and sprinkle on the ulcer after it has been thoroughly washed. Cover loosely with a clean bandage.

Any one of the following herbs may be taken internally with benefit, or mix equal parts of two or three of these herbs thoroughly: bayberry, golden seal, ragwort, lady's slipper, chickweed, sage, wood sanicle, slippery elm, bogbean, ground ivy, bittersweet, agrimony, and raspberry leaves. Use a heaping teaspoonful to a cup of boiling water, strain, and drink four cups a day, one an hour before each meal and one upon retiring.

Bedridden patients should be turned at regular intervals to prevent the formation of skin ulcers.

URINARY PROBLEMS — See also BLADDER IN-FLAMMATION (CYSTITIS)

Scalding (burning) urine. Burning on urination is usually associated with pain, frequency, and urgency. There are many causes for this problem, but the most common one is an infection in the bladder, prostate, or urethra. Tumors, stones, allergies, female troubles, and strictures are other causes. The condition may be overcome by cleansing the system, and by taking the following herbs. Mix equal parts of fennel, burdock, and slippery elm, or milkweed. Steep a teaspoonful in a cup of boiling water for twenty minutes and drink cold, one cup before each meal and on retiring. Teas made of cubeb berries, gravel root, or a combination of equal parts of buchu and uva-ursi are also excellent when used in the same way. One of the most important things you can do is to drink plenty of pure water, as much as two or three quarts a day, if possible. This will help to flush out the kidneys and bladder. Also, go on a fruit diet for a few days to rid the system of uric acid.

Inability to urinate. Retention of urine is caused by inflammation and swelling inside the bladder. The prostate gland, which surrounds the male urethra near the bladder, frequently becomes enlarged or inflamed and causes an obstruction, with inability to pass the urine. The pain caused by retention of urine may be so intense that the patient will break out in a cold sweat, with the odor of urine being very prominent. In most cases, the inability to urinate develops gradually over a period of weeks or months, rather than appearing suddenly.

Give hot sitz baths repeatedly, followed each time by a short cold bath. If the patient is bedridden, apply alternate hot and short cold applications over the genitals, bladder, and along the entire length of the spine. Give a high enema of catnip tea; this is very necessary and may permit natural urination when other means have failed.

If possible, inject into the bladder, through a soft, sterile catheter, a tea made as follows: one heaping teaspoonful of golden seal, one-half teaspoonful myrrh, and one-half teaspoonful boric acid; steep in a quart of boiling water and strain through a fine cloth. THIS MUST BE DONE BY A GRADUATE NURSE, OR SOMEONE WHO IS COMPETENT TO TEACH YOU.

If the patient has not urinated for some time, let the urine drain out through the catheter before making this injection. Moisten the catheter well with slippery elm tea , this makes it slip in easily, is very healing, and will thus help the condition. A sterile lubricant may be used if slippery elm tea is not available. Retain the solution as long as possible. Enlargement of the prostate gland is very common in elderly men, and if the above treatment is not successful, appropriate medical help should be sought to relieve the obstruction and to make sure it is not caused by a cancer in the prostate gland or the bladder.

Suppression of Urine. A decrease in the amount of urine is caused when the kidneys do not excrete the usual amount into the bladder. In severe cases the urine is almost completely suppressed.

Symptoms: If no urine has been passed for several days, there will be severe symptoms such as convulsions, extreme pain in the back and bladder, and always a great desire to urinate.

Treatment: The patient should have perfect quiet. A very warm high enema of catnip tea will give great relief. Hot fomentations wrung out of smartweed tea, applied to the bladder and small of the back, will afford relief. Give two or three hot sitz baths a day.

Yarrow herb is especially recommended. Steep a heaping teaspoonful in a cup of boiling water for twenty minutes. Drink a cup before each meal and upon retiring. Drink cold.

An unfailing remedy for suppressed urine is to use a strong catnip tea, as hot as can be borne, as an enema; also drink this tea freely.

Any one of the following herbs may be used to good advantage. See their descriptions and use those best suited to your condition. Prepare and use them in the same way as described above for yarrow tea: hyssop, burdock, broom, cleavers, dandelion root, wild carrot, meadow sweet, gravel root, tansy, wahoo, corn silk, parsley, St. John's-wort, cubeb berries, milkweed, and buchu. If after using this treatment the urine continues to be suppressed, see your physician.

Involuntary flow of urine. When this disorder is not caused by some other disease such as gout, palsy, or stones in the bladder or kidney, it can be easily remedied by using the following treatment.

It will be helpful to sleep either on the side or face.

Take equal parts of white pond lily, sumach berries, white poplar bark, bistort root, and valerian. Mix together. Steep a heaping teaspoonful of this mixture in a cup of boiling water; take a cup one hour before each meal and on retiring. Drink at least four cups of this tea a day.

Plantain is also very good when taken by itself. The dose is the same as above. It is all right to increase the dose, if you find it necessary.

VARICOSE VEINS

Causes: Pregnancy, local obstructions, sluggish circulation, and standing for long periods of time on the feet. In some cases the tendency to form varicose veins is inherited.

Symptoms: The veins in the legs become enlarged and knotted. There is frequently a dull aching pain and sometimes sharp stabbing pains occur. Skin ulcers may develop.

Treatment: The diet should be simple and very nourishing. Be careful not to overeat so that waste matter will not accumulate in the system. Take high herb enemas if bothered by constipation. Keep the bowels carefully regulated. They should move at least once a day. Regulate them with food if possible; but if not, use laxative herbs.

Cold morning baths should be taken regularly, rubbing the entire body vigorously and thoroughly with first a wet cold towel and then a dry one. If cold morning baths were more widely used, varicose veins would not be so common. When the veins are very large, wear a special stocking, which you can buy in a medical supply or drugstore. It will give relief as the result of a redistribution of pressure. Bathing the limbs with white oak bark tea is very helpful.

I was once called to treat a very fleshy woman who was suffering with varicose veins. Every night in order to sleep, she let her legs hang down over the side of the bed. I made some strong white oak bark tea and had her bathe her limbs with it two or three times before retiring. It relieved her so much that she was able to sleep all night. I have seen some bad cases of varicose veins relieved when this treatment is used. A cleansing diet and thorough cleansing of the system are necessary to make pure blood and to help in obtaining relief from the pain that varicose veins are capable of producing.

Steep a heaping teaspoonful of golden seal and a small half teaspoonful of myrrh in a pint of boiling water for twenty minutes. Take a swallow six or seven times a day.

If there are open sores, apply the herbal salve, (the recipe for which is given in Section II, Chapter 3).

Take one teaspoonful each of powdered hyssop, white cherry bark, and yellow dock root. Mix thoroughly and take one-half teaspoonful in a fourth glass of cold water, followed by a glass of water as hot as can be taken readily. Take this four times a day, one hour before each meal and upon retiring. Tansy or coral may be used in this way with benefit. If this treatment is not successful after being given a thorough trial, the valves in the veins may be permanently damaged and a different type of treatment may be needed.

WHOOPING COUGH (PERTUSSIS)

Whooping cough is a contagious disease caused by a bacteria, and it can be prevented by proper vaccination. There are only about 3,000 cases of whooping cough reported every year in the United States. This marked decrease over the past several decades is due to improved living conditions, as well as to the widespread use of vaccination. Whooping cough is most frequent in infants and children, and is spread by direct contact with an infected person.

The disease begins about seven to ten days following exposure. The early symptoms resemble an ordinary cold, with runny nose, loss of appetite, tiredness, sneezing, and sometimes a mild fever. The disease is highly contagious during this period. After a week or so, severe coughing spells begin. Each coughing spell ends by the infant drawing air into the lungs, producing a peculiar sound that has been named the "whoop." This is often followed by vomiting. In most cases, if the cough were treated and the simple herbs taken as described under coughs and colds, the whooping would be prevented.

A splendid remedy for whooping cough is wild cherry bark used as a tea. The following is also good: one teaspoonful each of red raspberry leaves, cubeb berries, coltsfoot, and a small teaspoonful of lobelia herb. Put in a dish and pour on one pint of boiling water, allow to steep for one-half hour. Give a teaspoonful of this every hour until the cough is better.

Good nursing care and an abundance of fluid and nutritious food are important in treating whooping cough.

WORMS

Worm infestation is a serious worldwide health problem, but it is found much more frequently outside of the United States. The worms that infect humans are usually of three types: roundworms, tapeworms, and flukes. In the United States, roundworms or tapeworms are the most frequent, and these may range in length from less than an inch up to fifteen or twenty feet.

The most common worms in the roundworm family are: pinworms, roundworms, hookworms, and whipworms. Pinworms are found mostly in children. At night the female pinworms pass to the anal region and lay their eggs. This causes severe itching, and the eggs can be transmitted to the mouth when the hands become contaminated, either by scratching around the anal area or by coming in contact with the pinworm eggs on contaminated bed clothes. More than one member of the family may be contaminated. It is important that during treatment, all underclothes and bed clothes be changed and sterilized daily. Whipworm and roundworm infection can be prevented by proper disposal of human waste. Hookworm disease is contracted by walking barefoot on contaminated soil. Prevention of this disease depends on proper sanitary disposal of human feces and wearing shoes.

Tapeworm infestation is acquired by the ingestion of eggs or larvae in uncooked meat. To prevent infection with tapeworm it is necessary that all beef, pork, and fish be thoroughly cooked before eating.

Symptoms: Many persons infected with worms have few if any symptoms. With a heavy infection of the worms, anemia or weakness may develop. Trichinosis, which is acquired by eating improperly cooked pork, frequently causes muscle pains; the worms may also lodge in the heart, brain, or eyes. Abdominal pain and diarrhea may be present. Children are frequently restless during the night with gritting of the teeth, a dry cough, and a slight fever. Occasionally worms may cause convulsions.

Treatment: The cause must be corrected, and this usually means the correction of unhygienic living conditions and the proper cooking of all meat and fish. It is easy to remove the worms from the body, but this does not necessarily cure the disease. Do not eat food robbed of its life-giving properties such as white flour products, cane sugar products, vegetables cooked in lots of water and the water thrown away, peeled potatoes, candy, cakes, ice cream, and meats of all kinds. Constipation, if present, must be overcome by herbal laxatives or enemas.

Fast two or three days and eat raw pumpkin seeds generously. You can eat as much as one pound a day. After doing this two or three days, drink freely of fennel seed tea. Worms do not like this as it is sedative to them, and they will pass from the body if the bowels are kept loose. Slippery elm tea taken freely will remove worms from the body and it is also good for the entire system. White oak bark tea used as an enema will remove pinworms.

Cut up an onion and soak it for twelve hours in a quart of water; then squeeze the juice out and take for four days. This juice will kill and expel worms. Take as much juice as possible, fasting while taking it.

Any of the following herbs are beneficial to those suffering from any kind of worms: wild yam, tansy, bogbean, poplar bark, balmony, hyssop, wormseed, American worm root, meadowsweet, white oak bark, golden seal, bitterroot, fennel, and slippery elm. Use them singly or in any combination to suit the need. Read their descriptions and take according to directions given.

WOUNDS AND CUTS

If the body is in a healthy condition, a wound or cut will heal readily. Tie a bandage on the cut immediately, or properly apply a tourniquet, to stop the bleeding. Wash the cut or wound with a solution of powdered golden seal and myrrh, made by steeping a heaping teaspoonful of each in a pint of boiling water for twenty minutes. If the wound bleeds freely, tie the bandage tightly over it, which will cause it to heal readily. Apply herbal liniment (see Section II, Chapter 3) over and around the wound. After bandaging, moisten it thoroughly with liniment five or six times a day or oftener. This aids healing and relieves soreness and pain.

If the cut is large and gaps open, place it in the golden seal and myrrh solution as hot as can be borne. Continue this, keeping the solution hot until the wound closes. I have kept a wound in this solution for as long as two hours. When the wound is practically closed, press it together, sprinkle a little powdered golden seal on the outside and bandage, using strips of adhesive tape to hold the skin edges together. Apply liniment all around it. This will relieve the pain and inflammation. If the wound is on the hand, wear a sling to prevent tearing the wound open again. If on the foot, it will be necessary to stay off the feet, or use crutches until healed.

I have seen many bad wounds healed in this way without stitches and without leaving a scar, and the patient does not suffer nearly as much. Be sure to apply the liniment freely; it will work like magic. If proud flesh should develop, it can be killed by sprinkling on burnt alum.

Wood sage is an excellent remedy for old wounds or anywhere where there is inflammation. Use as a poultice.

Wood sage, self-heal, chickweed, golden seal, myrrh, and slippery elm; these herbs can be effectively used as poultices and washes.

SPECIAL NOTICE

In Section IV, Your Body and Its Needs, and Section V, Your Foods, you may find several references to animal products (milk, eggs, cheese) as sources of calcium, vitamins, and other minerals. Our mentioning them in this revised edition is not to be considered a recommendation for their use, but only as a source of reference and information. While listing these items as nutrient sources, we are not advocating their use. In fact, we recommend that you do not use them at all. (Jethro Kloss did not eat meat or use animal products of any kind, and most of his immediate descendants also follow this dietary plan.)

I believe, as did my father, Jethro, that the very best foods were those given to our first parents in the Garden of Eden — fruits, grains, nuts, herbs, and vegetables. In recent years there has been a great deal of study and research in regard to diet and nutrition and it has now been adequately demonstrated that a diet high in carbohydrates and low in fat and protein (no sugar or salt) is by far the most healthful. If adopted, it would help protect you from the debilitating and degenerative diseases of old age. Your blood cholesterol and triglycerides will remain at normal levels — a necessity for a strong heart, healthy blood vessels and normal blood pressure.

Section IV
Your Body and Its Needs

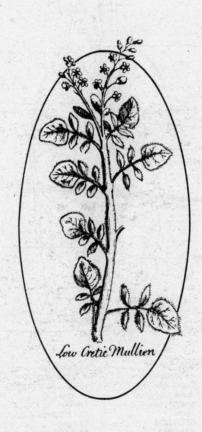

Low Cretic Mullien

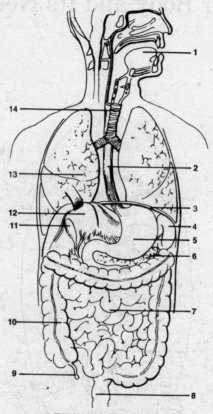

THE DIGESTIVE SYSTEM

1. **TONGUE**
2. **ESOPHAGUS**
3. Diaphragm (separates chest from abdomen)
4. Spleen
5. **STOMACH**
6. **PANCREAS**
7. **SMALL INTESTINE**
8. **RECTUM**
9. **APPENDIX**
10. **LARGE INTESTINE (COLON)**
11. **GALL BLADDER**
12. **LIVER** (lifted up)
13. Lung
14. Trachea (windpipe)

(Those parts belonging to the digestive system are in bold face letters.)

1

THE IMPORTANCE OF GOOD NUTRITION

The true science of eating should be thoroughly understood by all — what elements the system requires in order to build and repair, how best to supply them, and how to prepare them in the most appetizing manner without destroying their life-giving properties.

The human body is a finely constructed machine and transforms the food supplied to it into energy. As the automobile burns gasoline, the human body burns food. All the parts on every machine are constantly wearing and require renewal; just so, the body must have proper food to build new tissues and to repair worn-out ones.

The best way to obtain the nutrients that are needed by your body is from natural foods the way nature prepared them, and not from pills. Nearly 40 percent of Americans over the age of 16 regularly take some form of dietary supplement.

God in his infinite wisdom neglected nothing, and if we would eat our food without trying to improve, change, or refine it, thereby destroying its life-giving properties, it would meet all the requirements of the body.

Several recent surveys that included thousands of American families revealed several potential or real areas of nutritional deficiency. The vitamins that tended to be low were vitamin A, B6 (pyridoxine), and C. The minerals that were often deficient were iron, calcium, and magnesium.

In order to insure the proper function of the nearly limitless and complicated reactions that are necessary for our body's optimum health, good nutrition is absolutely essential. This means not only supplying the body with a sufficient amount of food, but just as important is eating the right kinds of food and eating them in the proper proportions. Strangely enough, many overweight persons, although they look well fed, are not getting the proper kind of nourishment.

In all the food we eat, whether it comes from plants or secondhand from animals, there are roughly 50 different nutrients — substances necessary for life and growth. These nutrients can be conveniently arranged into six basic groups, as follows:

BASIC NUTRIENTS

1. Carbohydrates
2. Fats
3. Proteins
4. Minerals
5. Vitamins
6. Water

The first three of these six — carbohydrates, fats, and proteins — provide energy that is used by the body to perform all the functions of daily living. This energy is measured in small units called calories. Calories are used to measure not only the energy used by the body, but also to tell us the amount of energy present in food.

Even when a person is lying down completely relaxed, awake, and with an empty stomach, a large amount of energy is necessary just to maintain life. This energy is known as the basal metabolic rate (BMR). In the average person the BMR is 1200 to 1800 calories per day. This represents more than half of the daily expenditure of energy. A rough estimate of your BMR can be found by multiplying your body weight in pounds by 10. The brain is responsible for about one-fifth of our total basal metabolic rate. But, unlike most other parts of the body such as the muscles, the amount of energy used by the brain stays about the same throughout the day, even when we are mentally very active.

While carbohydrates, fats, and proteins all supply energy, they are not all equal in this respect. As can be seen in Table 1, for any given weight fat supplies 2 1/4 times as much energy (calories) as the same amount of protein or carbohydrate — 9 calories per gram compared to 4 calories per gram.

Incidentally, alcohol gives 7 calories of energy per gram; but it is almost totally lacking in any of the other nutrients.

TABLE 1

	Calories per gram	Calories per ounce *
Fat	9	250
Protein	4	110
Carbohydrate	4	110

* approximate weight: 28 grams = 1 ounce

Carbohydrates are frequently condemned as being the main culprit responsible for obesity, one of America's most common and serious health problems, when fat actually contains more than twice the number of calories. Today, in the average American diet, 45 percent of our energy supply comes from carbohydrates, 43 percent comes from fat and 12 percent from protein. This pattern of eating is not the way it used to be in the United States, nor is it the way it is at the present time in less affluent countries, where most of the energy in the diet comes from carbohydrates — in some countries even as much as 80 percent. Although no definite daily requirement in grams has been suggested for fat or carbohydrates, as there has been for protein, it would certainly be much better for our health if we increased the amount of carbohydrate in our diet so that it provided about 55 or 60 percent of our daily energy needs. At the same time we should lower our fat intake from the present level of 43 percent down to 30 percent or even less of our energy supply, specially since we know that a high fat diet is strongly associated with coronary artery disease as well as colon, breast, and possibly prostate cancer.

One sure way to know if you are getting too many calories is to watch your weight. Excess calories are mainly stored in the body as adipose tissue, more commonly known as fat. It takes 3500 calories to make one pound of fat. So, if every day for one week you take in 500 more calories than you burn up as energy, by the end of the week you will have stored those excess 3500 calories as one pound of fat. The reverse is also true, so that for every 3500 calories you use in excess of what you take in, there will be a loss of one pound in weight.

Foods that are high in energy value (calories) tend to be those with a low water or high fat content, such as nuts, dried fruit, butter, etc. Fruits and vegetables are low in calories, except for avocados and olives, which are high in fat. A contrast between the amounts of some high and low calorie foods, showing how much of each it takes to produce the same number of calories, is shown in Table 2.

TABLE 2

AMOUNTS OF VARIOUS FOODS NEEDED TO GIVE 100 CALORIES

HIGH CALORIE FOODS	AMOUNT
Chocolate cake with icing	1 ounce
Almonds	16 nuts
Peanut butter	1 tbs.
Butter or mayonnaise	1 tbs.
Sugar	1 3/4 tbs.
American cheese	1 1/2 inch cube

LOW CALORIE FOODS	AMOUNT
Tomatoes, raw	4 medium
Strawberries, fresh	2 cups
Pear, fresh	1 average size
Peas, frozen	1 cup
Lettuce	2 heads
Peach, fresh	2 average size

Foods rich in protein: These foods repair and build tissue. Peas, beans, nuts, lentils, milk, eggs, cereals, cow peas (black-eyed peas), soybeans, peanuts, and nut preparations.

Foods rich in fat: These foods are used mainly for furnishing fuel and energy. Butter, cream, egg yolk, milk, cheese, cereal, ripe olives, olive oil, vegetable oils, all nuts, and avocados.

Foods rich in carbohydrates: These foods also furnish energy and fuel. Malt sugar, malt, honey, ripe fruit, starchy vegetables (such as potatoes), cereals, refined white sugar. (Sugar removes mineral salts as well as vitamin B from the body and should not be eaten.)

Foods rich in protein and carbohydrates: Peas, beans, lentils, peanuts, milk, oatmeal, wheat, natural grains.

Although protein is one of the three energy producers, the body is best suited to obtain its energy supply from carbohydrates, with fat as its second choice. Protein is used by the body as a source of energy only when there is more of it present than is necessary for normal growth and the repair of tissues, or when there is not enough carbohydrate and fat to meet the body's energy demand. Protein foods are the most costly way to obtain energy, while carbohydrates are the least expensive.

These three energy-producing constituents of food, plus water, are needed by our bodies in large amounts, and all are present in various amounts in nearly all the food we eat. Vitamins and minerals, on the other hand, though also essential for the maintenance of good health, are needed only in comparatively very small amounts.

2

CARBOHYDRATES

Carbohydrates are the cheapest, most efficient, and most readily available source of food energy in the world, since they are the main constituents of the foods that are the easiest to produce and that can be obtained throughout the world, namely, grains, legumes, and potatoes. In many of the less industrialized nations, carbohydrates supply 80 percent or more of the daily calories in the diet, while in the more affluent, highly industrialized countries the calories supplied by carbohydrates in the daily diet are usually much less. For example, in the United States only between 40 and 45 percent of the daily calories are obtained from carbohydrates. Nearly three-fourths of the carbohydrate in the average American diet comes from grains and refined sugar. The rest is divided about equally among potatoes, vegetables, fruit, and dairy products.

As the name implies, all carbohydrates consist of three basic elements — carbon, hydrogen, and oxygen. Carbohydrates vary markedly in their structure, from simple sugars such as glucose, to very complex carbohydrates such as starch, which contains thousands of simple sugars all joined together.

Carbohydrates can all be divided into three groups: *simple sugars or monosaccharides* such as glucose, fructose, and galactose; *disaccharides,* which are made from two simple sugars linked together, such as sucrose, lactose, and maltose; and *complex carbohydrates,* which are made up of hundreds or thousands of simple sugars connected together. Some examples of complex carbohydrates are starch, dextrin, glycogen, and fiber.

The carbohydrates we eat consist mostly of starch, sugar, and fiber. When carbohydrates are eaten either as complex carbohydrates or disaccharides, they must be broken down by the digestive processes in the body to simple sugars before they can be used for energy. Fiber is an exception. Although fiber is a complex carbohydrate, it passes through the body nearly unchanged, since humans have no enzymes that are able to break down fiber to simple glucose.

The digestion of starch begins in the mouth, where it is acted on by amylase, an enzyme in the saliva. Depending upon the length of time the saliva is in contact with the starch, before it is inactivated by acid in the stomach, it reduces the starch to simpler carbohydrates, thus preparing it for further digestion in the small intestine. The complete breakdown of starch to simple sugars is accomplished by other enzymes in the small intestine. Some of these enzymes are made in the pancreas and some in the wall of the small intestine itself. After the simple sugars are formed, they are absorbed through the wall of the small intestine into the blood and are carried to the liver. In the liver they are all changed to glucose. The glucose reenters the blood and is readily available to all the body cells for the production of energy. As the cells use the glucose to make energy, heat is produced as well as water and carbon dioxide. The water is removed from the body by the lungs, kidneys, and skin and the carbon dioxide is given off by the lungs as we exhale.

A small amount of the glucose is changed by the liver to a form of sugar called glycogen, also known as animal sugar. Some of the glycogen, about 100 grams, is stored in the liver in case of a need for emergency energy by the body. The rest of it, about 200 grams, is stored in the muscles and used when they contract. These stores of glycogen will last only 12 to 24 hours, depending on the amount of physical activity. Any extra carbohydrate that is not used by the body cells or changed to glycogen is stored as fat. Remember that it takes about 3500 excess calories to form one pound of fat, and that each gram of carbohydrate supplies four calories.

In case the body does not receive enough carbohydrate to meet its energy needs, some fat and protein can be changed to carbohydrate, although this is not the ideal situation.

Ideally the body should obtain its energy supply directly from carbohydrates.

Glucose (dextrose, grape sugar, corn sugar) is the only form of sugar that can be used by the body for energy. It is specially vital to the brain and nervous system, which use about 140 grams of carbohydrate a day. Glucose is found in most fruits, some vegetables, honey, and in a nearly pure form in corn syrup.

Sucrose (table sugar) is present in sugar cane, sugar beets, maple syrup, fruit, and some vegetables, especially sweet potatoes. Granulated table sugar is 99.5 percent carbohydrate and, if eaten in large amounts, it will cause fermentation in the intestines. Brown sugar is actually regular table sugar with a small amount of molasses or burnt sugar added for color. It is about 97 percent sucrose and although it has a slight amount of iron, the amount is negligible. Sucrose consists of a combination of glucose and fructose, the same as honey.

Fructose (levulose, fruit sugar) is found in fruits, some vegetables, honey, and berries. Fructose has 70 percent more sweetening power than sucrose, so it takes fewer calories to produce the same degree of sweetness.

Lactose (milk sugar) is found only in the milk of humans and other mammals. Lactose assists in the absorption of calcium from the intestines. It is composed of glucose and galactose.

Maltose (malt sugar) is present only to a very limited degree in most foods. It is produced during the malting process of grains and is found in beer, malted foods, and sprouted grains.

Starch is the form in which carbohydrates are stored in

plants. It is not soluble in water like the other sugars and it does not have a sweet taste. Starch is slowly broken down by the body to many units of the simple sugar glucose before it is absorbed, and because of this it supplies calories to the body at a slower rate than when the simple sugars themselves are eaten. Starch is found in whole grains, legumes, nuts, potatoes and other tubers, lentils, sesame and sunflower seeds, yams, sweet potatoes, and some other vegetables.

In their natural state, cereals contain starch and fiber as well as various important vitamins and minerals. When cereals are refined, however, most of these important nutrients are lost and it is mainly starch that remains. Some examples of the refining process are seen when sugar beets or sugar cane is refined to table sugar (sucrose) or when whole wheat flour is refined to white flour. Refined sugar gives only calories and little else in the way of any nutrients, and for this reason the term "empty calories" is used. Refined sugar is present not only in the foods where we expect to find it — candy, ice cream, jam, syrup, pastries, canned fruit, especially those in heavy syrup, etc. — but also in many other foods such as soup, salad dressing, TV dinners, fruit drinks, breakfast cereal, baby food, peanut butter, tomato catsup, fruit yogurt, granola bars, etc.

A new law beginning in 1994 requires that most foods in the grocery store must now have a nutrition label and an ingredient list. The new label has the title NUTRITION FACTS. Claims like "low cholesterol" and "fat free" can be used only if a food meets new legal standards. Read the label to help choose foods that make up a healthful diet. Eating a healthful diet can help reduce your risk factors for some diseases. For example, too much saturated fat and cholesterol can raise blood cholesterol (a risk factor for heart disease). Too much sodium may be linked to high blood pressure. High blood pressure is a risk factor for heart attack and stroke. No one food can make you healthy. In addition to eating healthful foods, stay active, don't smoke, and watch your weight.

As a good example of the use that may be made from nutritional labeling, Table 1 lists the percentage of calories that result from adding refined sugar to the usual serving of various popular ready-to-eat breakfast cereals. Also given is the cost per serving as of 1988 (this will vary in different localities and in different stores). The amount of sugar added to breakfast cereal ranges from 0 to 16 grams per serving. There are approximately 4 grams (16 calories) of sugar in a level teaspoon. This means that the cereal highest in sugar content has had four teaspoons of sugar added to an average serving during the manufacturing process, before any honey, sugar, etc. is added at the time it is eaten.

The amount of carbohydrate in the average American diet has decreased from 68 percent during the early 1900s to 47 percent at the present time, due mainly to eating less starchy food. During this same period of time, sugar consumption has increased from 30 percent to 53 percent. The average American now eats about 380 grams of carbohydrate a day; that is, between 13 and 14 ounces. The consumption of refined sugar and corn syrup in the United States is now nearly 127 pounds per person each year. This figure includes all sugar in the diet, both natural and refined. If food sweeteners containing calories are added, the total comes to about 143 pounds per year. Sugar and sugar substitutes account for more than $8 billion in sales every year. Our annual candy bill is now over $2 billion. A special note for former President Reagan and others who like jelly beans: one-half cup of jelly beans contains the equivalent of approximately 27 teaspoons of sugar. There are about 10 calories in one jelly bean. Soft drinks are now the number one national drink, over 30 gallons for each person per year for a total cost of over $9 billion.

TABLE 1
SUGAR CONTENT AND COST OF
VARIOUS BREAKFAST CEREALS

CEREAL NAME	ADDED SUGAR*	SUGAR CALORIES**	CALORIES PER SERVING	COST PER SERVING***	COST PER OUNCES
Shredded Wheat	0	0	90	8.5	10.2
Cheerios	1	4	110	13	13.2
Rice Chex	2	7	110	15	15
Corn Flakes	2	7	110	8	7.7
Fiber One	2	8	60	11.5	11.5
Corn Chex	3	11	110	13	13
Wheaties	3	11	110	12	11.6
Total	3	11	110	16	16
Special K	3	11	110	15	14.8
Product 19	3	11	110	16.5	16.5
Rice Krispies	3	11	110	13	13
Grape Nuts	3	12	100	9	8.7
Team	5	18	110	13	13
Life	6	20	120	12	11.9
Bran Chex	5	22	90	9	9.2
40% Bran Flakes	5	22	90	11	10.8
Raisin Grape Nuts	6	24	100	10	10.3
Frosted Mini Wheats	7	26	110	12	12.1
All Bran	5	27	120	12.5	11.8
Marshmallow Krispies	10	29	140	24	16.5
Fruit and Fiber	7	31	90	13	12
Golden Grahams	9	33	110	15	14.6
Honey Nut Cheerios	10	36	110	13.5	13.5
Nutri-Grain	13	37	140	24	15.8
Frosted Flakes	11	40	110	11	10.9
Honey Comb	11	40	110	16	16.3
Bran Buds	7	40	70	10	9.6
Cocoa Krispies	10	44	110	16	15.9
Pac-Man	12	44	110	17	17.1
Post Raisin Bran	9	45	80	10	10.2
Fruity Pebbles	12	44	110	15	15.3
Apple Jacks	14	51	110	18	18
Honey Smacks	16	58	110	14	13.8

---

*	In grams: 4 grams equals about 1 tsp.
**	As percent of total calories
***	In cents per serving

In 1984, for the first time in history, people drank more soft drinks than water. During 1986 the average person drank 42.2 gallons of soft drinks — 1.4 gallons more than in 1985. The sales of soft drinks increased from $1,857,000,000 in 1960 to $9,426,000,000 in 1975, and the per capita sugar consumption for soft drinks nearly doubled during this same period from 11.3 pounds to 21.5 pounds. A regular 12-ounce can of a cola drink has about 150 calories as well as caffeine, coloring, and other additives, but practically no other nutrients are present. This 150 calories represents 9 to 10 teaspoons of sugar, since there are about 4 grams (or 16 calories) of sugar in a level teaspoon. Twenty-one percent of our sugar intake now comes from soft drinks.

In 1930, 64 percent of the table sugar produced in the United States was purchased by the consumer and 30 percent was used in prepared food. These percentages have now been practically reversed so that in 1970 only 24 percent of the total production of 9,000,000 metric tons of sugar was used as table sugar and 65 percent was used by the food industry, about one-third of this being used in beverages.

As in most of the rest of the world, the largest source of carbohydrate in the United States is grain, with the average American's share being 22,000 pounds. Most of this grain, however, goes to feed animals, and nearly all the nutrients in the grain that are removed during refining are also used as animal feed.

Remember that carbohydrates in themselves are not nutritionally bad or necessarily fattening. In fact, Americans should increase the amount of carbohydrate in their diet and at the same time reduce the intake of fat. But the carbohydrate should be of the most nutritious kind, rather than refined sugar and devitalized grains.

Several health problems have been linked with an excessive intake of "empty calorie" carbohydrates. Probably the most common and best publicized is obesity.

Heart disease and diabetes have also been connected with excess sugar in the diet, although this connection has not yet been proven with certainty.

Undoubtedly, tooth decay is largely the result of eating refined sugar, specially if it is eaten frequently, between meals, or in a form that sticks to the teeth. There are several things you can do to cut down on cavities. Don't eat between-meal snacks containing refined sugar. Brush your teeth, or at least rinse your mouth, after eating. Finish your meal with a carrot stick, apple, etc., rather than with a dessert filled with refined sugar. Floss your teeth daily. Have regular checkups with your dentist and a thorough twice-a-year cleaning by a dental hygienist.

In summary, here are some ways to improve the use of carbohydrates in your diet.

1. Eat more whole grain bread and cereal. This will also add vitamins, minerals, and fiber to your diet.
2. Eat raw fruits as often as possible.
3. Cut down on all processed foods. Nearly 70 percent of the sugar we consume is hidden in these foods.
4. Eliminate refined sugar and refined cereals as completely as possible.
5. Pay attention to food labels. Any word ending in "-ose" is a form of sugar.

Watch out also for corn syrup, corn sugar, molasses, honey, brown sugar, and other forms of sugar.

The closer any sugar is to the beginning of the list of ingredients on a nutritional label, the greater is its percentage in the product.

Artificial sweeteners have now been around for nearly 100 years, and at the present time nearly 69 million Americans over age 18 consume products containing these noncaloric sweeteners. Nearly $4 billion is spent yearly on diet soft drinks, and the prediction is that by the year 1990 half the soft drinks sold will be sweetened with artificial sweeteners — a $15 billion market. The cost of the sweeteners for that many soft drinks will be nearly $1 billion.

It was as long ago as 1879 that an intensely sweet compound was accidentally discovered by a chemist working at Johns Hopkins University. This compound had originally been developed as a preservative and antiseptic. Around 1905 it was offered for sale to the general public as Saccharin, and although it was slow to gain acceptance at first, today 7 million pounds of saccharin worth $3 billion are consumed yearly in the United States.

During the 1960s and 1970s several studies claimed to show an increased incidence of bladder cancer in rats that were fed very high doses of saccharin. Because of these reports, in 1977 the FDA proposed a ban on the sale of saccharin. But because of the great public outcry as well as pressure from the manufacturer, Congress imposed a temporary moratorium on the proposed ban. This moratorium has been extended to the present time. Congress also agreed to have a label placed on all saccharin products warning of the possible risk of cancer.

In 1980 a large research program was started that cost over $1 million and involved the use of 2,500 rats. This study was intended to give a definite answer as to whether saccharin produced an increased incidence of bladder cancer. The final results, published in 1983, were not much different from earlier studies and showed that at very high doses, an amount that would be equal to a person drinking 750 to 1,000 cans of soft drinks a day, saccharin does have a strong connection with bladder cancer.

Cyclamate was also discovered by accident, at the University of Illinois by a chemist seeking to develop fever-reducing agents. By 1950 it had won FDA approval and was marketed as Sucaryl. It grew rapidly in popularity, since it does not have the bitter aftertaste that saccharin has. By 1967 cyclamate consumption was 18 million pounds a year and it was being nationally promoted as a noncaloric weight reducer; a substitute for sugar. In 1970 this rapid growth in consumption was suddenly brought to a halt when studies showed that cyclamate caused bladder cancer in mice and the product was banned by the FDA.

While working with some amino acids in 1965, James Schlatter, a chemist at the G.D.Searle Company, happened to lick his fingers and noticed an amazingly sweet taste. This discovery led to the formulation of Aspartame from 2 amino acids. It was approved for public use in 1973 by the FDA. Aspartame, marketed under the names of Equal and NutraSweet, has no bitter aftertaste. It does have about the same number of calories per gram as sugar, but because Aspartame is 200 times sweeter than sugar, the amount that is used in a 12-ounce can of soft drink adds up to less than 1 calorie. Since it is made from two naturally occurring amino acids, and not from synthetic materials as saccharin is, it can be digested as a protein. Aspartame is more than 20 times as expensive as saccharin, so while it costs over 4 cents to sweeten a 12-ounce can of soft drink with aspartame, eight 12-ounce cans can be sweetened using saccharin for only 1 cent. In 1984 sales of aspartame totaled $585 million.

Aspartame cannot be used in bakery products as it is not stable at high temperatures, nor can it be used by people having the inherited metabolic abnormality called PKU, or phenylketonuria, since its consumption may cause brain damage in such persons.

Another sweetener, acesulfame K, will likely be on the market soon. FDA approval is expected shortly. It has no calories; is about the same sweetness as aspartame; has some aftertaste; and is not metabolized by the body.

Recently certain plants growing in Africa and Latin America have been discovered that have been used as natural sweeteners by the people living in these countries for hundreds and possibly thousands of years. An African plant called katemfe appears to be the world's sweetest product. On a weight basis it is 3,000 times sweeter than sugar.

In Paraguay the leaves from a small shrub, stevia rebaudiana, contain a substance 300 times sweeter than sugar. The local population uses it to sweeten a popular but bitter drink called mate.

Scientists from the University of Illinois, following the

description given by a Spanish physician during the conquest of the Aztecs, tracked down a plant known as Lippia dulcis. Its sweetening power is 1,000 times that of sucrose and so far no toxic effects have been found.

Licorice, a well-known sweet root, has very few calories and is 50 times sweeter than cane sugar.

None of these sweet substances from plants are carbohydrates, as sugar is, but before any of them can be used on a commercial basis much more testing for safety needs to be done.

Following is a brief review of artificial sweeteners.

1. *Saccharin.* 300 times sweeter than sucrose. No calories. Inexpensive. Slightly bitter aftertaste. Known to cause cancer of the bladder in experimental animals when very high doses are given. Should not be used by children or pregnant women.

2. *Cyclamate.* 30 times sweeter than sucrose (table sugar). Has no calories. Is excreted unchanged by the kidneys. Banned by the FDA.

3. *Aspartame.* 200 times sweeter than sucrose. Same caloric content as sugar but because of its sweetness only a very small amount is needed, which makes the number of calories used very small. Cannot be used in cooking or by those having phenylketonuria. Marketed as Equal and NutraSweet. Approved by the FDA. Is relatively expensive.

4. *Acesulfame K.* 200 times sweeter than sucrose. Contains no calories. It is not metabolized by the body and does have some aftertaste. Not yet approved by the FDA.

3

FATS

Whenever we hear the word "fat," the first picture that comes to mind is often that of an overweight person. Certainly the amount of fat we eat is responsible for much of the extra weight that millions of Americans carry around and that millions of others constantly strive to either keep off or take off. It is estimated that 34 million Americans from 20 to 75 years of age are overweight. Child obesity is also becoming much more prevalent, particularly in those children who spend hours a day watching television. These children tend to get less exercise and to snack more than other children. The weight reduction business in the United States has grown to a billion dollar industry. When all the diet plans, exercise and aerobic clubs, books, magazines, reducing products, exercise equipment, etc. are taken into account, Americans spend over 10 billion dollars a year in usually unsuccessful efforts to permanently lose weight. At any one time throughout the United States, about 28 million persons are on some sort of a weight reduction program, and more than three-fourths of these will regain the weight they lost within one year of stopping their special weight-reducing diets.

In the early part of the twentieth century, the amount of fat in the average American diet accounted for about 30 percent of the total daily calories, whereas now it has increased to between 40 and 45 percent. This increase is largely due to the greater consumption of cooking oils, salad dressing, vegetable shortening, and hydrogenated fats. The average American now eats about 155 gm of fat every day.

This is much more than necessary. Most authorities on nutrition are now advocating a diet in which the calories provided by fat are no more than 30 percent of the total daily calories. For a person on a 2000 calorie per day diet this would be about 67 gm of fat and for a person on a 2800 calorie

473

diet, about 93 gm of fat. In the Orient, the amount of fat in the diet is only one-fourth as much as in the United States and consequently the amount of heart disease and colon cancer is much less.

About one-third of our dietary fat intake consists of foods that are obviously high in their fat content. Such things as butter, cream, cooking oil, salad dressing, and fatty meat would fall into this category. But about two-thirds of the fat that we eat is sometimes referred to as "hidden fat," since it is mixed in with our food. Some examples would be whole milk, luncheon meats, avocados, olives, nuts, cheese, and chocolate.

Fats, like carbohydrates, are composed of carbon, hydrogen, and oxygen, but the amount of oxygen in fat is much less than the amount of hydrogen and carbon. This is what makes fat such a concentrated source of energy, providing more than twice the number of calories per gram than carbohydrates or protein.

Fats are made up of a combination of fatty acids and glycerol. The most common form of fat in our food, and also composing over 90 percent of the fat that is stored in our bodies, is called a triglyceride. This type of fat consists of three fatty acids connected to one molecule of glycerol. The predominant type of fatty acid contained in the fat is what determines its taste and also whether it will be in a solid or liquid form. There are approximately 20 different fatty acids in the food we eat. Each fatty acid contains a long line (chain) of carbon atoms with hydrogen atoms attached to them. If all the potential spaces in the chain are filled, it is called a saturated fatty acid, since it is completely saturated, or filled, with hydrogen. If there are two empty spaces in the chain that could be filled by hydrogen atoms, the fatty acid is called a monounsaturated fatty acid. If there is room for more than two hydrogen atoms, the name polyunsaturated fatty acid (PUFA) is used. All natural foods contain a mixture of saturated and unsaturated fatty acids. The distribution of fatty acids in the average diet is about 38 percent saturated, 12 percent polyunsaturated, and 40 percent monounsaturated.

A.   SATURATED FATTY ACIDS

Most saturated fatty acids are solid at room temperature. They are found mainly in meat. Other sources are whole milk, cream, butter, cheese, chocolate, and coconut and palm oil. It is important to remember that saturated fatty acids raise the blood cholesterol level and are therefore a contributing cause to atherosclerosis, more commonly called "hardening of the arteries," which leads to coronary artery disease and strokes.

B.   MONOUNSATURATED FATTY ACIDS

These fatty acids are found in peanuts, peanut butter and oil, avocados, olives and olive oil, most nuts including cashews, pecans, and Brazil nuts, regular margarine, and vegetable shortening. It was believed until very recently that monounsaturated fatty acids had no affect on the level of cholesterol in the blood. Recent studies, however, suggest that monounsaturated fats, especially olive oil, not only reduce the total cholesterol level by about the same amount as polyunsaturates, but tend to mainly reduce the level of damaging low-density lipoproteins (LDL) while leaving the protective high-density lipoproteins (HDL) nearly untouched. They do not turn rancid nearly as fast as polyunsaturated fats.

C.   POLYUNSATURATED FATTY ACIDS

Polyunsaturated fatty acids are usually liquid at room temperature. They are abundant in plant oils such as corn, safflower, cotton seed, and sunflower oil, and in salad dressings made from these oils. Exceptions to this rule are coconut and palm oil, which are high in saturated fatty acids. Other sources include walnuts, and special margarines.

When hydrogen gas is bubbled through a polyunsaturated fatty acid, hydrogen atoms are added to the vacant spaces in the carbon chain, thus changing the fatty acid from the unsaturated to the saturated form. This makes the fat more solid and also makes it more resistant to turning sour or rancid. This process is known as hydrogenation and the fatty acids that result are called hydrogenated or partially hydrogenated fatty acids. Hydrogenation is used commercially to change the less expensive plant oils to more expensive margarine or shortening. Nearly 3 billion pounds of hydrogenated fats are consumed each year in the United States.

Hydrogenation also decreases the amount of linoleic acid present in the fat. Linoleic acid is the only essential fatty acid; that is to say, it is the only one that *must* be present in the diet as it cannot be made by the body as can the other fatty acids. Fortunately it is so abundant and widely distributed in our foods that to find a person in the United States with a deficiency of linoleic acid is a rarity. When a deficiency does exist, it causes a lack of normal growth and dry scaly skin.

Polyunsaturated fatty acids tend to lower the level of blood cholesterol and thus help prevent atherosclerosis, coronary artery disease, and strokes.

D. CHOLESTEROL

Cholesterol, a yellowish, wax-like substance closely related to fat, is obtained ONLY from eating animal products. It is a normal part of all our body cells and is specially abundant in the brain and nervous system. It is also present in large amounts in the liver and adrenal glands. The body produces about 1000 mg of cholesterol a day, while the average American diet supplies another 500 to 900 mg. This is two or three times more than should be eaten. The amount of cholesterol you eat every day should be no more than 300 mg at the very most. Even if there were no cholesterol in our diet, the liver, and to a lesser degree the body cells, would produce sufficient cholesterol for all of the normal body functions. Cholesterol is well-known for its connection with the buildup of waxy plaques in the walls of the arteries. When these plaques grow large enough to seriously interfere with the necessary flow of blood to vital structures, such as the heart and brain, the result is heart attacks and strokes. If the plaques obstruct the arteries supplying blood to the intestines, severe abdominal pain may result.

Less well-known to most people are cholesterol's important and, in fact, indispensable functions. Much of the cholesterol in our body is used to help in the formation of bile salts, Vitamin D, and several of the adrenal and sex hormones. It is also an essential part of every cell membrane.

While cholesterol is found only in animal products, the amount present varies greatly, depending on the type of food eaten. Some common foods and their cholesterol content are given in Table 1.

While persons with high levels of cholesterol in their blood are more prone to develop atherosclerosis, other factors also play an important part. Some of these are:

1. Cigarette smoking.
2. Lack of proper exercise.
3. Emotional stress.
4. Obesity.
5. A diet high in saturated fatty acids.
6. Heredity.
7. Coffee drinking, which has recently been found to elevate blood cholesterol levels.
8. Sugar — high intake of sucrose.
9. Diabetes.
10. Age and sex — higher cholesterol levels are found in males and older people.
11. High blood pressure.

Since cholesterol is insoluble in water, it must be attached to a protein in order for it to be carried in the blood. This combination of cholesterol linked to a protein is called a lipoprotein. Some lipoproteins contain a large amount of protein and are called high-density lipoproteins (HDL). Others contain a large amount of cholesterol and are called low-density lipoproteins (LDL). There are other groups of lipoproteins, but most of the cholesterol in the blood is in one of these two forms. In fact, about 25 percent of the blood cholesterol is HDL. Persons who have high levels of HDL have less coronary artery disease than those who have high LDL. It is, therefore, very important not only to determine the amount of total cholesterol in the blood but also the relative amounts of HDL and LDL. Persons who have a normal or low total cholesterol level may still have a high risk of coronary heart disease if they have a low level of HDL. In order to increase your HDL level, you should stop smoking, get regular exercise and maintain a normal weight.

TABLE 1
CHOLESTEROL CONTENT OF COMMON MEASURES OF SELECTED DAIRY AND ANIMAL FOODS

FOOD	Amount	Cholesterol (in mg.)
Milk, skim, fluid or reconstituted powdered milk	1 cup	5
Cottage cheese, uncreamed	1/2 cup	7
Lard	1 tbs.	12
Cream, light	1 fluid oz.	20
Cottage cheese, creamed	1/2 cup	24
Cream, half and half	1/4 cup	26
Ice cream, regular, about 10% fat	1/2 cup	27
Cheese, cheddar	1 oz.	28
Milk, whole	1 cup	34
Butter	1 tbs.	35
Oysters, salmon	3 oz. cooked	40
Clams, halibut, tuna	3 oz. cooked	55
chicken or turkey, light meat	3 oz. cooked	67
Beef, pork, lobster, chicken or turkey, dark meat	3 oz. cooked	75

Lamb, veal, crab	3 oz. cooked	85
Shrimp	3 oz. cooked	130
Heart, beef	3 oz. cooked	230
Egg	1 yolk or 1 egg	250
Liver (beef, calf, pork, or lamb)	3 oz. cooked	370
Kidney	3 oz. cooked	680
Brains	3 oz. raw	over 1700

From *Fats in Food and Diet.* Agricultural Information Bulletin No. 361, 1974. Washington, D.C., U.S. Department of Agriculture.

On the front cover of *Time* magazine of March 26, 1984 is a picture of a plate containing two fried eggs and a piece of bacon, with the caption "Cholesterol — And now the bad news...." The cover story, beginning on page 56 and entitled "Hold the Eggs and Butter," begins with the subtitle "Cholesterol is Proved Deadly, and Our Diet May Never Be the Same."

This article is summarized in the introduction as follows:

This year began with the announcement by the federal government of the results of the broadest and most expensive research project in medical history. Its subject was cholesterol, the vital yet dangerous yellowish substance whose level in the bloodstream is directly affected by the richness of the diet. Anybody who takes the results seriously may never be able to look at an egg or steak the same way again. For what the study found, after 10 years of research costing $150,000,000, promises to have a profound impact on how Americans eat and watch their health.

Among the conclusions:

1. Heart disease is directly linked to the level of cholesterol in blood.
2. Lowering cholesterol levels markedly reduces the incidence of fatal heart attacks.

Basal Rifkind, Project Director of the study, believes that research "strongly indicates that the more you lower cholesterol and fat in your diet, the more you reduce your risk of heart disease."

There are two other factors that seem to have an influence on blood cholesterol levels. The first of these is dietary fiber, which tends to lower blood cholesterol, and the second is coffee drinking, which tends to elevate it.

Considering the fact that a high fat diet has been linked with such potentially serious ailments as coronary artery disease, generalized atherosclerosis, cancer of the colon, prostate, and breast, and obesity — which leads to strokes, high blood pressure, heart disease, diabetes, and kidney failure — does fat have any real value in the diet, and if so what are some of its most important functions and uses in the body? The body must have a certain amount of fat to survive, but the *proper amounts* and the *right kinds* of fat are very important. Some important uses of fat in the body are as follows:

1. Energy: stored fat acts as highly concentrated form of energy, which can be used in place of carbohydrates. Producing energy from fat, however, is a complicated process and carbohydrates are by far the best source.
2. Fat is an essential part of every cell in the body.
3. Since vitamins A, D, E, and K are fat-soluble; fat is necessary for their proper utilization in the body.
4. The essential fatty acid, linoleic acid, is supplied abundantly in dietary fat.
5. While not an essential function, fat does increase the palatability of many of our foods.
6. The fat under our skin, called subcutaneous fat, provides insulation and helps our body maintain its proper temperature. About one-half of our total body fat is used in this way.
7. The other half is used inside our body and forms a cushion around many of the organs to protect them against sudden blows.

8. Fat is necessary for many of the body's metabolic functions.

The amount of fat in some of our common foods is shown in Table 2. Some general rules to guide you in your use of fat are as follows:

a. Reduce your total intake of fat. All fats, whether saturated or unsaturated, contain the same number of calories, 9 per gram, which is more than twice the number in carbohydrates and proteins.

b. Eat more foods containing unsaturated fatty acids and fewer foods with saturated fatty acids.

c. Omit high cholesterol foods, specially meat, and lower your consumption of eggs to no more than 2 a week.

d. Stay alert for hidden fats. Read the food labels. Don't forget that hidden fat accounts for two-thirds of the total fat you eat.

e. Be on your guard against foods containing coconut or palm oil or completely hydrogenated vegetable oils. These foods contain large amounts of the unhealthful saturated fatty acids.

In summary, while a certain amount of fat in our diet is essential, recent scientific data makes it clear that an excessive intake of fat is directly connected to heart disease and cancer, the No.1 and 2 killers in the United States. It would only seem to make good sense then, to shift the main emphasis of your eating to a more plant-oriented diet of fruits, vegetables, and whole grain products.

TABLE 2

FAT CONTENT AND MAJOR FATTY ACID COMPOSITION OF SELECTED FOODS*

FOOD	Total Fat Percent	Total Saturated Percent	Total Monoun-saturated Percent	Total Polyun-saturated Percent	Lino-leic Percent
Salad and cooking oils:					
Safflower	100	9	12	74	73
Sunflower	100	10	21	84	84
Corn	100	13	25	58	57
Soybean, unhydrogenated	100	14	24	57	50
Cottonseed	100	26	19	51	50
Sesame	100	15	40	40	40
Soybean, hydrogenated‡	100	15	43	37	32
Peanut	100	17	47	31	31
Palm	100	48	38	9	9
Olive	100	14	72	9	8
Coconut	100	86	6	2	2
Vegetable fats -shortening, household	100	25	44	26	23
Table spreads:					
Margarine, first ingredient on label:					
Safflower (liquid) - tub	80	13	16	48	48
Corn Oil (liquid) - tub	80	14	30	32	27
Corn oil (liquid) - stick	80	15	36	24	23
Soybean oil (hydrogenated) -stick	80	15	46	14	10
Butter	81	50	23	3	2

FATTY ACIDS†

TABLE 2 (Con't)

FAT CONTENT AND MAJOR FATTY ACID COMPOSITION OF SELECTED FOODS*

			FATTY ACIDS†		
FOOD	Total Fat Percent	Total Saturated Percent	Total Monoun-saturated Percent	Total Polyun-saturated Percent	Lino-leic Percent
Animal fats:					
Chicken	100	32	45	18	17
Lard (pork)	100	40	44	12	10
Beef tallow	100	48	42	4	4
Lamb tallow	100	52	43	5	3
Fish, raw:					
Salmon, sockeye	9	2	2	5	1
Tuna, albacore	8	2	2	3	0.5
Mackerel, Atlantic	10	2	4	2	0.5
Herring, Atlantic	6	2	2	1	0.5
Nuts:					
Walnuts, English	63	7	10	42	35
Walnuts, black	60	5	11	41	37
Brazil	68	17	22	25	25
Pecan	71	6	43	18	17
Peanut butter	52	10	24	15	15
Peanuts	48	9	24	13	13
Egg yolk	33	10	13	4	4
Avocado	15	2	9	2	2
Milk fats:					
Human		46	46	8	7
Goat		62	32	6	5
Cow		50	23	3	2
Cereal oils:					
Rye		16	14	70	62
Wheat germ		16	25	59	52
Whole Wheat flour		15	34	51	47
Oatmeal		22	36	42	40
Rice		17	45	38	37
Cocoa butter (chocolate)		57	41	2	2

* Modified from U.S. Department of Agriculture: Bulletin No. 361, *Fats in Food and Diet*. Washington, D.C., U.S. Government Printing Office, 1977, and from Keys, Ancel, and Keys, Margaret: *Eat Well and Stay Well*. New York, Doubleday, 1963.
† Total is not expected to equal "total fat."
‡ Common salad and cooking oil for commercial and household use.
< less than.

4

PROTEIN

Proteins are very complex substances that contain the same three basic elements as carbohydrates and fat — carbon, hydrogen, and oxygen — but in addition protein contains about 16 percent nitrogen. Sulfur is also present in many proteins, and other minerals such as iron, copper, iodine, and phosphorus, are present in smaller amounts. The word protein is derived from a Greek word meaning "to be in first place," and thanks to a strong advertising and public relations effort, the majority of Americans have been led to believe that they must eat large amounts of animal protein each day in order to have sufficient strength to do their work, especially if this work includes hard physical labor. The average American now consumes approximately 100 grams of protein a day.

The individual units, or building blocks, which join together to form a protein molecule, are called amino acids. There are about 22 different kinds of amino acids. A small protein molecule may consist of only about 50 amino acids, while a large protein molecule may contain hundreds or even thousands. For each particular protein, the amino acid "building blocks" are always present in exactly the same arrangement. Any variation from this arrangement results in a different protein. There are about 30,000 different proteins in the body, but only a very small percentage of these have been identified. A single liver cell contains nearly 1000 different enzymes and each one of these is comprised of a different protein.

When a protein is ingested, it is broken down in the intestinal tract into its individual amino acids. These then enter the large body "pool" of amino acids. From this "pool" each body cell selects the specific amino acids it needs to build a particular protein for its own special use.

Amino acids are divided into two groups — ESSENTIAL and NONESSENTIAL. Essential amino acids are those that must be provided in our food. There are 9 essential amino acids. All the others, the 13 nonessential amino acids, can be manufactured in the body so they do not have to be supplied in the diet.

It is the amino acids that are the really meaningful part of the protein. So it is not unreasonable to divide proteins into two main groups, depending on the presence or absence of the essential amino acids.

Complete proteins, sometimes referred to as high quality proteins, contain all the essential amino acids in sufficient quantity to support the growth of new tissue. These include all the proteins of animal origin except gelatin. Nonfat dry milk is probably the cheapest source of complete protein. Complete proteins contain about 33 percent essential amino acids, compared to 25 percent in the less complete proteins.

In less complete proteins, also called incomplete or low quality proteins, one or more of the essential amino acids is present in an insufficient amount to supply our bodily needs. Proteins present in plants are considered to be less complete and in general this is true, specially for fruits and vegetables (except legumes), which contain very little protein. Legumes, however, contain proteins rated nearly as high as those found in animal products. Soybeans, lima beans, navy beans, pinto beans, kidney beans, chick peas (garbanzos), black-eyed peas, and peanuts are all legumes. Nuts, seeds, and grains, while not as high in protein as the legumes, contain some amino acids that are either lacking or present in only small quantities in the legumes. For instance, legumes are rich in the essential amino acid lysine, but they are low in another one, methionine. Just the opposite is true for grains, nuts, and seeds, which are rich in methionine but low in lysine. These two groups of less complete proteins, therefore, complement each other; that is, when they are eaten together, an adequate supply of all the essential amino acids is provided for the body to use.

Some examples of this complementary activity are beans, peas or lentils eaten with rice, a peanut butter and whole wheat bread sandwich, or corn and lima beans. Complementary proteins need not be eaten during the same meal, but should be eaten the same day, so that the amino acids will be available for use by the body at approximately the same time. Combinations of plant protein sources that can be combined with each other to produce high quality protein are shown in Table 1. The best way for vegetarians to be certain of getting enough complete protein is by eating a large variety of plant foods daily from the three groups: grains, legumes, and nuts and seeds.

TABLE 1
COMBINING VEGETABLE PROTEINS

Combine LEGUMES With
Barley Corn Oats Rice Sesame seeds Wheat

Combine RICE With
Legumes Sesame seeds Wheat

Combine WHEAT With
Legumes Rice and Soybeans
Soybeans and Peanuts
Soybeans and Sesame seeds

All body cells and tissues contain protein, even bone, hair, and nails. Protein comprises about 20 percent of the total weight of the body and about 50 percent of the body's dry weight. The muscles and liver contain large amounts of protein. In fact, nearly one-half of the protein in the body is located in the muscles. The only components of the body that do not contain protein are bile and urine. There is constant renewal of the cells in the body, but the rate of renewal varies greatly among the different tissues. For example, the cells that line the intestinal tract are replaced by new ones every few days, the red blood cells every 120 days, the cells that make up the muscles take even longer, while the cells in the brain are rarely replaced. When tissue breaks down, the amino acids are released from the cells and added to the large pool of amino acids that are available in the body for the building of new protein.

Approximately 33 grams of protein are lost each day by the average adult male and must be replaced in the diet. The body has no means of storing amino acids, so the reserves are depleted in only a few hours. That is one of the reasons why we should try to eat some complete protein at each meal. If no protein is supplied in the diet, the body will continue to use up its protein in order to maintain all the vital body functions.

The diet of the average American contains two or three times the required daily amount of protein, and 60 to 70 percent of this is obtained from animal sources. Unlike some of the developing countries, where 70 to 80 percent of the protein in the diet is from cereals, protein deficiency in the United States is almost unheard of, even in those who follow a vegetarian diet. The protein requirement of the body is at its highest during infancy and childhood, the time of greatest growth.

A rough measurement of the daily requirement of protein in grams can be obtained by dividing your body weight in pounds by 3. A more accurate way is to multiply your weight in kilograms (Kg.) by 0.8. If you do not know your weight in kilograms, it can easily be found by dividing your weight in pounds by 2.2. The result (in Kg) is then multiplied by 0.8 to obtain the daily requirement of grams of protein. For example, a 150-pound man would weigh about 68 kg. This multiplied by 0.8 gives 54 grams of protein as his daily requirement. Additional protein must be supplied to growing children under the age of 18, following severe burns, hemorrhage, surgery, or serious illness, during pregnancy and lactation, and in the elderly. However, a person doing hard physical labor uses no more protein than the office worker, despite the many rumors to the contrary. Increasing the amount of protein in the diet does not mean that the body will make more protein if it already has a sufficient supply. Any excess protein in the diet is either burned for energy or stored as fat. In order for this to occur, however, nitrogen must first be removed from the protein. This nitrogen is changed to a waste product, urea, in the liver and is then excreted in the urine. This places an extra work load on the kidneys.

Protein is an expensive food and only in affluent industrialized countries are such large amounts of animal protein consumed. Following are some examples that illustrate the excessive use of plant protein that is necessary to provide food for those who believe they must have meat to eat. One acre of farm land will produce enough soybeans to yield 500 pounds of protein; however, if this same acre is used to grow feed for cattle, only 50 pounds of animal protein will result. Only about 15 percent of the protein is finally available to humans in the form of meat, milk, and eggs. It takes about 10 pounds of feed to produce one pound of beefsteak and about 6 pounds of feed to produce one pound of turkey protein.

Protein has many important uses, as follows:

1. It is essential for the growth, repair, and maintenance of all body tissues.
2. It takes part in the production of enzymes and hormones, which help to regulate nearly every important function in the body.
3. Proteins regulate the body's water and acid-base balance; they also help to maintain the body fluids in their normal, slightly alkaline state.
4. Protein is essential in the formation of antibodies, which are the first line of defense against disease.
5. They are a supplementary but very expensive source of energy, particularly when they are obtained from meat or meat products.

5

MINERAL ELEMENTS IN THE BODY

The following is a list of the essential mineral elements normally found in the body. All of these minerals are bountifully supplied to us in natural foods, if they are not lost or destroyed during meal preparation. All of the bodily functions are operating continuously and must be supplied by the essential minerals found in foods. Natural minerals, especially, are needed for the purifying, cleansing process.

ESSENTIAL MINERALS

Macrominerals	Microminerals	
Calcium	Iron	Molybdenum
Phosphorus	Iodine	Chromium
Potassium	Zinc	Fluorine
Sulfur	Selenium	Silicon
Sodium	Manganese	Vanadium
Chlorine	Copper	Nickel
Magnesium	Cobalt	Tin

Macrominerals are those needed in the diet in amounts exceeding 100 mg per day. *Microminerals* are also called "trace elements," because they are needed in only very minute amounts. If all the minerals in the body were collected and weighed together they would make up only 4 percent of the body weight. Oxygen, hydrogen, carbon, and nitrogen, the elements in carbohydrates, fats, and protein, comprise 96 percent of the body weight and contribute 99 percent of all the atoms that are present in the body. If the body was completely burned, there would be about five pounds of minerals remaining. About one-half of this five pounds would be calcium and another 25 percent would be phosphorus, the two major minerals that are in the bones.

About 60 different minerals have been identified in the body, but so far only those in the preceding list have been found to be essential. An essential mineral, like an essential amino acid, is one that must be supplied to our body in the food we eat. It performs a function that is necessary for the maintenance of life, for growth, or for reproduction. Minerals are necessary both for regulating body processes and for building tissue.

In comparison with the two and a half pounds of calcium in the body, all the trace elements (microminerals) together weigh only about one ounce. But they are just as necessary to the proper functioning of the body as those elements that are present in larger amounts. Cobalt, for instance, the mineral that is associated with vitamin B_{12}, is present in only two parts per trillion of body weight. A large amount of research is now in progress, and with new techniques it is possible to isolate elements in tissue that are present in very tiny quantities, about one part per billion; therefore, other trace elements will probably soon be discovered.

Minerals are widely distributed in our food supply. They are found in whole grains, nuts and seeds, dark green leafy vegetables, fruit, milk and milk products. There are substances in plants that combine with some of the minerals to form insoluble salts, thus rendering them less available for absorption into the body. For example, some of the iron, zinc, and magnesium we eat is made unavailable to the body by combining with phytates in whole grain. Calcium is rendered insoluble by oxalates that are found in some of the green vegetables. Minerals are not readily affected by acid or alkaline solutions nor by heat or oxygen. But, although minerals cannot be destroyed they can be dissolved in the cooking water and then discarded. Moreover, nearly all the minerals are removed during the processing of refined flour and sugar .

There are three minerals that tend to be low in the average American diet; these are calcium, iron, and zinc .

Some minerals are acid-forming when they are in solution,

while others are alkaline. Those that are acid-forming are chlorine, sulfur, and phosphorus. These minerals are found mostly in meat, fish, poultry, cheese, cereals, prunes, plums, cranberries, rhubarb, cocoa, tea, and certain nuts (Brazil nuts, peanuts, and walnuts). Those minerals that are alkaline-forming are calcium, sodium, potassium, and magnesium. They are found in fruits, vegetables, milk, olives, almonds, coconuts, and chestnuts.

The body functions best in a neutral or a slightly alkaline medium and if too much acid is present, as it is in most American diets that are high in meat and animal products, it is given off by the lungs as carbon dioxide and is also excreted in the urine. Several other mechanisms are built into the body that maintain the proper acid-base balance. Various minerals contribute greatly to this important function.

A. CALCIUM

When a wide variety of food is eaten, an adequate supply of most minerals is obtained. But because dairy foods contain the largest amount of calcium, those on a strict vegetarian diet (vegans, who eat no meat or animal products) should be sure they get an adequate supply of calcium from other sources. Calcium is the most abundant mineral in the body, accounting for roughly two percent of the total body weight. Ninety-nine percent of the calcium is located in the bones and teeth and most of the remainder is in the blood. One eight-ounce cup of milk will provide about one-third of the daily calcium requirement. To get an equal amount by eating whole wheat bread, you would need to eat 18 slices.

It is not so much the quantity of calcium that we eat that is important; what really counts is the amount that is absorbed from the intestines and utilized by the body. Although calcium absorption varies under different circumstances and in different people, as is true of many of the other mineral elements, on the average only 20 to 40 percent of the calcium we eat is absorbed from the intestines. The absorption of calcium is increased by the following.

1. Adequate amounts of vitamin D in the diet.
2. Lactose (milk sugar) in the diet, which increases the calcium absorption by as much as 20 percent.
3. An adequate supply of fluorine.
4. Proper exercise.
5. An acid environment of the upper intestinal tract.
6. Periods of need, such as rapid body growth or low body stores of calcium.

The less calcium there is in the diet, the greater will be the percentage absorbed.

The absorption of calcium is hindered or decreased by the following.

1. Oxalic acid in some foods unites with calcium and prevents its absorption. Some foods with high levels of oxalic acid are rhubarb, spinach, beet greens, peanuts, parsley, Swiss chard, and cocoa. But the oxalic acid in these foods binds only the calcium in that particular food and does not interfere with calcium from a different food that is eaten at the same meal. Thus, the overall effect of oxalates on calcium absorption is probably quite small.
2. Phytic acid, a form of fiber found in the outer coats of grain, also binds calcium; however, under most circumstances this has little effect on the overall calcium absorption.
3. A high protein diet causes increased excretion of calcium in the urine, so that the body cannot use it. Eating too much protein also inhibits calcium absorption from the intestines.
4. A lack of exercise. Anyone that is immobilized for a period of time, such as invalids or even astronauts.
5. Emotional instability.
6. Laxatives and other medicines that cause the intestinal contents to pass rapidly through the body.

7. Some antacids and diuretics cause decreased calcium absorption.
8. Excessive phosphorus intake. Some soft drinks are high in phosphorus.

Recommended daily allowance:
800 to 1200 mg
1200 mg — teenagers and during pregnancy and lactation
1500 mg — women over 52

Uses:
1. Development and maintenance of strong bones and teeth. Protects against osteoporosis.
2. Ensures proper clotting of the blood.
3. Needed for the contraction and relaxation of muscles, specially the heart.
4. Needed for the proper utilization of iron.
5. Acts as an enzyme activator.
6. Assists in the absorption of vitamin B_{12}.
7. Helps to regulate cell permeability.
8. Helps to maintain the neutrality of the body fluids.
9. Possibly helps in lowering the blood pressure.
10. May help ward off colon cancer.

Sources:
1. Dairy products, including yogurt. These provide 75 to 85 percent of the calcium in the average American diet. There is about 300 mg of calcium in one eight-ounce cup of milk.
2. Legumes; some dark green vegetables such as broccoli, collards, kale, mustard, and turnip greens.
3. Enriched cereals.
4. Citrus fruits, figs.

OSTEOPOROSIS

Osteoporosis, which literally means "porous bones," is a painful and potentially crippling disease caused by a loss of calcium from the bones. This loss results in thinning and softening of the bones with frequent fractures of the spine, hips and wrists, loss of body height, and the formation of a "dowager's hump." About 150,000 persons in the United States, mostly women, suffer from hip fractures each year due to osteoporosis and 40,000 of these people will be dead within one year of the fracture. Osteoporosis affects 15 to 20 million people in America for an annual health bill approaching $4 billion. One of every four women will eventually become a victim of this largely preventable disease. Its greatest incidence is in women past the menopause or in those women who have lost the normal estrogen production of their ovaries, usually as the result of surgery. The loss of estrogens leads to decreased intestinal absorption of calcium and an increased loss of this important mineral through the kidneys. The average age for the menopause is 52 years and the average life expectancy for women in the United States is now a little over 78 years. Fifty percent of women over the age of 75 suffer from the symptoms of osteoporosis. While osteoporosis is far more common in women than in men, elderly men may also suffer from this condition. It is also more common in whites and Asians than in blacks. Vegetarians have been shown to have a lower incidence of osteoporosis than those who eat meat, probably due to a lower intake of protein and phosphorus.

A healthy life style and proper treatment can go a long way towards the prevention of osteoporosis. Without a doubt, the ideal way to get all the calcium you need is from your food, but if a calcium supplement becomes necessary it should preferably be taken as calcium carbonate, the form in which calcium is most readily absorbed. Taking part at least 3 times a week in some form of weight-bearing exercise, such as walking, jogging, tennis, bicycling, jumping rope, etc., helps to maintain the normal bone structure. Cigarettes. alcohol, and excessive caffeine intake should be eliminated. Recent studies have shown that taking low dosages of estrogen together with a 1500 mg daily intake of calcium is much more effective in preventing bone loss in postmenopausal women than when large amounts of calcium are taken by itself. In fact, the number of fractures due to osteoporosis after the menopause has been shown to be just about the same in those who take only calcium supplements as in those who do not. If you have a tendency to form kidney stones, you should consult your family doctor before taking calcium supplements. Anyone taking calcium supplements should be sure to drink at least 8 cups of fluid a day.

Calcium supplements usually come in the following forms:

Percent calcium by weight

Calcium carbonate 40

Calcium citrate 22

Calcium lactate 18

Calcium gluconate 9

Dolomite, bone meal, or oyster shells are sometimes used, but the first two are not recommended because they may contain lead or other toxic substances. Read all labels carefully to see what form of calcium you are taking. For instance, a 1000 mg tablet of calcium carbonate contains 400 mg of calcium, while a 1000 mg tablet of calcium gluconate has only 90 mg of calcium.

In order to know if you need additional calcium, either in the form of food or supplements, you must first know about how much you already consume each day in your diet. The following chart gives several common food sources that are high in calcium and the amount of calcium each contains.

CALCIUM CONTENT OF SOME
COMMON FOODS

Dairy Products	mg	Fruits	mg
1 cup Yogurt*	415	5 medium Figs	126
1 cup Milk, nonfat	303	1 large Orange	96
1 cup Milk, low fat (2%)	314	4 large Prunes	45
1 ounce Swiss cheese	259	4 ounces Raisins	45
1 cup Cottage cheese, low fat	154	*Vegetables*	
1 cup Soymilk, fortified	150	1 cup Collards, cooked	152
1 cup Soymilk, regular	55	1 cup Turnip greens, cooked	139
Breads and Cereals		1 cup Mustard greens, cooked	138
1 cup Total, General Mills	200	1 cup Kale, cooked	125
1 cup Oatmeal, inst. Quaker	120	1 cup Rhubarb, cooked	105
1 each Buckwheat pancake, 4"	99	1 cup Spinach, cooked	83
1 cup All-Bran, Kellogg's	70	1 cup Broccoli, cooked	66
1 6-inch Tortilla, corn	60	1 cup Rutabagas, cooked	59
1 cup Cream of Wheat, inst.	40	1 cup Artichoke, cooked	51
1 piece Cornbread, enriched	28	*Legumes and Nuts*	
1 cup Oatmeal, rolled	21	1 cup Boston baked beans	85
1 slice Whole wheat bread	17	1 cup Soybeans	73
1 cup Cream of Wheat, reg.	13	1 cup White beans	50
Miscellaneous		1 cup Kidney beans	48
1 tbsp. Molasses, blackstrap	116	12-15 Almonds	38

Vegetarian Meat Analogs

1 each Stakelet (Worthington)	80	1 each Grillers,	
1 each Griddle Steaks, frzn	67	(Morningstar Farms)	67
(Loma Linda Foods)		2 each Breakfast Patties,	45
		(Morningstar Farms)	

*Note: The amount of calcium in yogurt varies from brand to brand and also depends on whether it is plain or fruit-flavored.

Notice the difference in calcium content between instant and regular Cream of Wheat and oatmeal: the instant varieties have calcium added.

While many other foods contain calcium, these are the best sources. Be careful about depending on multi-vitamin/mineral supplements to give you an adequate calcium supply. Most of them contain only small amounts of calcium. Check the label to find out the exact amount.

Many antacids contain calcium. For example, one regular Tums tablet contains 500 mg of calcium carbonate, which provides 200 mg of calcium.

It is extremely important to include adequate calcium in the diet during the growing years when the bones are developing. They will then be able to store a large amount of calcium that can be used later in life to help prevent osteoporosis. After about the age of 35 there is a gradual reduction in bone calcium that apparently cannot be prevented by any form of treatment. As mentioned in the preceding paragraphs, this loss accelerates considerably in women after the menopause. If you eat a well-balanced diet containing a good supply of calcium in early life and also form the habit of regular exercise, your bone mass will be increased and bone loss will be slowed during the middle and later years of life.

Teenagers in particular need to be taught why it is specially important for them to eat a good diet, including foods high in calcium, because so many in this age group frequently substitute soft drinks for milk, one of our best sources of calcium. The greatest benefits of following a healthy life style are obtained by those who develop good habits of eating and exercise early in life.

In a recent study of thousands of people around the country by the National Center for Health Statistics, it was found that teenage girls from 12 to 17 were eating an average of only 692 mg of calcium a day instead of the recommended 1200 mg. From 18 to 24 years of age, the calcium consumption was even lower. Girls and young women in these age groups who are not getting an adequate supply of calcium are not building up a good calcium reserve in their bones and are thus placing themselves in jeopardy for later developing osteoporosis. It cannot be emphasized too strongly that it is the adolescent years that are the most critical for building good strong bones. About one-half of the bone structure in an adult is formed during the rapid growth spurt of adolescence. This is not a matter of "What you don't know won't hurt you," for what you don't know (and do something about) may hurt you very much.

Another specially important period in which to get an abundant supply of calcium is during pregnancy and lactation, in order to promote good mineral formation of the infant's bone structure and baby teeth. The most critical period is during the last three months of pregnancy and the first few months of lactation, when bone development and growth is at its maximum. During the time of pregnancy and lactation, calcium intake should be 400 mg per day more than normal, or a total of about 1200 mg. If the mother is not getting enough calcium for the infant's needs, it will be withdrawn from the mother's bones, possibly leading to bone disease at some time in the future.

It should also be remembered that smoking, alcoholic beverages, and excessive intake of caffeine in coffee and soft drinks all seem to contribute to the development of osteoporosis.

B.   PHOSPHORUS

Next to calcium, phosphorus is the most abundant mineral in the body, comprising one percent of the total body weight. About 90 percent of the phosphorus is located in the bones and teeth and the rest is distributed in the cells throughout the body. No deficiency of phosphorus has been observed, for not only is it widely distributed in our food, but 50 to 70 percent of the phosphorus we ingest is absorbed. The average daily intake of phosphorus in the United States is 1500 to 1600 mg. If Amphogel, an antacid containing aluminum hydroxide, is taken with meals, it will react with the phosphorus and prevent some of it from being absorbed. Antacids containing aluminum hydroxide are not recommended.

Recommended daily allowance: 800 to 1200 mg.

Uses:
1. Development of strong bones and teeth.
2. A component of enzyme systems in the cells that govern the release and storage of energy.

3. Part of the RNA and DNA in the cells that controls protein production and the pattern of our genes.
4. Transportation of fatty acids to various parts of the body.
5. Helps to maintain the neutrality of the body fluids.
6. Enzyme formation.

Sources:

1. Whole wheat grains.
2. Nuts, legumes.
3. Dairy products, eggs.
4. Phosphate additives in carbonated drinks.

C. POTASSIUM

The word potassium comes from "potash," which is the ash that remains following the burning of vegetable substances. The average American diet contains 2000 to 6000 mg of potassium every day and it is readily absorbed from the intestines. The excess is excreted by the kidneys. A deficiency of potassium occurs in some illnesses in which there is prolonged vomiting and diarrhea. Certain medicines, such as diuretics, may cause a potassium deficiency. Poor circulation and constipation may indicate a lack of potassium. Foods that are high in potassium should be used in abundance in female troubles. A dietary deficiency of potassium occurs only rarely.

Recommended daily allowance: 1825 to 5625 mg.

Uses:

1. Release of energy from the cells.
2. Manufacture of glycogen and protein.
3. Regulates fluid balance.
4. Helps to regulate acid-base balance.
5. Transmission of nerve impulses.
6. Important in maintaining normal heart beat.

7. Muscle contraction.

Sources:
Widely distributed in a large number of foods. Specially good sources are bananas, dried fruit, potatoes, avocados, milk, whole grain, dark molasses, broccoli, and legumes.

D. SULFUR

Some sulfur is present in every cell of the body. It is a part of several amino acids, B vitamins, insulin, and other essential body compounds. It is found most abundantly in our hair, nails, and skin.

Recommended daily allowance: None known.

Uses:
1. Maintains healthy hair and nails.
2. Needed in eliminating blood diseases.
3. Helps to eliminate some skin diseases such as acne.
4. Stimulates the liver and increases the flow of bile.
5. Important in maintaining normal body metabolism.
6. Detoxifies some poisons in the body.
7. Part of some enzyme systems.

Sources:
1. Protein foods.
2. Cabbage and other members of the cabbage family —
    cauliflower, broccoli, and brussel sprouts.

E. SODIUM

Sodium is one of the two elements that make up salt (sodium chloride), which is one of the oldest known chemical preservatives. Regular table salt contains 40 percent sodium. About two-thirds of the sodium is in the body fluids outside of the cells. The other one-third is in the bones. There is rarely a deficiency of sodium in the diet unless it is self-imposed by a person that is on a very low salt diet. In fact, the average diet has two or three teaspoons of salt each day, more than twice the amount needed. The amount of sodium in the body may be lowered by ervere diarrhea or by excessive sweating.

About 18 percent of the population has high blood pressure. In about one-half of these the blood pressure rises as the sodium intake is increased. In the other half eating sodium seems to have little effect on the blood pressure.

Recommended daily allowance: 1500 to 2500 mg per day.

Uses:

1. Maintains normal fluid balance.
2. Transmission of nerve impulses.
3. Muscle contraction.
4. Increases the permeability of the cell wall.
5. Helps to regulate and maintain osmotic pressure and acid-base balance.
6. A good supply of sodium should be available in those who have rheumatism, hardening of the arteries, kidney stones, gallstones, stiff joints, acidosis, and diabetes. It should be restricted in those with high blood pressure and heart disease.

Sources:

1. Table salt.
2. Processed foods, baking powder, baking soda.
3. Milk, cheese, egg white.
4. Strawberries, apples, huckleberries, gooseberries, cucumbers, carrots, beets, okra, cauliflower, spinach, asparagus, celery, Romaine lettuce, and watermelon.

F.   CHLORINE

Chlorine is found abundantly throughout the body, both in the cells and in the body fluids. It is specially plentiful in the fluid that circulates around the brain and spinal cord and in the hydrochloric acid produced by the stomach. When sodium is lost by sweating, diarrhea, or excessive vomiting, there is a similar loss of chlorine.

Recommended daily allowance: 1700 to 5100 mg.

Uses:
1. Helps to maintain water balance, acid-base balance, and osmotic pressure.
2. Increases the capacity of the blood to carry carbon dioxide to the lungs for excretion.
3. Produces the normal acid environment in the stomach. This aids in the absorption of iron and vitamin B_{12}.
4. Helps to cleanse both the intestines and the body of toxins.

Sources:
1. Watercress, raw white cabbage, spinach, lettuce.
2. Tomatoes, radishes, asparagus, celery, cucumbers, parsnips, carrots, onions and turnips.
3. Pineapple.

G. MAGNESIUM

There is a total of about one ounce of magnesium in the body. Sixty percent of this is located in the bones, and the rest is in muscle, blood, soft tissues, and cells. Between 30 and 70 percent of ingested magnesium is absorbed by the small intestine, depending on the amount eaten. The amount that is absorbed is decreased by the presence in the intestines of calcium, phytates, and fat. It is increased by vitamin D and lactose.

Recommended daily allowance: 300 mg.

Uses:
1. Helps to form strong bones and teeth.
2. Helps to regulate muscle relaxation and contraction.
3. Proper function of the nerves.
4. Activates enzymes controlling energy metabolism.
5. Acts as a laxative.
6. Foods containing magnesium are helpful in people who suffer from constipation and autointoxication and may be of help in stiff joints.

Sources:
1. Green leafy vegetables.
2. Nuts, seeds, whole grain cereals. During refining of the grain, about 80 percent of the magnesium is removed.
3. Soybeans, peas, green beans, brown rice, apples, cherries, figs, raisins, prunes, lemons, alfalfa, and celery.
4. Milk.

H. IRON

If it were possible to collect all of the iron in our body into one place and weigh it, it would weigh about as much as a penny. About two-thirds of this iron is located in the hemoglobin of the red blood cells and the rest of it is in the liver, spleen, bone marrow, and muscles.

The most widespread nutrient deficiency of early childhood in the United States is not a lack of vitamins or protein, but rather a lack of iron. Nearly 10 percent of toddlers in the United States have been found to be iron deficient. Milk is a poor source of iron, even mother's milk, and a baby is born with only enough iron to last for about six months. Iron-fortified formulas and infant foods are therefore necessary starting when cow's milk is substituted for breast milk or at about 4 months of age for breast-fed infants. Cow's milk has less than 1 mg of iron per quart, and of that amount only 10 percent or less is absorbed. Other groups of people who may develop iron deficiency anemia are preschool and adolescent children, women during their childbearing years, women who are pregnant, and for two or three months following delivery. For these groups, an iron supplement in the form of ferrous sulfate or ferrous gluconate may be required. Because of its possible effects on the intestinal tract of nausea, constipation, and diarrhea, the iron should be taken either an hour before or with meals. Start with one pill daily and increase to several. Do not take them all at the same time, but spread them throughout the day. Iron supplements will turn the stools a very black color, which should not be mistaken for blood.

Another caution about taking iron is that it can be dangerous or even fatal if taken in large doses. It is the fourth most common cause of poisoning in children below the age of five years, so it must be kept well out of their reach.

Ordinarily only about 5 to 10 percent of the iron we eat is absorbed. But if for some reason the body needs more iron, as much as 30 to 35 percent can be absorbed. The body keeps using the iron that it has and very little is excreted, perhaps 1 mg a day in men and 1 1/2 mg in women. Men are able to store about 1000 mg of iron but women can store only about 300 mg .

Cooking in the old time cast-iron pots and kettles gave a good supply of iron, specially when acid foods were being cooked. The longer the food was allowed to simmer in the iron pot, the higher the iron content became in the food.

The absorption of the iron in our food is increased by:

1. The presence of vitamin C (ascorbic acid) taken at the same meal. Vitamin C has no effect on the absorption of iron supplements.
2. The hydrochloric acid in the stomach.
3. The form of iron that we eat.
4. An increased need of iron by the body.

The absorption of iron is hindered by:
1. The presence of tannic acid, which is found in tea, cola drinks, and coffee. Drinking tea, even iced tea, with a meal or within an hour after a meal, may reduce the iron absorption by as much as 87 percent.
2. Phytic acid, found in grain and fiber.
3. Excess phosphorus and calcium in our diet.
4. Phosvitin, present in egg yolk.
5. Some antacids that contain calcium and phosphate salts.
6. Inorganic iron. This is the form of iron in all plants and eggs and about half of the iron in meats. Only 3 to 5 percent of this kind of iron is absorbed, but this amount can be increased two to three times by eating a good vitamin C source at the same time as the other foods.

Recommended daily allowance: 10 mg for males. 18 mg for females.

Uses:
1. Iron is a vital part of the hemoglobin that carries oxygen to the tissues.
2. Iron is part of the enzyme system present in all cells that is responsible for energy production and release.
3. An important constituent of the muscles.

Sources:
1. Whole grain cereal products.
2. Nuts, legumes, raisins, molasses.
3. Green leafy vegetables, yellow vegetables, potatoes.
4. Dried fruits.
5. Boiled lentils or kidney beans.

6   One ounce of any of the following Kellogg's cereals will provide 18 mg of iron, 100 percent of the recommended daily allowance of iron for women: Product 19, Fruitful Bran, Raisin Bran, Bran Flakes.

I.   IODINE

About 15 to 30 mg of iodine is present in the body; this is just about equal to the size of a match head. Sixty percent of this is in the thyroid gland and the rest is in the blood. Iodine is readily absorbed from the intestines and it is also absorbed from the skin, where it is sometimes used on cuts, etc. as an antiseptic. About one-third of the iodine we eat is used by the thyroid gland and the rest is excreted in the urine.

If there is not enough iodine in the diet, the thyroid gland enlarges, causing a swelling in the neck. This enlargement of the thyroid gland is called a goiter. A goiter, which was treated with seaweed, was recorded as early as the year 3000 B.C. in Chinese literature. If the thyroid gland is too active, hyperthyroidism (Grave's disease) results. This causes a rapid pulse, weight loss, nervousness, excessive sweating, and protruding eyeballs.

Recommended daily allowance: 150 micrograms.

Uses:
1.   An important part of the thyroid hormone, thyroxine, that is responsible for total body metabolism.
2.   Essential for the normal function of the thyroid gland.

Sources:
1.   Iodized salt.
2.   Food that is grown near the ocean.
3.   Kelp.

J.   ZINC

Of the body's total of two grams of zinc, about 70 percent is in the bones. The rest is distributed in the blood, hair, skin, and testes. About one-half of the zinc that is eaten is absorbed. The amount absorbed is increased when the supply in the body needs to be increased and also during pregnancy and lactation. Fiber and phytic acid, found in whole grains, decrease the availability of zinc for absorption, as does the taking of oral contraceptives. There are large areas in the United States where the soil is low or lacking in zinc and in these areas some people have been found with a possible zinc deficiency. Vegetarians also have a tendency to be deficient in zinc, so they must be sure to eat some foods with a high zinc content. Large doses of zinc can prevent the proper absorption of copper and may lead to anemia. It also reduces the amount of good HDL-cholesterol in the blood.

Recommended daily allowance: 15 mg.

Uses:
1. Proper growth of the body.
2. Helps with the proper healing of wounds and maintains healthy skin.
3. Needed in enzymes concerned with metabolism and digestion.
4. Helps maintain proper sense of taste and smell.
5. For utilization of vitamin A.
6. Transportation of carbon dioxide.
7. Carbohydrate metabolism.

Sources:
1 Whole grains .
2 Legumes, nuts.
3 Vegetables and fruits are, in general, poor sources of zinc.

K. SELENIUM

In 1957 it was discovered that selenium was an essential mineral and that certain diseases in animals, which were thought to be caused by a lack of vitamin E, could readily be cured by giving selenium. The amount of selenium in the soil and water varies considerably throughout the United States, as well as the entire world, and this in turn causes a variation in the amount of selenium in our food. The section of the country from which our food originates is probably more important in determining the amount of selenium we get than the type of food we eat. But because the food we buy at the market comes from various parts of the country, the average American does not need to worry about obtaining enough selenium. The average diet contains 1.3 mg of selenium per day.

Several recent studies seem to indicate that in areas where there is an abundance of selenium in the soil, the rate of cancer is less. In an article published in the prestigious medical journal, *Diseases of the Colon and Rectum* in July 1984, Richard Nelson M.D. believes that a decreased consumption of selenium may be a cause for a recently noted change in the location of colon cancer in the United States and other western countries. This change has taken place gradually over the past 30 years. Whereas 30 years ago cancer was much more frequent in the last 10 or 12 inches of the colon, it is now becoming more common in the first part of the colon, which is located in the right side of the abdomen.

An investigation into the possible causes for this change suggested that it was not only the result of decreased selenium consumption, but also that an increased intake of zinc and fluoride may play a part by opposing the action of selenium.

When colon cancer was experimentally produced in rats, a 90 percent reduction in right-sided colon cancer was noted if the rats were given a selenium supplement. This did not occur if the selenium supplement was withheld.

It has been noted for some time that people living in areas with a deficiency of selenium in the soil have an increase in the amount of cancer in general, but specially of colon and breast cancer.

Why should there be a deficiency of selenium?

1. During the past 30 to 40 years there has been a gradual increase in the consumption of meat at the expense of grains and vegetables. The amount of selenium in meat is quite low compared with the amount in whole grain cereals. There is strong evidence that an increased rate of colon cancer is associated with a high consumption of meat and beef fat and a decreased intake of dietary fiber.

2. Meat is also very high in zinc, which prevents the utilization of selenium. The zinc in plant foods is bound to phytates and excreted in the stool, but all the zinc in meat is available for absorption. Increased zinc levels in the blood have been associated with colon and breast cancer.

3. The artificial fluoridation of water supplies may be linked to an increase in right-sided colon cancer. Fluoride is also a potential selenium antagonist.

Cancer is the second most common cause of death after heart disease, and cancer of the colon is the second most frequent cause of cancer deaths. Cancer of the colon is next in frequency only to lung cancer in men and to breast and lung cancer in women. About 62,500 deaths will occur from colon and rectal cancer in 1991, and approximately 157,000 new cases will be diagnosed. The lifetime risk of developing a cancer of the colon is about 4 percent, and 6 million Americans now living will die of colon cancer if the present trend continues.

The *FDA DRUG BULLETIN* of August 1984 reported 12 cases of toxic overdose of selenium that occurred when it was discovered that some selenium tablets contained 182 times the amount indicated on the label. The estimated doses that were taken ranged from 27 to 2310 mg. Symptoms of a toxic overdose consisted usually of nausea and vomiting, nail changes, fatigue, and irritability. Less commonly experienced were loss of hair and nails, diarrhea, abdominal cramps, dry hair, sensory changes on the skin, and garlic odor on the breath.

Recommended daily allowance: .05 to 0.2 mg (over age seven years).

Uses:
1. Selenium, along with vitamin E, protects the body tissues from oxidative damage. This is specially true of the cell membranes.
2. Helps to protect normal body cells against radiation damage.
3. Assists in the prevention of cancer.
4. Required by the body for maximum immune response.
5. Retards the rancidity of unsaturated fatty acids.

Sources:
1. Grains, nuts, cereals. Eighty percent of the selenium is lost in the refining and processing of food.
2. Foods grown in high-selenium areas, such as the Dakotas, Montana, and Wyoming.

L. MANGANESE

Most of the 10 mg of manganese that we have stored in our body is in the liver, pancreas, bones, and kidneys. About 30 to 50 percent of the manganese in our food is absorbed into our body, but calcium and iron inhibit the absorption of manganese from the intestines. No deficiency of manganese has been reported in humans.

Recommended daily allowance: 2.5 to 5.0 mg.

Uses:
1. Necessary for the normal development of bones and connective tissue.

2. Part of the enzyme systems involved in fatty acid, cholesterol, and carbohydrate synthesis.
3. Maintenance of normal reproductive functions.

Sources:
1. Whole grain cereals, nuts, rice.
2. Green vegetables.
3. Kelp.

M. COPPER

Almost half of the copper in the body is found in the bones and muscles, but the most concentrated source is in the liver. Vitamin C and phytic acid both act to hinder the absorption of copper.

Recommended daily allowance: 2 to 3 mg.

Uses:
1. Prevents anemia by controlling the storage and release of iron to form hemoglobin.
2. Energy and connective tissue metabolism.
3. Part of the tissue that acts as a covering for the nerves.

Sources:
1. Widespread in most foods.
2. Nuts, dried peas and beans, dried fruit, whole grains, leafy vegetables.

N. COBALT

In 1948 it was discovered that cobalt is an essential part of vitamin B_{12}, the vitamin that is necessary for the prevention of pernicious anemia.

Recommended daily allowance: None has been determined.

Uses:
1. Necessary for the formation of vitamin B_{12}.

Sources:
1. Widespread in food. The average American diet contains far more cobalt than is required for the formation of vitamin B_{12}. No deficiency has ever been reported.
2. Grains, seeds, green leafy vegetables.

O. MOLYBDENUM

Recommended daily allowance: .15 to 0.5 mg.

Uses:
1. Component of essential enzymes.

Sources:
1. Legumes, cereal, yeast.
2. No deficiency in the diet has been recognized.

P. CHROMIUM

Recommended daily allowance: .05 to 0.2 mg.

Uses:
1. Essential for the maximum utilization of glucose.
2. Synthesis of cholesterol and fatty acids.
3. An essential part of other enzyme systems.
4. May help to prevent atherosclerosis.

Sources:
1. Whole grains. Much of the chromium is lost during the refining of grain.
2. Brewer's yeast.

Q. FLUORINE

In the early 1930s it was noted that many children living in Colorado and some of the adjoining states had a very dark, mottled discoloration of their teeth. It was also found that these teeth had far fewer cavities. Further studies showed that this was due to the high content of fluorine in the drinking water. Mottling of the teeth did not occur unless there was more than 2.5 parts per million of fluorine in the water. Since that time, many communities in the United States have added small amounts of fluorine to the drinking water supply in amounts of 1 part per million. This has reduced the incidence of dental cavities from 50 to 60 percent in children. Although no definite harmful effects have been noted, there is still much controversy over whether this mineral should be added to the public water supply.

Recommended daily allowance: 1.5 to 4.0 mg.

Uses:
1. The main function of fluorine appears to be the prevention of cavities and to help build strong teeth.
2. Recent studies have shown that fluorine may help to prevent osteoporosis.

Sources:
1. Fluoridated water.
2. There are not many good food sources of fluorine.

R. SILICON

Recommended daily allowance: Not known. Because of its widespread distribution, a deficiency is rare.

Uses:
1. Promotes the formation of connective tissue.
2. Hardens teeth and bone.
3. Stimulates growth of the body.

Sources:
1. Whole grain cereal.
2. Green vegetables, tomatoes, figs.

S.   VANADIUM, NICKEL, TIN

These minerals have been found to be essential for the normal growth and development of animals. Their exact function in humans has not been determined at the present time but a deficiency is not likely, since they are widely available in foods.

6

VITAMINS

A. GENERAL INFORMATION

Hundreds of years ago it was found that some foods could prevent or even cure certain diseases, such as scurvy, beri-beri, rickets, and pellagra. Even in ancient Greece, Hippocrates gave liver as a treatment for night blindness without realizing that he was using a good source of vitamin A. It was not until the twentieth century, however, that the substances in food that were capable of producing these cures were discovered, isolated, and produced in the laboratory. Dr. Casimir Funk, in 1912, gave these compounds the name of "Vitamine," or vital amine. He wrote the first book on *Vitamines* in 1914. Later on, in 1920, after it was discovered that not all of these compounds were amines, the "e" was dropped from the end of the word. The name vitamin, now a household word, has been used ever since.

The last vitamin to be discovered was vitamin B_{12} in 1948. Perhaps others will be discovered some day.

In general terms, all vitamins are body regulators. They are complex organic substances that are essential for growth, reproduction, maintenance of health, and regulation of nearly all metabolic processes in the body by their association with enzymes and coenzymes.

The total weight of all the vitamins in the body is only about one-fourth of an ounce. An average person eats two to three pounds of food a day and in this amount of food the vitamins weigh only about 1/150th of an ounce. Vitamins cannot be produced in the body so they must be supplied as they are used up or eliminated. When several vitamins are needed for the proper operation of a certain function in the body, this function is impaired if even one of the necessary vitamins is lacking.

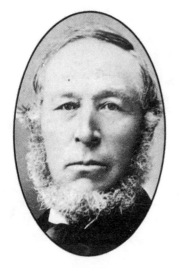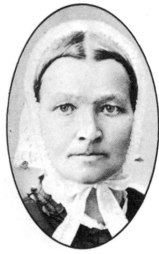

Wilhelm and Sofia Kloss, parents of Jethro Kloss

KLOSS FAMILY RECORD

*Names and birth dates of the children of
Wilhelm and Sofia Kloss*

1. Elnathan – January 7, 1848
2. Lydia – July 5, 1850
3. William – March 9, 1852
4. Theophilus – August 8, 1853
5. Jason – June 6, 1855
6. Ida – April 28, 1857
7. Sarah – February 2, 1859
8. Thirsa – February 2, 1861
9. **Jethro – April 27, 1863**
10. Achsa – March 6, 1865
11. Athniel – November 25, 1868

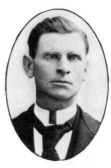

Jethro Kloss in 1900, as a young minister, healer and teacher.

Jethro Kloss married Carrie Stilson, his first wife, in 1901. Tragically, she died in 1905.

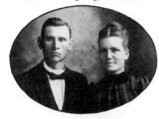

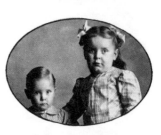

Promise, born to Carrie and Jethro in 1903 is shown here with her father.

Children of Jethro and Amy. Lucile Kloss, (1908-1929). Eden Pettis Kloss, born in 1910.

Amy Pettis Kloss, Jethro's second wife. They were married in 1907.

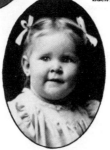

Naomi Joan Kloss at 17 months of age, Jethro's youngest child, born in 1913.

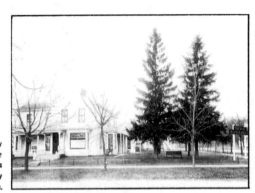

In 1907 Jethro and Amy opened this comprehensive health and medical center in St. Peter, Minnesota which they named The Home Sanitarium.

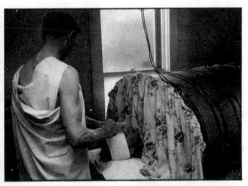

Jethro Kloss giving a hydrotherapy treatment at The Home Sanitarium. The Home Sanitarium was open from 1907 to 1912.

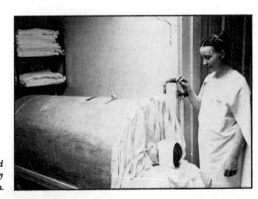

Amy operated the women's hydrotherapy treatment room.

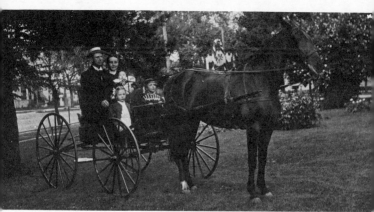

Jethro and Amy Kloss in St. Peter, Minnesota with her daughter Mabel (left) and his daughter Promise (right). Amy is holding Lucile, their first child.

In 1915, from their food factory in Nashville, Tennessee, the Klosses shipped foods throughout the United States and Canada.

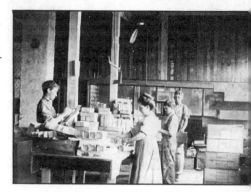

Patients, family, and friends enjoyed health foods canned by the Klosses in this outdoor "factory," which was a commercial enterprise as well.

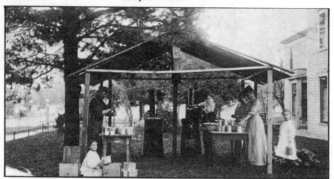

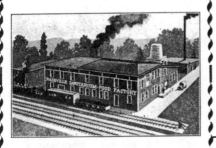

Jethro Kloss Health Food Company

BROOKE, VA. U. S. A.

Hand and Power Grinder for Flour and Nuts

Hand Grinder for Flour and Nuts

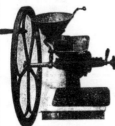

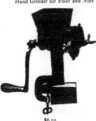

$6.50

$28.00 and up.

We manufacture a large line of Health Foods. Sell High Pressure Canners, Cookers, Sealers, Grinders, etc., for Health Food Making in the home. A few of these are shown in this circular. We are now completing a book on cooking, baking, health food making and home and emergency treatment.

Food canned in a high pressure canner will keep in any climate without preservatives.

Send for price list. Do not fail to get one of these most valuable books, will soon be off the press.

Jethro Kloss Health Food Company

Brooke, Va.

Gasoline Pressure Canner

Pressure Canner

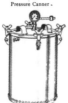

$60.00 and up.

$20.00 and up.

PRICE LIST
OF
NONPOISONOUS
HERBS and HERBAL
PRODUCTS

JETHRO KLOSS
Washington, D. C.

A 1920 advertisement for items sold by Jethro Kloss at his Brooke, Virginia Health Food Company.

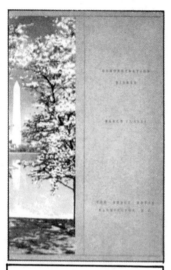

MENU

Herb Broth

Celery Hearts   Radishes

* * * * * * * *

French Toast   Malt Honey

* * * * * * * *

Sweetbreads a la Kloss

Sprouted Soy Beans   Potato Puff

Fresh Asparagus Milanaise

Corn Pone

* * * * * * * *

Raw Vegetable Salad

* * * * * * * *

Pumpkin Pie   Strawberry Sundae

* * * * * * * *

Sanka

A demonstration vegetarian dinner given by Jethro Kloss at the Dodge Hotel in Washington D.C. on March 27, 1933.

A 1940s BACK TO EDEN advertisement and order form.

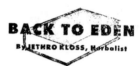

BACK TO EDEN
By JETHRO KLOSS, Herbalist

THE WAY TO INDEPENDENCE
from medical drugging, cutting and burning.

SIMPLE NATURAL REMEDIES
from garden, field and forest often work like miracles. yet leave no evil after-effects.

HERBS IN HISTORY
Primitive peoples have known and used them successfully from pre-historic times.

The Bible and secular history contain many favorable references to them.

The American Indians and our early pioneers had an effective knowledge of them.

THE BEST OF ALL THIS
has been brought together and made readily accessible to you in this marvelous book — BACK TO EDEN.

NEARLY 700 PAGES
of priceless information relating to the health of your family, written in homely style by the man whose exploits with the simple home remedies amazed and confounded his more orthodox contemporaries.

IT CONTAINS:
The secrets your great-grandparents employed in their survival, back in the days when the "going was really tough," and the nearest doctor was days or weeks distant.

- OVER PLEASE -

ORDER TODAY FROM

MESSAGE PRESS
PRINTERS AND PUBLISHERS
COALMONT. TENNESSEE

Add state tax if any.

$ ....   enclosed herewith for which

send to me prepaid .... COPY COPIES

of your book BACK TO EDEN, by Jethro Kloss, Herbalist, at $6.50 per copy.

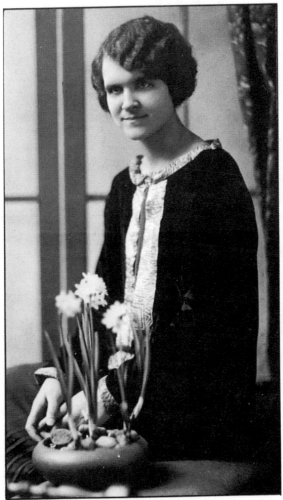

Promise Kloss

A 1926 photo of Promise Kloss (Moffett) at age 23.

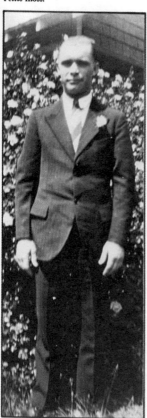

A 1935 snapshot of Jethro's only son, Eden Pettis Kloss.

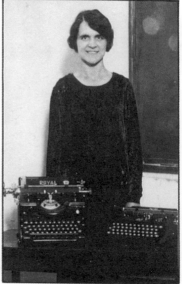

Jethro's daughter, Promise, with typewriters won in typing contests during the 1930s.

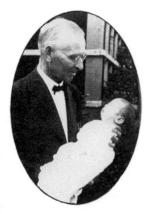

*Proud grandfather, Jethro, with his only
grandchild Doris Joyce, in 1929.*

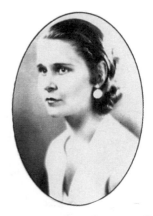

*Jethro's youngest child, Naomi Kloss Engelhard,
mother of Doris Joyce.*

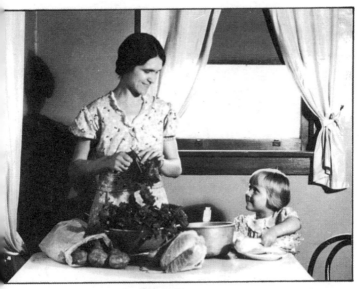

*Promise Kloss Moffett, Jethro's first child, shares food preparation tips with Doris Joyce,
his granddaughter, in 1934.*

Milk From Soy Beans Is New Economy Food

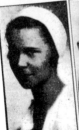 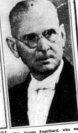

Wash. Post May 21, 1933.

nventor Claims Product More Nutritious Than Dairy Article.

Mrs. Naomi Engelhard, who was raised entirely on nut milk manufactured by her father, Jethro Kloss. She is feeding her daughter, Joyce Joan, on soy bean milk made by Mr. Kloss' process.

The Washington price of milk, which has been the target of a campaign by The Washington Post, provides no budget problem for the family of one Washington man, who has perfected a process of extracting a milk of equal value from soy beans.

Jethro Kloss, the inventor, points out that soy bean milk has certain advantages over the bovine product and that it is excellent for children. His own daughter, Mrs. Harry C. Engelhard, was raised on nut milk before he perfected the soy bean milk. Her daughter, Joyce Joan Engelhard, has been raised exclusively on the soy bean milk.

The bean milk has been used for many years in the Orient, but the strong flavor of its origin clung to it.

By Mr. Kloss' method of manufacture this taste is removed. The milk is pressed from the dried raw beans after they have been soaked in water overnight and then ground. The method is practicable for use in the home, and the cost of the product is only about 2 cents for three quarts.

Mr. Kloss, who lives at 100 Varnum street northwest, says that the soy bean milk may be handled exactly like

cow's milk. It will sour in the same time at the same temperature. Buttermilk and cheese may be made from it, although Mr. Kloss says he has never tried to make it into butter. He also claims that it tastes better when combined with other foods than cow's milk does.

The bean milk has a little more carbohydrates than cow's milk and little less fat. Its protein content is also a little lower, but .t has more vitamines than the nat.ral product. Because of its hith alkalinity, it is better for ba.ies, he says.

Soy beans have been fed to animals in this country for many years, but attempts to use them for human food have failed because of their taste. Mr. Kloss has demonstrated his method that there is nothing to prevent making the milk at home.

In feeding the milk to babies, it must be diluted with one-fourth water. The feeding can begin on the first day, Mr. Kloss says. In some instances it may be necessary to dilute it with more water than this. At the age of 6 months it can be given full strength, with the addition of a few spoonfuls of whole wheat flakes.

CIENTIST EXTRACTS MILK FROM SOY BEAN

ethro Kloss of Washington, D. C., Says Product Tests 3.15 Per Butter Fat and Can Be Obtained Much More Cheaply Than n Cow; Soy Bean Products To Be Exhibited.

rom contented soy beans. This ads like a joke, or prophetic ct, according to Dr. Jethro Washington, D. C., who has years to the study of the nd from it has derived so lds that an enumeration nds like a dairy menu.

"Milk so pure that it can hardly be detected by the taste alone can be taken from the soy bean," Dr. Kloss said. "From this milk more than 30 products already have been made, and have stood the test of careful analysis.

"Soy milk tests 3.15 per cent butter fat against 4.50 butter fat for the best of cows milk. It will sour just as the cows milk, and after this it may be made into cheese, butter-milk or anything else for which cows milk is used. And it may be produced for about 2 cents per quart."

Dr. Kloss said that he first became interested in the soy bean when he noted its fattening effect on cattle. He began an intensive study of the bean, and after many years of research perfected processes by which the milk could be extracted. From this the b,° products developed.

"The milk can hardly be detecte y taste alone. Most people expect to be slightly bitter, but it isn't," r. Kloss said. "My own 4-year-old randdaughter has never tasted cow's milk, and she has been pronounced an most perfect specimen of childhood."

Dr. Kloss will exhibit the products of the soy bean in Bayfront park to-morrow evening after the band con-

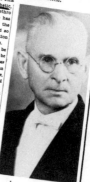

DR. JETHRO KLOSS

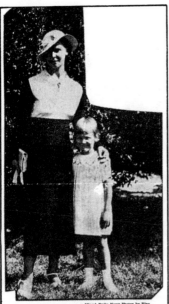

—Miami Daily News Photos by Rine

insert, Dr. Jethro Kloss, who is devoting his life to the dissemina-
tion of knowledge pertaining to soy bean milk, together with his
daughter, Mrs. Harry C. Engelhard, and her daughter, Joyce. Both
were reared on this milk.

Miami Daily News apr 8 1934

Food Products of Soy Bean
Urged for Daily Table Use

Milk, Cheese, Roasts, Bread and Other
Preparations Made From Herb Claimed
to Have High Nutrition Values

If the United States were at war and due to some disease
introduced by the enemy lost every cow or even goat, the
entire county still could have fresh milk, butter, cheese and
similar products derived from soy beans according to Dr.
Jethro Kloss of Washington, now in Miami.

*Newspaper articles during the 1930s
reporting Kloss's work with soybeans.*

chukos ʼ............ ʼ........ ʼ. pper live on soy
beꞏt milk delivered at the door by
"milkmen" as cows' milk is delivered
here is not known to many. Dr. Kloss'
married daughter and her five-year-
old daughter were reared on this milk,
which looks and tastes much like
cow's milk.

Dr. Kloss prides himself on having
once been a "farmer." He is credited
with having spent a fortune in phil-
anthropic work, the greater part having gone toward introducing a bean
which he feels is destined to eventually
revolutionize the economic structure
of this country and become of incal-
culable value in time of war.

Approximately 6,000 persons recently heard Dr. Kloss in Bayfront
park explain how he apparently performs miracles when he transmutes
beans into 24 or more different foods
which in addition to being delectable
also retain various life-giving elements usually attributed to cow's milk.

Dr. Kloss contends soy bean milk
is superior to milk from a cow or goat
due to an entire lack of bacterial contamination, besides being extremely
cheap. Children fed on this milk are
perfectly developed in every way, he

said. Comparative analysis of various milks as made by the bureau of
chemistry in Washington is as follows:

Milk	Water	Ash	Pro-tein	Fat	Carbo-hydrate
Human	89.95	0.25	1.30	2.50	6.00
Cow's	87.30	0.80	3.20	3.50	5.20
Goats'	87.00	0.50	4.00	4.50	4.00
Soy bean	87.00	0.52	3.40	3.15	6.00
Nut Milk	87.00	2.03	2.60	3.50	7.20

Dr. Kloss during his demonstration
makes a soy bean "roast" which many
compared favorably with beef steak.
For this he claims a higher food value
than meat. The protein being of
vegetable origin is not acid forming,
he said.

He exhibited 21 articles made from
soy beans and invited the public to
taste them. These were soy bean
milk, bread, pie, cakes, buns, cookies,
roast, buttermilk, coffee, cottage
cheese, cream cheese, yellow cheese,
soy bean sauce, pancakes, broth, butter, "mashed potatoes," mayonnaise,
soy bean roast not like that from
meat, ice cream, sprouted beans. None
of these contained white flour nor
cane sugar, making such foods especially valuable for diabetics. Soy
bean foods are also recommended for
arthritis.

He advocates the teaching of edible
food preparation from soy beans as
part of school curriculum and drew a
parallel tending to show how the government spends millions to spread hog
and other stock-feeding knowledge
while almost ignoring the phases
which would create well-fed humans.

Dr. Kloss pointed out that he was
merely in this country revealing something which for centuries has been
common knowledge throughout the
Orient. He cited China as the soy
bean milk products nation having endured not one but hundreds of economic depressions, floods, earthquakes,
famines and wars without number. He
quoted Dr. S. Hovarth of Rockefeller
institute as one of the world's leading authorities on soy beans, who
said: "The Chinese nation exists today because of the use of the soy bean
as a food."

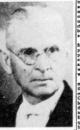

By the request of thousands who heard
Dr. Kloss speak in Bayfront Park, he
has consented to give further instructions in the preparation of the wonderful Soy Bean Products.

He will give two food demonstrations
in the Miami School of Applied Arts,
400 N. E. 2nd Ave. Monday afternoon
at 3:30 and Monday evening at 8, April
9th.

Dr. Kloss makes more delicious table
foods from the soy bean than any one
else knows. The soy bean is a complete food, and is highly alkaline.
Following is a partial list of the foods
he makes:

Soy bean milk, soy bean buttermilk,
cottage cheese, ice cream, bread, buns,
pies, cake, cookies, roast, coffee, pancakes, butter, macromaise, broth.
These foods do not contain any cane
sugar or other harmful ingredients.
They are most economical, simple to
prepare, and very healthful and invigorating. The use of the articles would

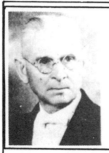

Back to EDEN

By JETHRO KLOSS

JUST OFF THE PRESS

The following is a partial description of my new book, "Back to Eden." The entire book is simplicity itself and is written from my actual experiences.

"Back to Eden" is the result of almost a half century of study, experience, investigation and experimentation by one who is a living demonstration of the virtue of obedience to nature's laws. It is written in language easily understood by anyone who may read its pages. Its suggestions and counsel on procedure in treating the sick, in the preparation of foods, and many other features that are presented are available and practical for every home, whether it be in the mansions of the rich, or in the homes where poverty reigns.

It is veritable encyclopedia on Nature's Path to Health and Healing.

HOW to restore health when you are sick.

HOW to enhance health when you are well.

HOW to co-operate intelligently with nature and nature's laws in building up bodily resistance to disease: — *Nature's Preventive Medicine.*

HOW to use the endless array of nature's methods and remedies in the treatment of disease: — *Nature's Curative Medicine.*

"Back to Eden" should be in every home in America, because it presents to all who are sick Nature's three-point program in the healing art —

1. *Dietotherapy* — The use of foods as provided in the great laboratory of nature in sickness and in health.

2. *Hydrotherapy* — The use of water in the treatment of disease.

3. *Herbotherapy* → The use of herbs in various forms, in contrast with poisonous drugs in the treatment of disease.

DO YOU KNOW THAT —

Heart failure leads all other human maladies as the contributing cause in the United States every year.

Cancer of various types follows us that one out of every seven women cancer.

800,000 people spend some time i

Excerpts from Jethro Kloss's four-page brochure describing his new "just off the press" book, BACK TO EDEN, in the year 1939.

There is a remedy for every disease in the natural products of the earth

JETHRO KLOSS

920 ALLSTON STREET
HUSTON, TEXAS

WASHINGTON, D. C. ADDRESS
TAKOMA PARK, STATION, D. C.

CONSTITUTION HALL

WASHINGTON D. C. EIGHTEENTH and D. STS. N. W.

Wednesday Evening - January 3rd. 8:00 P. M. *1940*

FREE TO THE PUBLIC!

**Elaborate Musical Program, Furnished by
ALFRED MANNING, Harpist and Organist
and a special, all - Soloist Choir JUSTIN LAWRIE, Director**

JETHRO KLOSS

Author of a new book "BACK to EDEN"

Will lecture and demonstrate his formulas, recipes, and remedies for the treatment of the four greatest scourges of mankind--Cancer. Heart Disease, Tuberculosis, and Infantile Paralysis.

**Entirely Free to the Public, Given as an
Educational Feature**

DOORS OPEN AT 7:00 P. M. PROGRAM BEGINS AT 8:00 P.M.

COME EARLY TO SECURE A GOOD SEAT

1940 handbill announcing health lecture by Jethro Kloss in Constitution Hall, Washington, D.C.

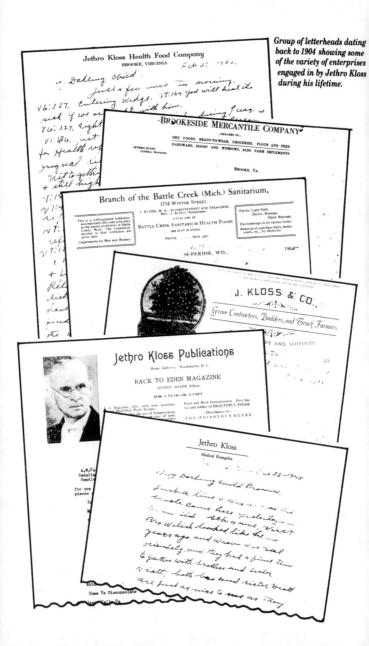

Group of letterheads dating back to 1904 showing some of the variety of enterprises engaged in by Jethro Kloss during his lifetime.

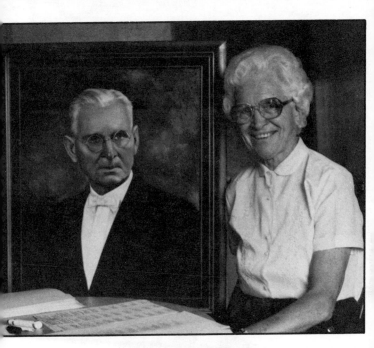

Promise Kloss Moffett, with photograph of her father, Jethro Kloss, taken on her 80th birthday, August 16, 1983.

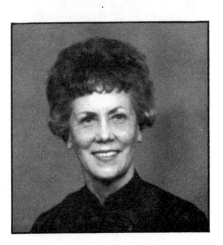

Doris Joyce Engelhard Gardiner, only grandchild of Jethro Kloss.

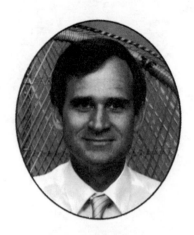

Stephen Kloss Gardiner

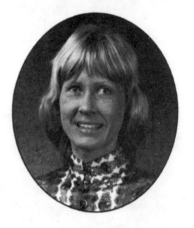

Nancy Kloss (Bramlett)

Great-grandchildren of Jethro Kloss dedicated to continuing his life work and philosophy.

Vitamins are made by plants. Humans get their vitamins either by eating the plants or by eating meat after the animals have eaten the plants and incorporated the vitamins into their own bodies. Vitamin supplements can be purchased nearly anywhere. The total amount of money spent on vitamins yearly in the United States is about 1.2 billion dollars, and this is increasing at the rate of about 10 percent a year. The F.D.A. estimates that 40 percent of the U.S. population aged 16 or over takes vitamin and mineral supplements.

There are some groups of people in the United States that most likely should be taking vitamin and mineral supplements. These include the following.

1. Those who are not eating an abundant and well-balanced diet; such as the elderly, specially those living alone, or teenagers and others eating out a lot and not taking care to get a good variety of foods.
2. Women who are pregnant or breast-feeding their babies.
3. Those who are recovering from a severe illness or surgery.
4. Alcoholics.
5. People who eat a lot of refined or processed foods.
6. Those in low income groups where a wide variety of food from the different food groups cannot be obtained.
7. Those who are suffering from severe debilitating diseases of various kinds.

Several recent surveys of thousands of American families showed that there were some deficiencies in the average diet. The vitamins that were found to be low were vitamins A, B_6 (pyridoxine), and C, while the minerals that tended to be deficient were iron, calcium, and magnesium.

Vitamins can be separated into two groups depending on whether they are soluble in fat or in water. While some characteristics are common to the members of each group, they are not related chemically nor do they have similar effects on the bodily functions.

Fat-soluble Vitamins A, D, E, and K:
1. Soluble in fat but not in water.
2. Stored in the body. Because there is no good mechanism for their excretion, taking large doses over a prolonged period of time may result in toxic symptoms and can even prove fatal. This is true of vitamins A, D, and K, but not of vitamin E.
3. They are stored mainly in the liver, where the supply is sufficient to last for several months.
4. They are absorbed from the intestines in the same way as fat.
5. They are not easily lost by cooking or storage, but are destroyed by rancidness.
6. Symptoms due to a deficiency of these vitamins appear slowly.
7. Mineral oil in the intestines hinders their absorption.

Water-soluble Vitamins B-Complex and C:
1. Soluble in water but not in fat.
2. Not stored in the body so a fresh supply is needed daily.
3. Easily destroyed by heat, normal cooking, and storage.
4. Any excess beyond the amount that is needed by the body is excreted in the urine.
5. Deficiency symptoms develop rapidly.

B. FAT-SOLUBLE VITAMINS

VITAMIN A: (Retinol)
Vitamin A deficiency is common throughout the world in underdeveloped, overpopulated countries. It is estimated that worldwide, 80,000 children a year become blind as a result of vitamin A deficiency and about one-half of these children die.

Vitamin A is present in our food in two forms. In food of animal origin it is found as the active vitamin (retinol), while in plant foods it is found as provitamin A carotenes, a precursor of vitamin A. Carotene is an orange-yellow pigment that is present in green vegetables, but is masked by the green color of the chlorophyl in the leaves. A precursor, or provitamin, is a substance that is changed in the body to a vitamin. Only a portion of the carotene that we eat is changed to vitamin A. This takes place in the wall of the small intestine. The amount that is changed varies between 30 and 70 percent, depending on the type of food and the form in which it is eaten. Carotene itself is not active in the body.

In most of the food we eat about half of the vitamin A is in the form of retinol and the other half is provitamin A. The liver stores about 90 to 95 percent of our vitamin A, enough to last months or perhaps even years under normal circumstances.

Functions:

1. Gives the ability to see in dim light.
2. Maintains normal skin.
3. Needed for growth and development of strong bones and teeth.
4. Needed for the secretion of mucus by the cells lining the respiratory, urinary, and intestinal tracts that helps keep them moist and healthy.
5. Aids the normal reproductive processes.
6. Needed for carbohydrate metabolism in the liver.
7. Essential for proper smell, hearing, and taste.
8. Aids in the prevention of certain types of cancer.
9. Beta carotene is a non-toxic antioxidant and helps prevent disease by neutralizing free radicals.

Deficiency:

1. Poor vision in dim light (night blindness).
2. Dry, scaly, itching skin.

3. Increased susceptibility to infections, specially in the respiratory tract.
4. Changes in the eyes that may lead to blindness. The eyes become dry, swollen, and infected. This condition is called xerophthalmia.
5. Slow wound healing.
6. Poor bone growth in children.
7. Defective enamel on teeth and an increased number of cavities.
8. Loss of taste and smell.
9. Stunting of body growth.

Toxicity:

Because vitamin A cannot be excreted from the body in any significant amount, toxicity results from prolonged daily doses in excess of 50,000 IU in adults and less in children. The symptoms of an overdose are nausea, diarrhea, headache, dizziness, loss of hair, bone pain, dry itching skin, drowsiness, and cessation of menstruation. These symptoms will clear up in a few days if the excess intake is stopped. Toxicity only occurs with retinol and not with carotene. An excess intake of carotene will cause the skin to turn yellow. This can be seen in those who drink large amounts of fresh carrot juice.

Sources:

1. Deep yellow vegetables such as carrots, pumpkin, sweet potatoes, winter squash, yellow corn, tomatoes.
2. Dark green vegatables such as broccoli, chard, spinach, beet greens, collards.
3. Yellow fruits such as apricots, cantaloupe, peaches, persimmons, oranges, mangoes.
4. Watermelon

Dosage:
5000 IU (1000 RE): Males 11 years and over.
4000 IU (800 RE): Females 11 years and over.
5000 IU (1000 RE): During pregnancy.
6000 IU (1200 RE): During lactation.

Since 1974 the designation RE (retinol equivalent) has been the preferred method for indicating the dose of vitamin A. Most food value charts at the present time give both the IU (International Units) and the retinol equivalent.

Stability:
Very little vitamin A is lost during cooking or processing. It is stable to heat and alkali, but not when it is exposed to acids, light, or oxygen.

VITAMIN D: (Calciferol)
Vitamin D, the "sunshine vitamin," is produced by the ultraviolet rays of the sun reacting with a cholesterol-like chemical that is naturally present in the skin. But the older one gets, the less vitamin D can be made in this way. The skin of a person in his or her eighties can only make about one-half the vitamin D of a 20 year old. Over a period of several days this chemical is changed to vitamin D by the liver and kidneys. Recent studies suggest that exposing only your arms, hands and face to the noonday sun for 10 to 15 minutes twice a week will allow enough vitamin D production to meet the average requirements. Fog, smog, clouds, clothing, and skin pigment are effective in filtering out part of the ultraviolet rays and thus reducing the amount of vitamin D that is produced. Window glass and sun-blocking agents with a protective factor over 8 totally stop vitamin D production. For the most part, vitamin D is stored in the liver, but it is found also in the bones, skin, brain, and fat. There is no good way for the body to eliminate an excess amount of this vitamin.

Functions:
1. Regulates the absorption and metabolism of calcium and phosphorus to produce strong bones and teeth.
2. Necessary for the proper absorption of calcium and phosphorus from the intestine.
3. Maintains normal blood levels of calcium and phosphorus.

Deficiency:
1. Rickets in children. The bones become soft and bend easily, causing bowed legs and knock-knees. The teeth make their appearance late and they decay easily. The chest is usually deformed and the growth stunted.
2. Osteomalacia in adults. The bones lose their strength and tend to become painful and may even break.

Toxicity:
Because the body does not excrete excess vitamin D, toxicity is not uncommon. Symptoms consist of failure to grow normally, kidney stones, high blood pressure, weight loss, loss of appetite, irritability, vomiting, excessive thirst, diarrhea, and weakness.

Toxic symptoms may be caused by amounts of 2000 IU in children or 75,000 IU in adults, taken daily over a long period of time. The amount necessary to produce these symptoms of toxicity varies considerably from person to person.

Sources:
1. Vitamin D is the least available vitamin in food. Fruits, vegetables and grains are poor sources of this vitamin. The best sources are egg yolk, milk, butter, and cheese.
2. Formed in the skin when exposed to sunlight.

Dosage:
400 IU to age 18 (10 micrograms of cholecalciferol).
200 IU in adults (5 micrograms of cholecalciferol).
200 IU added to the usual dose during pregnancy and lactation.

Stability:
Vitamin D is stable to heat, storage, oxidation, acids, and alkali but is sensitive to light.

VITAMIN E: (Tocopherols)
Vitamin E was first recognized as essential in the diet in 1922, when it was found to be necessary for normal reproduction to take place in certain laboratory animals. Because of this initial connection with the reproductive process, it soon became known as the "antisterility factor." In fact, the word "tocopherol" comes from the Greek and means "to bring forth offspring." Eight natural forms of vitamin E are found in our foods and alpha-tocopherol is the most active form.

Approximately 40 to 60 percent of the vitamin E in our diet is absorbed and stored in the fat, muscle, and liver.

Functions:
1. A strong antioxidant. Vitamin E neutralizes free radicals, preventing them from producing disease by injuring the normal cells in our body.
2. Protects vitamins A and C and unsaturated fatty acids from undergoing oxidation.
3. Protects the red blood cells from destruction.
4. Regulates the release of energy from glucose and fatty acids.
5. Takes part in the normal reproductive process by helping to prevent recurrent spontaneous abortions.
6. Slows down the aging process.

7. May be useful in treating persons exposed to air pollution, particularly if there is a high ozone content.
8. Useful to those who develop pain and cramps in the legs while walking.
9. Has been felt to be helpful in cases of sterility, impotence, decreased sexual drive, heart disease, certain psychiatric disorders, and to increase the performance of athletes.
10. May help to prevent the formation of nitrosamines, some of which cause cancer.

Deficiency:

1. A deficiency has sometimes been found in premature babies, causing a special type of anemia, and in persons who have deficient fat absorption over a long period of time.
2. In general, deficiency is not a problem as vitamin E is so widely distributed in food. However, to help prevent damage from free radicals 150 to 400 I.U. should be taken as a daily supplement.

Toxicity:

None has been identified. Large doses have been reported to interfere with the action of vitamin K, thus causing an increased tendency toward bleeding.

Sources:

1. Wheat germ and wheat germ oil are the richest sources.
2. Soybeans.
3. Whole grain cereal, legumes, corn, nuts, seeds. Up to 90 percent of the vitamin E in cereals is lost during the refining process.
4. Green leafy vegetables, peppers, carrots.

Dosage:
15 IU in males (10 mg alpha-tocopherol equivalents).
12 IU in females (8 mg alpha-tocopherol equivalents).

Stability:
Vitamin E is not affected by normal cooking, acid, alkali, or heat. Deterioration of vitamin E occurs with exposure to light or oxygen, and it is also caused by rancidity. Deep fat frying destroys vitamin E because of the long periods of high temperature, which results in the fat turning rancid. The freezing of vegetables may cause considerable loss of vitamin E. This is not true of any of the other vitamins, which show no appreciable loss during the freezing process.

VITAMIN K: (Menadione)
Vitamin K is the last of the four fat-soluble vitamins. It has also been called the "anti-hemorrhagic" vitamin. Like the other fat-soluble vitamins, it is not a single entity but a group of chemically related substances that, in the case of vitamin K, are called quinones. These include both the naturally occurring vitamin K that is in plant and animal foods, and also the synthetic vitamin K (menadione).

Functions:
1. Necessary for the proper clotting of blood.

Deficiency:
1. There is normally a deficiency of vitamin K in newborn babies, since vitamin K cannot reach the baby in any significant amount while it is still in the uterus. Furthermore, for the first few days after birth vitamin K cannot be produced in the intestine of the newborn baby, because no bacteria are present. This results in a condition called hemorrhagic disease of the newborn. Therefore, to prevent this

from occurring, all newborn infants are routinely given vitamin K.

2. In adults a deficiency of vitamin K is always due to a lack of absorption. This may be due to various diseases, including any condition that causes chronic diarrhea or bile duct obstruction. Certain drugs may also result in a vitamin K deficiency, such as antibiotics, sulfonamides, salicylates, and dicoumarol.

Toxicity:

Toxicity only results from an excess of the synthetic forms of vitamin K, and may result in jaundice and anemia in infants.

Sources:

1. Dark green leafy vegetables.
2. Cauliflower, alfalfa, peas, and cabbage — specially the outer leaves.
3. Cereal.
4. Soybean oil and other vegetable oils.
5. Synthesis by bacteria in the intestines.
6. Both cow's milk and mother's milk are low in vitamin K. Mother's milk contains only about one-fourth as much as cow's milk.

Dosage:

10 to 20 micrograms: newborn to one year.

15 to 100 micrograms: increasing dose from one to eleven years.

70 to 140 micrograms: adults.

Stability:

Vitamin K is destroyed by light, some oxidizing agents, acids, and alkali. It is stable to heat, air, and ordinary cooking.

C. WATER-SOLUBLE VITAMINS

VITAMIN B COMPLEX

Several different vitamins compose what is commonly known as vitamin B complex. These vitamins are different from all the others vitamins, in that they all contain nitrogen in addition to carbon, hydrogen, and oxygen. Two of the B complex vitamins, thiamine and biotin, also contain sulfur, and vitamin B_{12} contains cobalt and phosphorus.

The B complex vitamins are very closely associated in their functions in the body and they all tend to be found in the same food groups. If there is a deficiency in one of these vitamins, the others in the group will not function properly. They are all concerned with the proper functioning of some of the coenzyme systems in the body. Perhaps the most important of the group are thiamine, riboflavin, and niacin. When these three are present in adequate amounts in the diet, there is not likely to be a serious deficiency of vitamin B. During the milling process, cereals loose nearly all of their vitamin B as well as other important nutrients. Enriched cereal has thiamine, riboflavin, niacin, and iron added.

VITAMIN B1: (Thiamine)

The first description we have of a disease resembling vitamin B deficiency is found in ancient Chinese writings dating as far back as 2600 B.C. A lack of this vitamin results in a disease called beriberi, which means "I can't, I can't." It was apparently called this because those who had a severe thiamine deficiency that affected their nervous system eventually were unable to move.

Little is then recorded of beriberi until about the middle of the nineteenth century, when refined grains and cereals came into common use. This is specially true in some countries where rice was the main food. During the 1800s many Japanese sailors developed beriberi and many of them died. When fish, meat, and vegetables were added to their diet, the disease immediately disappeared. In Java a Dutch prison physician noted that chickens fed with polished rice left over from the prisoners' meals developed a disease with symptoms that were very similar to those in beriberi. He found that this disease was cured by feeding the chickens whole rice instead of the polished rice that the prisoners were eating. Later it was thought that beriberi was caused by some unknown factor that was present in the outer coat of grains and beans, but was lacking after the grain was milled. This finally led to the discovery of thiamine as well as other members of the vitamin B complex family.

Even with the knowledge that we now have available, beriberi is still a problem in some countries such as the Philippines, where a large percentage of the rice that is eaten is highly polished and not enriched. Additional vitamin B_1 is also lost during the washing and cooking of the rice.

Raw fish is frequently eaten in some countries, and it is interesting to note that there is an enzyme present in certain raw fish that divides the vitamin B_1 molecule, making it unavailable for use by the body. This, however, usually does not result in a vitamin B_1 deficiency, since this enzyme is destroyed by cooking the fish.

The body stores enough vitamin B_1 to last for about one or two weeks, and any excess is excreted in the urine.

Functions:
1. Necessary for energy production.
2. Stimulation of the appetite.
3. Essential as part of the coenzyme system for carbohydrate metabolism.
4. For proper functioning of the nervous and cardiovascular systems.
5. Prevention of beriberi.

Deficiency:
A lack of this vitamin results in beriberi. In infants of two to five months of age, this may be a rapidly fatal disease

unless treated immediately with thiamine. This occurs more often in breast-fed babies.

Beriberi was first noted when polished rice was eaten in place of brown rice. Now we know that since thiamine is located mostly in the outside layer of the rice (the bran layer), it was being removed during the milling process.

The nervous system is severely affected in cases of beriberi because it depends upon glucose for its normal function, and thiamine is intimately involved in glucose metabolism. Symptoms that may occur are fatigue, depression, irritability, moodiness, inability to concentrate, confusion, headaches, leg cramps, numbness and tingling in the feet, problems with walking and finally paralysis of the legs.

The gastrointestinal system may also be involved with loss of appetite, constipation, nausea, and weight loss.

Heart failure may occur with accumulation of fluid in the tissues. This is known as "wet beriberi."

In the United States, beriberi is seen mainly in chronic alcoholics.

Toxicity:
None known.

Sources:
1. Wheat germ, whole grain bread and cereal.
2. Dried peas and beans, peanuts and peanut butter, legumes.
3. Nuts.
4. Green leafy vegetables.
5. Protein-rich foods are generally good sources of vitamin B_1.

Dosage:
0.5 mg per 1000 calories in the diet. The total amount of thiamine should not be allowed to fall below 1.0 mg per day in adults.

Stability:

Since this is a water-soluble vitamin, cooking must be done with care. Use as little water as possible at as low a temperature as possible and for as short a time as possible. Reuse the water, since much of the thiamine is leached out into the water. Alkali, such as in baking soda and some antacids, destroys thiamine. The destruction of thiamine begins at temperatures over 100°C. The smaller the pieces of food that are being cooked the greater will be the loss of this vitamin. Although vitamin B_1 is stable in the dry state, in the wet state it is the most unstable of all the vitamins except for vitamin C.

RIBOFLAVIN: (Vitamin B_2, Vitamin G)

Recent studies have shown that between 6 and 26 percent of persons in America have either a definite or borderline deficiency of this vitamin. This is specially true among those who drink little if any milk. Other groups in which there is an inadequate intake of riboflavin are alcoholics, the aged, women during pregnancy and lactation, and women taking oral contraceptives. An increased intake of this vitamin is needed during periods of growth or physical stress.

One quart of milk a day supplies all the necessary riboflavin. Milk in general supplies about 40 percent of all the riboflavin consumed by Americans. The safest course, if you use milk, is to sterilize it by sufficient boiling. (See Special Notice, end of Section III)

Functions:

1. Production of energy.
2. Tissue growth, maintenance, and repair.
3. Red blood cell production.

Deficiency:

Cracks appear at the corners of the mouth. The lips become inflamed and also split and crack. The tongue becomes smooth and purplish-red in color and the skin gets dry and scaly. The eyes become very sensitive to light, water easily, and become irritated. There is impairment of vision, diminished reproductive capacity, and the general growth pattern of the body is retarded.

Toxicity:
None known.

Sources:
1. Wheat germ.
2. Leafy vegetables, nuts, legumes.
3. Whole grains.

Dosage:
1.2 mg — women.
1.4 mg — men.
A minimum dose of 1.2 mg per day should be taken by everyone.

Stability:
Riboflavin is slightly soluble in water. It is stable to heat, acid, and oxidation, and only a small amount is lost during ordinary cooking. It is destroyed by sunlight, ultraviolet light, and alkaline solutions.

It was discovered that when milk in clear glass bottles was delivered on the doorstep by the milkman and allowed to sit in the sun, 50 to 70 percent of the riboflavin was lost in two hours.

NIACIN: (Nicotinic acid, vitamin B3)
Niacin is the only vitamin that can be manufactured in the body, where it is made from tryptophan, an essential amino acid, in the presence of other nutrients. Sixty mg of tryptophan gives about one mg of niacin.

It was not until 1937 that niacin was found to be the cure for pellagra. This deficiency disease was widespread in the United States in the early part of the twentieth century. It was specially common in some cities in the south, where many of the people lived largely on a diet of corn (maize), molasses, and salt pork. In 1918, 100,000 cases of pellagra were reported in the United States, resulting in 10,000 deaths.

Niacin occurs both as nicotinic acid and nicotinamide. Neither one should be confused with nicotine, which occurs in tobacco.

Functions:
1. For proper functioning of the nervous and digestive systems.
2. Energy metabolism.
3. Maintains a healthy skin.
4. Production of fatty acids, steroids, and cholesterol.

Deficiency:
Pellagra's symptoms are the "four D's" – diarrhea, dermatitis, depression, and dementia or death. Pellagra affects primarily the skin, nervous system, and gastrointestinal tract.

Skin. The name "pellagra" comes from the Italian words meaning "rough skin." A reddish rash appears on the skin of the feet, hands, and face. This rash becomes much worse when these parts of the body are exposed to the sun. Later the skin may become dark, rough, and dry.

Nervous system. Headache, confusion, irritability, dizziness, delusions, severe depression, and sometimes death.

Gastrointestinal tract. Sore mouth and tongue, mild intestinal upset, loss of appetite and weight, diarrhea.

General symptoms of fatigue, weakness, backache, and anemia may also be present.

Toxicity:
None has been reported for nicotinamide.

Nicotinic acid in large doses produces flushing of the skin, stomach upset, dizziness, and nervousness.

Sources:
1. Legumes, peanut butter.
2. Whole grain or enriched bread and cereals.
3. Seeds and nuts.
4. Broccoli, potatoes, tomatoes, collards.
5. Avocados, figs, prunes, bananas.

Dosage:
13 niacin equivalents (NE) per day is the minimum dose.

Stability:
Niacin is stable to heat, acids, alkali, light, and oxidation. It is lost in the water to some degree during cooking.

PYRIDOXINE: (Vitamin B6)
Pyridoxine has been used in large doses in the treatment of many conditions. It has attained some success in the treatment of nausea that occurs commonly during the early months of pregnancy and also in the reduction of dental cavities, if the pyridoxine is sucked in the form of lozenges.

Functions:
1. Active in the metabolism of protein, glucose, and fat.
2. Red blood cell production. Synthesis of hemoglobin.
3. Aids in the manufacture of niacin from tryptophan.
4. Normal functioning of the nervous system.
5. Production of antibodies.
6. Production of regulatory substances.

Deficiency:
It has been discovered that many people in this country have a borderline or low intake of pyridoxine.

While the symptoms of pyridoxine deficiency are not commonly seen, they do occasionally occur and consist of anemia, nausea, sore mouth, smooth red tongue, kidney stones, dermatitis around the eyes and at the corners of the mouth, poor growth, vomiting, abdominal pain, depression, and confusion. In infants there are sometimes convulsions.

Toxicity:

Usually none. Recently several people taking extremely large doses ranging from 500 to 5,000 mg per day have had symptoms of difficulty in walking, tingling sensation in the hands, lips, and tongue, numbness in the feet, and clumsiness in the handling of objects.

Sources:

1. Whole grain cereals, yeast, nuts.
2. Legumes, bananas, potatoes, green vegetables, yellow corn.
3. Wheat germ, seeds, avocados.

Dosage:

2.2 mg per day in males.

2.0 mg per day in females.

This dose should be increased during pregnancy and lactation, in the elderly, in alcoholics, and in women taking oral contraceptives.

Stability:

During the milling process of wheat 75 to 90 percent of the pyridoxine is lost and is not replaced in enriched flour. Up to 50 percent can be lost during the cooking and processing of food.

It is stable to heat and acid, but destroyed by oxidation and light.

FOLACIN: (Folic acid)

Functions:

1. Formation of hemoglobin and red blood cells.

2. Normal growth and reproduction.
3. Protein metabolism.
4. Treatment of sprue and pernicious anemia.
5. Prevents neural tube defects in the fetus.

Deficiency:

A deficiency of folacin is common throughout the world, even in the United States, but is found mostly in the tropics. There is an increased need for folacin during infancy, pregnancy, and in conditions where the food is not properly absorbed. A folacin deficiency leads to a special type of anemia called "pernicious anemia." Symptoms of diarrhea, weakness, and fatigue are noted. The tongue and mouth become sore and the tongue itself appears smooth and reddish in color. The daily needs of an adult male could be supplied for 6 years by only one teaspoon of folic acid.

Toxicity:

None known.

Sources:

1. Green leafy vegetables, broccoli, asparagus, okra, parsnips, cauliflower, brussels sprouts.
2. Nuts, legumes, whole grain cereals, yeast.
3. Oranges, carrots, cantaloupe.

Dosage:

400 micrograms (0.4 mg).
800 micrograms during pregnancy.
500 micrograms during lactation.
During her childbearing years, every woman should take 0.4 mg Folacin daily.

Stability:

Folacin is destroyed by processing, light, and improper cooking and storage of foods.

COBALAMIN: (Vitamin B_{12})

This vitamin was synthesized in 1948, the last of the B complex vitamins. The crystals are a bright red color, so vitamin B_{12} is sometimes referred to as the "red vitamin." Plant foods contain none of this vitamin. In order for vitamin B_{12} to be absorbed from the intestine, it must be united with a special protein in the gastric juice called "intrinsic factor." The average person absorbs about 30 to 70 percent of vitamin B_{12} in the diet. Persons who are deficient in the "intrinsic factor" are not able to absorb this vitamin properly and subsequently develop pernicious anemia. Strict vegetarians (vegans), who eat no animal products of any kind, may also develop a vitamin B_{12} deficiency. Some of this vitamin is made in the human intestinal tract, but this occurs in the colon where no absorption of the vitamin can take place.

Functions:

1. Normal functioning of all the body cells.
2. Proper functioning of the nervous system.
3. Normal growth.
4. Protein, carbohydrate, and fat metabolism.
5. Production of red blood cells.

Deficiency:

1. Pernicious anemia with a sore mouth and tongue, loss of appetite and weight, weakness, difficulty in walking, mental disturbances.

Vitamin B_{12} is found only in animal foods: therefore, those on a total vegetarian diet, who eat no meat or animal products of any kind, should take a supplement or eat some type of vitamin B_{12} fortified food such as fortified soybean milk.

In adults a rather large amount of vitamin B_{12} is stored in the liver. This is sufficient to last for several years with no further intake. Children, however, will show a deficiency of this vitamin after two to three years, since their storage capacity is low. The stores of the vitamin in the liver seem to increase with age.

Toxicity:
None.

Sources:
1. Animal products only.
2. Dietary supplements.

Dosage:
3 micrograms per day over age seven.

The average diet contains about 5 to 15 micrograms per day.

Adults take a B12 (50 micrograms) tablet once a week.

Stability:
Destroyed by alkali. About 30 percent of vitamin B12 is lost in normal cooking.

PANTOTHENIC ACID:
This vitamin, once called vitamin B3, is present in every cell in the body and is a component of all living matter.

Functions:
1. Metabolism of protein, fat, and carbohydrate.
2. Synthesis of hemoglobin, hormones, and cholesterol.
3. Energy metabolism.
4. Production of antibodies.
5. Essential for numerous chemical reactions in the body.

Deficiency:
An actual deficiency of pantothenic acid is difficult to document, but persons who are found with low values seem to have a decreased resistance to infection and an inability to withstand stressful situations.

Experimental deficiencies have been produced that show symptoms of tiredness, headache, insomnia, nausea and vomiting, abdominal pain, numbness and tingling in the hands and feet, and muscle cramps.

Toxicity:
None.

Sources:
1. Yeast, green leafy vegetables.
2. Broccoli, whole grain cereals and bread, legumes, yams.

Dosage:
4 to 7 mg per day.

Stability:
Only a small amount of this vitamin is lost during normal cooking.

VITAMIN C: (Ascorbic acid)

Nearly everyone who completed a high school or college history course remembers studying about the events concerning British sailors, scurvy, and lime juice that took place during the seventeenth and eighteenth centuries. The story goes back much further than this, however, and descriptions of a disease resembling scurvy have been found on papyrus tablets in the city of Thebes, dating back as far as 1500 B.C. Hippocrates, in 450 B.C., described symptoms resembling scurvy in Greek soldiers. Scurvy was also noted during the time of the Crusades, particularly in the winter when fresh fruits and vegetables were not available. In 1497 when Vasco de Gama sailed around the Cape of Good Hope, almost two-thirds of his crew died from scurvy, and Magellan lost many of his crew when he sailed around Cape Horn in the 1520s. This disease was particularly prevalent among British sailors during this time, and usually appeared about three months after the ship had left the home port. In 1753 Dr. James Lind published his experiments on British seamen, showing that giving them oranges or lemons prevented scurvy. Even though those in positions of responsibility in the British Navy at that time seemed to officially ignore the results of these experiments, when Captain Cook made his long voyage in 1775, he stocked his ship with as much fresh fruit and vegetables as possible and replenished them at every port where such supplies were available. None of his crew came down with scurvy. It actually takes only one-tenth cup of orange juice a day to prevent scurvy. By 1795 lime juice was regularly supplied on all British ships. This is why the British sailors were called "limeys," a name that has persisted to this day. As recently as the American Civil War, some soldiers died from scurvy, and even today there are still areas in the United States where the intake of vitamin C is border-line or inadequate. This is specially true among the lower income groups.

At the present time fresh fruits and vegetables contribute over 90 percent of the vitamin C in the American diet.

Functions:

1. Essential for collagen formation. Collagen is the protein material that binds the tissue cells together and is necessary for healthy teeth, bones, skin, and tendons.
2. Increases the absorption of iron and calcium from the intestines.
3. Promotes the healing of wounds.
4. Converts the inactive form of folic acid, a vitamin of the B complex group, to the active form.
5. Protects the body from infections.
6. Regulates many essential body processes.
7. Essential for the integrity of the blood vessel walls.
8. The synthesis of red blood cells and some hormones.
9. An antioxidant vitamin.

Deficiency:

A deficiency of vitamin C results in scurvy, probably the oldest recognized vitamin deficiency disease. When this vitamin is totally eliminated from the diet, the symptoms of scurvy begin to appear in about 90 days and consist of dryness of the skin, bleeding into the skin around the hair follicles, bleeding in the eyes, loss of hair, bleeding and swollen gums, fatigue, pains in the bones and joints, cavities in the teeth, sore mouth and gums.

If vitamin C is not completely eliminated from the diet, but the amount is less than adequate, the symptoms of scurvy take a longer time to develop and may be somewhat different. These symptoms are irritability, listlessness, swollen and tender joints, loss of appetite, weakness, fatigue, restlessness, bleeding under the skin and in the mouth around the gums, and in children a failure to grow normally.

Those requiring a greater than normal intake of vitamin C are smokers, women taking birth control pills, and elderly people.

Toxicity:

No toxic effects have been noted with doses moderately over the recommended allowance. With sustained high doses, there is an increased risk of kidney stones developing due to the conversion of excess vitamin C to oxalic acid. There may be some interference with the normal metabolism of vitamin B_{12}, and symptoms of anemia, skin rash, diarrhea, and low blood sugar have occasionally been reported.

Sources:

1. Citrus fruits and juices, either fresh, frozen, or canned.
2. Green peppers, broccoli, brussels sprouts, tomatoes and tomato juice, cabbage, greens, potatoes, yams, cauliflower, asparagus, and cabbage.
3. Strawberries, cantaloupe, guava, mangoes, papaya.
4. Rose hips, acerola (a West Indian cherry).

Dosage:
35 to 50 mg to age 14.
60 mg over age 14.
80 mg during pregnancy.
100 mg during lactation.

Stability:
Vitamin C is the *most unstable* of all the vitamins. When exposed to air, vitamin C is rapidly lost. The loss is not as great if the foods are stored in a refrigerator. It is easily destroyed by alkali, so baking soda should not be used while cooking vegetables. Other methods of preserving vitamin C are as follows.

1. Avoid excess chopping and cutting of foods.
2. Cook the vegetables in a steam pressure cooker or use as little water as possible.
3. Cook potatoes with the skin on.
4. Don't use copper cooking utensils.
5. Add the food to be cooked to water that is already boiling.
6. Keep the pot covered.

Vitamin C is preserved by freezing. Microwave cooking preserves slightly more of the vitamin C than cooking with steam pressure. Both of these methods preserve about twice as much of the vitamin as boiling the vegetables in water.

WATER

The best 6 doctors anywhere,
And no one can deny it,
Are sunshine, water, rest and air,
And exercise and diet.
These 6 will gladly you attend,
If only you are willing.
Your ills they'll mend
Your cares they'll tend,
And charge you not a shilling.

Water is the most abundant of the essential nutrients in our body, the total amount being about 45 quarts. Between 50 and 75 percent of our total body weight is water; fatter people have proportionately less water than thin people. Water is present in all the tissues of the body as well as in every cell. Even our bones are made up of nearly one-third water, while our muscles and our 10 to 12 billion brain cells contain 71 percent water.

It is possible to live for several weeks without food, but we can survive for only a few days without water. Next to oxygen, it is the most essential substance for the preservation of life. None of the nutrients we eat would be of any value without the presence of water. Thirst occurs when we lose only about one percent of our total water; if we lose as much as 20 percent, death results.

About two-thirds of the body's water is located inside the cells, and the remainder is outside the cells in the tissues. Water, as well as nutrients and waste material, continually passes in and out through the cell walls by a process called osmosis.

The two most important functions of water are: (1) to act as a solvent for the essential nutrients, so that they can be used by the body; and (2) the transportation of nutrients and oxygen from the blood to the cells and the return of waste material and other substances from the cells back to the blood so they can be removed from the body. Other important functions are:

1. To give shape and form to the cells.
2. To regulate the body temperature.
3. As a lubricant in joints and other areas.
4. To cushion certain body organs.
5. As a body builder, and to maintain peak physical performance. A loss of only 5 percent of our body water results in a 30 percent decrease in work performance.

The intake and output of water must balance each other, and in the normal person the body has wonderful ways of maintaining this important balance. Most of our water comes from what we eat and drink, although some of it is made in the body. We eliminate water normally through our lungs, skin, urine, and intestines.

The following outline gives the approximate amount of water gained and lost from each of these sources every day.

WATER LOSS

Skin	550 cc.
Lungs	440 cc.
Urine	1550 cc.
Stool	150 cc.
Total	2650 cc.

WATER INTAKE

Liquids	1500 cc.
Solid foods	750 cc.
Produced in the body	400 cc.
Total	2650 cc.

1,000 cc. equals 1 quart
500 cc. equals 1 pint
240 cc. equals 1 cup

Some foods, especially fruits, contain large amounts of water while others have very limited amounts. Table 1 gives the water content of various foods.

We should drink 6 to 8 eight-ounce glasses of pure water daily. This will provide enough water for all of the essential bodily functions and will help to maintain normal elimination.

Here is a helpful suggestion for the millions of Americans who are constantly troubled with constipation; perhaps it is caused by not including enough roughage and liquid in the diet, or sometimes because the colon just becomes lazy from the overuse of laxatives. Shortly after rising in the morning, drink some lukewarm water. Start by drinking half a glass or less and over a week or two slowly increase the amount until you can take two glasses without your stomach rebelling. It is best not to use ice water at this time of day, since energy is needed to warm it to body temperature and also because cold water tends to slow down the emptying time of the digestive tract. Two additional glasses of water (not warm) can be taken between breakfast and lunch and two more between lunch and dinner.

TABLE 1

WATER CONTENT OF VARIOUS FOODS

Food	Percent Water
White sugar	0.5
Nuts and dry cereals	2-3
Crackers	5
Gelatin	13
Butter	15
Dried fruits	25
Bread	36
Cheese, cheddar	37
Beef	47

Food	Percent Water
Chicken	63
Veal	66
Bananas	75
Cottage cheese	79
Potatoes	80
Oranges, apples	86
Milk	87
Fruit juice, vegetables	90
Lettuce	96

Adapted from Adams, C.: *Nutritive Value of American Foods*, USDA Handbook No. 456, Washington, D.C. 1975.

FRESH AIR, EXERCISE, AND SLEEP

Through the lungs, the body receives life-giving air. One may live for many days without solid food and for several days without any liquid, but death comes in a few moments without air. The capacity for using air can be greatly increased by properly exercising the lungs, as has often been demonstrated in the treatment of those with tuberculosis (consumption). Air is a simple mixture of numerous gases, but it is composed chiefly of oxygen and nitrogen. Life is more dependent upon the regular and adequate supply of oxygen than upon any other element. Fortunately for us, the nitrogen in the air dilutes the oxygen, for in an atmosphere of pure oxygen we would be so overactive as to be very short-lived. Experiments have shown that prolonged inhalation of air in which the proportion of oxygen is much greater than that in which it naturally occurs in the atmosphere causes such great disturbance in the body metabolism that death finally results. Therefore, we know that the mixture called air did not happen accidentally, but has been perfectly and admirably formed for the needs of human beings as well as for those of animals and plants.

The water vapor present in the air is necessary to enable the lungs to use the oxygen readily, as is shown by the fact that dry oxygen is not as readily absorbed as that which contains the proper amount of moisture.

A very important change takes place in the blood as it passes through the lungs. The blood is returned in the veins from all parts of the body to the right side of the heart. At this point the blood has a dark purplish color because it is low in oxygen and contains a large amount of carbon dioxide and other impurities. Next it is pumped through the pulmonary arteries to the lungs. In the lungs, the pulmonary arteries carrying the impure blood keep branching and getting smaller and smaller until they are only about the width of one red blood cell. When they reach this size, these very tiny blood vessels are surrounded by the air sacs in the lungs so that the red blood cells are able to give off their carbon dioxide and take on a fresh supply of oxygen. There are about 300 million of these tiny air sacs (alveoli) in the lungs, and if we could lay them out on a flat surface they would cover an area roughly 700 square feet in size. When the blood leaves the lungs with a fresh supply of oxygen it flows back to the left side of the heart and is pumped all through the body. It is then a bright red color, due to the increased oxygen. The oxygen is taken up by the hemoglobin in the red blood cells, and is supplied to every part of the body.

There are about 25 to 30 trillion red blood cells in our bodies, but each one lives only about 120 days. This means that in order to provide an adequate supply of oxygen to the many millions of tissue cells, 2.5 million new red blood cells must be produced every second. In adults, these new cells are manufactured mainly in the bone marrow.

As the blood passes through the tiny capillaries — the smallest channels that carry blood to every tissue in the body — each red cell gives up a portion of its oxygen, takes in carbon dioxide, and returns to the lungs to be cleansed again. The blood is slightly cooled and loses some of its water as it passes through the lungs. The amount of carbon dioxide that is released by the blood while digestion is taking place is greatly diminished by the use of such items as stimulating foods, sugar, animal foods, and even more by wine, rum, beer, ale, cider, tea, and coffee. Strenuous exercise increases the removal of carbon dioxide gas up to six times the ordinary amount.

The lungs are greatly improved by regular exercise. Ancient peoples also recognized this fact, as shown by Fig.1, a page of illustrated breathing exercises from an old Chinese book dating back several thousand years. When the lungs are not exercised and expanded to their limit on a regular basis, they lose to a greater or lesser degree their elasticity. In many persons there is almost a total loss of the power to really expand the chest, which is very necessary for perfect health.

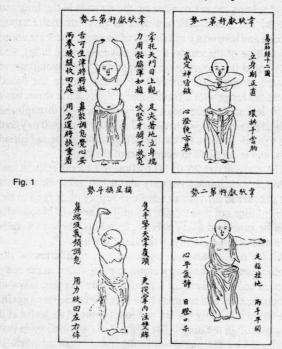

Fig. 1

Forming the habit of deep breathing will make you sleep better, think more clearly, have better circulation, and make you feel better all over because of the increased supply of oxygen that will be provided to every organ in your body.

A. DEEP BREATHING EXERCISE

The following exercise is most beneficial when it is done in the fresh air.

1. Stand straight, placing your hands along your lower ribs, with the fingers pointing down and inward.
2. Take in a slow deep breath through your nose, making sure you feel the lower ribs move outward.
3. When you have filled your lungs with as much air as possible, force yourself to take another sniff of air. If your ribs have not moved outward, give them a slight tug by hooking your fingers beneath them.
4. Now let the air out slowly through your mouth, keeping the lips partly closed so there will be some resistance. When you feel like all the air has been let out, push the lower ribs in with your hands to force out the last little bit.

Start doing this exercise once three times a day and gradually work up to four or five deep breaths three times a day.

You may vary this routine by breathing in rapidly and exhaling slowly or vice versa. Musicians and public speakers are often benefitted by taking these deep breathing exercises, as it helps them to develop better breath control. When a person feels weary and exhausted from sedentary employment, the practice of deep breathing in the manner just described, with the body erect and the chest well expanded, will prove very refreshing and will help induce a restful sound sleep. The great advantage of an abundance of lung exercise can be seen from the fact that professional singers suffer less from lung disease than others and their chests are always better developed than are those of most other persons.

The detrimental effects of breathing impure air, especially in a room where there are several people, are headache, nervousness, dullness, and aggravation of all diseases pertaining to the lungs. Current scientific studies show that there is an increase in lung cancer in nonsmokers who are constantly subjected to an atmosphere polluted with cigarette smoke. It is interesting to note that the cells that are the most sensitive to a lack of oxygen are the cells of the brain. The headaches with which school children are sometimes afflicted are often caused by breathing foul air. Tuberculosis (consumption) is most frequent in those whose habits, vocations, or occupations are sedentary, as they usually spend much time in an atmosphere of impure air.

An old army surgeon, who was in charge of large hospitals during World War I, related a very interesting experience illustrating the importance of providing the sick, especially persons suffering with fever, with an abundance of pure air. He said that in a large hospital he had 320 cases of measles at one time during the winter season. The hospital caught fire and burned to the ground, and the patients had to be placed outdoors on the hospital grounds in tents. All but one or two recovered. He said he had no doubt but that the number of deaths would have been thirty or forty at least, if the patients had remained in an indoor environment.

Walking increases the inhalation of oxygen threefold and has recently become one of the most popular forms of exercise in the United States. Participation in this wonderful and inexpensive exercise is possible by nearly everyone. Regular exercise in the open air is one of the most important factors for the preservation of health and the prolongation of life. The greater the degree of activity, the larger the amount of oxygen taken into our bodies. In cold weather we get a larger supply of oxygen than in hot weather. This makes us more active, both mentally and physically. Outdoor life in the cool fresh air of temperate zones helps us to develop a strong constitution and increases our resistance to disease. It is a well-known fact that the inhabitants of temperate zones have more energy than those who live in the tropics. A sound and vigorous body can only be produced by pure blood and healthy nerves.

Proper exercise in the open air and sunshine is among God's greatest gifts to man. It gives good form and strength to the physical body and — all other health habits being equal — is one of the surest safeguards against disease and premature death. It gives buoyancy and strength and maintains a healthful mental balance, free from the extremes that result from artificial living.

Oxygen, the elixir of life, is one of the best blood purifiers and one of the most effective nerve tonics. It is freely provided by nature for all. Useful work in the open air will bring new strength and vitality, and produce a happy and cheerful attitude of mind. If the poisonous waste matter that should be thrown off by the lungs is retained, the blood becomes impure and not only the lungs but the stomach, liver, and brain are affected. The digestion is retarded, the skin becomes sallow, the brain clouded, the thoughts confused, the heart depressed, and the whole system inactive and very susceptible to disease.

B. WELL-VENTILATED HOUSES

Every room, and especially every sleeping room, in the house should be well-ventilated throughout the year, both day and night. Have plenty of light, sunshine, and air, which has been wisely provided by our gracious God, in your houses to make you strong, healthy, and happy.

ANNOTATION: The statements about the bad effects suffered from breathing impure air in enclosed quarters is certainly medically and scientifically correct today. Consider the following item that recently appeared in a leading science journal.

The men who built the beige and brick one-story house in rural Mount Airy, Maryland, boast that they can heat the whole place with a hair dryer. It is a veritable fortress against the loss of energy. There are leakproof, triple-glazed windows, a weather-stripped, magnetically sealed front door, and plastic sheets in the walls, floors, and ceilings that keep the homes living space as airtight as the inside of a sandwich bag.

But a funny thing happened when these conservation-minded men from the National Association of Home Builders Research Foundation bottled things up so tightly. Without the drafts of fresh outside air typical in most homes, the indoor air went bad. Investigators found high levels of formaldehyde gas throughout the house and they detected indoor radioactivity more than 100 times the natural outdoor background level.

The Mount Airy house dramatically demonstrates an environmental problem that has only lately attracted governmental and scientific attention. The problem is indoor air pollution.

In the new breed of energy-efficient homes, as well as in more typical "leaky" homes around the United States, recent air sampling has established that pollutants are more concentrated indoors than out. In some residences — both old and new — these pollutants exceed national health limits. (Michael Gold, "Indoor Air Pollution," *Science,* Vol 80, March/April, 1981, pg 30.)

C. GETTING A GOOD NIGHT'S SLEEP

The usual causes for a lack of sleep are pain, headache, cold feet, painful stomach or colon, nervous tension, worry, lung congestion, emphysema, mental illness, and inability to relax.

The following 10 suggestions will help you get a good night's sleep.

1. Engage in some form of physical activity during the day, but not just before retiring. Don't take a midday nap.

2. The room should be dark, but not necessarily pitch black.

3. A comfortable bed; if the bed is too soft, it may produce various muscle aches, and especially may cause or increase back pain.

4. Usually the quieter the better. Some people get used to sleeping with certain noises such as traffic, trains, music, clocks, etc. and have a hard time going to sleep if these sounds that they are used to are not present.

5. Relaxation is very important. Before going to bed, try reading or listening to some soothing music for an hour. One of the best positions for relaxing tense muscles is lying on the back with pillows under the head, arms, shoulders, and knees. Try to think of each muscle group. Tighten the muscles and then purposely relax them, starting with the toes and working up to the head. Be sure the facial muscles, including the eyelids and jaws, are all relaxed.

6. Try to have your stomach empty. Your evening meal should be light and should be eaten 3 to 5 hours before you retire. Avoid any drinks with caffeine, especially coffee, tea, colas, cocoa, or chocolate. If you really feel you need something to drink, take warm herb tea.

7. Take a warm bath for 10 to 20 minutes immediately before retiring. The temperature of the water should not be over 95°F. If the water is too hot, it will have a stimulating effect and keep you awake. If your feet are still not warm, use a heating pad or hot water bottle.

8. Don't smoke cigarettes before going to bed; the nicotine acts as a stimulant.

9. The best temperature in the bedroom for most people to sleep is 60° to 70°F.

10. See herbs to use for insomnia as listed in the index. "The sleep of a laboring man is sweet, whether he eat little or much: but the abundance of the rich will not suffer him to sleep." Ecclesiastes 5:12. (Adapted from J.D. Hendrickson, M.D., "Sleep Soundly," *Life and Health,* November 1971, p. 18.)

Section V
Your Foods

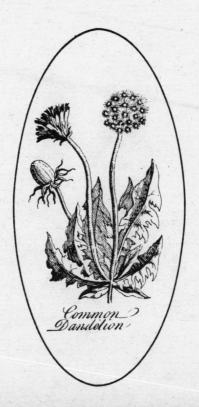

*Common
Dandelion*

1

FRUITS

God planned in the beginning that fruit should form a large part of our diet, and if we would follow that plan today, it would add much to our health. While it is true that fruit, like other things, has deteriorated significantly since Creation, yet if we would take care of the trees and eat fruit in the proper way, it would prove an untold blessing today.

In the beginning, man was told to dress the trees. This was for a purpose. Every tree should be pruned and dressed so that the sun will shine on the fruit for at least part of the day, if not all day. If there are too many limbs and leaves, and the fruit grows completely in the shade, it will have much less food value, flavor, and life-giving properties. The seed of fruit and vegetables grown in the shade for two or three years will not germinate. It will, to a great extent, lose its quality and life-giving properties. Therefore, all fruit trees should be pruned so that sun and air have free access to the branches.

Another thing that should be remembered is that fruit, before it is ripe, is in the starchy state, and while in this condition it has but little food value and is hard to digest. But as fruit ripens it turns into grape sugar, especially when ripened in the air and sun, and is very easily digested. Fruit that is grown in the shade or is picked before it is ripe is better eaten cooked than raw. A great deal of the fruit that is shipped is picked before it is ripe. While it does ripen to some extent after it is picked, it is never the same as when it ripens on the tree.

A. SELECTING FRUIT

If fruit is picked before it is fully grown, it is practically worthless as far as real food value is concerned, except perhaps for the banana, which is a very peculiar fruit. It can be picked green and will continue to ripen and develop its sugar. It should never be eaten until every particle of green has disappeared, the outer skin begins to turn brown, and the pulp has become mellow. Most bananas are eaten altogether too green while they are still in the starchy state. When the banana is fully ripe, it contains twenty-five percent grape sugar, which requires very little or no digestion. Any infant or invalid can eat mashed ripe bananas.

Some time ago I was in a fruit store looking for a bunch of bananas that suited me. The storekeeper said: "I like bananas, but I cannot eat them. Yesterday about eleven o'clock I got very hungry and ate two bananas, and they made me so sick that I had to go to bed." I asked him to point out what kind he had eaten. He had eaten bananas that were in the starchy state, and had probably not masticated them properly. Without proper mastication, bananas will form gas, putrefy, and cause trouble.

In buying prunes, buy a large size, since the large prunes have practically no larger pit than the small ones. The smaller the prunes, the less fruit you have, and the more pit. A large prune, when soaked overnight in cold water, can be eaten without any cooking and is very delicious. You can do the same thing with figs, apricots, or peaches when you get a good grade. When you do cook them, only very little cooking is needed .

Unripe grains are the opposite of unripe fruits. The grain before ripening is in the milky state, or the grape sugar state, and can be digested without any cooking. That is the way grain was eaten in the beginning and no doubt that is the way the disciples and Jesus ate it. But when it ripens, grain turns into starch. Therefore, ripe grain should be thoroughly cooked before it is eaten.

The juice of oranges, grapes, pineapples, and grape fruit may be taken when ripe with no sugar added. These juices can be used to quench the thirst with good results if they are used as a drink between meals.

Citrus fruits in particular, but also strawberries, cantaloupes, and cherries, are high in vitamin C. All the yellow-colored fruits are also high in vitamin A. Dried fruits, such as apricots, prunes, and raisins, contain little if any vitamin C but they are extremely rich in minerals, specially iron.

There are several reasons why we should not eat so much soft food or drink with our meals. First we hear so much about alkaline foods and that they are all right to eat, but the fact is that the saliva is more alkaline than any of these foods. Another fact is that if we eat our food in its natural state and thoroughly mix it with saliva before we swallow, it will alkalinize the system more than all of the known alkaline foods combined. When the food reaches the stomach, it is mixed with the digestive juice known as the gastric juice. In order for the gastric juice to do its work properly, it needs the help of the saliva. The food leaves the stomach in a semi-liquid form and in the small intestine it mixes with the pancreatic juice and the bile, which cannot perform their functions satisfactorily without the prior work of the saliva and the gastric juice.

If many of these little points were observed, you would see a marvelous improvement in your health. When you take so much fluid and soft foods with your meals, it dilutes these various digestive juices so that they become weak and do not have the proper power to digest the food as God had planned they should. There is perfect law and order in our system, and when we violate these principles we suffer the consequences.

Many years ago when we made tests on these things, we found that half a good-sized lemon would destroy typhoid germs in a glass of water; the healthy gastric juice in the stomach is four times as strong as lemon juice. Here is where the Scripture is fulfilled, that when we eat or drink any deadly thing, it shall not hurt us. Of course, I would not advise anyone to take carbolic acid or any concentrated poison and think they would be protected by what the Scripture says and that our digestive fluids would counteract the impurity. But nevertheless it is true that if you see to it that your blood-

stream is pure and you eat the foods that make your digestive
fluids pure or normal, then your system will be better able to
resist typhoid, diphtheria, smallpox, tuberculosis, and other
deadly germs .

God has provided still further preventive, nonpoisonous,
remedies like gentian root, calamus root, valerian root, black
currant juice and leaves, and many others. These are God's
harmless preventives and anyone can take them in abundance. God never intended that man should take any poisons
that are Satan's production. God cannot answer our prayers
for recovery when we continue to use poisonous remedies
that always do the system harm. God's remedies never leave
a harmful effect on the system.

Nature is God's physician for suffering humanity, healing
without money and without price. There is no law against
anyone being his own doctor and going into the garden and
eating the right fruit and then plucking some of the leaves
and making a tea of them and drinking it.

B. GRAPES AND GRAPE JUICE

I have experimented with grape juice a great deal, with
gratifying results. Combining grape juice with a nut milk,
about half-and-half, quickly furnishes the system with new
blood of the purest kind. It is an excellent remedy for anemia.

Much of the grape juice found on the market is not good
because it is adulterated. But good grape juices are available
that are pure and unadulterated and are good medicine. The
best way is to make your own, drinking it immediately after
it has been squeezed. Then you know it is pure and you lose
nothing of the flavor or food value. If it stands for any length
of time after being squeezed, it loses something of the flavor
and food value. The same rule applies to all fruit juices —
drink them at once after squeezing. If left standing, they
undergo a change. You may also can your own fruit juices.

The very best way is to eat the grapes fresh from the vine
when they are in season. A grape diet for a week or so is

beneficial to the system. I have known people who thrived on eating the entire grape: skin, seeds, and all. But those who have weak digestion, and others with whom this would not agree, should not swallow the skin or seeds. In cancer cases grape juice is particularly recommended.

A grape drink may be made as follows: two-thirds cup grape juice, one-third cup water, and one heaping teaspoon of soybean flour. This is very nourishing.

C. ORANGES

The orange is one of Nature's finest gifts to man. Orange juice contains predigested food in a most delicious and attractive form, ready for immediate absorption and utilization. The amount of food value contained in a single large orange is about equal to that found in a slice of bread. But orange juice differs from bread in that it needs no digestion, while before bread can be used for energizing and strengthening the body, it must undergo digestion for several hours. A glass of orange juice has more vitamin A, thiamine, niacin, vitamin C, and more iron and potassium than a glass of milk. This is the reason oranges are so strengthening and refreshing to invalids and feeble persons, as well as to those in good health.

Orange juice is rich in salts, specially in lime and alkaline salts that counteract the tendency to acidosis. In such serious diseases as scurvy, beriberi, neuritis, anemia, or any condition in which the tissues are bathed in acid secretions, the alkaline mineral salts of fresh fruits will be of great benefit. The orange, lemon, and grapefruit are invaluable.

Orange juice has a general stimulating effect on the peristaltic activity of the colon. It should be taken about one hour before breakfast.

Orange juice is perfectly suited to those who are suffering from a fever. Four to six quarts of liquids should be taken daily to relieve and quench the fever's fire and to eliminate poisons through the skin and the kidneys, as fever is Nature's effort to rid the body of accumulated poisons. Acid fruits satisfy the thirst; and the agreeable flavor of orange, lemon, and other fruit juices makes it possible for the patient to obtain the large amount of liquid needed.

During the time of the severe epidemic of influenza this country suffered following World War I, a doctor published a paper saying that if people would use large quantities of orange juice, fever would be allayed and the patient would recover. It was found by practical experience to bring good results. This caused the price of oranges to jump from $3 or $4 per box to between $18 and $25. This price jump caused the growers and shippers much alarm, as they feared they would be prosecuted for raising prices when in fact they were not to blame. It was simply due to the increased demand. It so happened that it was just in between seasons for oranges and the supply was small in the States. The growers offered all they had on hand to the government and the hospitals. Their offer was not accepted, however, because the officials of the food commission said that due to the small supply it would not be worthwhile. They said it was better to let the individuals that could afford to buy the oranges have them, for they would not go far in large institutions. But there was a great lesson in this for the people; if they would only use fruit juices to help cure all fevers, what a blessing it would be to mankind.

Orange juice is indispensable for feeding bottle-fed babies. The use of orange juice will help prevent scurvy, pellagra, and rickets.

The acid and sugar in the orange aid digestion and stimulate and increase the activity of the glands in the stomach .

Orange juice is capable of serving more useful purposes in the body than any of the other fruit juices. The sweeter the orange the greater its food value. As people become better educated in nutrition, oranges will be much more freely used and appreciated.

D. LEMONS

Medicinally, lemons act as an antiseptic — an agent that will prevent infection or putrefaction. They are also anti-scorbutic, which means a substance that will prevent scurvy. They also assist in cleansing the system of impurities. The lemon is a wonderful stimulant to the liver and is also a solvent for uric acid and other poisons. It liquefies the bile and is very good in cases of malaria. Sufferers from chronic rheumatism, rickets, tuberculosis, and gout will benefit by taking lemon juice, as will those who have a tendency to bleed or have uterine hemorrhages. During pregnancy it will help to build strong bones in the child. We find that the lemon contains certain elements that help to build a healthy system and then to keep that system healthy. The lemon, owing to its potassium content, will nourish the brain and nerve cells. Its calcium strengthens the bony structures and makes healthy teeth.

The minerals found in lemons have an important part to play in the formation of plasma — the fluid portion of the blood. A single average-sized lemon contains phosphorus, 16 mg; sodium, 2 mg; calcium, 26 mg; potassium, 138 mg; vitamin C, 53 mg and iron, 0.6 gm. Lemons are useful in treating asthma, biliousness (gas), colds, cough, sore throat, diphtheria, influenza, heartburn, liver complaints, scurvy, fevers, and rheumatism.

For diphtheria, use pure lemon juice every hour, or more often if needed. Use either as a gargle or swab the throat with it. Swallow some until it cuts loose the false membrane in the throat.

For sore throat, dilute lemon juice half-and-half with water and gargle frequently. It is better to use it full strength if possible.

A slice of lemon tied over a corn overnight will greatly relieve the pain.

A slice of lemon tied over a felon will not fail to bring the pus to the surface where it can be easily removed.

To relieve asthma, take a tablespoon of lemon juice one hour before each meal.

For liver complaints, the juice of a lemon should be taken in a glass of hot water one hour before breakfast every morning.

To break up influenza, take a large glass of hot water with the juice of a lemon added, while at the same time keeping the feet in a deep bucket or other vessel of hot water. Have the water deep enough so that it comes almost to the knees. Keep adding water as hot as the patient can stand it for about twenty to thirty minutes, or until the patient is perspiring freely. Be sure there is no draft on the patient while this is being done. The patient should be near the bed so he can get into bed without moving around, thereby avoiding any danger of getting chilled. If it is convenient, a full hot tub bath would be good in place of the foot bath. The lemon water should be taken every hour until the patient feels that all symptoms of the cold are gone .

A teaspoon of lemon juice in one-half glass of water will relieve heartburn.

Lemon juice is an agreeable and refreshing beverage in fevers if the bowels are not ulcerated.

For rheumatism, one or two ounces of lemon juice freely diluted should be taken three times a day, one hour before meals and at bedtime. In cases of hemorrhage, lemon juice diluted and taken as cold as possible will help stop it.

Scurvy is treated by giving one or two ounces of lemon juice diluted with water every two to four hours. In excessive menstruation, the juice of three or four lemons a day will help check the bleeding. It is best to take the juice of one lemon at a time in a glass of cold water.

The question may be asked: "How can one with an inflamed or ulcerated stomach partake of lemon juice? Would not a strong acid like that of the lemon act as an irritant?"

That would depend on how it was taken. If in quantity — yes, but if taken very weak at first, diluted with water, it will eventually cease to burn. The sufferer afflicted with an ulcerated stomach has to use great perseverance to effect a cure, but it can be cured if care and patience are used.

The gastric juice in the stomach is four times as strong as lemon juice.

I wish that humanity would understand the real value of the lemon and learn to make a real medicine of it.

It should be especially remembered that it is a wonderful remedy for colds, influenza, and all kinds of fever. Always take without sugar.

There are many household uses for lemons. For example, lemon juice will sour sweet milk, making it suitable for cooking. Add a few drops or a small teaspoonful to each cup of milk. The addition of one teaspoon of lemon juice to a quart of very hot soybean milk will make it curd to make soybean cheese. (See the index.)

Lemon juice is excellent to use in the place of vinegar. Use it just as you would use vinegar.

The addition of a little lemon juice and some of the grated lemon rind adds greatly to the flavor of dried fruits, figs, prunes, peaches, etc. Add while stewing the fruit.

To bleach linen or muslin, moisten with lemon juice and spread in the sun.

For the hands, after washing dishes and to remove vegetable stains, rub them well with lemon juice. It will keep the hands white and soft, and will also remove any strong odor, such as onions.

To remove ink stains, iron rust, or fruit stains, rub the stain well with lemon juice, cover with salt, and put in the sun. Repeat if necessary.

2

VEGETABLES

A.   NUTRITIONAL VALUES

Vegetables, along with fruits, are a wonderful source of vitamins and minerals, and at the same time they are low in calories. One-half cup of such vegetables as broccoli, tomatoes, green beans, and carrots, among many others, has only about 25 calories.

According to the *U.S. News and World Report,* December 8, 1980, the amount of fresh vegetables consumed per person in the U.S. decreased 1.2 percent between 1960 and 1979 to 144.3 pounds, while the percentage of processed vegetables increased 29 percent to 65.0 pounds. The same magazine in its February 4, 1985 issue gives the total vegetables consumed per person as 207 pounds, up from 187 pounds in 1963. Such items as fruit, grains, meat, fish, and poultry also showed an increase in consumption while coffee, milk, and eggs decreased.

A survey reported in the Summer 1985 Newsletter of the American Institute for Cancer Research showed that the percentage of fruits and vegetables consumed by Americans over the past 3 years increased by 25 percent. Strangely enough, however, 21 percent of American households reported eating no potatoes, 22 percent no fresh fruits, 23 percent no canned fruits or vegetables, and 72 percent no dried fruits or vegetables.

As a general rule, the darker the color of the vegetable, the richer it is in nutrients. Leafy vegetables are exceptionally good sources of calcium, iron, vitamin A, vitamin C, and riboflavin. The leaves are the most active part of the plant and the greener the leaves the higher the vitamin and mineral content will be. The outer, darker-colored leaves of cabbage and lettuce contain much more nutrient value than the inner, lighter-colored leaves. Broccoli and cauliflower are also very good sources of minerals and vitamins. Broccoli, along with the other cruciferous vegetables, cauliflower, cabbage, and Brussels sprouts, may also play a part in the prevention of cancer. Broccoli is a member of the cabbage family and was brought to the United States from Italy. It once was called "Italian Asparagus." One cup of cooked broccoli gives up to 300 percent of the daily needs of vitamin C for an adult, 4.5 grams of protein, only 50 calories, and hardly any fat. One stalk of broccoli, if properly cooked, contains 30 percent more vitamin C than an eight-ounce glass of orange juice. In addition broccoli contains significant amounts of pantothenic acid, folic acid, thiamine, niacin, riboflavin, potassium, phosphorus, iron, and calcium.

While the calcium in some dark green vegetables, such as spinach and beet greens, is rendered largely unavailable to the body because of a high level of oxalates, the oxalic acid level in broccoli is low, making it a much better source of calcium. Of course, you don't have to worry about the high oxalates in some vegetables interfering with the absorption of calcium from other sources, such as other high calcium foods, when they are eaten at the same meal.

The dark-orange vegetables, such as carrots, yams, and winter squash, are a rich source of vitamin A and the deeper the color the more vitamin A is present. Light yellow vegetables like corn and wax beans are not as high in vitamin A.

Growing your own vegetables is the surest way to get the most nutritional value, provided they are prepared properly. The sooner vegetables are eaten after being picked the more nutrients will be present. If you let vegetables or fruit sit around the house at room temperature for a few days after bringing them home from the market, there will be a large loss of vitamins A and C due to the action of destructive enzymes. In fact, 50 percent of the vitamin C can be lost from some vegetables after only one day. It is best not to buy more vegetables than you can use in a few days, but what you do purchase should be kept cool and away from light and air. The best place for them is in the refrigerator in a plastic bag.

Eating a wide variety of vegetables daily is best, including at least one serving each of a yellow and a green leafy vegetable.

Starchy vegetables include potatoes, lima beans, peas, corn, parsnips, winter squash, pumpkin, and yams. Even these starchy vegetables have only about 100 calories in half a cup.

Starchless vegetables are carrots, young beets, celery, cucumbers, tomatoes, soybeans, squash, turnips, onions, okra, Brussels sprouts, and artichokes. Starchless and sugarless vegetables are lettuce, spinach, all greens, tomatoes, celery, radishes, string beans, cabbage, cauliflower, eggplant, endive, and asparagus.

Another advantage of eating an abundance of vegetables and fruits is the presence of fiber, which helps to keep the digestive tract functioning properly and is an excellent aid to prevent constipation. See Chapter 3, Fiber, following.

Many people are concerned about the effect that processing has on the nutritive value of vegetables, and rightly so. Freshly picked vegetables, of course, are most nutritious, with frozen next and canned last. There may not be as much difference, however, as you would think between these methods of preparation. Vitamin A losses are minimal during processing and one study showed 44 percent of vitamin C remaining in freshly cooked peas, 39 percent in frozen, and 36 percent in canned. The best way to be sure of getting a good supply of nutrients from vegetables, if you can't always get properly cooked fresh ones, is to eat as wide a variety of fresh, canned, and frozen vegetables as you can.

During the cooking process, minerals as well as the water-soluble vitamins B complex and C are lost to varying degrees in the cooking water. This water should be saved and used in soups, stews, and the like. Heat, light, and exposure to air are other causes for the loss of vitamins while preparing vegetables. These losses affect vitamins A, C, E, K, and many members of the B complex family of vitamins. In order to preserve as much of the nutrient value as possible, the suggestions for cooking given in Section VI, Chapter 1 should be followed as closely as possible.

B.   POTATOES

We hear so much about mashed potatoes not being good to eat. It is true that the ordinary mashed potatoes that are eaten everywhere are a very unwholesome product. When potatoes are peeled, boiled, and then mashed with a large piece of butter or other fat, they become unwholesome food. When potatoes are peeled there is practically nothing left but starch. The alkaline part of the potato is cut away when they are peeled, and the starch is acid-forming.

The Irish potato is a very valuable food, but not after it has been peeled and boiled in a quantity of water that is drained down the sink, leaving the potato lifeless, without minerals, and acid-producing. The eyes and the peeling of the Irish potato contain its life-giving properties. When the skin of the potato is not eaten, the best part of it is lost. Also, when the skin is baked too brown, the life-giving properties are destroyed.

Baking is the ideal way to cook a potato, but it must be properly baked. When properly baked, the skin should be a little crisp, but not too dark brown or black. Before putting potatoes in the oven to bake, scrub them thoroughly and prick the skin all over with a fork. This causes some of the moisture to evaporate, and helps to make the potatoes dry and mealy.

Another excellent way to prepare potatoes is to steam or pressure-cook them. All vegetables may be excellently prepared in the steam pressure cooker under a low temperature, as the original food flavors are then preserved in an economical way. They can also he improved by placing them in a warm oven and allowing them to dry out for a few minutes after pressure cooking. Many who have found it impossible to eat potatoes prepared in any other way are able to eat them when they are prepared in this way.

3

FIBER

A great deal has been written during the past several years about fiber in the diet, both in scientific journals and in lay publications. Plus, people who are interested in their health, which includes most of us, want to know more about fiber; what it is, what it's good for, where to get it, etc. Even several well-known cereal manufacturers are promoting the large amount of fiber that is contained in some of their products. Drugstore counters display many bulk and fiber-type laxatives, and there are even high-fiber cookies and wafers to "help keep you regular."

Sometime you may hear the term "bulk" or "roughage" used, but these really mean essentially the same thing, so we will refer to them all as fiber. Fiber is the tough, structural part of plants, such as the stems, leaves, coverings of the seeds and fruits, etc. , that undergoes little if any digestion as it passes through the intestinal tract. This is because humans, unlike some animals, do not possess the enzymes necessary to break down fiber to any degree.

The beneficial effect of fiber is nothing new. About 2400 years ago, Hippocrates said, "wholesome bread clears up the gut and passes through as excrement." Dr. John Harvey Kellogg, a vegetarian who founded the famous Battle Creek Sanitarium in Michigan in the late 1800s, was one of the early American advocates of a high-fiber diet. His brother, W. K. Kellogg, established the world-famous cereal company based on Dr. Kellogg's corn flakes, which he had developed for the patients at the sanitarium.

The average American diet contains only about half the fiber that it should. The reason is quite simple. Most Americans eat large amounts of refined food, specially refined cereals and bread from which the bran has been removed during the milling process. The bran, which is the outer covering of the grain, is where the fiber is located. We also eat a lot of overcooked vegetables and drink a lot of fruit juices instead of eating the fruit raw.

The benefits of a diet containing adequate fiber are no longer in doubt. At the top of the list would probably be the help received by those who are troubled by chronic constipation. According to some recent statistics, this would include a large percentage of those living in Western countries. Walk down the aisle of nearly any drugstore and see for yourself how many preparations are available for the treatment of constipation—pills, oils, powders, liquids, granules, suppositories, and enema kits, to name but a few. Most people have found it necessary to take a laxative at some time during their lives and this does no harm. It is, however, entirely possible to become "addicted" to some types of laxatives and after using them daily over a period of years, it becomes impossible for the bowels to move normally by themselves.

When eating the average Western-type highly-refined diet, it takes the food about three days to pass completely through the intestinal tract. This results in a small, hard stool that requires much straining and therefore develops a very high pressure in the colon in order for the bowels to move. This increased pressure is responsible for other problems in the colon and elsewhere, which we shall mention shortly.

How does fiber help? In the first place it increases the bulk of the stool and this makes it pass through the digestive tract in about half the time. The increased bulk results in decreased pressure buildup in the colon. Fiber also attracts and holds water like a sponge, making the stool much softer and easier to pass, and this also contributes to a lowering of the pressure. If you are one of the millions who suffer from constipation, following are some helpful suggestions.

1. Increase the amount of fiber in your diet.
2. Drink one or two glasses of water in the morning about 30 to 60 minutes before breakfast. Use the water as it comes out of the tap or try heating it slightly. Take your time. Don't gulp the water down

in a hurry. Your stomach, like your body, requires a daily morning bath.
3. Eat lots of fresh fruits and vegetables.
4. Drink 6 to 8 glasses of water a day between meals.
5. Exercise daily for at least 30 minutes. Walking is good.
6. Use whole grain bread and cereals.
7. Do not resist the natural urge for your bowels to move.

Besides constipation, there are many other physical problems that appear to be related to a low-fiber diet. Dr. Dennis Burkitt of London, England, is the person who has done more than anyone else in recent years to investigate and promote the use of fiber in the diet. He had this to say in a recent article: "There is now a fairly well-defined list of diseases that are recognized as characteristic of modern Western culture. All of them have their minimum presences in economically more developed countries and are rare in rural communities in the Third World. ...These diseases include ischemic heart disease, gallstones, diabetes (Type II), obesity, varicose veins, deep vein thrombosis, hiatus hernia, colorectal cancer, appendicitis, diverticular disease, and hemorrhoids. ...There is evidence to suggest that all the diseases in this list are diet-related. The reduction in intake of dietary fiber, and in cereal fiber in particular, is the diet change that has been predominately incriminated in the increased prevalence of certain gastrointestinal diseases, in Western countries mainly, during the past half-century." (From "Fiber as Protective Against Gastrointestinal Diseases," Dennis Burkitt, C.M.G., F.R.S., M.D., F.R.C.S., *The American Journal of Gastroenterology,* April 1984, pp. 249-252.)

Diverticulosis is a very common disorder of the large intestine that is found in Western countries. In fact, it is present in nearly half the population over the age of 50 years. Diverticula are pockets that are found on the outside of the colon when the high pressure in the colon forces apart the lining of the colon through a weak place in the wall. Everyone has these areas of weakness. They are located where the small blood vessels that nourish the intestine pass through the wall. These pockets, which look like bubbles on the outside of the colon (Fig. I), may connect with the colon by a rather narrow opening. The pockets may be large or small, few or many, and are one of the most common causes of bleeding from the intestines. They are most numerous in the portion of the colon that is located in the left lower abdomen, but they do not occur in the rectum. Diverticulosis is rarely seen in some parts of the world, such as Africa, where a high-fiber diet and large stool volume are typical.

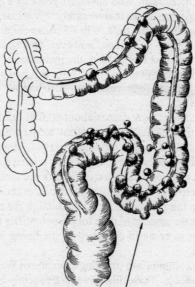

Fig. 1 – Colon with many Diverticula

Most people who have diverticula never develop any serious problem, although some may have a nagging lower abdominal pain, cramps, or suffer from constipation. Some may have a "spastic" or "irritable" colon. In about 20 percent of persons with diverticulosis, an infection with an abscess or even a perforated diverticulum may occur. If this should happen, the term diverticulitis is used, and at times it may develop into a life-threatening situation where surgery is urgently needed. There are usually fever and severe pain in the left lower abdominal region. About 200,000 persons are hospitalized each year in the United States with diverticulitis. It has been shown recently that not only will a high-fiber diet prevent the formation of diverticula, but it will also improve the symptoms of diverticulosis that have already developed.

Appendicitis has also been linked with the amount of fiber we eat. Dr. Burkitt, who spent 20 years as a physician in Uganda, Africa, states that he rarely saw a case of appendicitis during this entire time. When African children were sent away to school in Europe, however, and started eating a Western-type diet low in fiber, the incidence of appendicitis began to increase dramatically. Those children that remained at home and ate their customary diet had no trouble with appendicitis.

Colon cancer now causes about 60,000 deaths each year in the United States. It is one of the most common cancers, with 157,500 new cases estimated in 1991. More evidence is accumulating daily that it is not only related to the amount of fat but also to the amount of fiber in the diet. A diet high in fiber helps to protect against colon cancer because the fiber speeds up the passage of the stool through the colon, which decreases the amount of time for the potentially cancer-causing toxins to come in contact with the lining membrane of the colon.

A very common and irritating affliction of Western society is hemorrhoids. These dilated veins frequently become painful and irritated, and often bleed. They are very frequently seen in those with chronic constipation and are thought to be caused by excessive straining while attempting to move the bowels. Hemorrhoids are rarely seen in those who regularly eat a high bulk diet. As an interesting sidelight, Dr. Burkitt mentions that "the Emperor Napoleon was suffering from hemorrhoids during the battle of Waterloo, and it is interesting to cogitate on whether the outcome of the battle might have been different had he been given bran sometime before the conflict, in which case his attention might have been more on the battle and less on his bottom!"

The amount of fiber in the average American diet is about 15 to 20 grams a day. This should be increased to 30 to 40 grams. This can be accomplished quite readily by observing a few simple rules, as follows.

1. Read the nutrition labels on bread and eat only bread that is made from 100 percent whole grain.
2. Eat breakfast cereals that are high in fiber content, such as All Bran, Fiber 1, Shredded Wheat, oatmeal, Wheatena, or add a few spoonfuls of unprocessed oat bran to your favorite cereal.
3. Use brown instead of white rice.
4. Eat fruits fresh instead of cooked, canned, or juiced whenever possible. Also eat the skin whenever possible.
5. Cook vegetables as little as possible.
6. Eat legumes such as beans, lentils, and garbanzos (chick peas) often.
7. Sunflower seeds and most nuts are high in fiber content. Use nuts moderately, however, as they are high in fat.

There are some precautions to observe when starting to increase the fiber in your diet.

1. Drink plenty of liquid; 6 to 8 glasses a day is best.
2. Increase the amount of fiber in the diet gradually over a period of several weeks.
3. Some gas or bloating may occur as the amount of fiber is increased, but this will slowly improve over a period of several months.

FIBER CONTENT OF FOODS

The following list of rich and moderately rich sources of fiber was originally published by the National Cancer Institute. NCI advises that to increase the amount of fiber, choose several servings of foods from this list. The dietary fiber content of many foods is still unknown, so this is not a comprehensive list. Also, with regard to cereals, the brand name products listed are representative of the fiber content of similar types of cereal products. Other cereal would be expected to have similar amounts of dietary fiber.

RICH SOURCES OF FOOD FIBER

4 grams or more per serving. Foods marked with an * have 6 or more grams of fiber per serving.

Breads and Cereals	*Serving*
All Bran*	1/3 cup-oz.
Bran Buds*	1/3 cup-1 oz.
Bran Chex	2/3 cup-1 oz.
Corn Bran	2/3 cup-1 oz.
Cracklin' Bran	1/3 cup-1 oz.
100% Bran*	1/2 cup-1 oz.
Raisin Bran	3/4 cup-1 oz.
Bran, unsweetened*	1/4 cup
Wheat germ, toasted, plain	1/4 cup-1 oz.

Legumes (Cooked portions)	
Kidney beans	1/2 cup
Lima beans	1/2 cup
Navy beans	1/2 cup
Pinto Beans	1/2 cup
White beans	1/2 cup

Fruits	
Blackberries	1/2 cup
Dried prunes	3

MODERATELY RICH SOURCES OF FOOD FIBER

1 to 3 grams of fiber per serving

Breads amd Cereals	*Serving*
Bran muffins	1 medium
Popcorn (air-popped)	1 cup
Whole wheat bread	1 slice
Whole wheat spaghetti	1 cup
40% Bran Flakes	2/3 cup-1 oz.
Grapenuts	1/4 cup-1 oz.
Granola-type cereals	1/4 cup-1 oz.
Cheerio-type cereals	1-1/4 cup-1 oz.
Most	1/3 cup-1 oz.
Oatmeal, cooked	3/4 cup
Shredded wheat	2/3 cup-1 oz.
Total	1 cup-1 oz.
Wheaties	1 cup-1 oz.
Wheat Chex	2/3 cup-1 oz.

Legumes (cooked) and Nuts	
Chick peas (Garbanzo beans)	1/2 cup
Lentils	1/2 cup
Peanuts	10 nuts
Almonds	10 nuts

Vegetables	
Artichoke	1 small
Asparagus	1/2 cup
Beans, green	1/2 cup
Brussels sprouts	1/2 cup
Cabbage, red and white	1/2 cup
Carrots	1/2 cup
Cauliflower	1/2 cup
Corn	1/2 cup
Green Peas	1/2 cup
Kale	1/2 cup

Parsnip	1/2 cup
Potato	1 medium
Spinach, cooked	1/2 cup
Spinach, raw	1/2 cup
Summer squash	1/2 cup
Sweet potato	1/2 medium
Turnip	1/2 cup
Bean Sprouts (soy)	1/2 cup
Celery	1/2 cup
Tomato	1 medium

Fruits

Apple	1 medium
Apricot, fresh	3 medium

Fruits

Apricot, dried	5 halves
Banana	1 medium
Blueberries	1/2 cup
Cantaloupe	1/4 melon
Cherries	10
Dates, dried	3
Figs, dried	1 medium
Grapefruit	1/2
Orange	1 medium
Peach	1 medium
Pear	1 medium
Pineapple	1/2 cup
Raisins	1/4 cup
Strawberries	1 cup

From *FDA Consumer*, June 1985, page 32.

4

OATMEAL

Common oatmeal, which can be purchased in every grocery store in the land, is a most wonderful food. However, it is not properly prepared by many and is terribly abused by the majority of people. It is one of the finest foods for growing children that we have, but the way the oats are eaten many times spoils the real quality of the oats. When milk and sugar are put on the oatmeal, they cause it to ferment in the stomach and thus its benefit is lost. There also is a great misunderstanding among some people about steel-cut and finely flaked quick-cooking oats. There is not a hair's breadth of difference between the steel-cut oats and the finely flaked oats as far as food value or life-giving properties are concerned.

"The chemical analysis of rolled oats and steel-cut oats is identical, because quick-cooking rolled oats is nothing more than steel-cut oats run through heavy rollers revolving at a great rate of speed. We guarantee a minimum of 15 percent protein and of 7.5 percent fat, and a maximum of 1.9 percent fiber, 66 percent nitrogen free extract, and 77 percent carbohydrate.

"Rolled oats is one of the few — if not the only — cereal food that carries the germ of the grain, and that is important."

The above is taken from a letter by G. M. Hidding, General Manager of the Purity Oats Co., of Keokuk, Iowa, May 27, 1936.

The food value in one cup of cooked rolled oats is as follows:

Calories 148
Protein . . . . 5.4 grams
Fat . . . . 2.8 grams
Carbohydrate . . . . 26.0 grams
Fiber (crude) . . . . 0.5 grams

MINERALS		VITAMINS	
Sodium	1 mg	Thiamine (B₁)	.17 mg
Potassium	130 mg	Riboflavin (B₂)	.07 mg
Calcium	21 mg	Niacin	0.5 mg
Magnesium	0 mg	Ascorbic Acid	0 mg
Phosphorus	158 mg	Iron	1.7 mg

A. BENEFITS OF EATING OATMEAL

Flaked oats are much more easily handled by most people because they digest quicker and take less time to cook. The steel-cut oats ought to cook at least four hours in a double boiler, while the finely flaked oats take only three minutes — a great saving in fuel and a great saving to our old weak stomachs. A fine way to prepare oats is just the way it is given on the package. I eat it just that way with some zwieback and some nice soybean butter on the zwieback. I enjoy it very much, more so than many years ago when I used milk and sugar on it. Something dry, like zwieback or some whole wheat crackers should be eaten with the oatmeal, so that plenty of saliva is produced to mix with it.

Cook the oatmeal this way to increase the fiber in your diet: combine equal parts of steel-cut oats and sterilized bran with water according to the directions on the package. Cook six to ten minutes, then set aside five minutes before serving. A considerable part of this will be imperfectly cooked; therefore, it is not readily acted upon by the saliva and intestinal juices, but passes on into the colon where it will aid in the destroying of putrefactive poisons caused from the decomposition of proteins and other foods.

Oatmeal can be used in many ways. When oatmeal is not spoiled in the preparation or used in wrong combinations, it is one of the finest foods we have to prevent disease. I read in a daily paper many years ago that the Great Northern Railroad had a very urgent piece of road to make. They hired a big crew of men and worked them fourteen hours a day. Instead of giving them ordinary water to drink, they gave them oatmeal water and the paper stated that not one man was laid off on account of sickness. It stated that never before had there been such a wonderful experience in the history of railroads.

Oatmeal water should be more frequently used than it is. It is a very good medicine for the sick. To make oatmeal water, use the finely flaked oats and put two heaping teaspoonfuls in a pan with a quart of water. You can make it stronger or weaker to suit your taste. Put it on the stove and let it simmer for half-an-hour. Then beat it with a spoon or eggbeater and strain it through a fine sieve. This makes an excellent drink for anybody, especially the sick. If desired, you can add just a pinch of salt and a little soybean milk.

Another recipe for making oatmeal water is: take a heaping tablespoonful of oatmeal to a quart of water and let it simmer for two or two and a half hours in a tightly covered pan, and then strain it. This makes a very refreshing, cooling drink after it is cooled off in the icebox.

I quote the following from *Diet, The Way to Health,* by R. Swinburne Clymer, M.D.: Oats, steel-cut or Scotch: silicon 24.0; phosphorus 18.2; potassium 13.6; magnesium 5.2. Oats is one of the richest silicon carriers known and if properly combined with fruit or vegetable eliminants, is the ideal basic food for children during the winter months to prevent infection from all zymotic diseases.

It is not too much to say that oatmeal, if combined with other foods so as to prevent congestion and the formation of toxins and acids due to the acid reaction, would do more to prevent contagious diseases than all the serums thus far invented. Oatmeal is neither artificial nor a substitute. It is a natural agent that supplies those elements that, by their antiseptic properties, help to combat contagious infections.

Besides this antiseptic quality, oats are rich in phosphorus, which is required by the child for the formation of strong bones and teeth and also for brain and nerves — tissues required by the mind in study.

Wherever a large amount of silicon is required, prescribe

oatmeal, or if this is not practical due to digestive disturbances, then use the extract, "Avena Sativa."

The following are extracts from a letter dated April 21, 1936, which I received from F. L. Gunderson, biochemist in the Nutrition Laboratory of the Quaker Oats Co., Chicago, Illinois.

We are very glad to enclose a description of the manufacturing process for both standard and quick-cooking rolled oats flakes. Many people have the erroneous idea that the hulls of the oat grain are comparable to the bran of wheat. That is not correct. The hulls (or flowering glumes) of the wheat grain envelop the whole kernel rather loosely and consequently go into the straw stack at threshing time. In contrast, the glumes of the oat grain are wrapped a bit more securely around the kernel, and remain on the oat kernel as an individual wrap until they are removed in the rolled oats mill. After removing the hull from the oats, the kernel from which rolled oats are made possesses all of the bran, middlings, endosperm, and germ portion natural to the grain. Whole oat kernels (oat groats), steel-cut oats, large or "standard" type rolled oats flakes, and small or "quick" type rolled oats flakes are all whole grain products. In the sense that "refined" is sometimes used as an antonym for "whole grain," there are no refined oat foods. The very botanical and physical structure of the oat grain together with the universal oat milling processes are such that all oat foods are whole grain products. The composition of steel-cut oats, large flaked oats, and small flaked rolled oats is identical if made from the same type of grain.

With regard to the vitamins in oats, our own tests, as well as those of other well-known research people, indicate that there is no destruction in the manufacturing process.

B. MANUFACTURING PROCESSES FOR QUAKER OATS, MOTHER'S OATS, QUICK QUAKER OATS, OR QUICK MOTHER'S OATS

DESCRIPTION: Flaked oats made from the best quality

of large oats with the hulls removed.

METHOD OF MANUFACTURE: The oats go through an extensive cleaning process in which corn, wheat, barley chaff, and wheat seeds are removed. The oats are then carefully sized to uniform diameter by grading in special machines, the light oats, double oats, and pin oats being removed for feed. The oats are again graded to uniform length, about five grades being obtained. Only the plump sound oats of good size go into either of these four products. The clean, graded oats are roasted and partially dried, after which they are cooled and passed to a large burr stone where the hulls are torn from the groats. The oats mixture is next bolted to remove any flour and the hulls are then removed in special machines and the cleaning process is continued until the groats are free of hulls and unhulled oats.

For production of the two brands of "quick" rolled oats, the groats are at this stage steel cut. The clean groats pass to the steaming chamber, where they are partially cooked with live steam and from which they pass to the rollers, where the groats are formed into flakes. The rolled oat flakes are cooled in a current of air to about 110°F., following which the product is immediately weighed and packed by automatic mechanical equipment.

5

NUTS

Nuts take the place of meat in nearly every respect. With the exception of the peanut (which is really a legume) and chestnuts, the average nutritive value of nuts is about 160 to 200 calories per ounce. This is double the value of an equal quantity of sugar or starch. The large amount of fat in nuts and seeds makes them very high in calories. They have a relatively large amount of protein and are good sources of iron and the B vitamins. All nuts except walnuts, peanuts, and filberts produce an alkaline reaction in the body.

Nuts should be purchased in the shell when possible. In this form they are probably fresher, since the shell protects the nut, and they are very likely to be cheaper, depending on the quantity purchased. Of course, shelling the nuts takes time. Brazil nuts are particularly difficult, but the task may be made easier by soaking these nuts in water anywhere from 30 minutes to 2 hours before shelling them. If you do elect to purchase nuts already shelled, buy them whole and break them up yourself. Don't forget that salted nuts turn rancid much faster than unsalted ones and that shelled nuts should be kept in the freezer in a plastic bag away from light, heat, and moisture.

Almond: One-fifth of the weight of the almond consists of protein and it is of the very finest quality. The almond yields a most delicious oil, which is highly digestible. Almond butter can be made into a milk or cream which, with the addition of a little sweetening, resembles cow's milk in appearance and in nutritive properties.

Hickory Nut: A pound of hickory nut meat is equal in nutritive value to more than four pounds of average meat.

584

Two-thirds of the weight of the hickory nut is easily digested oil.

Pecan: The pecan is a valuable nut, high in nutrition.

Walnut: One pound of black walnuts contains more than 100 percent more protein than the same quantity of Salisbury steak. The English walnut differs slightly from the black walnut in that it contains more fat and less protein.

Butternut: The butternut also contains more fat than the black walnut, but has the same amount of protein. The butternut is low in carbohydrates; therefore, it is very valuable for persons suffering from diabetes.

Peanut: When thoroughly dried, the peanut contains 50 percent or more protein than the best beef steak. Further, half of its weight is an excellent oil. Emphasis must be placed on the fact that salted roasted peanuts, found on the market are over-roasted and indigestible. Unroasted peanut butter is easily digested and highly nutritious. The protein of the peanut is nearly equal to the protein of milk and eggs as a tissue-building element. A very fine milk can be made from unroasted peanut butter. Peanuts are also used extensively in malted nuts and vegetable meats.

Coconut: A most excellent substitute for butter can be prepared as follows: cut the meat of the coconut in strips, grate or grind it with a meat grinder. Soak it in several times as much warm water as you have coconut and let it sit for two or three hours. A rich cream will rise to the top. Skim off the cream and work it into a butter with an ordinary butter ladle. Coconut oil is high in saturated fatty acids, so it should be avoided.

It is better to eat nuts in an emulsified form such as nut butters. Otherwise they must be thoroughly masticated, so that no little hard pieces enter the stomach.

Small particles of such concentrated foods cannot be acted

upon by the digestive juices and often pass undigested through the alimentary canal.

Nut butters prepared without roasting are superior in nutritive and hygienic value to the best cuts of meat and to dairy butter and cheese.

The protein of nuts is of greater value for the renewal of the body cells than the protein derived from the muscular tissues of a dead animal with all its waste products.

The pecan, filbert, English walnut, almond, hickory, and chestnut are abundant in growth-promoting vitamins. Chestnuts should never be eaten raw because of their tannic acid content.

The nut should not be used as a dainty but as a staple article of diet. The popular idea that nuts are hard to digest has no foundation as long as they are thoroughly masticated when eaten. The habit of eating nuts at the end of a meal, when in all probability more food of a highly nutritious nature has been eaten than is necessary, is very injurious. It is an equally injurious habit to eat nuts between meals. Improper mastication is a common cause of indigestion from the use of nuts.

Peanuts should be heated slightly to remove the skin. Other nuts may be blanched and crushed without roasting. Over-roasting makes the nut very difficult to digest.

Nuts should be eaten as a part of every heavy meal, and made a part of the bill of fare. But because nuts are so highly concentrated, only a few ounces should be eaten at a time.

Nuts contain more iron than other foods; they also contain a high content of calcium, particularly almonds, Brazil nuts, and filberts. Nuts are high in fat, but contain no cholesterol. Most nuts have an alkaline reaction on the system except for peanuts, walnuts, and filberts, which are acid-forming.

ANNOTATION: The statement that "A pound of walnuts contains almost 50 percent more protein than the same quantity of beef" is not accurate. At the time this statement was made (in the 1930s), there were no specific nutritive values assigned to edible foods by the United States Department of Agriculture. But now such values are available and

NUTRITIVE VALUE OF NUTS
(usual serving – 100 grams or 3½ ounces)

	VITAMINS (MG)			MINERALS (MG)				CARBOHYDRATE GRAMS	PROTEIN GRAMS	FAT GRAMS	CALORIES
	B₁	B₂	NIACIN	CALCIUM	PHOSPHORUS	IRON	POTASSIUM				
ALMONDS	.25	.67	4.6	254	475	4.4	—	597	18.6	19.6	54.1
BRAZIL NUTS	.08	—	—	186	693	3.4	660	646	14.4	11.0	65.9
BUTTERNUTS	—	—	—	—	—	6.8	—	629	23.7	8.4	61.2
CASHEWS	.63	.19	2.1	46	428	5.0	—	578	18.5	27.0	48.2
CHESTNUTS	.22	.22	.6	27	373	3.8	—	377	2.9	—	4.1
COCONUT	.10	.10	.2	21	98	2.0	—	359	3.4	14.0	34.7
FILBERTS (HAZEL NUTS)	.46	—	.9	209	337	3.4	—	634	12.6	16.7	62.4
HICKORY NUTS	—	—	—	TR.	360	2.4	—	673	12.6	12.8	62.4
MACADAMIA NUTS	.34	.11	1.3	48	161	2.0	—	691	7.8	15.9	71.6
PEANUTS	.30	.13	16.2	74	393	1.9	337	559	26.9	23.6	44.2
PECANS	.72	.11	.9	74	324	2.4	300	696	9.4	13.0	73.0
PISTACHIOS	.22	.11	.7	—	—	—	—	594	19.3	19.0	53.7
SUNFLOWER SEEDS	1.96	.23	5.4	120	6	7.1	—	560	24.0	19.9	47.3
WALNUTS, ENGLISH	.48	.13	1.2	83	380	2.1	225	654	15.0	15.0	64.4

they show that one pound of black walnuts (chopped or broken kernels) contains about 86 grams of protein. The same weight (one pound) of oven-cooked relatively fat roast beef contains 85 grams of protein; one pound of oven-cooked relatively lean roast beef contains 112 grams of protein; one pound of broiled relatively lean and fat sirloin steak contains 100 grams of protein; and one pound of broiled relatively lean sirloin steak contains 144 grams of protein.

Nuts are very high in potassium and magnesium content.

The percentage of protein content of some nuts, dairy products, and meat, is as follows: peanuts, 26.9; walnuts, 15.0; turkey, 24.0; cured ham, 16.9; fresh ham, 15.2; beef (meaty and fat), 18.6; beef (regular hamburger), 16.0; cheddar cheese, 23.2; dried nonfat milk, 35.6.

Dairy products and meat are very high in cholesterol, which is now implicated as one of the major causes of heart attacks (coronary occlusion). Nuts have no cholesterol content.

It should be remembered that the statement, "Nuts perfectly take the place of meat" was written by my father in the 1930s. It is now a well-known fact that a total vegetarian diet (vegan) is lacking in Vitamin B_{12}. This vitamin was not discovered until 1948, at least a decade after this book was first published. Therefore, persons on a total vegetarian diet must seek a Vitamin B_{12} supplement.

The statement that "nuts contain more iron than any other foodstuff" is true for certain nuts, but not all of them. Parsley is extremely high in iron; however, an equal weight of black walnuts contains more iron than parsley. Most of the other nuts, however, including English walnuts, contain somewhat less iron than parsley does for an equal weight. These figures are from the USDA Home and Garden Bulletin #72, 1981.

6

BREAD AND REFINED FLOUR

A. IMPORTANCE OF BREAD

Bread is a most important health food. "There is more religion in a loaf of good bread than many think." (*Ministry of Healing*, p. 302.) Properly baked bread made from the right material, whole grain flours, has been the staff of life from the earliest Bible times, and has always been one of the principal foods that God gave to man; but it has indeed been made the staff of death by the modern invention of milling.

Bread made with milled white flour cannot impart to the system the nourishment that is found in whole grain bread. The use of refined flour aggravates the difficulties under which those who have inactive livers labor.

Most of the wheat breads purchased in the grocery stores are unhealthful, for they contain various percentages of white flour and are seldom thoroughly baked. Make sure that you purchase 100 percent whole wheat bread. Bread is more healthful if eaten when it is at least one day old. It should be baked clear through the center of the loaf so that no part of it is soft or gummy.

God never intended that wheat and other grains should be separated into their different parts, presented to the people as a wonderful invention, and then sold for a big price. It is indeed an invention, but one that may destroy both soul and body. Untold harm is done by the bakery goods that are found on the market today. They are baked just enough to stand up, but not enough to kill the yeast germ; nor are they baked enough so that the starch is changed to an easily digested form. The baking process was instituted by God Himself to prepare the grains and starchy foods so they could be eaten by humans and provide proper nourishment.

From the earliest times a great deal of unleavened bread was used; more, in fact, than leavened bread. The bread that Abraham's wife baked for the strangers who were angels was unleavened bread, for it took her just a short time to make this bread. In the sacrificial offering no leavened bread was ever used. Leaven was looked upon as a symbol of sin (Luke 12:1). If leaven or yeast of any kind is used in bread, it needs to be thoroughly baked so that the yeast germ is entirely destroyed.

Lately yeast has been widely advertised to be eaten raw as a stomach remedy, but yeast should never be eaten unless it is first cooked. Yeast is a highly nourishing and wholesome product when it is cooked until the yeast germ is destroyed. The analysis of yeast is just the same as the analysis of Vegex, which is sold for such a high price on the market.

In recent times a myth has been spread that no one over the age of 35 or 40 years should eat bread. This is correct when applied to most of the bread that is sold on the market, as it should not be eaten by anyone at any time. But one can live very well on a diet of only whole wheat bread, whole rye bread, or whole barley bread, with vegetables and fruit added.

Oats also make an excellent bread. Delicious bread can be made by taking part whole wheat flour, whole corn flour, whole oat flour, and whole soybean flour. Add a little malt honey or Karo syrup. This will make a bread that anyone can live and work on by eating just a little fruit with it.

Before any of the grains are ripe, when they are still in the milky state, they can be eaten raw. They are then in the grape sugar state and are like the sugar that is found in thoroughly ripe fruit. After the grain ripens, it turns to starch, and before starch can be used by the body, the outer cellulose wall must be broken by grinding or cooking. Animals have digestive fluids that are different from those of humans and thus they are able to digest this cellulose (fiber).

The baking process is very similar to the ripening of the fruit on the tree. Before it is ripe, fruit is in the starchy stage and unfit to eat, but after it ripens in the sun the starch turns to grape sugar. It is then ready for assimilation, and requires very little digestion. When bread is put in the oven, it goes through the same process. To a large extent, the prolonged baking gradually changes the starch into a form that the digestive juices in the body can properly act upon to renew the body.

B. REFINED OR MILLED FLOUR

Unlike the refining of gold, which removes impurities and makes the product much more valuable, the refining of cereal grain (wheat, rice, corn) removes most of the valuable nutrients and makes the grain much less valuable from a nutritional standpoint. Perhaps instead of calling it refined flour, which to many people suggests improvement in the product, it should be called milled or devitalized flour. This type of flour has a definite advantage to all those who are engaged in the distribution, storage, and baking processes, since not only does refined flour not spoil and turn rancid, but it is also much less likely to be infested with insects. The real loser, then, is actually the consumer. Refining cereal, however, also removes phytates and phytic acid, which bind some of the iron, calcium, and zinc, resulting in a loss of some of these minerals to the body.

All of the commonly used cereal grains are the seeds of grasses and each one has a structure somewhat similar to the grain of wheat shown in Fig.1. Notice that the essential vitamins and minerals are located in the bran, aleurone, and germ layers; and that the endosperm, which is the portion remaining after the milling process, contains only starch and a little protein. Whole grain contains the entire seed except for the outer layer or hull, which is inedible and therefore discarded. It should be remembered that whole grain cereals and breads must be kept in the refrigerator since the fat,

A KERNEL OF WHEAT

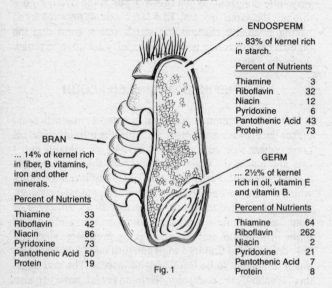

ENDOSPERM

... 83% of kernel rich in starch.

Percent of Nutrients

Thiamine	3
Riboflavin	32
Niacin	12
Pyridoxine	6
Pantothenic Acid	43
Protein	73

BRAN

... 14% of kernel rich in fiber, B vitamins, iron and other minerals.

Percent of Nutrients

Thiamine	33
Riboflavin	42
Niacin	86
Pyridoxine	73
Pantothenic Acid	50
Protein	19

GERM

... 2½% of kernel rich in oil, vitamin E and vitamin B.

Percent of Nutrients

Thiamine	64
Riboflavin	262
Niacin	2
Pyridoxine	21
Pantothenic Acid	7
Protein	8

Fig. 1

which is present in the germ portion, tends to turn rancid quickly.

The refining of grain began in the United States around the year 1910. Enrichment of refined white flour was made mandatory by the U.S. government during World War II. This enrichment program consisted of adding thiamine, riboflavin, niacin, and iron in sufficient quantity to bring the grain almost back to its original content of these four nutrients. The addition of calcium and Vitamin D was optional. Table I shows the effect of enrichment on three types of wheat flour.

TABLE I

Nutrient Mg Per lb	Unenriched	Flour Enriched	Whole Grain
Iron	3.6	13.0	15.0
Niacin	4.1	16.0	19.7
Thiamine	0.28	2.0	2.49
Riboflavin	0.21	1.2	0.54
Calcium	73.0	73.0	186.0

Source: *Nutritive Value of American Foods in Common Units,* Agriculture Handbook No. 456, Agricultural Research Service, U.S. Department of Agriculture, Washington, D.C., 1975, p.274.

Following World War II, the decision regarding the enrichment of grains was left to the states, and about 34 states now require the enrichment of bread and flour. It is very important, therefore, that consumers, specially those who do not live in states that require enrichment, read the labels on bread, cereals, pasta, rice, etc. to make sure they are enriched. It costs the manufacturer the paltry sum of less than 1/10 of a cent for the vitamins and minerals that are needed to enrich one loaf of bread. Even though approximately 90 percent of the bread sold in the United States is enriched, refined foods still comprise approximately 50 percent of the American diet, and while the consumption of enriched bread and flour is decreasing, the consumption of nonenriched foods is increasing.

Another, and perhaps more important, fact to remember is that 17 other minerals and vitamins, as well as fiber, that are removed during the milling process are *not* replaced and are therefore absent even in enriched bread and flour. A list of these nutrients with the approximate amount that is lost is shown in Table II.

TABLE II
NUTRIENTS LOST DURING MILLING
OF WHEAT FLOUR

	Percentage Lost by Milling	Loss Replaced by Enrichment
Bran (fiber)	100%	–
Vitamins		
Thiamine (Vitamin B_1)	77	Yes
Riboflavin (Vitamin B_2)	80	Yes
Niacin	81	Yes
Vitamin B_6 (Pyridoxine)	72	–
Pantothenic acid	50	–
Folacin	67	–
Alpha–tocopherol (Vitamin E)	86	–
Choline	30	–
Minerals		
Calcium	60	–
Phosphorus	71	–
Magnesium	85	–
Potassium	77	–
Sodium	78	–
Chromium	40	–
Manganese	86	–
Iron	76	Yes
Cobalt	89	–
Copper	68	–
Zinc	78	–
Selenium	16	–
Molybdenum	48	–

Adapted from: Henry A. Schroeder, M.D., "Losses of Vitamins and Trace Minerals Resulting from Processing and Preservation of Food," *The American Journal of Clinical Nutrition,* Volume 24, pages 566-569, May 1971.

What happens to all the valuable minerals, vitamins, and bran that are removed during the milling process? These nutrients are used as animal food, mainly for cattle and hogs.

Following is the nutritional information for frequently purchased loaves of "supermarket" bread. These figures are for an average serving size of two ounces, which is approximately two slices of bread.

The ingredients in a loaf of *enriched white bread* are as follows: enriched flour (barley, malt, iron, niacin, thiamine mononitrate, riboflavin), water, corn syrup, yeast, partially hydrogenated animal and/or vegetable shortening, (may contain lard and/or beef fat and/or soybean oil and/or cotton seed oil and/or palm oil), salt, wheat gluten, dough conditioners (contains one or more of the following: calcium, stearoyl lactylate, mono- and diglycerides, ethoxylated mono- and diglycerides, mono- or dicalcium phosphate), potassium bromate (soy flour, calcium sulfate, whey).

The ingredients listed on a loaf of *enriched wheat bread* are as follows: enriched flour (barley, malt, iron, niacin, thiamine mononitrate, riboflavin), water, whole wheat flour, sugar, corn syrup, partially hydrogenated animal and/or vegetable shortening (may contain lard and/or beef fat and/or soybean oil and/or cotton seed oil), yeast, salt, wheat gluten, soy flour, calcium sulfate, dough conditioners (contains one or more of the following: calcium stearoyl lactylate, mono- and diglycerides, ethoxylated mono- and diglycerides, mono- or dicalcium phosphate), potassium bromate (caramel color).

The ingredients listed on a loaf of *generic white enriched bread* are as follows: flour, water, corn syrup, salt, yeast, soy bean oil, calcium propiniate (preservative), mono- and diglycerides, lecithin, ethoylated mono- and diglycerides, barley, malt, ammonium sulfate, potassium bromate, niacin, azodicarbonamide, iron, fungal enzymes, thiamine mononitrate, riboflavin.

In comparison with these commercially available loaves of bread, the ingredients listed on two loaves of bread baked at the Loma Linda Market Bakery are as follows:

Sprouted Whole Wheat Bread — ingredients: sprouted wheat, whole wheat flour, water, yeast, salt, honey, soy oil, malt, and lecithin.

100% Whole Wheat Bread — ingredients: whole wheat flour, water, yeast, sugar, soy bean oil, malt, salt, and lecithin.

As mentioned before, it must be remembered that since the last two loaves of bread listed above contain the entire grain of wheat, including the *fat* in the germ layer, they will become rancid if left in the open air for very long and therefore they should be kept in the refrigerator.

Bread is really not a particularly fattening item of food, as most people think. A slice of nearly any kind of bread contains about 70 calories, and an important point is that about 75 percent of these calories is supplied by the carbohydrates. Bread is low in fat. If you use 100 percent whole-grain bread, you will find it to be a good source of fiber, minerals, vitamins, and complex carbohydrates.

7

MEAT AND VEGETARIANISM

Meats of all kinds are unnatural food. Flesh, fowl, and seafoods are very likely to contain numbers of bacteria that infect the intestines, causing colitis and many other diseases. They always cause putrefaction.

Research has shown beyond all doubt that a meat diet may produce cancer in some cases. I have treated patients who have suffered from severe headaches for many years. Every remedy had been tried without relief, but when meat was excluded from the diet they obtained most gratifying results.

Excessive uric acid is caused by eating too much meat and may result in rheumatism, Bright's disease, kidney stones, gout, and gallstones. A diet of potatoes is an excellent way to rid the system of excessive uric acid. Increased uric acid excretion in the urine comes from the following two sources.

1. Uric acid taken into the body in meat, meat extracts, tea, coffee, etc. A pound of steak contains about 14 grains of uric acid. This accounts for the stimulant effect of eating a steak, since uric acid is a close chemical relative to caffeine.

2. Uric acid formed in the body from nitrogenous foods.

It is an established fact that meat protein causes putrefaction twice as quickly as vegetable protein. There is no ingredient in meat (except vitamin B_{12}) that cannot be procured in products of the vegetable kingdom. Meat is an expensive second-hand food material and will not make healthy, pure blood or form good tissues. The nutritive value of meat broths is practically nothing. They always contain uric acid and other poisons.

The argument that flesh must be eaten in order to supply the body with sufficient protein is unreasonable. Protein is found in abundance in beans, peas, lentils, nuts of all kinds, and soybeans.

Whereas, before the flood when no flesh was eaten, men regularly lived over 900 years; after the flood, when flesh was added to man's diet, the life expectancy soon decreased to a little over 100 years.

The meat we eat is composed mainly of part of a muscle from an animal, along with varying amounts of fat and other tissues such as nerves and blood vessels, as well as many toxic substances that we cannot see. At the time of slaughter, all the vital processes that were taking place in the animal came to an abrupt halt and the toxins that were in the tissues at the moment of death remained there. Some of these products are urea, uric acid, creatinine, creatine, phenolic acid, adrenalin, possibly various bacteria and parasites, either alive or dead, various hormones, antibiotics, pesticides, herbicides, and other elements the animal had been exposed to or eaten while still alive.

Chemicals occasionally found in fish in some areas are lead, mercury, calcium, cadmium, zinc, antimony, and arsenic. Pesticides such as DDT are only very slowly degradable in the body, so it accumulates in the fat and muscles of animals. Meat, fish, and poultry contribute 13 times more DDT to the average diet than vegetables do.

Dr. Wynder of the American Health Federation stated: "It is our current estimate that some 50 percent of all female cancers in the Western world, and about one-third of all male cancers, are related to nutritional factors." As the consumption of animal fat and protein increases, the incidence of breast cancer increases in females and the incidence of colon cancer increases in both sexes. Women who eat large amounts of meat have a tenfold greater chance of developing breast cancer than those who eat little animal fat.

A one-pound charcoal-broiled steak, well done, contains 4 to 5 micrograms of benzopyrene, an amount equal to what a person would get from smoking about 300 cigarettes. During broiling, fat from the meat drips onto the charcoal, producing benzopyrene that distills back up onto the meat. Benzopyrene is one of the main cancer-producing agents found in tobacco smoke. In Iceland, where large amounts of smoked fish containing benzopyrene are consumed, there are large numbers of patients with cancer of the stomach and intestinal tract.

Food additives also add to the cancer danger. Nitrites, added to some meat to help it keep a healthy, fresh, pink color, may be changed to nitrosamines that are highly carcinogenic.

Animal proteins somehow alter the way that some bacteria act in our intestines. These bacteria change bile acids into potential cancer-forming compounds, and a low-fiber (meat) diet promotes constipation and prolongs the contact of these toxic compounds with the lining membrane of the colon, in this way promoting the development and growth of colon tumors.

The fat content of chicken has more than doubled in the past 20 years because of modern production techniques. In 1960 raw chicken contained 5 grams (about one teaspoonful) of fat in every 100 grams of edible meat. By 1980 this had tripled to 15 grams of fat in every 100 grams of meat. During the same 20 years the consumption of chicken increased from 23 pounds per person per year to 56 pounds per year. Sixty-three percent of the calories in a fast-food chicken dinner, with extra crispy dark meat, deep fried, and with mashed potatoes, gravy, and cole slaw come from the high fat content. This is enough to supply the recommended amount of fat for an entire day. Dark meat contains two to three times as much fat as light meat. Most of the fat is just beneath the skin and should be removed along with the skin if this meat is eaten.

The typical American diet with its high intake of fat and nearly twice the necessary amount of protein, has the following ill effects on the body.

1. An increased risk of colon, breast, and possibly prostate cancer.
2. Increases the formation of atherosclerosis in the arteries.

3. Causes softening of the bones by increasing the excretion of calcium.
4. Alters the normal immune mechanism.
5. Decreases stamina and depletes energy reserves.
6. A low-fiber diet results in constipation, diverticulosis, and hemorrhoids.
7. Increases the blood cholesterol and triglyceride levels.
8. Toxins found in the animals before they are slaughtered are eaten with the meat.
9. The risk of ingesting parasites, such as beef and hog worms, and bacteria.
10. Possible allergic problems from substances added to the food.

In the 1940s most nutritionists felt that it was not possible to obtain a nutritionally adequate diet without the use of meat. They have now had to revise these ideas, since numerous scientific studies have verified the fact that a well-planned vegetarian diet can be nutritionally adequate, with a supplemental source of vitamin B12 needed by strict vegetarians who use neither milk nor eggs.

Since deficiency diseases have been found in those eating meat as well as in vegetarians, it is clear that a nutritionally adequate diet involves much more than whether or not a person eats meat. In America today, it is not difficult to obtain a diet with all of the needed nutrients without eating meat, provided that a wide variety of food is eaten. This is very important since the greater the variety of food that is used in the diet the more likely it is that all the necessary nutrients will be supplied.

There are many reasons why some people choose not to eat meat. Among these are religious, ethical, economic, and ecological reasons; but the main reason is to have better health.

One concern of ecologists is that the world's food supply will not be able to keep up with the rapid increase in population, which amounts to about 208,000 persons a day. We have recently been made keenly aware of how close millions live to starvation every day, by the recent worldwide publicity given to the severe famine in Ethiopia, and other North African countries, where untold thousands have died of starvation.

In 1974 the President's Science Advisory Committee stated: "The world food problem is not a future threat. It is here and now." At the time this report was given, many hundreds were starving daily in India, Africa, and other underdeveloped areas of the world. The full impact of this statement was not felt, however, until 1985, when the severe famine in Ethiopia and some surrounding countries, during which hundreds of thousands of children and adults starved to death, was dramatically brought to the attention of the entire world.

It has been estimated that in 1974 there was about one acre of agricultural land for every person. This is far more than enough to provide an adequate food supply for a vegetarian, who requires only about one-fourth of an acre. Those who depend on animal protein for food, however, require about 3 acres of land per person. This is a very significant difference; about twelve times more land is needed to feed a meat-eater than a vegetarian. As the population of the United States increases, more and more good agricultural land is disappearing, as urban areas continue to expand further into the surrounding countryside.

Another way to look at it is this. If a man chooses to use his acre of land to feed cattle, he would be able to produce enough meat to supply his protein requirement for 77 days; if he used his acre to produce milk, his protein requirement could be met for 236 days; for 877 days if he grew wheat; and for 2,224 days if he used his acre to grow soybeans.

This comparison is emphasized even further when you realize that 21 pounds of protein must be fed to cattle in order to get one pound of protein in return. This difference between the amount of protein fed to cattle and the amount returned comes to 48 million tons, enough to meet 90 percent of the world's protein deficiency if it were fed to them as cereal.

At the present time, nearly one-half of all land that is harvested in the United States is planted in crops that are fed to animals. These crops include corn, oats, wheat, barley, soybeans, rye, and sorghum. Add to this a million tons of fish products, and you get some idea of the amount of our food resources that are used to produce meat. This is taking place at a time when millions around the world are either starving or are undernourished, and even though the vast majority of Americans get too much protein in their diet, starvation in the United States remains a daily threat for thousands.

Even though in Russia only 28 percent of their crops are used to feed animals, compared to 78 percent in the United States, their daily intake of protein is nearly the same as ours.

Is it any wonder, then, that the President's Science Advisory Committee states later in the same report that "the production of animal foods cannot be justified on an economic basis except in special cases."

While the heart-rending pictures of children dying from starvation have been projected by television into millions of homes around the world, another substance that few people give much thought to, but that is just as essential for maintaining life, has also been gradually getting more scarce. That substance is water. While our population continues to grow, and there seems to be an endless need for more water for industry, agriculture, drinking and other uses, more and more of our water supply is becoming contaminated and unfit for use.

But how is this connected with meat eating? Simply in this way: 2,500 gallons of water a day are required to provide food for a meat-eater, but only 300 gallons a day are needed for a vegetarian.

The name "vegetarian" was coined in 1842 by English vegetarians, and it was not very long ago that vegetarians were still looked upon as rather odd, even fanatical individuals. They were often called "grass eaters" and many other even less complimentary names. It was generally felt what was needed to do a "man's work" was lots of meat and potatoes.

TABLE I

THE AVERAGE DAILY PROTEIN INTAKE OF VEGETARIANS AND NON-VEGETARIANS

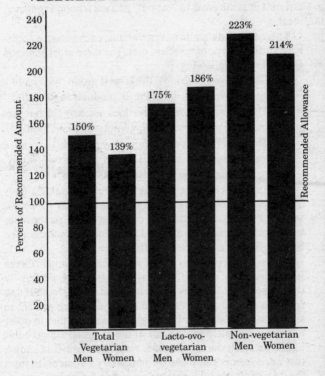

Taken from *Food For Us All-The Vegetarian Diet*, American Dietetic Association, 1981.

Today more and more people, especially in the younger generation, are turning to a vegetarian diet. With nearly three-quarters of a billion vegetarians in the world and about 7 million of them living in the United States (1 in every 32 Americans), being a vegetarian no longer carries the stigma that it once did. More restaurants are now providing for those who do not choose to eat meat, but even so it can still be difficult in some areas to "eat out" and get a good vegetarian meal.

There are many kinds of vegetarians, each eating a somewhat different type of meatless diet. The three most common groups are the following.

1. *Lacto-ovovegetarians,* the largest group, who include eggs as well as milk and milk products in their diet.

2. The *lacto-vegetarian,* who does not eat eggs but uses milk and milk products in addition to plant food.

3. The *total (pure) vegetarian, or vegan,* who eats no animal products of any kind. Fewer people follow this type of vegetarian diet than the other two.

Vegetarians who eat eggs, milk, and milk products have no difficulty in obtaining all the components that are necessary for a nutritionally adequate diet. The vegan, on the other hand, must be much more careful in the foods he selects. (See Special Notice, end of Section III).

The most practical way to make sure that our protein intake is adequate, not only in quantity but also in quality, is by supplementation of food proteins; that is, by combining foods so that all of the essential amino acids are present in sufficient amounts. It was thought at one time that in order to form a complete protein, all of the essential amino acids had to be eaten during the same meal. But now it is known that our systems can make up temporary deficiencies from the pool of amino acids that are present in the body. Combining the protein in eggs and milk with the protein from vegetable sources — grains, nuts, seeds, legumes, vegetables — raises the protein in the plant foods to a good biological value. With the vegan, however, supplementation of foods becomes more of a problem, but one that can and must be dealt with if a nutritionally adequate diet is to be obtained. For example, some grains such as corn, wheat, and polished rice, are high in the essential amino acid methionine but limited in lysine. These grains can be combined at the same meal with legumes such as lentils, beans, and peas that are low in methionine but high in lysine, and in this way good high quality proteins can be obtained.

Some other good supplementary food combinations for the vegan are as follows:

1. Combining grains with legumes.
2. Combining nuts and seeds with legumes.
3. Combining grains with vegetables.
4. Combining legumes with vegetables.

Grains combined with nuts and seeds may not furnish high quality protein.

In the United States today few cases of protein deficiency are seen. When they are found, they usually occur in those people who are not getting enough to eat. One problem with most American diets is that there is too much protein and not too little. The typical American eats about twice the amount of protein required by the body. The excess is either burned for fuel or stored in our body as fat. This places an increased work load on the kidneys and liver. A diet persistently high in protein and low in carbohydrates may cause permanent damage to the kidneys. It may also cause a loss of calcium from the bones resulting in osteoporosis (softening of the bones).

Since the turn of the century there has been a marked increase in the consumption of animal fat and protein, which now provides over two-thirds of the total protein consumption. In 1975 each person in the United States consumed 99 grams of protein a day, nearly twice the recommended dietary allowance. While it is true that animal foods in general provide a higher concentration of protein than plant foods, Table I clearly shows that even total vegetarians obtain more protein than the daily amount needed.

Vegans have to be especially careful to obtain enough of the following nutrients in their diet.

1. *Calcium*. Vegetarians in general need less of this mineral than those who eat meat, since less calcium is required when there is a reduced intake of protein. Calcium is present in dark green leafy vegetables; however, both spinach and chard contain oxalic acid, which combines with calcium to make it largely unavailable to the body. Soybeans, sesame seeds, dried fruit, citrus fruits, black strap molasses, and cauliflower are also good sources of calcium. Children may need to take fortified soy milk to be sure of developing strong bones and teeth.

2. *Riboflavin*. Found abundantly in green leafy vegetables. Also in mushrooms, squash, and almonds.

3. *Vitamin D*. This vitamin is obtained either by exposure of the skin to sunlight for 15 to 20 minutes each day or by drinking fortified soy milk if daily exposure to sunlight is not possible. Vitamin D increases the absorption of calcium and phosphorus from the intestinal tract.

4. *Zinc*. Found in legumes and whole grains. Wheat germ is high in zinc.

5. *Iron*. Iron is found in legumes, dried fruits, and green leafy vegetables. It is also present in whole grains, especially if eaten in yeast bread. The yeast destroys the phytates in the grain so that they cannot combine with the iron and zinc and render them unavailable to the body. The 10 mg of iron required daily in males is readily obtained in a vegetarian diet if a variety of foods high in iron is eaten. But the 18 mg of iron required by females is much more difficult to obtain without the use of fortified foods. An iron deficiency anemia is frequently found in women throughout the world. This may result from

an inadequate intake of foods containing iron, the improper absorption of iron from the intestines or from an increased blood loss. The increased fiber and phytates in a vegetarian diet may also result in the decreased absorption of both iron and zinc from the intestines: taking some vitamin C at the same meal increases the absorption of these two minerals and tends to counteract the action of the phytates. Cooking in a cast-iron pot will also increase your iron intake. A recent study has shown that the iron nutritional status of vegetarians and meat eaters is essentially the same. Vegans must be sure to eat foods with a high iron content every day. If this is not possible, they should take an iron supplement. Others who may need an iron supplement are infants, women that have an unusually heavy menstrual flow, and women who are pregnant.

6. *Vitamin B_{12}.* The question of vitamin B_{12} always comes up when vegetarianism is discussed. This is the vitamin of which we need the smallest amount — only three millionths of a gram per day. Vitamin B_{12} is not found in plant sources. Only the total vegetarian has any difficulty in obtaining enough vitamin B_{12}, since large amounts are found in milk and eggs. Perhaps the best way for a vegan to obtain a sufficient amount of this vitamin is to take a B_{12} supplement or use fortified soy milk, breakfast cereal, or meat analogs. Comfrey is also a source of vitamin B_{12}; twelve comfrey tablets a day are necessary, however, to fulfill the body's need for this vitamin. Miso, a fermented soybean product used as a flavoring agent, can also be used as a source of vitamin B_{12}. If children on a total vegetarian diet have difficulty in eating enough of this type of food, soy milk that is fortified with calcium, riboflavin, and

vitamins D and B_{12} can be used. Some people who have been total vegetarians for 15 or 20 years are still found to have normal blood levels of vitamin B_{12}, while others have low blood levels after being on the same diet for only three or four years. The reason for this difference is not known, but it is known that vitamin B_{12} may be stored in the liver for many years. It is also recognized that the reabsorption of vitamin B_{12} from the intestines is very efficient.

A recent study reported in the *New England Journal of Medicine* showed that a low protein, largely vegetarian diet could stop the advance of various kidney diseases in many persons. Such diseases included diabetes, high blood pressure, and chronic glomerulonephritis. Many persons with these diseases were saved from a kidney transplant operation or from going on renal dialysis treatments by using a nearly totally meat-free diet.

Research on the relation of diet to coronary artery disease, reported in the *Journal of the American Medical Association,* June 3, 1961, by Dr. W.A. Thomas, showed that a vegetarian diet can prevent 90 percent of clots from forming in arteries and veins and 97 percent of coronary heart attacks.

The American Heart Association in 1961 issued a report on dietary fat and its relation to heart attacks and strokes. This report, which was updated in 1965, recommends the following.

1.   To eat less animal (saturated) fat.
2.   To increase the intake of unsaturated vegetable oils and other polyunsaturated fats, substituting them for saturated fats wherever possible.
3.   To eat less food rich in cholesterol.
4.   If overweight, to reduce caloric intake so that a desirable weight is achieved and maintained.
5.   To start to apply these dietary recommendations early in life.

6. To maintain the principles of good nutrition that are important with any change in the diet. Professional nutritional advice may be necessary in order to assure that correct adherence to the diet will not result in any imbalance or deficiency.

7. To adhere consistently to the above dietary recommendations, so that a decrease in the concentration of blood fats may be both achieved and maintained.

8. To make sound food habits a "family affair," so that the benefits of proper nutritional practices — including the avoidance of high blood fat levels — may accrue to all members of the family.

In summary, some of the important benefits of following a vegetarian diet are the following.

1. Less colon, breast, and possibly prostatic cancer.
2. Greater bone strength.
3. Lower blood pressure.
4. Lower serum cholesterol and triglyceride (blood fat) levels.
5. Less obesity.
6. Less expense.
7. Less heart disease.
8. Fewer problems with constipation, diverticulosis, and hemorrhoids.
9. Less chance of developing varicose veins.
10. Less exposure to toxins present in meat.
11. Conservation of the world's food supply.
12. No danger of ingesting parasites, bacteria, carcinogens, or other toxic substances found in meat.
13. Vegetarianism doesn't require the cruel treatment and slaughter of animals.

8

MILK

For many people, drinking cow's milk is like taking a poison. Half the invalids in the world suffer from dyspepsia and milk may be the cause. In some people, milk causes constipation, biliousness, coated tongue, and headache. All these are the symptoms of intestinal autointoxication. Soybean milk and nut milks are excellent substitutes and have practically the same nutritional analysis, but with the danger of autointoxication removed.

ANNOTATION: A large number of adults, and some children as well, have either an absence or a deficiency of the enzyme lactase that is normally present in the intestinal tract. Lactase breaks down the lactose (the sugar in milk) to simple sugars so that they can be absorbed. If the milk sugar remains unchanged as it passes through the digestive tract, it causes gas, bloating, cramps, and diarrhea. If you find that drinking cow's milk or eating milk products causes you to have these symptoms, they should be eliminated from the diet to see if you get relief, and special milk that already has lactase added should be used.

It is probably true that more people are allergic to cow's milk than to any other food. Infants and children seem to be especially susceptible and may develop severe diaper rash or some other type of skin rash, diarrhea, breathing trouble, asthma, or irritability. These symptoms may begin shortly after cow's milk is first used, or they may not show up for several years.

Milk is an excellent source of calcium and also supplies good amounts of phosphorus, riboflavin, vitamin D, and high-grade protein (refer to Table I). One-and-one-half pints of milk a day provides 855 mg of calcium, which is more than the recommended daily allowance of 800 mg. One cup (8 ounces) of milk supplies 300 mg or about one-third of the daily requirement. It also supplies 20 percent of the protein and 5 percent of the vitamin D requirement. Women who have passed the menopause need more calcium, because of weakening of the bones with the consequent possibility of fracture. The recommended daily intake of calcium for such women is 1200 to 1500 mg.

The disadvantage of whole milk is its high content of cholesterol and saturated fats. Low fat or nonfat milk should be used instead (See Table II). Since this form of milk does not have the fat-soluble vitamins, it is usually fortified with vitamins A and D. In a cup of whole milk there are over 8 grams of fat, while in the same amount of nonfat milk there is less than half a gram of fat.

Nondairy creamers have about 30 calories per tablespoon and in addition they usually contain coconut oil, which is very high in saturated fats.

While modern methods of milk processing have eliminated most of the serious diseases once spread by contaminated milk, it is true that even today pasteurized cow's milk can be the source of bacteria that cause serious illness. (See Section VII, Chapter 3, Danger from Disease in Animals.)

TABLE I

THE NUTRITIONAL VALUE OF VARIOUS KINDS OF MILK COMPARED WITH ORANGE JUICE

1 cup (8 ounces)	GRAMS					MINERALS - MG						VITAMINS - MG						
	CALORIES	PROTEIN	CARBOHYDRATE	FIBER	FAT	SODIUM	CALCIUM	PHOSPHORUS	POTASSIUM	MAGNESIUM	IRON	THIAMINE	NIACIN	A (I.U.)	RIBOFLAVIN	C	D
Orange juice	111	1.7	25.8	0.3	0.6	3	27	42	496	—	0.5	.22	1.0	496	.07	124	—
Whole Milk 3.25% fat	150	8.1	11.5	—	8.1	120	291	228	370	33	0.1	.09	0.2	307	.39	2	100
Low-fat Milk 2% fat	122	8.1	11.7	—	4.7	122	298	232	374	34	0.1	.10	0.2	500	.40	2	100
Skim Milk	89	8.0	11.9	—	0.4	128	303	251	418	27	0.1	.10	0.2	502	.34	2	100
Soybean Milk	87	8.9	5.8	—	3.9	51	55	126	310	57	2.1	.21	0.5	105	.08	—	—

From Bowes and Church's *Food Values of Portions Commonly Used*; Thirteenth ed., 1980; J.B. Lippincott Company.

TABLE II

FAT CONTENT AND CALORIES IN MILK AND DAIRY PRODUCTS

	Percent Fat	Calories per Cup
Whole milk	3.3	150
Low-fat milk (2%)	2.0	120
Low-fat milk (1%)	1.0	100
Nonfat (skim) milk	trace	85
Buttermilk	trace	100
Chocolate milk	3.3	210
Chocolate drink (low fat)	2.0	180
Plain yogurt (low fat)	2.0	145
Flavored yogurt (low fat)	2.0	230

Source: Nutritive Value of Foods. U.S. Department of Agriculture, Home and Garden Bulletin No.72, Washington, D.C. 1977, p.5-7.

9

SALT

Salt should be used sparingly. It is sodium chloride, which is an inorganic mineral and cannot be used by any cell structure in the body. It irritates the stomach and the bloodstream, is indigestible, and hinders the digestion of other foods. It is one of the causes of high blood pressure and should be restricted in the diets of patients with heart disease as well as those with certain types of kidney and liver disease.

Sodium salts are plentiful in fruits and vegetables such as tomatoes, asparagus, celery, spinach, kale, radishes, turnips, carrots, lettuce, strawberries, and many others.

When no salt is added to food, a person soon learns to enjoy the flavor more. The main taste of people who use any quantity of salt is a salty one. But without salt, more food flavors may be enjoyed. Salt must not be used by patients with dropsy, which is a swelling of the soft tissues due to an abnormal collection of fluid and is commonly seen in those who have heart failure or kidney disease. Swelling of the ankles may be an early sign of heart failure. Salt should also be restricted in persons who have hyperacidity, Bright's disease, gastric ulcer, obesity, epilepsy, and high blood pressure.

The word salt comes from the Latin word "salus," meaning health. Salt has been used as a preservative for centuries. Roman soldiers at one time received their pay in salt, not in coins, and from this custom the word "salary" originated.

During the past 10 to 15 years, salt has been so widely proclaimed as a health hazard that 40 percent of adults are now trying to cut down on their salt consumption and another 20 to 30 percent are worried lest they get too much salt in their food.

The sodium in our diet comes from three approximately equal sources:

1. Salt that is naturally present in food.
2. Salt that is added to food by commercial processors.
3. Salt that we add to food, either during cooking or at the table.

Table salt is composed of sodium (40 percent) and chloride (60 percent). The sodium is responsible for fluid retention in the tissues of persons with some types of heart, liver, or kidney disease.

But sodium is an indispensable mineral in our bodies. It helps maintain the proper water balance, assists in muscle contraction, aids in the proper functioning of the nervous system, maintains the correct balance of acids in both the blood and urine, and aids in the absorption of nutrients through the cell membranes.

The recommended daily allowance of salt is 3 to 8 grams, or 1100 to 3300 mg of sodium.

The average daily intake of salt is 6 to 17 grams, or 2300 to 6900 mg of sodium.

One teaspoon of salt has about 2000 mg of sodium.

Following are some ways to reduce the amount of sodium in your diet.

1. Remove the salt shaker from the dinner table. This may be done gradually over two or three weeks.
2. Cut down by one-half the amount of salt added to food while cooking.
3. Omit or limit salty foods.
4. Eat fresh fruit and vegetables when possible. Canned vegetables may have up to 10 times as much sodium as fresh vegetables.
5. Eat unsalted frozen vegetables rather than canned.
6. Cut down on the consumption of prepared foods.
7. Avoid foods with MSG on the label. Oriental food is high in MSG (monosodium glutamate), which has been reported to cause mental confusion and/or headaches in some people. This has been termed the "Chinese Restaurant Syndrome."

Probably the best-known harmful effect of salt is its propensity to cause high blood pressure, particularly in susceptible individuals.

Some processed foods contain quite large amounts of sodium. If you are concerned about the amount of sodium you are eating, be sure to check the food labels. If you must reduce your salt intake, look for foods with "low sodium," "salt free," or "no added salt" on the label.

Foods High in Salt

Cheese
"fast foods"
Processed meat:
  luncheon meat
  corned beef
  franks
  sausage
  salami
  cured ham and bacon
Canned soups
Canned fish:
  herring
  sardines
  anchovies
Bouillon broth
Canned Vegetables

Frozen dinners
Bread
Celery salt
Garlic salt
Onion salt
Salted snacks and nuts
Sauces:
  Worcestershire
  ketchup
  soy sauce
Pickles, olives
Frozen entrees
Sauerkraut
Drinking water, specially
  if water softener is used.

Most Common Food Additives Containing Sodium

1. Table salt (sodium chloride)
2. Monosodium glutamate (MSG)
3. Baking powder
4. Baking soda

Sodium Content of Some Selected Foods

Food	Portion	Sodium (mg)
Coffee, instant:		
regular	1 cup	1
with flavoring	1 cup	124
Cheese, natural:		
cheddar	1 ounce	176
Swiss	1 ounce	74
Roquefort	1 ounce	513
cottage cheese	1 ounce	114
Milk, whole or		
low-fat	1 cup	122
Buttermilk	1 cup	257
Fish:		
herring, smoked	3 ounces	5234
halibut	3 ounces	114
shrimp, canned	3 ounces	1955
Meat:		
chipped beef	1 ounce	1219
cured ham	3 ounces	1114
frankfurter	1 frank	639
Prepared dishes:		
beef and macaroni	1 cup	1185
chili con carne	1 cup	1194
Frozen dinners:		
beef	1 dinner	998
meat loaf	1 dinner	1304
chopped sirloin	1 dinner	978
Corned beef hash	1 cup	1520
Swedish meat balls	8 ounces	1880
Veal parmigiana	7 ounces	1825
Fast foods:		
cheeseburger	1 each	709

Food	Portion	Sodium (mg)
chicken dinner	1 portion	2243
fish sandwich	1 sandwich	882
hamburger	1 each	461
taco	1 each	401
pizza, cheese	1/4 pie	599
Grains:		
bread:		
white	1 slice	114
whole wheat	1 slice	132
Cereals:		
Cream of Wheat:		
regular	3/4 cup	2
quick	3/4 cup	126
All-Bran	1/3 cup	160
Raisin Bran	1/2 cup	209
Cheerios	1 1/4 cup	304
Rice Krispies	1 cup	340
Corn flakes	1 cup	256
Pancake mix	1 cup	2036
Legumes and nuts:		
almonds, salted	1 cup	311
beans, baked, canned		
Boston style	1 cup	606
kidney, canned	1 cup	844
pinto, cooked	1 cup	4
cashews, salted	1 cup	1200
peanut butter	1 tbsp	81
Soups:		
beef broth (cube)	1 cup	1152
chicken noodle	1 cup	1107
minestrone	1 cup	911
pea	1 cup	987
tomato	1 cup	872

Food	Portion	Sodium (mg)
vegetable beef	1 cup	957
Vegetables:		
asparagus:		
frozen	4 spears	4
canned	4 spears	298
lima beans, cooked	1 cup	2
lima beans, canned	1 cup	456
corn, cooked	1 ear	1
corn, canned, cream	1 cup	671
peas, green, cooked	1 cup	2
peas, green, canned	1 cup	493
potatoes:		
baked or boiled	1 medium	5
canned	1 cup	753
au gratin	1 cup	1095
sauerkraut, canned	1 cup	1554
spinach, cooked	1 cup	49
spinach, canned	1 cup	910
tomatoes, raw	1 tomato	14
tomatoes, canned	1 cup	584
tomato juice	1 cup	878
Condiments, Fats, Oils:		
baking powder	1 tsp	339
baking soda	1 tsp	821
catsup	1 tbsp	156
garlic salt	1 tsp	1850
meat tenderizer	1 tsp	1750
olives, green	4 olives	323
onion salt	1 tsp	1620
dill pickle	1 pickle	928
salt	1 tsp	1938
soy sauce	1 tbsp	1029
French dressing	1 tbsp	214

Food	Portion	Sodium (mg)
Thousand Island dressing:		
regular	1 tbsp	109
low calorie	1 tbsp	153

10

GARLIC

For nearly as long as there has been a written record of history, garlic has been mentioned as a food. It probably originated in central Asia, but now it is cultivated in many countries and grows wild in Italy and southern Europe. The garlic bulb is divided into 10 to 20 smaller sections called cloves, and the entire bulb is covered with a rather scaly membrane.

During the time of the Pharaohs, when Egypt was at the peak of its power, garlic was given to the laborers and slaves who were building the great pyramids in order to increase their stamina and strength as well as to protect them from disease. In the fifth century A.D., the Greek historian Herodotus wrote that on an Egyptian pyramid there are inscriptions in Egyptian characters describing the amount of garlic, onions, and radishes consumed by the workers and slaves who were building the great pyramid of King Khufu (Cheops).

It was not until centuries later that certain substances were isolated from garlic and onions that were found to be effective against such constantly present Egyptian scourges as cholera, typhoid fever, and amebic dysentery. Garlic was also used by the Egyptian soldiers as a way to increase their courage during battle. The Ebers Papyrus, an Egyptian medical papyrus dated sometime around 1500 B.C., mentions garlic twenty two times as a remedy for a variety of diseases. Hippocrates, the father of modern medicine, used garlic as a laxative, a diuretic, for tumors of the uterus, leprosy, epilepsy, chest pains, toothaches, and for wounds incurred during battle. Aristotle also mentions the value of garlic and Aristophanes used garlic as a treatment for impotence.

The Bible clearly states that for 400 years (probably around 1730 to 1330 B.C.), while the Israelites were slaves in Egypt and no doubt being forced to help build some of the pyramids, garlic, as well as some of the other herbs in the same family, was a part of their diet. Shortly after they had been delivered from slavery by Moses, and were traveling through the bleak desert country of the Sinai peninsula, they began complaining of their food and wishing for the same things they had been eating while they were slaves: "Oh, that we had some of the delicious fish we enjoyed so much in Egypt, and the wonderful cucumbers and melons, leeks, onions, and garlic!" Numbers 11:5, *The Living Bible.*

Garlic is mentioned in the literature of all of the great ancient world kingdoms: Babylon, Medo-Persia, Greece, and Rome. The great Roman naturalist Pliny the Elder recommended garlic for intestinal disorders, dog and snake bites, asthma, tuberculosis, convulsions, tumors, and scorpion stings in his "Historia Naturalis." Garlic was probably introduced into Japan from Korea along with Buddhism in about 30 B.C. Dioscorides, the chief medical officer in the Roman army in the first century A.D., used garlic to treat intestinal worms.

Down through the centuries garlic has been used as a treatment for all sorts of diseases. Some of the most common of these are: lung problems, including pneumonia, asthma, and bronchitis; various skin disorders such as leprosy, acne, athlete's foot, dandruff, and ringworm; intestinal illnesses such as gastric ulcer, gastritis, constipation, diarrhea, worms, hemorrhoids, pinworms, cholera, amebic dysentery; arthritis, rheumatism, high blood pressure, tuberculosis, some forms of cancer, diabetes, anemia, heavy metal poisoning, epilepsy, whooping cough, colds, typhus, conjunctivitis, cold sores, hypoglycemia, spinal meningitis, diphtheria, and snake bites.

Because of its strong, disagreeable odor, garlic is most often used today only in small amounts, either mixed with other foods or as a seasoning, so even though it does contain vitamins A, C, and B1 as well as the minerals copper, iron, zinc, tin, calcium, potassium, aluminum, sulphur, selenium, and germanium, the limited amount that is eaten prevents these nutrients from being a significant factor in our diets. The assimilation of vitamin B_1 (thiamine) is reportedly enhanced by the presence of garlic.

Garlic, whose scientific name is allium sativum, belongs to the lily family and is closely related to onions, leeks, scallions, and chives. All of these are known for their pungent, irritating, and unpleasant odor.

Garlic is one of the best plant sources of sulphur. There are about 67 mg of sulphur in every 100 grams of garlic. It is mainly the sulphur-containing compounds in garlic that are responsible for its medicinal effects.

Garlic may be eaten raw, but most people can eat only small amounts of raw garlic, and even then it is usually mixed with other foods. In some of the countries in southern Europe, however, larger amounts of garlic are a common ingredient in the food.

Raw garlic, when eaten to excess, is not completely harmless; it may cause anemia as well as various digestive problems. It may also result in burns in the mouth, throat, esophagus, and stomach. Garlic can be taken in tablet form, either with or without parsley. The parsley is added to the tablets in an attempt to neutralize the offensive garlic odor. Odorless capsules are also available at most health food stores.

During the 1940s Dr. Arthur Stoll, a chemist working in Switzerland, was able to extract an oil from garlic that he named alliin. He also discovered an enzyme in the garlic, to which he gave the name of aminase. Aminase was found to change the alliin to allicin when the garlic was cut or crushed. It is the allicin that is responsible for the garlic odor as well as for the antibacterial properties used during both World Wars. It is an oxidizer and a strong disinfectant. In fact, even when it is diluted with water 1/80,000 or even as much as 1/120,000, it is still able to kill the germs that cause cholera and typhoid fever.

Garlic contains more allicin than any of its close relatives —onions, leeks, chives, or scallions. The allicin can be destroyed by heating the garlic, but unfortunately heat also destroys the other nutrients that are present. Allicin is also slowly destroyed by aging: it takes nearly two years for all of the allicin to become inactive. The other nutrients survive the aging process.

Interest in the possible medicinal uses of garlic has increased markedly within the last decade or so, and during this time numerous experiments have been conducted in animals as well as in humans. The effect of garlic on the cardiovascular system (the heart and blood vessels) has been the subject of much recent investigation. Studies show that animals fed garlic extract have increased physical endurance, decreased blood pressure, and less buildup of fatty deposits in the walls of the blood vessels. There has also been considerable study given to garlic acting as an antibiotic and also as an anticancer agent.

As discussed in Section IV, Chapter 3, Fats, the heart muscle is supplied with blood and oxygen by the coronary arteries. If these arteries become narrowed by plaques forming on their inner lining, the heart muscle cannot obtain as much oxygen as it needs to function properly, particularly during times of increased activity or stress, and the well-recognized pain of angina pectoris results. If an artery should become completely blocked, a fatal heart attack may occur. Coronary artery disease is still the number one killer in the United States, and will result in over half-a-million deaths in 1985, with more than twice that number surviving a heart attack. Over $60 billion is spent each year in treating this disease.

Our blood cholesterol level is an important indicator of the risk we run of having a heart attack. A total cholesterol level below 150 mg is best, and the simplest way for most people to keep their blood cholesterol level down is to reduce the amount of cholesterol and saturated fats in their diet.

In order for cholesterol, a fat-like substance normally produced in the liver and essential for several important body functions, to be transported in the blood, it must be connected to a special protein. This union of cholesterol, which itself is a fat (lipid), with a protein is known as a lipoprotein. The total cholesterol in the blood is made up of several of these lipoproteins. The two most important are low-density lipoproteins (LDL) and high-density lipoproteins (HDL).

The LDL is bad. It promotes the formation of cholesterol deposits, called plaques, on the inside of the arteries, causing them to become narrow or sometimes completely blocked. When the total blood cholesterol is elevated, the LDL is almost always increased also.

HDL is good. It opposes the LDL and tends to prevent the formation of cholesterol plaques in the arteries. Since women in general have higher levels of HDL than men, this is probably the reason they have fewer heart attacks.

The importance of both lowering the total blood cholesterol and LDL and raising the HDL is clear. The simplest and least expensive way for most people to do this is to cut down on the total fat in the diet, use more unsaturated and less saturated fat, stop smoking, get regular exercise, and maintain a normal body weight.

Now what is the connection between garlic and all that we have just been saying? Simply this. Recent studies have shown that garlic prevents or slows down the formation of plaques in the blood vessels. It does this by lowering the total amount of cholesterol in the blood as well as the amount of injurious low-density lipoproteins, while at the same time increasing the amount of protective high-density lipoproteins.

A well-controlled study was recently reported in the *American Journal of Clinical Nutrition* written by A. Bordia, MD. He gave capsules of garlic oil each day for six months to healthy volunteers. The amount given was equivalent to eating 10 average-sized garlic cloves each day. At the end of 6 months, he found that the total blood cholesterol level had dropped 14 percent, LDL-cholesterol dropped 17 percent, while the beneficial HDL-cholesterol rose by 41 percent. Triglycerides were also significantly decreased.

Garlic has been used for centuries in China and Japan to treat high blood pressure. In 1948 Piotrowsky published a paper showing that he was able to lower the blood pressure in nearly one-half of 100 patients that he treated with garlic. The blood pressure decreased 20 mm Hg or more after only one week of treatment. He felt that this beneficial effect was due to dilatation of the blood vessels caused by the garlic.

Some studies have shown that garlic acts to prevent the blood from clotting so readily. The compound responsible for this action has been named ajoene, and has just recently been isolated from garlic by Dr. Eric Block and his co-workers at New York State University. In 1979 Sainani, at the University of Poona, India, studied three groups of people living in the Jain community in India. All of these people were vegetarians and their diets were all essentially the same except for the amount of garlic and onions that were eaten daily. One group ate garlic and onions liberally every day; the second group ate a lesser amount every day; the third group never ate either garlic or onions. It was found that those who ate the most garlic and onions (the first group) had the least tendency for the blood to clot; that is, they had the longest blood clotting time. This study also revealed that the fasting cholesterol blood levels for the three groups was respectively: 159, 172, and 208 mg percent. The total triglycerides in the blood were 52, 75, and 109 mg percent. This clearly demonstrated that those who never ate garlic or onions had the highest blood levels of triglyceride and cholesterol.

An experiment using two hunting dogs was reported in *Runner's World* of December 1979 by D. Gasque. The two dogs were initially found to run equally well behind the trainer's truck. Fresh garlic was then added to the diet of one of the dogs for two weeks, but otherwise there was no difference in the diets. After two weeks, the dogs were again allowed to run behind the truck, and it was found that the dog that had been fed the garlic showed much less fatigue after running for a distance of three miles, and was several hundred yards ahead of the other dog.

Garlic has been regarded by some as having the effect of a broad spectrum antibiotic, the active ingredient being allicin. Garlic was reported to have saved many lives during the great plagues of the Middle Ages that swept through Europe killing millions. Even as early as 1858, Louis Pasteur noted the mild antibacterial action of garlic. Near the turn of this century, several reports indicated that garlic was remarkably effective in the treatment of tuberculosis. During both world wars garlic was used successfully as an antiseptic and disinfectant to prevent infection and gangrene in wounds. Dr. Albert Schweitzer, while working as a medical missionary in Africa, used garlic to treat cholera, typhus, and also amebic dysentery with apparent good results. In Russia today garlic is used extensively in treating various infections; in fact, it has earned the name of "Russian penicillin." Garlic juice has been found to be active against many fungi and yeasts as well as bacteria; it even inhibits the growth of several bacteria that are found to be resistant to some antibiotics.

Garlic has also been studied as a possible cure for cancer. During the 1950s and 1960s, several animal studies were published that gave encouraging results. Germanium and selenium, which are both present in garlic, have also been investigated as possibly having a beneficial effect on cancer.

While the majority of studies have given encouraging results, a few problems have arisen. When raw garlic was fed to rats in high doses it was found to cause anemia, weight loss, and failure to grow properly. The nearly universal agreement regarding the unacceptable odor of garlic, that affects not only the breath but also the perspiration, is another problem. Moreover, an occasional person will be found who is allergic to garlic and will develop a contact dermatitis, with redness and itching of the skin.

11

HEALTHFUL DIETS

The fundamental principal of true healing consists of the return to natural habits of living. Proper diet is of much more value than medicine in the production and maintenance of good health. There is today a greater menace to civilization than that of war. This menace is malnutrition.

We eat too much and most of what we eat is poison to our system. Half of what we eat keeps us alive, and the other half keeps the physicians alive. As well as eating too much, we do not masticate our food thoroughly. Since many of our diseases can be traced to improper diet, the cure for these ailments is a correct, well-balanced diet.

A true diet is not based on calories but on the organic and inorganic elements that promote and sustain life. Many of our most common and serious diseases are caused by wrong habits of eating and drinking, including the use of tobacco, alcohol, and drugs. This has been proven by numerous scientific experiments in recent years. When food is absorbed by the body, it will nourish, repair, and furnish life force and heat to the body, but if in its preparation and refining the life-giving elements are taken away, it cannot furnish life force, but instead it will clog the normal functions of the body and result in many disorders.

Many diseases are nature's effort to free our system of poisons that result from wrong habits of eating and drinking. When we assist nature in expelling impurities and in reestablishing right conditions in the system, we can overcome disease.

The whole nation needs more vitamins, better cooks, more care exercised in the preparation of our food, and smaller hospitals.

The human race has been growing more and more self-indulgent until health is being sacrificed on the altar of appetite.

God gave our first parents food that He designed for the human race to eat. Only after the world was destroyed by a flood did He give permission to eat flesh foods, since all vegetation was dead, but then only the clean animals, as given in the Bible in Leviticus, Chapter 11. Animal foods are not, however, the most healthful foods for humans. Recent scientific research and experiments have proven this beyond a doubt. The diet given to Adam and Eve in the Garden of Eden did not include flesh meats. We should learn how to avoid and overcome sickness by correct eating and living.

A. NORMAL DIET FOR THE AVERAGE PERSON

First, observe the following rules for eating.

Diet Rules

1. Do not eat fruits and vegetables together.
2. Do not eat between meals.
3. Do not drink any liquid with meals.
4. Allow five hours between meals.

Second, more care must be exercised in the cooking of food every day so as not to destroy during preparation the vitamins, minerals, and other life-giving properties.

Third, 75 to 85 percent alkaline food should be used in the everyday diet. If you have any ailments, your diet should be at least 90 percent alkaline base-forming foods. Eating acid foods brings on disease, while alkaline foods overcome disease and help to prevent it.

Fruits

all berries	apricots	apples	pears
grapefruit	cherries	lemons	plums
pineapple	raisins	grapes	figs
quinces	bananas	prunes	dates
peaches	oranges	melons	limes

Do not use cane sugar on fruits. Do not eat bananas unless they have dark spots on the skins and the ends are not green. Dried fruits are good if they are not sulphured. Do not mix more than two kinds of fruit at a meal. It is best to eat fruits raw. Applesauce is very good if the whole apple is cooked - skin, core (unless wormy), and seeds-then strained through a colander or sieve. Raisins added to applesauce make a very delicious dish.

Vegetables

asparagus
beets
beet tops
celery
cabbage (uncooked)
cauliflower
carrots
cucumbers
turnips
tomatoes
dandelions
Irish potatoes (unpeeled)
kale
lettuce
onions
okra
parsley
greens of all kinds
watercress
parsnip
pumpkin
rutabagas
sweet potatoes
squash
Swiss chard
all sprouts
spinach
beans

Legumes

soybeans
green beans
dried beans of any kind
split peas
lentils
lima beans
garbanzos (chickpeas)
peanuts
wax beans
navy beans
string beans
peas

Legumes are very high in protein and therefore are useful

as meat substitutes. As an example, peanut butter contains four grams of protein per tablespoon. The proteins contained in legumes are an adequate substitute for meat proteins if they are combined with the proteins in wheat or corn products.

B. RAW DIET

I believe in eating everything in its raw and natural state as far as possible, of the foods that can be digested. I just read an article by a man who thinks we should never cook anything, but eat it raw as people did in the beginning of time. But this fact is generally overlooked: foods are not as they were in the beginning.

In the beginning, fruits, grains, and nuts grew all the year around, and there was no need to can, cook, and bake as there is today. The wheat, rye, barley, oats, beans, and nuts were never hard and dry as they are now. There were fresh fruits and grains the year around, and they were eaten in their milky or grape sugar state, in which they needed scarcely any digestion. When our green corn is in the grape sugar state, it can be easily digested and requires very little cooking. After it matures and gets dry, it has turned into a starchy state, and will take a longer time to digest. Therefore, we need to grind and bake it. If properly baked, it turns the starch back into grape sugar, to a great extent.

Starch comes only from plant foods but there is an abundance of it in our food supply. Some foods rich in starch are nuts, grains, peas, corn, lentils, dried beans, sunflower seeds, potatoes, parsnips, and winter squash.

Much impurity is produced in the system by too much protein. Now we know how to prepare our food, and also what foods to eat to balance the amount of protein with other foods. Too much protein overtaxes the system. The corn, wheat, peas, and beans in their milky state, before they are full-grown, contain three or four percent protein, but are high in minerals and life-giving properties. When they mature, the wheat has from eight to fourteen percent protein; the dried corn a little less; while the beans have from twenty to thirty percent more. All beans, lentils, and corn may be picked and canned in the milky state. Being thus very low in protein, all can eat freely of them. Peas, beans, lentils, and grains can be sprouted, which turns the protein into peptogen to a great extent, and starches and sugars into dextrose and grape sugar. They are then very easy to digest. Moreover, the sprouts have a very good flavor, and are high in life-giving properties. Sprouting increases the amount of protein and also the water-soluble vitamins, B complex and C. Leafy vegetables, such as spinach, lettuce, celery, and cabbage, are good when eaten in their natural state.

Clean, freshly prepared raw vegetable juices are excellent to supply the body with natural minerals, salt, and vitamins. Of course, it is necessary that they be properly macerated so that the life elements are released into the liquid.

APPROXIMATE TIME REQUIRED FOR DIGESTION (in hours)

Rice, boiled	1
Barley, boiled	2
Carrot, boiled	3 1/4
Beets, boiled	3 1/2
Egg (soft-boiled)	3
Egg (hard-boiled)	3 1/2
Egg (fried)	3 1/2
Egg (raw)	2
Butter	3 1/2
Bread, whole wheat	3 1/2
Bread, corn	3 1/4
Vegetable, hash, warmed	2 1/2
Parsnips, boiled	2 1/2
Green corn and beans, boiled	3 3/4
Milk, boiled	2
Milk, raw	2 1/2

Turnips, boiled 3 1/2

Potatoes, Irish 2 1/2
(baked)

Potatoes, Irish 3 1/2
(boiled)

Cabbage, raw 2 1/2

Cabbage, boiled 4 1/2

Apples, hard and sour, raw 3

Apples, sweet and mellow, raw . . . 2

C. FRUIT DIET

All fruits contain acids, which are necessary for the proper elimination of various toxins, poisonous acids, and other impurities. These natural acids are highly alkaline after they have been reduced in the body.

The value of a fruit diet cannot be overestimated, especially in sickness, ill health, or whenever the body is filled with poisons. Germs cannot grow and live in fruit juices. The germs that cause typhoid fever and cholera cannot resist the action of fruit juices such as lemon, orange, pineapple, strawberry, apple, and grapefruit. A fruit diet will disinfect the stomach and alimentary canal. Fresh fruits are more effective for this purpose than stewed or canned fruits.

Malic, citric, and tartaric acids are powerful germicides found in fruits.

Malic acid is found in pineapples, apples, quinces, pears, apricots, plums, peaches, cherries, currants, gooseberries, strawberries, raspberries, blackberries, elderberries, grapes, and tomatoes.

Citric acid is found in strawberries, red raspberries, cherries, red currants, cranberries, lemons, limes, grapefruit, and oranges.

Tartaric acid is obtained from grapes and pineapples. Tartaric acid is important in treating all diseases that have hyperacidity, such as lung diseases, sore throat, indigestion, peptic ulcer, etc.

Oxalic acid is found in plums, tomatoes, rhubarb, sorrel, yellow dock, and spinach. It is especially good for both constipation and an inactive liver. But a word of caution should be given about eating foods high in oxalates. About 10 percent of Americans will, at some time during their lives, develop a kidney stone, and most kidney stones are at least partly composed of oxalates. Therefore, if you have trouble with kidney stones you should not eat foods that have a high content of oxalates.

Lactic acid is found in buttermilk, clabber milk and soybean buttermilk. It is good for the treatment of fermentation and putrefaction, and in treating hardening of the arteries it is especially good.

It is best to use fruits uncooked. Never sweeten them with cane sugar.

A fruit diet is an excellent cure for chronic constipation, and is also good for reducing. Fruit gives the body strength and energy. Fruits are solvents. and should always be used abundantly while on an eliminating diet.

Fruit is an ideal food. It grows more slowly than other foods, and therefore it receives the beneficial effects of the sunlight and air for a longer time.

Dates, raisins, figs, and many other dried fruits have become staple foods in many countries. Dates and raisins are high in natural sugar, so they are very easily assimilated. Dried figs, especially Black Mission figs, are rich in the bone-building elements, calcium and phosphorus, as well as iron.

D.   ORANGE CLEANSING DIET

Drink from 5 to 8 glasses of orange juice daily. Drink the juice immediately after the oranges have been squeezed or the container opened. Keep orange juice tightly covered even when in the refrigerator. Do not let it stand exposed to the air as it rapidly loses its vitamin C content.

Take a high enema every night while you are on this diet.

Herbal enemas are preferable, especially if there is colon or intestinal trouble: it is excellent to use slippery elm, because it is very cleansing, nourishing, and healing to all the mucous membrane surfaces in the body.

After taking the orange juice from 5 to 10 days, eat a very plain, simple, and nourishing diet. This will improve anyone's health. If the person who wishes to take a cleansing diet is undernourished and weak, and feels that a little something else is necessary, eat apples, masticating them thoroughly; a few nuts might also be eaten.

If you are troubled with skin diseases of any kind, boils, carbuncles, etc., a most helpful treatment is to eat 8 or 10 oranges a day, and drink 3 or 4 glasses of sanicle tea each day. Take the tea after the orange juice has left the stomach, which usually takes an hour or so. Take a high herbal enema with white oak bark every evening for 8 or 10 days. This will bring results beyond all expectation.

Some will find that the orange juice itself acts as a strong cathartic so that the bowels may move several times a day. If you find this to be true, the enemas may be omitted after the first or second day.

E. THE ELIMINATING DIET

All the good food that may be eaten cannot do the body any good until you have first cleansed the body by eliminating excess acid and mucus. The intestines retain these poisons, and they are one of the main causes of disease and premature aging. By eating an abundance of alkaline or base-forming foods, one can rid himself of these poisons and acids. To correct these unnatural and unhealthful conditions and make it possible for the food that is eaten to be assimilated and absorbed by the system, the body must be flushed and cleansed. Eating these foods will bring about a natural rejuvenation by constantly supplying the bloodstream with its original elements. These elements are found in natural foods, which should be either eaten raw or cooked as little as possible so as not to destroy the minerals or life-giving properties. You will be feeding the entire body, not starving it. Leviticus 17:11, "The LIFE is in the blood," and in the same chapter, fourteenth verse, "For the life of all flesh is in the blood." Health and happiness depend upon the bloodstream containing all of the necessary elements; when one is missing, disease in some form often results. To make the bloodstream pure and healthy, eat food in its natural state as far as possible, drink freely of pure water, bathe frequently, exercise in the pure air and sunshine, and use nonpoisonous herbs that were given for the "service of man." Psalms 104:14.

In most of the civilized world we are able to do this almost any time of the year, as we have citrus fruits and fresh vegetables available the year around.

We repair our homes, buy new parts and have our automobiles repaired, and give regular care to other machinery that we may be using. Just so, we must take care of our bodies by supplying them with natural elements and minerals to build and repair the parts that are constantly being worn out.

If pure and alkaline, the bloodstream, which provides nutrition to every cell in the body, will dissolve all poisons and carry them away. No disease can exist with a pure bloodstream.

Fruit:

Use all kinds of fruit liberally. All fruits must be ripe before being picked or else they will not have the eliminating qualities.

Eat at least 2 grapefruit a day, 6 oranges, and 3 lemons. Do not use cane sugar with your fruit or lemonade as it destroys the benefit of the fruit.

Fresh pineapple, ripe peaches, cherries, plums, pears, apples, ripe strawberries, blueberries, and raspberries are excellent.

If fruits do not seem to agree with you, take one-fourth teaspoon of golden seal in one-half glass of water twenty minutes before you eat.

Persons wishing to eliminate who have an ulcerated stomach and cannot take fruits should drink two quarts of potassium broth a day. This is also excellent for invalids.

Vegetables:

The best vegetables to use are spinach, celery, carrots, parsley, tomatoes, asparagus, mild green onions, red or green cabbage (best raw), lettuce, cucumbers, radishes, okra, eggplant, etc. Eat a large raw vegetable salad each day. Have one meal of properly cooked vegetables each day.

Cook all vegetables in as little water as possible, and if salt is necessary, use only a small amount for seasoning.

General Rules While on the Eliminating Diet:

All the above foods, when taken in abundance, will cleanse the bloodstream. Therefore, the greater the quantity taken of these foods, the sooner the body will be cleansed.

The eliminating diet is not a fast. It is a feeding process. It feeds the body through the blood with the necessary life-giving minerals that everybody needs. The eating of fresh fruits and vegetables in large amounts prevents shrinkage of the stomach and intestines, and also prevents lines and wrinkles from forming on the face and body.

Drink water copiously between meals.

Take moderate exercise in the open air.

Eat nothing but fruits and vegetables.

When taking the eliminating diet, do not use any of the following: milk, cane sugar or cane sugar products, gravies, butter, free fat of any kind, macaroni, spaghetti, tapioca, corn starch, meat, tea, coffee, chocolate, ice cream, pastries of any kind, white flour products, any kind of liquor or tobacco, bread, oils of any kind, canned fruits or vegetables, potatoes, cakes, eggs, or any food that is not mentioned in the eliminating diet.

It is highly important that the bowels move freely. If they do not completely evacuate at least once a day, it is wise to cleanse them once or twice a week with an herbal enema.

We have 5 organs of elimination — skin, lungs, bowel, kidneys, and liver.

The bowels will be greatly improved by these foods and the help of nonpoisonous herbs.

The lungs eliminate poisons freely when we practice deep breathing and exercise.

The skin cannot eliminate poisons when it is dry and inactive. There are millions of pores that breathe and eliminate poisons. Therefore, a daily bath should be taken by everyone and, during the eliminating, it is excellent to take an Epsom salts bath every other day to stimulate the skin and open the pores.

Use 3 pounds of Epsom salts to a tub full of water. Drink plenty of water or broth while in the tub. Massage the body while in the tub. Salt glows are also highly beneficial. Rub the body thoroughly all over with half common and half Epsom salt. This increases the activity of the skin and stimulates the circulation. Finish with a cool shower or sponge-off, rubbing vigorously with a Turkish towel.

Many people do not understand why they cannot eat other good wholesome natural foods while on the eliminating diet. This is because they would upset the reaction of these cleansing foods. Do not take any starchy foods, sugars, or proteins as these things congest and clog the system.

When the cells of the body are clear, they function normally and harmoniously. Therefore, the whole body is rejuvenated and the vitality is restored.

Before beginning to eliminate, cleanse the system with an herbal laxative. This will rid the body of much waste matter and mucus and prevent such a great stirring up.

Immediately after taking the eliminating diet, eat sparingly of easily digested foods, such as baked potatoes, green lima beans, tender peas, corn, tomatoes, carrots, etc.

An abundance of oxygen assists elimination greatly. So above all things breathe deeply. Use grape juice, orange juice, grapefruit juice, and sweet apple juice liberally. Oxygen hastens elimination and burns up poisons.

How Long Should One Stay on an Eliminating Diet?

This depends entirely upon the individual. If you have been sick or eating unnatural foods for years, or almost a lifetime, you may have to follow the eliminating diet many times. Eliminate a week or longer if you are stout or overweight, and repeat if necessary. One pound a day may be lost by faithfully eating just the elimination foods and that which is lost is mostly waste and poisons. If one has taken patent medicines, drugs, serums, etc., it will take longer to eliminate these poisons from the system. When all pains and discomfort in the body are gone, the poisons will have been eliminated. Until they are, you will have to go on the eliminating diet again. Everyone could safely eliminate seven days in every month. Very little healthy tissue will be lost. The most that is lost is unhealthy tissues and waste, and the sooner you rid your body of these, the better it will be for your health.

12

OBESITY

Calories are not a sufficient foundation to determine the nutritive value of food. Foods that have a high caloric value are often deficient in nutrient elements and organic salts. In order to determine the true nutritive value of foods, it is important to study their composition in regard to the amount and type of vital elements they contain. For perfect health we must have perfect digestion, assimilation, and elimination. The ignorance of the average person regarding the laws of his being is appalling.

Overeating or too frequent eating produces a feverish state in the system and overtaxes the digestive organs. The blood becomes impure, and diseases of various kinds occur. It also produces excessive acid and causes the mucous membrane lining of the stomach to become congested. Hyperacidity is a common result. An excessive intake of food is much more common than a deficiency. Overweight people are much more likely to have a serious illness than those who maintain a normal weight. Cancer of the breast and womb, kidney disease, diabetes, gallstones, osteoarthritis, arteriosclerosis, high blood pressure, and apoplexy (strokes) are some of the consequences of overeating. Obese persons frequently have high levels of cholesterol and triglycerides in their blood and are much more likely to die suddenly of a heart attack.

It must always be remembered that what is enough food for a hard-working man would be a great excess for a person of sedentary habits of living.

The modern order in which food is served at meals is very destructive. The meal is arranged so that the most highly tempting dishes are presented last, such as pastries, ice cream, etc. This encourages excessive eating. After having eaten enough, a person adds this extra rich food, which becomes a burden and poison to the system.

When the intestines are already full of food, any additional food that is eaten is forced to remain in the stomach overtime and sour. When this food putrefies, its poisons are absorbed into the blood and consequently the whole system is affected. Overeating makes the work of the heart, stomach, liver, kidneys, and bowels much harder.

There is probably no other country in the world that has as many obese people as the United States. If obesity is defined as being more than 20 percent over the ideal weight (Table I), it has been estimated that 80 million Americans fall into this category. And it is not only adults that are affected. More and more children and adolescents are overweight, largely due to their poor diet that is high in refined, high caloric foods and also snacking between meals and during the many hours spent daily watching television.

The secret to losing weight is simple. Use more calories than you take in. For almost everyone this is easier said than done. Less than 10 percent of those who go on special diets or other types of reducing programs are able to keep the weight off. So they try a different diet, lose weight again, but then go back to their old way of eating and soon gain all the lost weight back. Dr. Mayer of Tufts University has aptly termed this "the rhythm method of girth control."

In order to lose weight you must first of all decide that you really want to and then you have to attack the problem sensibly, safely, and slowly. If you were trying to overcome a drinking problem, you wouldn't stop in at the neighborhood bar on the way home from work to say hello to your friends, or if you were trying to stop smoking you wouldn't purposely place yourself in a position where others all around you were smoking. The same principle applies when you are trying to lose weight. When you go shopping, don't linger in front of the candy counter or saunter slowly by the bakery, admiring all the beautifully decorated pies, cakes, and other desserts. Why make it harder on yourself than necessary? Learn what foods are fattening and avoid them. If there is a nutritional label on the food you are about to purchase, read it and see how many calories you will be getting in an average serving. It is amazing how quickly eating only a few extra calories a day will put on the extra pounds. Eating an excess of only 100 calories a day will cause a weight gain of about 10 pounds in a year. If you don't know your daily calorie requirement, you can figure it out roughly by multiplying your weight by 15 if you are a moderately active adult.

Remember that eating 3500 calories more than you use up in daily living puts on one pound of fat. So in order to lose one pound a week you must decrease your caloric intake by 500 calories per day. Table II shows how the calories in a simple nutritious meal can be more than doubled by adding or using high calorie items.

TABLE I
Desirable Weights for Men and Women
of Age 25 and Over

Height (in shoes)[a]	Weight in pounds (in indoor clothing)		
	Small frame	Medium frame	Large frame
Men			
5'2"	112-120	118-129	126-141
3"	115-123	121-133	129-144
4"	118-126	124-136	132-148
5"	121-129	127-139	135-152
6"	124-133	130-143	138-156
7"	128-137	134-147	142-161
8"	132-141	138-152	147-166
9"	136-145	142-156	151-170
10"	140-150	146-160	155-174
11"	144-154	150-165	159-179
6'0"	148-158	154-170	164-184
1"	152-162	158-175	168-189
2"	156-167	162-180	173-194
3"	160-171	167-185	178-199
4"	164-175	172-190	182-204

Women

4'10"	92-98	96-107	104-119
11"	94-101	98-110	106-122
5'0"	96-104	101-113	109-125
1"	99-107	104-116	112-128
2"	102-110	107-119	115-131
3"	105-113	110-122	118-134
4"	108-116	113-126	121-138
5"	111-119	116-130	125-142
6"	114-123	120-135	129-146
7"	118-127	124-139	133-150
8"	122-131	128-143	137-154
9"	126-135	132-147	141-158
10"	130-140	136-151	145-163
11"	134-1444	140-155	149-168
6'0"	138-148	144-159	153-173

Reprinted with permission of the Metropolitan Life Insurance Company.

NOTE: Data are based on weights associated with lowest mortality. To obtain weight for adults younger than 25, subtract 1 pound for each year under 25.

[a]1-in. heels for men; 2-in. heels for women.

TABLE II

Food	Calories	Added Item	Calories	Total Calories
Bread, whole wheat, 1 slice	56	Butter and Jam	110	166
Milk, skim, 1 cup	90	Milk, whole, 1 cup	150	
Salad, lettuce and tomato	40	Mayonnaise, 1 tbs	100	140
Peas, 1 cup	95	Butter, 1 tsp	60	145

Food	Calories	Added Item	Calories	Total Calories
Potato, baked, 1 avg. size	95	Butter, 1 tbs	108	203
Entree	150	Gravy	100	250
Baked apple	90	Apple pie, homemade		410
Total Calories	606		858	1464

Proper exercise is almost a must to include in any reducing program. It doesn't even have to be vigorous exercise like jogging, aerobics, or swimming. Just taking a *brisk* 20-to-30 minute walk three times a week will be very helpful and will increase the rate at which the excess calories are burned off. Table III gives a list of some common exercises and activities and shows about how many minutes it takes to use up 100 calories. Table IV gives the number of calories that are used during an hour of various kinds of vigorous exercise.

TABLE III

MINUTES NEEDED TO USE 100 CALORIES DURING CERTAIN SPORTS ACTIVITIES

Activity	Weight of person	
	155 lb	130 lb
Skiing	8	9
Swimming at 2 mph	10	11
Running	11	13
Football	11	13
Tennis	14	17
Horseback riding	16	19
Gardening	17	21
Skating	19	23
Walking, rapid	19	23
Bicycling	24	29
Walking, moderate, 3 mph	28	33
Golf	33	40

TABLE IV

EXERCISE AND CALORIE EXPENDITURE

Activity (for one hour) . . . . Calories

Activity	Calories
Bicycling 6 mph	240
Bicycling 12 mph	410
Cross-country skiing	700
Jogging 5 mph	740
Jogging 7 mph	920
Jumping rope	750
Running in place	650
Running 10 mph	1280
Swimming 25 yards per minute	275
Swimming 50 yards per minute	500
Tennis-singles	400
Walking 2 mph	240
Walking 3 mph	320
Walking 4 mph	440

From *FDA Consumer,* July-August, 1985, page 27.

Here are some positive suggestions to help you get down to and then maintain your weight within the ideal range.

1. Don't be in a hurry to lose weight. You should lose between one-half and two pounds a week; never more.
2. Don't eat or snack between meals.
3. Eat a good nutritious breakfast and lunch, but go easy on supper. Do not eat before going to bed.
4. Learn to recognize the foods that are high in calories, and avoid them.
5. Skip desserts; eat fresh fruit instead.
6. Don't take seconds; leave the table while you are still somewhat hungry.

7. Use lots of fruits, vegetables, and whole grains.
    These will give you a feeling of fullness while keeping the calories down.

8. Cut down on fatty foods such as fatty meats, meat products, mayonnaise, salad dressing, nuts, etc.

9. Purchase and learn how to use a calorie counter.
    Lower your caloric intake to a point where you are losing about one pound a week, never more than 2 pounds. Don't forget: *you lose weight by eating fewer calories than you use.*

10. Establish a regular exercise program that fits your needs, and stick to it.

13

FASTING AND HEALTHFUL EATING

There is much said throughout the entire Bible about fasting. We will consider some of its uses and benefits. God instituted fasting for both spiritual and physical blessings. The priests in Christ's day fasted twice a week. Throughout the history of the Old Testament the people fasted and prayed in order to gain victories. Fasting has two useful purposes — the upbuilding of the body and the spiritual upbuilding of the soul. Christ fasted 40 days to get the victory over appetite on man's behalf. On this point of appetite our first parents fell, and thousands have gone to an untimely grave because of indulgence.

I have made many experiments with fasting. I fasted for one day a number of times just to get the victory over appetite and to gain spiritual strength. I have also fasted a number of times for 3 days. Once I fasted for 21 days, and worked from early until late and never rested during the day. Another time I fasted for 23 days, and worked every day. I could have fasted 40 days, but was working too hard.

There are persons who advocate long fasts for health (and otherwise), but I WARN EVERYONE AGAINST LONG FASTS, as they do not benefit physically, and are not a spiritual requirement.

Short fasts for a day or two are very beneficial, both spiritually and physically. Make sure you drink plenty of water and take the deep-breathing exercises as outlined earlier in this book. To abstain from rich food, and to eat but very little plain food, even for days or weeks, would be very beneficial. This would give the system a chance to purify itself of poisonous substances. *But the weak, the lean, and the undernourished must be very careful about fasting.*

At one time I was with others eating dinner at an outing and we noticed a man who was not eating. I went to him and asked, "Friend, have you anything to eat? We have plenty and some to spare." This man replied, "I am fasting. I do not care for anything to eat." I then asked him his reason for fasting. He said, "I used to have rheumatism so bad that I was unable to do anything. All the doctors and their medicine didn't help me. One day a man came to me and said if I would fast two days a week my rheumatism would leave me." I asked him who the man was who told him this. He replied that he did not know, that he had never seen the man before, and had never seen him since. He said, "I followed his instruction, and it was but a short time until my rheumatism was gone, and I have never had it since. This was a number of years ago."

In Bible times when one fasted an entire day, it was counted that he had gained a victory. I know of different times when people fasted one day, and then in the evening after sundown they ate a lot of food. This should not be considered as fasting for one day. Fasting means to eat nothing all day until the next day. A serious mistake is often made when too much food is taken after the fast, and much injury to the system is the result. A great deal of the effect of the fast is thus lost.

There are several medical problems that may arise with fasting, and for this reason, even though fasting may be beneficial, if it is carried on for longer than a day or two you need to keep on your guard for the following possible complications.

1. Kidney stones
2. Low blood pressure
3. Irregular heart beat
4. Gouty arthritis
5. Headaches or light-headedness
6. Abdominal pain or nausea
7. Decreased urine output
8. Severe cramps

If any of these or other complications develop, the fast should be stopped immediately.

Aside from spiritual and health reasons, fasting is also used to treat obesity and certain convulsive disorders. It has also been used with varying degrees of success as a means of political protest. Gandhi in India, well known for his passive resistance, fasted as a political protest many times and for as long as three weeks, on at least three occasions. In quite recent times ten men from the Irish Republican Army died in prison, following fasts ranging from 45 to 61 days. The longest fast of which we have any record was that of an obese 27-year-old man. While under constant medical supervision, he fasted for 382 days and lost a total of 276 pounds.

I am thoroughly convinced that a great many people eat too much. Americans are the most overweight group of people in the world, but this does not necessarily mean that they are properly nourished. In fact, many eat food that does not give them proper nourishment. It is also true that many people are undernourished because they eat devitaminized (refined) food improperly prepared, and improper mixtures of food that ferment and make poor blood from what they do eat.

But if we eat food as God made it, containing all of its natural vitamins and minerals, we will not get nervous, irritable, unreasonable, and out of sorts. When the minerals, vitamins, and other nutrients that would keep the body healthy are removed from the food during its preparation, we become malnourished and subject to all kinds of diseases, of which there are as many as there are different concoctions made for us to eat. When we feel so tired all the time, it is because those nutrients that give us pep and make us strong have been removed from our food.

I have seen many herds of horses, cattle, sheep, and other animals, and they are all very much alike because they eat the food the way God made it for them. Just stop and think! There is not anything in any of the meats that is not in the grains, hay, and grass that the animals eat. Why eat it second-hand? Let's eat it in its pure original state. What do you say?

A diet of acid-forming foods and combinations causes

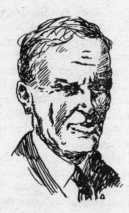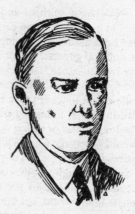

Fig. 1

waste matter in the system, which in turn causes wrinkles and makes us look old. I have seen just as radical a change in a person as you see in the accompanying picture (Fig. 1). The change occurred in a man with his skin wrinkled, yellow, and old-looking after he was put on a correct diet and given sweat baths and herbs to cleanse the bloodstream and intestinal tract. The change was so great that people who knew him said he looked 20 years younger. I have seen this change take place many times. I, today, am a living example of such a change.

There is so much written about foods today that it becomes confusing. They write about calories, acid-forming foods, alkaline foods, vitamins, minerals, etc.; and one writer who claims to be an authority says this, while another one says that. I have heard people say many times that they did not know what to eat any more. In the accompanying picture (Fig. 2), we see a cow with her calf. This cow raised the calf in this pasture. She was never out of the pasture and had nothing to eat but the grass that grew in that pasture. The calf had nothing but the milk she got from her mother until she was large enough to eat the grass too. This calf was beauti-

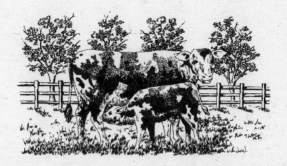

Fig. 2

fully developed, had a well-proportioned body, nice hair, good solid bones, good sound teeth, good hoofs, and good eyes. Now there was not anything in the milk that was not in the grass, and this milk produced this calf. That shows very plainly that all of the vitamins, minerals, protein, and carbohydrates were in the grass.

Now it is just the same with all of the food that God has given us. Of course it is true that different kinds of fruits, grains, and vegetables have somewhat different properties, and I would not recommend that anyone should choose a particular food and live on it to the exclusion of all others. As large a variety of food as possible should be eaten. This is very important.

But if the natural life-giving properties, which are in the foods as God made them, were not destroyed in their preparation, we wouldn't have to worry about calories, or alkaline and acid-forming foods. If a wide selection of food from the four basic food groups is eaten every day, the body will be kept in perfect health and there will be no need to wonder whether or not we are getting the proper amount of protein, carbohydrate, fat, vitamins, and minerals. I was born and raised on a farm in the northern part of Wisconsin, and we raised practically everything we ate, and we were a large family. We were never sick and we all lived to an old age.

Section VI
Food Preparation

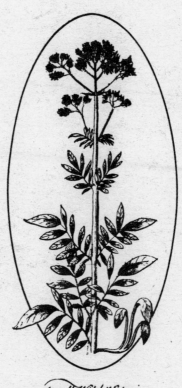

Small Wild Valerian

1

USEFUL HINTS TO PRESERVE VITAMINS

Many important nutrients are lost to a greater or lesser degree when food is cooked by ordinary methods. In particular, the water-soluble vitamins — B-complex and C — may be largely lost by careless cooking and storage. Vitamin C is the most unstable of all the vitamins and if, by observing the following rules for cooking, this vitamin can be largely retained, other important nutrients, including iron, will also be preserved in significant amounts. Fortunately, some of our food sources that are highest in vitamin C, the citrus fruits, are best eaten raw. Fruits and vegetables together supply well over 90 percent of our vitamin C. See also Section IV, Chapter 6.

Follow the practical suggestions listed below in order to retain the most nutrients while cooking your food, and remember the four nutrient robbers are air, water, heat, and light.

1. Use as little water as possible during cooking.
2. Have the water boiling for about one minute before adding the food.
3. Let the water simmer rather than boil vigorously.
4. Save the leftover water to use as vegetable stock for gravy or soup.
5. Cut the vegetables in large, uniform pieces just before cooking. Leave the peeling or skin on when possible. The smaller the pieces being cooked, the larger the area exposed to water, and therefore the greater the vitamin loss will be.
6. Use the shortest cooking time possible. Serve vegetables tender and crisp, not soggy and mushy.
7. Serve food immediately after preparation. Do not keep it hot for a long time before serving. Plan your

meals so that the reheating of food is done as seldom as possible. Cover and refrigerate leftover foods right away.

8. Keep cooking vessels tightly covered.
9. Cooking by steaming or pressure cooker will preserve about 30 percent more of the vitamins than boiling.
10. Do not add soda to cooking water, because this destroys vitamin C and some of the B-complex vitamins.
11. Food that is high in vitamin C should not be cooked in copper or iron vessels.
12. Store fresh fruits and vegetables in a refrigerator and prepare them immediately before they are to be used. Do not let them stand in water or remain exposed to air any longer than is necessary.
13. Place frozen food directly into boiling water after removing from the freezer. Do not permit the food to thaw first.
14. Keep orange juice covered and in the refrigerator. Drink fresh orange juice immediately after squeezing. Do not leave it exposed to the air.

A.   TIME TABLE FOR COOKING

Apples, sour	baked, medium hot oven, 30 minutes
Apples, sweet	baked, medium hot oven, 45 minutes
Asparagus, whole	boiled 10 to 15 minutes
Beans, dried	boiled until tender, about 2 to 3 hours
Beets, whole	boiled until tender, 20 to 30 minutes
Broccoli	boiled 10 to 15 minutes
Carrots, whole	boiled until tender, 15 to 20 minutes
Carrots sliced	boiled until tender, 10 to 15 minutes
Cauliflower, pieces	boiled until tender, 8 to 10 minutes
Corn on the cob	boiled 6 to 10 minutes
Eggplant	baked in hot oven, 30 minutes
	steamed, 15 to 20 minutes

Eggs, soft-boiled	put in boiling water, turn heat off, and allow to stand for 7 or 8 minutes
Eggs, hard-boiled	boiled 30 minutes
Gems and muffins,	quick oven, 375°F. for 25 minutes
Onions, small,	boiled 10 to 15 minutes
large	boiled 20 to 30 minutes
Parsnips, whole	boiled 20 to 30 minutes
Peas	boiled 10 to 12 minutes
Potatoes	boiled 15 to 30 minutes
Potatoes	baked in hot oven, 45 to 60 minutes
Rice, brown	boiled 40 to 50 minutes
Rolled oats	direct boiling, 15 minutes
	double boiler, 1 hour
Salsify (oyster plant)	boiled 2 hours
Squash	boiled, whole, 10 to 15 minutes
	boiled pieces, 8 to 12 minutes
String beans, whole	boiled until tender, about 10 minutes
Sweet potatoes	baked, hot oven, 45 to 60 minutes
	boiled 20 to 35 minutes
Tomatoes, whole	boiled 10 to 15 minutes
Turnips, whole	boiled until tender, 20 to 30 minutes
sliced	boiled 15 to 20 minutes
Whole grain rolls and biscuits	quick (hot) oven, 20 to 25 minutes

B. WAYS TO COOK VEGETABLES

The best way to cook vegetables is to bake them. Boiling is good if very little water is used and none of the liquid is thrown away. Waterless cooking, casserole baking, and low pressure steam cooking are also good.

When boiling vegetables, put them in just enough boiling water to cook them and don't overcook them. If there is any water left, save it to add to your soups or broths. The vegetables must boil or simmer continuously after placing them in the water; otherwise they will become water-soaked.

Add sea salt sparingly just before the vegetables are entirely done; if salt is added as they are beginning to cook, it has a tendency to toughen them. Cook vegetables only until they are tender; prolonged cooking destroys the life-giving properties. Do not add fat to the vegetables while they are cooking; add your seasoning just before they are done, and serve them at once.

Never peel or remove the eyes of Irish potatoes before cooking; the life of the potato is in the eyes and the peel. Do not peel any vegetable that can be used without peeling. Carrots, parsnips, salsify (vegetable oysters or oyster plant), rutabagas, and others may be scraped lightly, so as not to lose the minerals that are found just under their skins.

Green vegetables are very desirable during the winter months; if you think them expensive remember that they are far cheaper than the cost of an illness, and when properly prepared they are real medicine.

Canned or frozen vegetables, even if you get a good brand, are not as good as properly prepared fresh vegetables. But they are better than fresh vegetables that are poorly prepared.

To obtain protein with your vegetables, serve one of the many new meat analogs now on the market, or any nuts you like best. Nuts require thorough mastication, however, and they should be chewed to a creamy consistency in order to get the most good out of them. The meat substitutes that contain nuts are better for most people, because the nuts used in them have been ground.

Vegetables can be seasoned with soy mayonnaise that has been made without the lemon if desired. Either dilute the mayonnaise with cold water to the consistency of cream, or use it as is. Either rich soybean milk or one of the nut milks is good when added to hot vegetables; heat the vegetables for only a few minutes after the milk has been added, and serve at once. (See Sections C and D in the next chapter for soybean recipes.) Good soybean milk can now be purchased; thus, you can always have it on hand.

All the nonstarchy vegetables, such as carrots, cabbage, cucumbers, radishes, and parsley, should be eaten raw if they agree with you.

2

KLOSS'S FAVORITE HEALTH RECIPES

A. VEGETABLE RECIPES

Mashed Potatoes

Select the dry, mealy variety, such as the Idaho potato. Wash them thoroughly and boil or steam them until they are thoroughly done. Steaming is better than boiling. When done, peel the outer thin skin off, being careful not to remove the eyes. Mash, add rich soybean milk, salt to taste, and bake in a greased casserole dish for twenty minutes in a hot oven.

Boiled Cabbage

Select a head of cabbage that has many green outside leaves in good condition. Slice into eighths, put in cooking pan, and cover with sliced onions. Pour 1 to 2 cups of boiling water over it and cook for about twenty minutes, or until tender. Salt sparingly when about half done.

Carrots and Peas

Equal parts of sliced or cubed carrots and peas can be cooked together until tender; season with rich soybean milk or soybean butter if desired. Salt to taste.

String Beans

Wash, string, and break the beans about one inch long, or slice them lengthwise. Cover the bottom of a pan with a little vegetable fat and put the beans in the pan. Salt, and cover the pan with a tight lid, cooking over moderate heat until the beans are a bright green, stirring them often so they will not stick. Then barely cover the beans with boiling water, and cook until tender.

Mixed Greens

Use as many kinds of greens as you wish, having them all as near the same tenderness as possible. Wash and chop. Rub the cooking kettle with a little garlic, add enough fat to just cover the bottom of the kettle well, put the greens in, cover tightly and cook over medium heat for about ten minutes. Salt and serve at once.

Eggplant

1/2 cup chopped onions	1 or 2 cloves of garlic
1/2 cup green peppers	2-1/2 cups of tomatoes,
3 tbs. vegetable fat	chopped
3 cups raw eggplant,	salt
unpeeled, diced into	
1/2-inch cubes	

Put onions and peppers in hot fat and brown them lightly. Add eggplant and garlic and cook a few minutes. (Eggplant can be peeled very thinly if you prefer.) Then add tomatoes and salt to taste. Put in greased baking dish and bake for about 30 minutes in a 350° oven.

Beets

Always use young beets when obtainable. Cut the tops up fine and cook in hot water for about 5 minutes. Then dice the beets about 1/8-inch square, add them to the tops, and cook until tender; salt, and just before serving add a little soybean butter if you wish.

Okra

Select even-sized, tender pods of okra. Cook until tender in just enough water to keep from burning. Salt and season with soybean butter (optional) just before serving.

Spinach

Wash thoroughly. Put in a tightly covered kettle and cook until tender; from five to ten minutes. Salt when partly done. Add a little lemon juice if desired for extra flavor.

Beans with Tomato Sauce

Use any kind of dried beans. Soak them overnight in cold water, and the next morning drain them, cover with cold water and tomato sauce, or other seasoning if you prefer, and cook in a crock pot for about four hours. Those who cannot eat beans prepared in the ordinary way may be able to eat them when they are cooked in this fashion.

After soaking the beans overnight, they may also be put in cans. Fill the cans about three-quarters full of beans, and then fill to the top with water, salting the water before pouring it in the can; or use half tomato sauce and half water. Seal and cook in a steam pressure cooker, using ten pounds pressure for about an hour and a half. Some beans require a little less cooking and some a little more. Test them for yourself. Old beans require longer cooking than new ones, but all beans should be thoroughly soft and tender. When prepared properly, they will not produce gas and will digest more easily.

Another way to prepare beans is to boil them until almost dry, then put them in a baking dish, add some soybean milk, put in the oven, and bake thoroughly. This method adds to the flavor and digestibility of the beans, and makes them more alkaline.

The Great Northern bean is very fine and cooks easily. The lima bean is alkaline and therefore one can eat it more freely than the navy bean and some of the others.

Soybeans are, no doubt, the most nutritious of all beans, but the flavor is not as pleasant. This can be overcome by using various seasonings, such as tomato sauce, a little onion, and celery.

To Sprout Soybeans, Lentils, or Grains

Cover well one pint, or any amount you desire, of soybeans (or others) with water and let stand overnight. Pour off the water but keep the beans moist. Rewash two or three times daily, keeping them moist, and in a dark place, for approximately three days until well-sprouted. Allow to stand until the sprouts are about one-half inch long. Lentils are prepared in the same manner, but they do not take as long to sprout as soybeans. Soybeans may be allowed to sprout until they are an inch long, and then only the sprouts are eaten. The sprouts need only about ten minutes cooking.

The sprouting of any bean or pea turns the protein into peptogen to a great extent, and the starch into dextrose or maltose. The sprouts are very high in vitamins, more so than spinach, lettuce, or celery.

Cook sprouted beans or peas the same way you cook any fresh beans or peas; but be careful not to overcook. Salt to taste. A little tomato and onion added make a very palatable and wholesome dish.

Soybean Sprouts and Rice

Boil the sprouted soybeans until tender. Boil brown rice separately. Mix approximately equal parts, add tomato sauce and some cubes of nut roast or loaf (recipes given later in this chapter). Mix these all together and place in the oven at 350° for 30 to 60 minutes.

If the flavor of the soybeans is too strong, they may first be parboiled in strong salt water for a few minutes.

B.   SOYBEANS

A knowledge of the value of the soybean here in America is one of the greatest things that was ever launched in the food line in the history of the nation, and at this time of great poverty, want, and disease, it is the most important thing that could be given to the people.

Anyone with a piece of ground may raise his own soybeans. They will not only greatly improve the soil, making fertile soil out of worn-out soil, but at the same time they will supply the family with most delicious and nourishing food. Soybeans should be planted at different intervals throughout the summer in order to have shelled soybeans all summer. The green soybeans can be shelled just like any other bean or pea. Some varieties do not shell easily, but these can be easily removed from the shell by first boiling for just a few minutes.

Soybean milk can be made from soybeans at home for less than two cents a quart. The Yellow Mammoth, Dixie, Illinois, and Tokyo soybeans are among the best varieties for making soybean milk. There are other varieties that are better for green shelled beans. W. J. Morse, senior agronomist of the U. S. Agriculture Experimental Station, Washington, D. C, can give most valuable information along this line, as he has made, and is still making, extensive experiments with soybeans, and is thoroughly acquainted with that subject.

For stomach ulcers, duodenal ulcers, cancer, and diabetes, as well as liver, kidney, and bladder troubles, soybean milk in not only a good food, but a real medicine. It is easily digested, it does not curd, is highly alkaline, and is rich in mineral matter.

The soybean is one of the greatest and most complete foods that we have. In the Orient, it has been used for thousands of years, and in this country it has been used for some time for stock feed, and to improve the soil. But only recently has much effort been made to use it for human consumption. At the present time, there are many people in various sections of the United States who are experimenting with it to some extent with considerable success.

The objection to the soybean is that it does not have a flavor as pleasant as some of the other beans. The flavor can be improved, however, by preparing the beans for human consumption in a different way.

I have experimented with soybeans for fifteen years and

have produced a fine, acceptable soybean milk as well as many other soybean products.

I use soybeans in more than fifty dishes. I can make soybean bread, buns, pie, pones, roast, cottage cheese, and soybean cheese (which is very similar to both Philadelphia cream cheese and American yellow cheese); also soybean coffee and ice cream, without any cane sugar in any product. My soybean milk is simply delicious, very palatable, and both children and adults like it.

Soybean milk, properly made, is a wonderful food for the sick. Soybean milk does not form hard curds in the stomach and putrefy as cow's or goat's milk can do, and it can be used in the same ways they are used. Beans and peas cook quicker when they are boiled in soybean milk than when they are boiled in water. Soybean milk can sour and clabber like cow's milk, and after souring, can be beaten up into most delicious buttermilk. The beauty of it is that it is highly alkaline, and is well adapted for the human system, for both adults and children.

Many pay a big price for goat's milk, while soybean milk is infinitely better for human consumption. It does not have the contamination of the animal in it, nor the tendency to disease and putrefaction.

The following is an analysis of human, cow's, goat's, soybean, and nut milks as given by the United States Department of Agriculture, Bureau of Chemistry and Soils, Washington, D.C.

Type of milk	Water	Ash	Protein	Fat	Carbo-hydrates
Human	89.95%	0.25%	1.30%	2.50%	6.00%
Cow's	87.30	0.80	3.20	3.50	5.20
Goat's	87.00	0.50	4.00	4.50	4.00
Soybean	87.03	0.52	2.40	3.15	6.90
Nut	87.00	2.03	5.60	5.50	7.23

To the soybean milk used for the above analysis, I had added a little emulsified soybean oil and a little malt.

Soybeans are also used for industrial purposes in the manufacture of artificial petroleum, automobile steering wheel rims, cable insulators, candles, casein, celluloid, core oil, crude and refined oil, emulsifier, electric distributor parts, illuminant (for lamps), hard and soft soaps, horn buttons, glue, hard curd soap, cooking oil, glycerine, enamels, foundry sand-cores, linoleum, lard, lubricant, laundry oil-cloth, paints, photographic films, paper, plastic material, potassium soap, printer's ink, rubber substitute, silk-scouring soap, seawater soap, shampoo mixture, silver soap, soy vinegar, varnish, textile dressing, waterproof cement, etc.

The following quotation is from an address delivered by Dr. J. A. LeClerc before the annual meeting of the American Soybean Association, Sept. 15, 1936.

THE NUTRITIONAL VALUE OF THE SOYBEAN

The soybean is going to revolutionize the food of human-ity more than the potato did two hundred years ago, when it was a curiosity — and today is a staple food. It differs from the potato in the respect that it has been used for thousands of years as one of the principal foods of the Chinese. The Chinese nation exists today because of the use of the soybean as a food. China has survived five thousand years, its people have endured not only one, but hundreds of severe economic depressions, floods, earthquakes, famines, and wars.

Their recovery from these calamities is due largely to the use of the soybean, as it is a food which perfectly takes the place of disease-producing meat, milk, and eggs. It (the soybean) contains all the life-sustaining properties of meat, milk and eggs, and is far more economical and easier to produce than any of these.

If Americans were suddenly deprived of meat, milk, and eggs and no more thought was given to planning our diet than most of us do, the result would be a condition of malnutrition due to a shortage of protein in our food.

The Chinese under similar circumstances have gone on living normal lives, simply by eating soybeans in some form. The Buddhist priests in the Orient are forbidden meat by their religion; in place of it they eat tofu, a soybean curd, and other soybean foods. The Chinese coolies, whose strength and endurance are traditional for carrying heavy burdens, pulling rickshaws, etc., live chiefly on soybeans and rice. Chinese babies are dependent on the soybean for food, dairy products being rare in the Orient. Those babies that must be fed artificially are given milk made from soybeans. It is a scientific fact that physical development on a soybean diet is perfectly normal. History proves the value of soybeans as a food.

Food chemists have conclusively proven that soybeans cannot only be substituted for more expensive foods but are more wholesome than those articles of diet. Today soybeans are one of the most economical sources of nourishment.

Not only are soybeans suitable for all kinds of baked products but soya flour or soybeans can also be used in breakfast foods, diabetic and infant foods, in pancake and self-rising flours, macaroni, doughnuts, pretzels, soy sauce, pate de foie gras, potted meats, meat loaf, and sandwich spreads, mayonnaise, soups, confectionery, beverages, coffee substitutes, beer, milk, cheese, ice cream, dog food, besides numerous industrial products. It is understood, of course, that food products containing soya flour should be properly labeled.

Soya flour is considerably richer in protein than are the flours made from such other legumes as the navy bean, pea, lentil, lima bean, etc., and about four times as rich in this constituent as are the cereal flours. Soya flour protein is of especially good quality. Soya flour contains less than two percent starch, whereas starch is the main constituent in other cereal flour, containing as it does about thirty times as much.

Soya flour is especially rich in the vitamins and in minerals. The amount of calcium is twenty times greater than that in potatoes, twelve times that found in wheat flour, five times that in eggs, about two times the amount present in liquid milk, and one-fourth as much as in dried milk. Milk has always been regarded as the calcium food par excellence.

One pound of soya flour is equivalent to two pounds of meat in protein content. To the extent that people might consume one-half pound of soya bread per day instead of ordinary bread, the extra amount of protein in the soya bread is sufficient to replace a quantity of protein in over one-fourth of the daily intake of meat on the average. Meat protein costs five times that of soya protein.

Proteins are muscle-builders and are absolutely indispensable. There is a high quality protein content in soybeans, which makes them such a successful substitute for meat, milk, and eggs. They are the only natural food in the vegetable kingdom that contains a higher protein value than milk or eggs.

The soybean has life-giving properties that meat and other proteins do not have.

The soybean is king of the beans. It is a fine alkaline food, and there are many varieties of the soybean. For cooking purposes get the "easy cook" variety, as it cooks much quicker than other varieties. It is best to cook soybeans under a low steam pressure, five pounds pressure for forty to sixty minutes for most varieties. They should be cooked until tender, not mushy. Always soak the beans overnight before cooking. It is best to cook all beans under a low steam pressure.

C.   SOYBEAN RECIPES

Soy Patties

2 cups soybean pulp	1 onion, chopped fine
2 cups natural brown rice (cooked)	1 tbs. soysauce
	1/4 tsp. salt
2 tbs. vegetable fat	flavor with garlic, sage or whole wheat bread crumbs

Mix the first seven ingredients thoroughly together, and shape into patties. Roll the patties in whole wheat breadcrumbs. Bake in a greased pan until brown, or warm in a frying pan, but do not fry.

Soybean Loaf

2 cups soybeans, cooked and ground

2 cups pinto bean pulp

1 cup tomato juice

1 cup finely chopped nuts

salt to taste

1-1/3 cups whole wheat zwieback crumbs, toasted

1 onion, chopped fine

2 tbs. soy sauce

spices to flavor

Mix ingredients thoroughly together. Add sage, celery seed, thyme, or other flavorings you like. Put in greased baking dish and bake one hour in a moderate oven.

Soybean Cottage Cheese Loaf

1/2 cup celery

parsley

1 cup onion

1/2 cup green pepper

6 tbs. lemon juice

6 tbs. soy sauce

3/4 cup raw peanut butter

3 cups soybean cottage cheese (see Cheese section, following)

1 cup whole wheat bread crumbs (toasted)

1/4 cup peanut oil

1 tbs. chopped garlic

1 heaping tsp. sage

pinch cayenne pepper

salt to taste

Chop the celery, parsley, onion, and green pepper fine. Mix in the lemon juice, soy sauce, peanut butter, and cottage cheese. Then add the other ingredients and mix thoroughly. Put in a greased baking dish and bake in a moderate oven.

Soybean Milk No.1

Take one pound soybeans, cover with water, and soak them overnight. In the morning wash them thoroughly, cover with fresh water, and bring to a boil. If the water is changed again a couple of times and brought to a boil each time, it helps to remove the soybean taste after the milk is made. Then drain and grind the beans. Put the beans in a fine-meshed sugar sack or cheese cloth and tie the top securely. Put the sack of ground soybeans in a large dish or pail. Pour two quarts of water over them; warm water is preferable as the milk has fat in it. Knead the sack of ground beans well, washing and squeezing the milk out. Pour off the milk into a large pan or pail. Pour two more quarts of water over the beans, and knead and squeeze out well again. Combine the second two quarts of milk with the first two quarts in a large flat-bottomed pan, and boil twenty minutes or more, stirring constantly with a pancake turner from the bottom of the pan as it boils, so that it will not stick to the bottom of the pan. You may add a little malt honey, honey, or malt sugar, but do not make it too sweet. Add salt to taste. Do not cook in aluminum.

Addendum: The residue of the beans left in the sack or cheese cloth is called soybean mash or pulp. Today soybean milk may be purchased already mixed, or soybean powder may be mixed with water in a blender. Make only enough for one day at a time.

Soybean Milk No.2

Take one pound soy meal (do not have it ground too fine) and three quarts of cold water. Mix and boil 25 minutes.

Strain, sweeten, and salt to taste. It is best to use a flat-bottomed pan, and stir with a pancake turner, as it burns very easily. If you desire it richer, add some soy bean cream, the recipe for which is given later in this section.

These soybean milks may be used in the same way as cow's milk. When using for cooking, do not sweeten. You may add the sweetening to the milk as it is used: it keeps fresh longer if the sweetening is not added. This milk is highly alkaline. It must be handled in the same way as cow's milk. When cooled, keep in ice box or cool place, as it will sour in about the same length of time as cow's milk.

This soybean milk makes a more nourishing and healthful chocolate milk than dairy milk.

The best grinder to use for grinding the wet soybeans is Enterprise Grinder No. 69, manufactured by the Enterprise Manufacturing Company, Philadelphia, Pennsylvania.

How to Curd Soybean Milk

After making the soybean milk, while it is still boiling hot, add enough citric acid so it will curd at once. Use three or four tablespoonfuls of citric acid to the quart of boiling milk. Stir briskly and let set. The curds form within a few seconds, and it doesn't take long until the milk is curded. Skim the curd off the clear water and place in a double cheesecloth, squeezing out all the water, making the cheese as dry as possible.

If a smooth cheese is desired, use less citric acid. If a granular cheese is liked, use more citric acid.

Soybean Jelly
4 cups soybean milk (unsweetened)
2 rounded tbs. agar-agar (flaky)
4 tbs. malt sugar

Soak the agar-agar in the soybean milk one hour. Put in a saucepan, bring to a boil and simmer slowly until the agar-

agar is entirely dissolved. Add the sweetening and cool. Fresh fruit or fruit juice may be added for flavoring, if desired. Put on ice.

Soybean Butter
1/2 pint water
2 tbs. soybean flour
1 pint oil

Mix the water and flour together, put in a heavy iron frying pan, and boil five minutes, or until thickened. Strain into a mixing bowl. Pour in one pint of soybean oil, very slowly, as in making mayonnaise, beating constantly. (You may use any good vegetable oil, but preferably not palm or coconut oil.) Use a blender for easier mixing.

Soybean Cream
1 pint rich soybean milk
1/2 pint soybean oil (or any vegetable oil)

Place the milk in a mixing bowl, and pour in the oil in a very small stream, beating constantly, until it is the desired thickness; if you desire a thick cream use more oil; if a thin cream, use less.

If you do not have any soybean milk, use a heaping tablespoonful of soybean flour, and one-half pint of water. Mix and place in a frying pan, stirring with a pancake turner, and let it boil until thickened, five minutes or a little more. Then strain, and proceed as above, beating in the oil until you have the desired thickness.

Soybean Ice Cream
1 tbs. agar-agar
2 quarts rich soybean
  milk
2 lbs. malt sugar

1 tsp. vanilla, or to taste,
  or crushed fruit or fruit
  juice as desired to taste
1/2 pint soybean butter or
  soybean mayonnaise

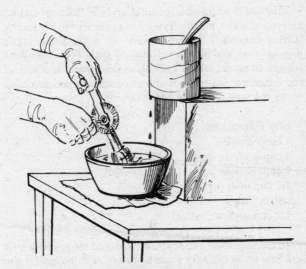

A Unique Arrangement for Pouring Oil in Making
Mayonnaise or Soybean Butter and Cream.

Soak the agar-agar in cold water until it swells. Drain and
put in soybean milk, add the malt sugar, and butter or
mayonnaise. Put on stove and let boil for five minutes. Strain
through a fine sieve or cheesecloth. Add vanilla or any
crushed fruit or fruit juice you desire. Put in a freezer and
freeze the same way as any other ice cream. Made in this way,
ice cream can be melted and fed to invalids and infants.

"Egg Yolk"

You may use the following "egg yolk" in any recipe that

calls for the yolk of an egg; it looks very much like egg yolk, tastes like it, and has very much the same properties, but no cholesterol.

Take one heaping tablespoonful soybean flour, mix with a half cup of water, put in a frying pan and boil until it thickens, stirring constantly so that it does not stick. Strain into a mixing bowl, and beat in soybean oil until it becomes thick enough to be cut with a knife. Use this wherever a yolk of egg is desired. Season with a pinch of salt, and use dandelion butter coloring for a little added color.

Soy Pancakes

1 cup cornmeal
1 cup soybean mash
1 cup soybean milk
1/2 cup malt sugar
salt to taste
1/2 cup soybean butter

To the corn meal and soybean mash add the soybean milk and beat up as ordinary pancake batter. Add the malt sugar, salt, and beat in the soybean butter.

If the batter is used when very cold, the pancakes can be made nicely without yeast or baking powder. If the pancakes are for breakfast, it is well to soak the cornmeal in the soybean milk the night before.

Some like these pancakes made with yeast. For raised pancakes, take one cake of Fleischmann's yeast, dissolve it in the soybean milk, and proceed as above, letting the batter rise about an hour before baking.

D.   CHEESES, NUTS, AND VEGETABLE PROTEIN DISHES

Soybean Cottage Cheese

This is made in the same way as ordinary cottage cheese.

Use unsweetened soybean milk. Allow the milk to sour or clabber, then heat to body temperature until it separates from the whey. Drain in a very fine sieve or through cheesecloth. When it has drained dry, add a little rich soybean milk to soften and flavor, as you would add cream to ordinary cottage cheese. The addition of a little Kloss's Mayonnaise also improves the flavor and makes a richer product. Salt to taste. Some add a little honey; this makes it a tasty spread for children, and is a splendid nerve builder.

Soybean Cheese
5 lbs. raw peanut butter
1 or 2 quarts tomato puree
5 quarts soybean milk

To five pounds of raw peanut butter add one quart of tomato puree, or if you prefer a strong tomato flavor, use two quarts. Stir in gradually five quarts of soybean milk, and put in a warm place until it develops lactic acid, or until it gets about as sour as cottage cheese. Then it is ready to use and can be placed in the refrigerator in a covered container. If you wish you may put it in cans (either No. 2 or No. 3), place in a large pan and cover with boiling water. Let this cook for four or five hours. If you have a steam pressure cooker, cook under five pounds pressure for two or three hours. The cheese is then ready for serving.

Soybean Cream Cheese

Use unsweetened soybean milk. Let stand until it thickens (not sour). Then put on the stove and boil a minute or two until the water separates from the whey. Put in a cheesecloth and wring dry. Run through a mill or blender until it is a smooth paste. Add a little rich soybean milk to soften and make a creamy consistency. Salt to taste. Kloss's Mayonnaise may also be added for richness.

Nut Cheese No.1

1 1/2 pints water or soybean milk
1 lb. raw peanut butter
1/2 lb. soybean butter
salt to taste

Pour the water into the peanut butter very slowly, stirring to a paste, gradually adding water until the entire amount has been used. If soybean milk is used instead of water, a better product is obtained. Let stand until it sours to suit the taste, thus developing lactic acid like the lactic acid found in buttermilk. Beat in the soybean butter and salt to taste. It is now ready to use. Keep it covered in the refrigerator. You may also put it in cans and prepare as for Soybean Cheese, preceding.

Nut Cheese No.2

1 lb. raw peanut butter
4 tbs. ground oatmeal flour
1 1/2 pints water
salt to taste

Prepare in the same manner as Nut Cheese No. 1.

Some of the Nut Cheeses which I make are much like the yellow American cheese, while others are similar to cream cheese. They are very agreeable to the taste, are high in food value and emulsified nut oils, are much easier to digest, and contain none of the harmful bacteria of ordinary cheeses found on the market. These nut cheeses may be put up in cans to keep them pure and sanitary. They are prepared in a way that develops lactic acid such as is found in yogurt, buttermilk, and cottage cheese.

Those who cannot eat ordinary cheese made with rennet can eat freely of nut cheese, and there is no exposure to disease, as is the case with other cheeses.

Nut cheese is more economical, and may be used in any way that the cheeses on the market are used. More food value is obtained for the money.

Malted Nuts

1 cup raw peanut meal or raw peanut butter (peanut meal
   is preferable)
1/2 cup malt honey
few grains of salt

Mix all ingredients well. Place in a slow oven until thoroughly dried out, but do not brown. Then run through a mill, but do not grind it too fine because it must remain in a powder form, and not be as a butter. If iron pans are to be used, lay heavy brown paper in the bottom so that the nut mixture will not come in contact with the iron. If the oven is too hot, the nuts will turn too brown. Another way is to dry the nuts in the sun and then put in the oven for a while, or just long enough to cook them.

Nut Milk

1 cup raw peanut butter
1/2 cup milk sweetening (malt sugar or honey)
1 cup boiling water
few grains of salt

Mix the peanut butter and the milk sweetening thoroughly together. Use a heaping teaspoonful of this mixture to a cup of boiling water. Thoroughly mix, adding salt.

This may be used as any other milk.

Uses for Kokofat

Kokofat is a trade name for the pure fat extracted from the coconut, one of the richest fats on the market. One-fourth less Kokofat than any other fat is needed in cooking. For instance, if a recipe calls for one pound of butter or Crisco in cooking or baking, you need only three-quarters of a pound of Kokofat to get the same results.

You can melt it, add some dandelion butter coloring, salt to taste, cool, and use in place of cow's butter. It can be used for baking and cooking in any way that you would use butter, makes very nice pie crust, is sweet, has no foreign taste, and keeps a long time without getting rancid.

Coconut Oil and Nut Butter

1 lb. coconut oil
1/2 lb. peanut oil
butter coloring
salt to taste

A fine butter is made by mixing these ingredients with an egg beater or an electric beater, beating until they are thoroughly blended. It is a wholesome butter with a delicious flavor.

Addendum: Coconut and palm oil are now known to be high in saturated fatty acids, and should be used sparingly if at all.

To Blanch Peanuts

Buy shelled nuts and steam them for 2 to 5 minutes. Rub the nuts between the hands, or place them on a table and lightly press with a rolling pin to loosen the skins sufficiently to enable one to blow them away. Place on a cookie sheet in the oven at 350° until they are a very light golden brown.

Peanut Butter

1 lb. blanched, raw peanuts
Run the peanuts through a peanut butter mill. This is a very excellent and wholesome butter. Peanut butter made this way can be diluted with water and used like cream, or spread on bread.

Mock Almond Butter

Take one pound blanched peanuts, cover with water, and boil until they just begin to get tender, but not mushy. Drain off the water and dry the peanuts thoroughly. This can be done in the sun, or in a very slow oven if they are stirred frequently, but the nuts must not be browned at all. Grind them fine. This makes an excellent butter, which can be used in many ways. To eat with vegetables or fruit, add water until it is of the consistency of milk or cream.

This same butter may be reduced with water, and lightly salted to taste, making a palatable and nourishing butter that is easy to digest.

Original Meat Or Vegetable Protein

Take five pounds of strong gluten flour, which is ordinarily called bread flour. The gluten flour to use is not like ordinary white flour. It has more food value and more vitamins. (It can be obtained at large mills, bakeries, or wholesale grocers.) Add two quarts of water, and make into a fairly stiff dough, about the consistency of bread dough. Let stand for one hour after mixing. Then put in a large pan and cover with water. Wash out the starch by working it with both hands. When the water becomes white with starch, pour it off, and put on fresh water. Repeat this until the water is clear; then all the starch will be washed out.

If it is desired to have it very tender, cover this gluten with water and let stand a day or two under water. If the weather is cool it should stand about two days, but in warm weather, a day will be sufficient time. Do not let it stand too long, however, for the gluten will dissolve.

Then cut the gluten mass in small pieces, dropping, as it is cut, into a pan of boiling water, containing enough water so that the gluten will float. Stir on the bottom of the pan with a pancake turner to prevent burning. Cook for half an hour.

Remove from the water what is desired for immediate use and add a little soy sauce. This gives it a meat flavor.

Always keep the gluten covered with water, both before it is cooked and afterwards.

It can be warmed in a frying pan with a little Mazola or

corn oil, seasoned with finely cut onions, if desired. Too much frying makes it tough, however.

This vegetable protein can be used in stews, pot pies, vegetable roasts, or any place where lean beefsteak is used. It is excellent in vegetable soup.

Vegetable Roast

8 oz. strong cereal coffee
1 lb. washed gluten
5 oz. raw peanut meal
salt to taste

Mix all ingredients in a blender and thoroughly blend. Put it in cans, seal, and cook in a steam pressure cooker for about four hours under five pounds of pressure; or if in an open kettle, cook for six hours. This can also be put in a stone crock, placing the crock in a dish of water, and baked four hours in a moderate oven. The placing of the crock in the dish of water is to prevent the meat from burning.

This vegetable roast will be found to be an excellent product when cut in cubes, to combine with any kind of a vegetable stew that the housewife may wish to prepare.

Vegetarian Roast No.1

2 tbs. ground onions
2 cups raw peanut butter
1/2 cup boiled kidney beans
3 cups water
ground celery seed to suit taste

Mix the ingredients, put in cans, seal, and cook for four hours under five pounds pressure. This can also be placed in a crock and baked in the oven, as described in directions for Vegetable Roast.

Vegetarian Roast No.1 can be used diced in casseroles, stews, and soups. It is also good sliced and browned for sandwiches.

Vegetarian Roast No.2

1 lb. raw peanut butter
1 1/2 pints water
salt to taste

Add the water to the peanut butter a little at a time, stirring continuously to make a paste free from lumps. Add salt to taste. Cook from one to four hours. Can be boiled in a double boiler or cooked in the oven by placing the dish containing the roast in a dish of water to prevent it from burning on the bottom and sides. May also be cooked in sealed cans.

This roast should be of such a consistency that when it is cold it can be sliced and eaten. Children and people with delicate digestions may eat this. This is good made up into sandwiches, also diced in casseroles, stews, and soups.

Gluten Patties

2 cups ground gluten
1 onion, finely chopped
2 cups crumbed zwieback, or cooked brown rice
1/2 cup soy sauce
1/2 tsp. salt

Flavor with garlic, Vegex, or sage. Mix thoroughly, make into patties, and brown in oven or frying pan.

Tomato Vegetarian Roast

Prepare it just like the Vegetarian Roast No.2, except use half water and half tomato juice; or you can use all tomato juice if you like.

Vegetable Salmon

1 lb. raw peanut butter
1 medium-sized carrot, ground very fine
1 No.2 can of tomatoes, put through a fine sieve
1 pint water

Mix ingredients thoroughly and salt to taste. It is then ready to be put in cans, if desired, and cooked under five pounds steam pressure for four hours. If cooked in an ordinary kettle, well covered with water, it will require one and a half to two hours longer boiling. This mixture can also be baked in the oven. First boil it a few minutes in an open saucepan, stirring constantly until it thickens, and then bake in a slow oven for one hour. It is then ready to serve. This is a very wholesome and palatable dish.

How To Cook Brown Rice

One cup brown rice will make 3 cups cooked rice. Bring 2 1/2 cups water to a boil. Add 3/4 tsp. sea salt. Stir in 1 cup of brown rice. Bring to a boil again. Cover tightly. Turn heat as low as possible. Steam for 50 minutes. Remove cover and leave over heat for a few minutes.

Nut Loaf
2 tbs. onions
2 tbs. celery
2 tbs. soy sauce
2 cups brown rice, cooked
1 cup nuts, chopped
1/2 cup whole wheat bread crumbs, toasted
soy milk to moisten
salt to taste

Chop onions and celery fine. Then mix all ingredients together thoroughly. Add more soy milk if too dry. Put loaf in a greased pan and bake in moderate oven 3/4 hour.

Gluten Roast
2 cups sprouted lentils
2 cups washed gluten

Mix lentils and gluten together and run through an Enterprise grinder two or three times. Season with a little tomato, Vegex, or sage. Salt to taste. Cook four hours in sealed tins under five pounds pressure. If cooked in an open vessel or double boiler, six hours cooking is required.

To cook in the oven, make the material into a loaf, put in a greased pan and just barely cover the loaf with water. Place this pan in another larger pan containing water and bake for 1 hour in a moderate oven at 350°. When done, pour the liquid off the loaf and use this for a gravy. It may be thickened with cornmeal and seasoned with Vegex or any vegetable extract.

E. SOUPS

Soups can be made from any combination of vegetables one likes, such as celery, carrots, potatoes, parsley, onions, and okra. Other good vegetables for soup are dried beans such as navy, lima, Great Northern beans, or green split peas, soaked overnight in water and cooked very slowly until thoroughly done, then put through a fine sieve or colander to remove any of the outside covering of the bean that may not have cooked up soft. If the sifted pulp is too thick, thin out with soy or nut milk, flavor with onion, garlic, or parsley, which should be cut very fine, added to the sifted pulp, and heated about ten minutes before serving. Soy sauce, Savorex, or Vegex is good for flavoring. Use salt sparingly. Never use black or white pepper. Read the description of cayenne (red pepper) in this book.

A good soy soup is made just as you make any other bean soup. Soybeans can be purchased in cans, which makes it easier for the average home to use them more freely. They are a wonderful food.

All nut milks may be used in place of soybean milk. Flavor with a little soy sauce if desired, to taste.

Much is said about vegetable juices, and they are good, but not everyone can digest raw vegetable juices. Make your own vegetable juices by using any vegetable or vegetables you wish. The dark leafy vegetables are very good. Cut the leaves fine, put them in cold water, bring to a boil and boil gently for a few minutes. Then pour the leaves into a fine-mesh bag and squeeze it to extract the juice. Then you have a real vegetable juice; use hot or cold. Flavor with soy sauce, onion juice, or any vegetable flavoring you like.

Vegetable Soup No.1

In a large soup kettle put about one cup each of the following vegetables: carrots, cabbage, celery, potatoes (do not peel the potatoes, but scrub with a wire brush, so the eyes will remain in the potatoes, as they are the life-giving part); and also one-half cup onions. Be sure to use the green leaves of the celery and the green leaves of the cabbage. The green leaves of the cauliflower are even better although they are generally thrown away. Add one gallon of water. After the soup has come to a boil, add one cup of brown rice, and simmer slowly from one to two hours, or more. Salt to taste.

When the soup is done, you may, if desired, add one quart soybean milk, more or less to suit the taste.

If the soup is to be fed to invalids, to small children, or to those who have ulcers or cancer of the stomach, let it simmer at least two and a half or three hours slowly. Then mash the vegetables with a wire potato masher and boil them a few minutes longer. Then strain the soup through a fine wire strainer, and add the soybean milk. Tomato juice may be added instead of the soybean milk if you like. This is a most wonderful alkaline dish and highly nourishing.

When the soup gets cold, it is a very nourishing drink and very high in vitamins and life-giving properties, far superior to sauerkraut juice or tomato juice.

One can add different kinds of green vegetables to suit his own taste, and may also use more of one kind and less of others if preferred.

Vegetable Soup No.2
2 large carrots, scraped
4 turnips

4 onions
parsley (use generously)
green leaves of cabbage, chopped
medium bunch of celery, using stalks and leaves
1 cup lima beans, fresh or frozen
1 cup green peas, fresh or frozen, or you may use a cup of
 puree made from the dried split peas and lima beans
soy sauce to taste

Cut the vegetables in small pieces, and do not boil hard. Let them simmer until cooked soft. Add a little salt and soy sauce when finished, if desired.

Potato and Onion Soup
6 medium-sized unpeeled potatoes, sliced fine
3 good-sized onions, cut fine
5 tbs. parsley, chopped
2 quarts water

Let simmer for one hour. Then add one heaping table-spoonful each of soybean flour and oatmeal flour, mixed thoroughly with a little cold water, and then added to the soup. Let boil five minutes, salt sparingly, and serve.

Fruit Soup
My parents used a great deal of fruit soup when I was a child.

2 cups raisins
2 cups prunes
4 quarts cold water
1 cup grape juice (unsweetened)
2 lemons
malt sugar or honey to sweeten to taste

Soak the raisins and prunes overnight. Then add them to the water and let them simmer until done. Add the grape juice and lemons, sliced very thin, and the sweetening to taste. This can be served hot or cold as you desire. This soup can be thickened with cornstarch or agar agar.

Do not serve this soup with a vegetable meal; use whole wheat toast, whole wheat zwieback, whole wheat crackers, or any of the whole grain products, soybean gems, and nut products, or nuts; used in this way it makes a fine luncheon or fruit meal.

Cream of Tomato Soup

6 cups very rich soybean milk
6 cups tomato juice
6 rounded tbs. soybean flour
  (make into a thin paste with cold water)

You may also use a milk made from any nuts in place of soybean milk. Milk made from raw peanut butter is excellent, and so is almond milk.

Heat the soybean milk. Then heat the tomato juice, add the soybean flour paste, stirring constantly. Do not let it boil, just simmer. After five minutes stir the thickened tomato juice into the hot milk, let heat a few minutes, add a pinch of salt and serve.

Oatmeal water, made by soaking four parts of water to one part of oatmeal overnight and then strained, is an excellent addition to any soup stock. It increases the vitamins and makes the soup creamy.

Tomato Soup No.1

3 cups tomato juice
3 cups cold water
3 heaping tbs. soybean flour

Mix the tomato juice and water, and bring to a boil. Make a thin paste of the soybean flour mixed with cold water, stir this into the hot tomato juice, and let simmer five minutes. A heaping tablespoonful of soybean butter may be added to this (dilute the butter in a little cold water and put through a fine sieve before adding to the soup). Let the soup get real hot, add a pinch of salt and serve.

Tomato Soup No.2
1 tbs. 3-minute oats
1 quart water
1 quart tomatoes
1 tbs. Kokofat
salt to taste

Cook the three-minute oats in boiling water ten minutes. Mash the tomatoes and put them through a flour sieve. Add the tomatoes to the water and then add the Kokofat. Boil five minutes. Salt sparingly.

Cream of Corn Soup
1 pint fresh or canned corn
3 pints rich soybean milk
salt to taste

Heat the milk. Put the corn through a sieve, and add to the hot milk. Salt to taste and serve.

Cream of Celery Soup
1 cup diced celery
1 pint soybean milk
1/2 pint water
1/2 tsp. salt
2 tbs. soybean butter

Cook the celery in the milk and water and when nearly done, add salt. Simmer until celery is soft. Add soybean butter just before serving.

Cream of Lentil Soup
3 cups cooked lentils
1 pint rich soybean milk
1 quart water

salt
1 small, fresh onion, chopped fine or 1/4 cup dried onion
vegetable extract such as Savorex or Vegex
parsley
2 tbs. soybean butter

Put the lentils through a sieve, add the soybean milk, and one quart of water; salt to taste. Season with onion, and a little vegetable extract. Just before serving, add finely cut parsley, and 2 tablespoonfuls soybean butter.

Lentil Soup
2 cups cooked lentils
1/4 cup chopped, cooked carrots
1/4 cup chopped green onions
1 cup tomato juice
2 cups lentil juice (the water that the lentils are cooked in)
1/2 cup finely cut parsley

Mix all the ingredients, heat to the boiling point, add one tablespoonful soybean butter, salt to taste, and serve.

Vegetable Oyster (Salsify) Soup
3 cups vegetable oysters (cut in small rings)
2 cups water
2 cups rich soy milk
1 tbs. soybean butter

Cook the vegetable oyster rings in the water until tender. Add the soybean milk and butter. Salt to taste and serve.

Cream of Spinach Soup
1 cup spinach pulp
2 cups rich soy milk
1 cup mashed potatoes
    (as given earlier in this chapter)
2 cups potato water
1 tbs. soybean butter

Mix the spinach pulp and soybean milk, add the mashed potatoes and potato water, salt to taste, bring to a boil, add one tablespoonful soybean butter and serve.

Potato Soup
3 cups mashed potatoes
2 tbs. chopped onions
1 pint rich soybean milk
1 quart parsley or watercress for seasoning

Make the mashed potatoes by following the recipe given in Section B, earlier in this chapter. Mix all the ingredients together, bring to a boil, add one tablespoonful soybean butter, and serve.

Split Pea Soup
Cook until tender either green or yellow split peas. Rub the cooked peas through a sieve. To the pea puree add rich soybean milk until it reaches the desired consistency. Some gluten meat, diced small, will add greatly to this soup. Season with onions, garlic, parsley, or soybean sauce. Vegetable extract may also be used. Simmer five minutes and serve hot.

F.   GRAVIES

Oatmeal Gravy
1 quart boiling water
4 oz. oatmeal flour or 3-minute oats
1 tbs. oil
seasonings such as bay leaf, onion, or desired flavoring
Vegex or vegetable extract (to taste)
salt

Into one quart of boiling water stir gradually the four ounces of oatmeal flour, or 3-minute oats. Boil until thickened. If 3-minute oats are used, a little longer boiling is necessary than when oatmeal flour is used. Add about one tablespoonful corn oil, or any other good oil. The gravy may be seasoned with a little onion, bay leaf, or other seasoning as desired. Also add 1 teaspoon Vegex or vegetable extract, which will give it a meaty flavor.

This makes a very wholesome and well-flavored gravy.

Soybean Gravy

Into one quart boiling soybean milk, add oatmeal flour or 3-minute oats (about 4 ounces) to make the desired consistency, or thickness. Oatmeal flour works quickest.

Let simmer until thickened, stirring constantly with a pancake turner so it will not burn on the bottom. Add a little soy sauce or vegetable extract to lend a meaty flavor.

This may be made with water instead of milk, and enriched with a little Kloss's butter, and a little fine cut onion to add to the flavor.

G.   SALADS AND SALAD DRESSINGS

Salads are refreshing and life-giving if made of any combination of vegetables that are fresh and crisp.

Do not combine fruits and vegetables in the same salad, as it is not a healthful combination. Have your vegetable salads with your vegetable meals, or make a good nourishing vegetable salad and eat with nuts or some good meat substitute for luncheon. Another time have a fruit salad with nuts or some good meat substitute for luncheon or with a fruit meal.

Do not use mayonnaise that has vinegar, mustard, black or white pepper, or cane sugar in it. If you wish to use mayonnaise, make your own. (See the recipe for soy oil mayonnaise later in this section.)

Vegetable Salad No.1

1 cup finely diced or grated carrots
1 cup finely diced celery

1 cup cabbage, chopped fine
1 green pepper, cut in thin rings or fine slices
1 cup finely cut parsley
finely chopped nuts
olives

Mix the carrots, celery, and cabbage together and put as large a serving as you wish of these on lettuce leaves, arranging the rings or slices of green pepper around the mixed vegetables and garnish with whole sprigs of parsley. Finely chopped or ground-up nuts sprinkled over this make a very nourishing salad or you can use the nuts whole. Ground-up nuts are the best, however, as very few people will chew the whole nuts enough to thoroughly emulsify them; thus they do not get the good of the nuts. Soy mayonnaise is very nice with this salad, and so are a few olives arranged around or over it.

Vegetable Salad No.2
green onions (spring)
green peppers
cucumbers
celery
parsley
radishes
watercress

Use equal parts of these vegetables. Chop or dice the green onions, celery, and green peppers; mince the parsley and watercress; mix and place a serving on lettuce leaves. If the cucumbers are nice, with a thin fresh skin, do not peel, but wash well. Cut in thin round slices or lengthwise and arrange with radishes around and over the other vegetables.

Potato Salad
potatoes
ripe olives

nuts
cayenne pepper

onions	soy oil mayonnaise
parsley	radishes
celery	
cucumbers	

Prepare the potatoes by boiling with the skins on, and drying them on the hot stove burner when done so they are dry and mealy. Cool the potatoes and skin them, making your salad for use immediately if you wish the best flavor.

Have the onions, celery, and ripe olives chopped quite fine, mince the parsley, and mix with your diced cucumbers and potatoes. Leave the skin on the cucumber if it is a nice thin skin. Salt moderately, add finely ground-up nuts or halves of walnuts, and a pinch of cayenne. Mix with soy oil mayonnaise, and garnish with radishes and parsley. Never use leftover potatoes in making potato salad; it is much better to have them fresh cooked.

Fruit Salads

In making fruit salads be careful of your combinations. Citrus fruits do not combine well with other fruits, such as dates and figs. Avocados may be used with citrus fruits. Combine these as you wish, using figs and dates as a garnish. When using avocados, sprinkle some lemon juice over them. Any kind of nuts may be used with a fruit salad. Finely ground nuts sprinkled over the salad make it more nourishing.

Good Combinations for Fruit Salads

1. Ripe bananas, fresh or dried coconut, shredded or ground, cherries, and pineapple
2. Apples, raisins, and walnuts
3. Bananas, apples, and pineapple
4. Ripe strawberries and ripe bananas

5. Red raspberries and bananas
6. Black raspberries and bananas
7. Ripe pears, strawberries, and bananas
8. Fresh peaches, cántaloupe, and Thompson seedless grapes

Fresh coconut is a good combination with fresh fruit.

All berries and fruits must be vine-ripened and tree-ripened to be really valuable for food. Be sure that bananas are fully ripened; they must not show any green on the ends and must be sprinkled with brown spots generously over the entire skin before they are really ripe and valuable for food.

Fruit salads look nice served on fresh crisp lettuce leaves. Soy oil mayonnaise diluted to the consistency of cream is delicious with fruit salads.

Fruit Salad

1/2 cup wheat flakes
1/2 cup diced or chopped raw apples
1/2 cup chopped raisins

It is best to soak the raisins overnight before using. More or less of any ingredient may be used to suit the convenience and taste. Mix ingredients together and serve. This makes a salad that anyone can live on.

Soy Oil Mayonnaise

1 heaping tbs. finely ground flour
1/2 pint cold water
1/2 pint soy oil
1 tbs. lemon juice (more or less to taste)
pinch of salt
paprika and cayenne
vegetable butter coloring

Mix the soy flour into the cold water, boil for five minutes. Cook in a smooth flat-bottomed dish, using a pancake turner for stirring to keep free from the bottom of the dish, as it burns very quickly. Strain through a fine sieve into a medium-sized mixing bowl. While beating rapidly and continuously, or using a blender, pour in the soy oil in a very fine stream. If the oil is poured in fast, the mayonnaise will separate after standing awhile. (If this should happen, pour the oil off, and beat again.) It will be very simple after you have made it a few times. Then add the salt, paprika, cayenne, and vegetable butter coloring and beat just enough to mix well. It needs only a small pinch of cayenne to make it taste snappy. Using more or less soy oil, you may make it any consistency you wish. Peanut oil may be used in place of soy oil, but I prefer the soy oil and soy flour.

A clove of garlic cut and rubbed on the bowl in which the mayonnaise is made greatly adds to the flavor.

Kloss's Mayonnaise

1/2 cup water
1/4 cup soy milk powder
1/4 tsp. sea salt
1/4 tsp. paprika
1/4 tsp. seasoning of your choice
1/2 cup oil
lemon juice

Blend the first five ingredients in a blender. Add 1/2 cup oil slowly while blending at high speed. Remove from blender. Add 3 tbs. lemon juice or according to taste.

This mayonnaise can be used anywhere that dairy cream is used. It makes a very fine dressing for cole slaw or any kind of greens.

A little cayenne pepper may be added if a snappy mayonnaise is desired. To add the cayenne pepper, sprinkle it a little at a time directly into the mayonnaise, beating until it is thoroughly mixed.

Red pepper or cayenne is a wonderful medicine, and does not injure the product. Cayenne pepper should not be classed with black and white pepper, or mustard and vinegar, which are found in the mayonnaise on the market and are highly injurious to the digestive tract and stomach. Look in the index for red pepper.

"Nut Mayonnaise"

Dilute one-half cup raw peanut butter or mock almond butter (see recipe given earlier in this chapter) with one cup of water. Then beat in one cup of oil, either corn or olive oil. Add about 1 tablespoonful lemon juice. Salt to taste.

This can also be boiled for two or three minutes, and then beaten thoroughly.

Milk Sweetening

1 cup malt honey
1 cup corn or olive oil

Pour the corn or olive oil into the malt honey, beating constantly. Pour slowly. In this way the fat is emulsified and easily digested.

H.   BREAKFAST FOODS

French Toast

Slice soybean or other bread about one-half inch thick and let dry in a moderately warm oven. When thoroughly dry, increase the heat in the oven enough to turn the bread a golden brown. This browning turns the starch into dextrose or grape sugar, making it practically like the juice in ripe fruit.

Now immerse the toast in soybean milk, being careful not to leave it too long. Lift out with a pancake turner, and spread a thin coating of Kloss's Mayonnaise on each slice. Have your frying pan hot with a little oil in it, place the toast in with the side down that has the mayonnaise on it. Now, spread the top side with mayonnaise, leaving until the under side is browned, then turn it over until the top side is browned.

Serve with diluted malt honey, honey, or maple syrup. French toast can be served with any meal, but is especially nice for breakfast. French toast, with a cup of hot soybean milk, is nice for a light supper.

This toast makes a wholesome and easily digested dish, containing all the necessary food elements.

Zwieback

Bread baked in the ordinary way is never entirely dextrinized, so that the starch turns into grape sugar. But zwieback, or twice-baked bread, is very wholesome and easy to digest.

To make zwieback, slice the bread about three-quarters of an inch thick, and let it dry in a slow oven until it is entirely dry. Increase the temperature of the oven and brown the bread to a golden brown. It must be carefully watched, as it burns easily.

Breakfast Wheat

1 cup natural whole grain wheat
3 cups water
salt to taste

Place all ingredients in a double boiler and cook until the kernels burst. Raisins, pitted dates, or chopped figs may be stirred into the wheat just before serving. These give a natural sweetness and are far better for the system than cane sugar.

This can also be cooked in a steam pressure cooker until the kernels are done, about one hour, or in a crock in the oven; set the crock in a pan of water to keep the wheat from burning and cook about 4 hours; or cook in an electric crock pot overnight.

Malt Honey

Take one pound of wheat or cornmeal. Add eight quarts of water. Let it come to a boil and boil it until it thickens so that the starch is cooked. Cool to between 140°F and 170°F. Then add two ounces of barley malt, either in powder or syrup form. Stir. Let stand until the starch is changed into dextrose or malt honey. When the water is clear, pour or siphon it off, being careful not to get any mash from the bottom, otherwise the malt honey will not be clear. Now boil it down to the consistency of syrup.

Old-Fashioned Granola

Take whole wheat flour and enough water to make a stiff dough. Roll it out about a quarter or half an inch thick. Put in oven and bake until it is partly dextrinized, nearly a golden brown. Take a hammer and break it up and grind through a Quaker City Mill made by the A. W. Straub Company of Philadelphia. After grinding, put in a baking pan and reheat to slightly dextrinize it.

Boiled Rice

1 cup natural brown rice
3 cups water
salt to taste

Put one cup of rice and one teaspoon of salt into a pan, pour on three cups of boiling water, cover tightly and simmer on low heat without stirring for 45 minutes, when the rice will be thoroughly cooked but not mushy.

Baked Rice

1/2 to 3/4 cup natural brown rice
2 cups soybean milk
1/2 tsp. salt

Wash and drain the rice. Pour the hot milk into a baking dish and add the rice. Cover and bake in a slow oven two to three hours without stirring, or until the milk is thickened and creamy with rice. If the milk boils out under the cover, the oven is too hot.

This makes a very delicious dish, and does not require any additions. If a dressing is desired, however, milk sweetening, the recipe for which was given earlier in this chapter, may be diluted with a little water or soybean milk and poured over the rice. Fig marmalade may also be used with rice: see the recipe for Fig Marmalade Pie in chapter 5.

An excellent rice pudding can be made by adding one-half cup malt honey and one cup of raisins just before placing the rice in the oven to bake.

Dixie Kernel

1 cup cornmeal
1 cup oatmeal
1 cup whole wheat flour
1 cup finely ground bran
1 tsp. salt

Mix all ingredients and add enough water to make a stiff dough. Roll out to about one-half inch thickness. Bake in a moderate oven until slightly browned. When a day old, grind up while still a little moist.

Add one cup of water to a cup of malt honey, mixing thoroughly. Sprinkle this over the ground cereal product. Do not let the mixture get too moist. Now spread out to partly dry, and then place in an oven to dextrinize, making a slight golden brown.

Old-Fashioned Dixie Kernel

Take various kinds of broken crackers, such as bran, whole wheat, oatmeal, graham and white, and grind them together.

Take equal parts each of malt honey and water, stirring well together, and sprinkle over the ground crackers, mixing them up thoroughly to slightly moisten them. Place in the oven, stirring frequently to prevent burning, and slightly dextrinize to a golden brown.

This makes a very delightful breakfast food.

3

COOKING UNDER STEAM PRESSURE

We hear much about cooking with steam pressure. Some condemn it and some recommend it. In this chapter I will give some of my practical experiences, which I believe prove its value. I have had much experience with steam pressure cooking for many years, and had the honor of securing the first patent on a home steam pressure cooker ever granted in the United States. This cooker is now used over practically the entire civilized world.

Some time ago I read a long argument against steam pressure cooking. The doctor who made this argument is well-known in the United States; therefore, I shall not mention his name. His experiment proves that he is not a competent judge of steam pressure cooking. He spoke of having cooked wheat, corn, oats, barley, rye, buckwheat, and sunflower seed two hours under thirty pounds of steam pressure. These cooked grains were fed to such animals as rats, guinea pigs, etc. These small animals became sick and paralyzed in a few weeks. From these facts the doctor concluded that steam pressure cooking is detrimental to food.

I have operated canning factories large and small, and have visited many other large canning factories, but have never yet heard of anyone cooking food under thirty pounds of steam pressure for two hours, nor even for one hour under any such pressure. People used to cook navy beans and corn under ten to fifteen pounds of pressure for one hour. Most all steam pressure cooking is done at about five pounds steam pressure, which is ideal. In California a law was passed forbidding certain foods to be cooked using more than five pounds steam pressure.

There is no kind of cooking, either in a kettle or in a baking oven, that preserves the life-giving properties better than closing the foods tightly in a steam pressure cooker and cooking them until thoroughly done. I have had the privilege at different times of feeding groups of people where everything was cooked under steam pressure. We use the steam pressure cooker in our home with most gratifying results.

Potatoes are very delicious cooked in this way. Medium-sized potatoes will cook in twenty minutes in a steam pressure cooker under five pounds pressure. When you take them out, they are dry and mealy and have an excellent flavor, providing of course that they had a good flavor to start with.

Spinach is wonderful when cooked under steam pressure. It retains all of its life-giving qualities when cooked under a low pressure, say five pounds for 2 to 5 minutes, depending somewhat on the condition of the spinach. A canning recipe book comes with every steam pressure cooker, giving all the details on how to cook each food and how to use the steam pressure cooker.

The following table shows the comparative amount of heat developed for each pound of pressure in the pressure cooker.

Steam Pressure (Lbs. per square inch as shown on steam gauge)	Degrees of Heat Fahrenheit (Boiling point of water is 212°F.)
1	216
2	219
3	222
4	225
5	227
6	230
7	233
8	235
9	237
10	240
11	242
12	244

Steam Pressure (Lbs. per square inch as shown on steam gauge)	Degrees of Heat Fahrenheit (Boiling point of water is 212°F.)
13	246
14	248
15	250

The steam pressure cooker is one of the finest cooking utensils that has ever been invented. You can cook everything without putting water on it. You can also put several different foods in the cooker, cook them all at the same time, and each food will retain its natural flavor. Another advantage is that breakfast food or any other food can be cooked in a steam pressure cooker without having to stir it. It does not have to be watched, for it will never burn.

There is no way to cook foods that will preserve the life-giving properties, vitamins, and flavor more perfectly than under steam pressure. At the same time, it is a great fuel saver. After the food starts to cook, only a little heat is required to keep up the temperature. It also requires less attention than any other way of cooking, because, as previously mentioned, food will not burn or stick to the cooker. After you have set the pressure where you want it, you can go away and let it cook as long as necessary.

4

ALUMINUM COOKING UTENSILS

Aluminum poisoning is so prevalent that I feel it is a part of my duty to give my experience and warn people against the use of aluminum.

Some years ago we bought a nice supply of aluminum cooking utensils. Among them was a tea-kettle, which was constantly standing on the stove with some water in it. I would drink two or three cups of this water every morning and then some more about an hour before dinner. I developed terrible bowel trouble. I tried all kinds of remedies that ordinarily effected a cure, but neither herbs nor anything else did lasting good. I tried to find the cause, but everything failed. The doctors made all kinds of explanations of my condition, but they were all far from the cause.

The condition grew worse until I said to my wife: "Unless something helps me, I will surely die." One day I described my condition to a person who told me that the description was similar to the distress aluminum poison would cause. I immediately began to search into the aluminum proposition. I read different books on aluminum poisoning. I also went to Washington to search for what the government had on the subject in the Food Department. In those books I found reports of experiments that different doctors had made on animals. I also learned that they held postmortems on those who had died from supposed aluminum poisoning, and found that organs, such as the liver, spleen, and kidneys contained aluminum. They found that everyone who had had any practical experience with aluminum cooking utensils condemned them. For example, in Jefferson College at Philadelphia, many experiments have been made on aluminum, the findings of which are available in the Food Department at Washington.

I have boiled water in aluminum kettles and then some in

granite ware. I poured some from each kettle into two different glasses. The particles of aluminum could easily be seen
in the water boiled in the aluminum kettle. Many others have
made the same experiment.

Everyone who knows anything about aluminum knows
that it is poison. It flakes off very easily when food is cooked
in it. I have seen heavy aluminum dishes that were all pitted
on the bottom. Of course this aluminum had all gone into the
food that was cooked in these utensils.

I asked Doctor Charles T. Betts, of Toledo, who has had
long practical experience with aluminum, to write the following article.

ALUMINUM COOKING UTENSILS
Dr. Charles T. Betts
320 Superior Street
Toledo, Ohio

Before I became ill, the question of poisoning by aluminum compounds never interested me. We had a splendid
assortment in our home of aluminum cooking utensils in
which we took great pride, thinking them the finest available.
It was not long, however, after we began using them that my
health was reduced to such a serious condition from some
kind of poisoning that a journey was made to Colorado,
seeking air, water, sunshine, or whatnot, in the hope that life
might be prolonged.

My first attention to the possibility of aluminum being
poisonous or probably not fit for cooking purposes came
when it was noted that the water from the soda spring at
Manitou was effervescent when in contact with an aluminum
cup that I used for drinking purposes, and that the same water
had no such chemical action in a glass container.

The above observation brought recollections regarding the
activity of aluminum, or what is better known as the chemical
action of the metal upon foods that had been prepared in our
home. I remembered that peeled potatoes, if allowed to stand

in an aluminum dish overnight, would become yellow and when cooked would look somewhat shriveled and have dark streaks through the inner part.

Cranberries changed to a darkened color when cooked in an aluminum dish, with quite a few of the berries turning black.

Bread or pie dough when mixed on a sheet of aluminum acquires a grayish color. An aluminum pot becomes darkened when cabbage is boiled in it. Tomatoes, applesauce, rhubarb, cherries, grapes, etc., will clean an aluminum dish beautifully within five minutes, or as soon as the food is brought to a boil.

Ordinarily, well water boiled two hours will look rather milky and cause a dark coating over the inside of the aluminum dish.

Another observation of particular note was that a butterscotch pie filling, boiled a few minutes in an aluminum dish, changed from a rich brown to a dark green color and that a mayonnaise dressing turned from a light yellow to a brown color.

Lemonade made in an aluminum container will have a very bad taste if allowed to remain standing in the metal for any length of time.

Coffee remaining in an aluminum coffee pot has a puckery or metallic taste.

When you drive your car with an aluminum throttle, your fingers or gloves will become blackened by the metal rubbing off.

Hydrogen gas is formed by boiling well water, or when heat is in contact with an aluminum dish. This can be noted on cold aluminum by the bubbles all around the sides of a pail. They form as far down as the bottom of the receptacle.

If the batter of an angel food cake is stirred in an aluminum dish a few minutes, the finished product will have dark streaks through it. Whites of eggs will turn green if stirred ten minutes in an aluminum pan.

A few other experiments brought to the writer's attention

more vividly the possibility of being poisoned by these utensils. It was found that ordinary foods other than protein (beans, etc.), will not adhere to the metal. Cake, pancakes, and waffles do not stick to aluminum, and the use of butter or oil is not needed. (Alum baking powder sprinkled upon an iron utensil will prevent sticking of the dough).

Tarnished silverware can be made bright and shiny within a few minutes by putting the ware in an aluminum dish. Partly fill with water, add a little bicarbonate of soda, and bring to a boil. It will be found that all bubbles on wild beer will instantly disappear when the beverage is placed in an aluminum dish.

When water is boiled in an aluminum dish for one-half hour and placed in a glass, a light, feathery substance can be seen with the naked eye, and precipitation takes place in the bottom of the glass after cooling. An interesting experiment can be noted by cleaning an aluminum dish with lye or bichloride of mercury. After this is done, a fine dust will cover the inside of the utensil within a few minutes. Aluminum chloride is produced when salted bacon is fried in an aluminum spider after the grease has congealed. Vegetables cooked until dry will be covered with a white dust.

It was further noted that it is impossible to make hard soap in an aluminum dish. Persons become sick after they eat seafoods that have been cooked with milk in aluminum ware. The same effect was noted after eating custard that had been allowed to stand in an aluminum dish for some hours before serving. The most frequent cases of group poisoning came from serving salted fricassee of chicken, pork, or veal that had been cooked and allowed to remain standing in the aluminum vessel for twelve hours.

Recipes are given in various papers apparently by aluminum organizations advising the public how to clean the utensil that has acquired a dark coating. The following is one that was found in the *Toledo Blade*, Toledo, Ohio.

Lightning Workers

"Cook your rhubarb or fresh tomatoes in a discolored aluminum pan. They will accomplish more in five minutes than you could do by scrubbing for an hour."

It was discovered that agents were selling 'Lightning Silverware Cleaners.' Investigation proved that the lightning workers were nothing more or less than a small piece of aluminum, which was to be inserted in boiling water together with the silver, with a little soda added. This does the trick beautifully.

Many persons throughout the land noted the effects of food upon aluminum and of aluminum upon food. These observations were made in various localities, so that a discussion of national prominence arose regarding the possibility of such culinary ware being unfit to use for cooking purposes.

Many believe the metal that dissolves from aluminum dishes is either filth or dirt. The metal is not a food substance and it cannot become a constituent part of the human body. It is evident that it contaminates food with poisonous effects. That food values are damaged or destroyed is noted by the best available scientists in America; that the color of cooked foods shows adverse chemical changes when cooked and stored in aluminum; that various chemical poisons are formed according to the kinds of foods cooked when their salts react with the metal or when seasoning agents are employed like salt, cooking soda, etc. It was observed that a poisonous gas, hydrogen, is formed by them, which permeates the room in which they are used.

The above observation caused the writer to investigate what is in the record at Washington upon the subject, particularly the physiological effects to the human when the drug called "alum" (an aluminum salt) is ingested. Alum is the generic term applied to any member of a class of double aluminum-containing compounds.

The government made a thorough investigation upon this particular point from 1925 to 1930. The Federal Trade Commission, Docket 540, took more than four thousand pages of typewritten testimony from 158 witnesses over a period of five years, after which an official report was made by Edward M. Averill. Many of the witnesses were professors, deans, biologists, and toxicologists from many colleges, some of which are the highest schools of learning in America.

Following are two comments by Averill as part of his findings:

"The evidence in this record does not prove that they (aluminum dishes and cookware) are harmless."

"The evidence in this record does prove that there are substantial grounds upon which to predicate an honest opinion that they are harmful."

We have evidence of a real nature, understandable by anyone, as a further proof that the aluminum, which dissolves from the utensils, has evil effects upon the body when consumed with foods. Our American people are banqueters. They love picnics and have extensive church gatherings at which they come to enjoy food, to worship, and have a good time. Often these are turned into places of grief, anxiety, and death. The following is a report of an extensive group poisoning at one of these church dinners held at Punxsutawney, Pennsylvania, reported in the *Sun-Telegraph,* Pittsburgh, Pennsylvania.

200 Church Diners Poisoned

Punxsutawney, PA., Dec. 3 — Two hundred people who attended a chicken supper at the First Baptist Church today are recovering from ptomaine poisoning. A dozen or more are seriously ill, but so far there have been no deaths.

Women of the church prepared the supper at their homes and served it in the church auditorium, and every person who partook of the supper became ill.

Physicians stated that the entire supply of gravy had been poisoned as the result of one of the women leaving the gravy in an aluminum container too long before taking it to the church. All the gravy was collected into one container to heat, and in that way the entire supply was contaminated.

The question is often asked, "Will aluminum cooking utensils cause gas in the stomach?" It was found that some American manufacturers of baking powder use a total of many thousands of tons of aluminum annually, mixed with an alkaline substance — soda. This combination does make gas. If aluminum will make gas in a dish on the table, as when baking powders are used, aluminum from cooking utensils will certainly make gas in the stomach or bowels when it comes in contact with the same kind of chemicals — the alkaline juices of the body.

Within eight weeks after I stopped eating the poison from our aluminum cooking utensils, I regained my health sufficiently to resume practice, and have enjoyed good health for many years since. All that is asked of the sick is that they do not use aluminum utensils or alum baking powders for a period of eight weeks and note results. If no improvement is observed, they can be used as before. This would surely not be a hardship on anyone seeking health.

ADDENDUM: In this chapter a clear-cut case against using any kind of aluminum cooking utensils whatsoever is presented. It is backed up by thorough research of the available material and scientific data current at the time in which this book was first published. But as the years and decades slipped by, these ideas became out-of-date and were relegated to the status of nutritional quackery by many food scientists and doctors.

But now these warnings, first sounded by Jethro Kloss nearly a half-century ago, are reappearing with additional evidence from the very community that had ignored and ostracized his ideas in the first place.

A number of important articles have appeared in medical and scientific journals within recent years citing the definite health hazards connected with the use of aluminum cookware. Two such articles discussed the association between aluminum cookware and Alzheimer's disease — a condition of mental deterioration experienced prior to the usual age when mental deterioration most commonly occurs. (Ref. Crapper, D.R. et al, "Brain Aluminum in Alzheimer's Disease and Experimental Neurofibrillary Degeneration," *Science,* 180:511-513, 1973. Trapp, G.A. et al, "Aluminum Levels in Brain in Alzheimer's Disease," *Biological Psychiatry,* 13:709-718, 1978.) Another article has demonstrated that the use of aluminum cookware can lead to kidney failure in the elderly as well as poor memory and eyesight. (Ref. Arieff, A.I. et al, "Dementia, Renal Failure, and Brain Aluminum," *Annals of Internal Medicine,* 90:741-747, 1979.)

In a Letter to the Editor published in the prestigious *New England Journal of Medicine,* Vol. 303, page 164, July 17, 1980, Stephen E. Levick, M.D., of the Yale University School of Medicine, cites his own experience with cooking in inexpensive aluminum pots and pans while he was a medical student and intern. He goes on to mention "the growing literature implicating aluminum as the causative agent in dialysis dementia and discussing the association between aluminum and Alzheimer's disease." He concludes: "Large numbers of people in our aluminum-using society may be the victims of slow aluminum poisoning from several sources. Corrodible aluminum cookware may be a nontrivial source.... In the meantime, out with my corroding aluminum pots!"

Essentially, then, what a Yale M.D. in 1980 has done is to underscore the truthfulness of Jethro Kloss's words, written some time in the 1930s: "Aluminum poisoning is so prevalent that I feel it is a part of my duty to give my experience and warn people against the use of aluminum." After nearly 50 years, this piece of unofficial folk-health wisdom is now becoming firmly established as a medical fact.

In 1939, the same year that *Back to Eden* was first published by Jethro Kloss in the United States, a small booklet entitled *Why Aluminium Pans are Dangerous,* by Edgar J. Saxon, was printed in London, England. (Aluminium is the English spelling for aluminum.) Aluminum was first used for making cooking utensils in England in the year 1887 and, according to Mr. Saxon, it was only a few years later that questions were being raised both in England and the United States as to the suitability of using aluminum for cooking vessels. Many persons who had chronic intestinal disturbances found that these problems disappeared promptly after they stopped cooking in aluminum pans.

Aluminum salts are produced when salt or soda is added when cooking vegetables in aluminum pans. Some of these aluminum salts exert a deleterious affect on proteins in the body, so that their use in baking powder or as a preservative was forbidden by law in England. Since vegetables and fruits contain their own acids and alkali, it is very likely that aluminum salts are formed when these foods are cooked in pans made of this metal.

Mr. Saxon tells of a report from the British Ministry of Health in 1935 that, while seeming to vindicate the safety of using aluminum cooking vessels, actually contained many statements that were contradictory and indirectly indicted aluminum as a potential health hazard.

In sum, Mr. Saxon stated: "If coffee prepared in an aluminium pot can produce obvious gastric disturbance, if a black deposit is left on the inside of an aluminium pan after cooking cabbage, beans, etc., without the presence of soda, and if the taste of an egg poached in an aluminium pan and then allowed to get cold is what it is, it would seem in the highest degree possible that this is not the way to bring salts into the marvelous world of human cells which, in the digestive organs, blood, and tissues are dealing all the time with mineral material in a highly attenuated form.

"If the facts and considerations advanced in this book leave any reader satisfied that it is safe to cook food in aluminium pans, he or she must have a truly touching faith in medical pronouncements and in the disinterested motives of the aluminium industry."

Presenile dementia, Alzheimer's disease, afflicts two to three percent of the United States population and many researchers now believe that aluminum, which has a predisposition to affect the brain tissues, is directly or indirectly responsible. Autopsies performed on those who die from this disease show an excessively high level of aluminum in some of the brain cells. Dr. Armond Lione presented a paper at the Aluminum and Alzheimer's Disease Symposium in Toronto in November 1981, giving a list of foods and drugs that contain aluminum. Among these are processed cheese, vaginal douches, baking powder, toothpastes, antiperspirants, bottled pickles, nondairy creamers, as an additive to drinking water supplies in some cities, antacids. (Nearly every antacid on the market today has as one of its components aluminum hydroxide.) He also states that "Alzheimer's disease is the most common form of senility and is....causing 60,000 to 90,000 deaths annually."

Dr. Furman, near the end of his article discussing the relationship of aluminum to Alzheimer's disease, makes this observation: "A careful review of available evidence clearly shows a close relationship between aluminum and Alzheimer's disease.

"Even though the final word is not in, we do know enough to make a concerted effort to avoid all sources of aluminum pollution. We must try not to add to the unavoidable aluminum contamination in our bodies." (Ref. "Aluminum Pots and Pans May Contribute to Alzheimer's Disease," Dr. Arthur F. Furman, *The Nutritional Consultant*, Feb. 1984, page 12.)

5

BAKING AND BREADS

A. GENERAL PRINCIPLES

Food must be prepared properly to be easily digested and thoroughly assimilated. Our physical well-being depends on this. Considering cooking's importance to health, we do not give it the attention it deserves. A thorough knowledge of healthful cooking is just as essential to health as is eating good food.

Successful cooking and baking depend largely upon using the best quality of food. But even the best food is often damaged during preparation. When food is not prepared in a wholesome, appetizing manner, it is more difficult for it to make good pure blood that is necessary to build up wasted tissues. For health's sake, food must be prepared in a simple manner and be free from grease.

Ninety percent of all human ills originate in the stomach, and are caused from overeating wrong combinations of food, or unwholesome, unnatural foods. Remember, properly cooked food is always much easier for the body to digest.

All food should be prepared in one of the following ways: boiled, steamed, simmered, stewed, braised, roasted, broiled, or baked. Do not eat fried foods; they are indigestible and harmful to the system.

B. MAKING BREAD

Breads are divided into two classes: fermented and unfermented. Fermented bread is made light by a ferment, yeast usually being employed. Unfermented bread is made light by the introduction of air into the dough or batter. This method will be discussed later.

712

Yeast or Fermented Bread. Fermented bread is generally made by mixing flour, water, salt, and yeast into a dough. A small amount of malt extract, malt honey, or honey may be added, if desired, as it increases the food value and hastens fermentation. This is the straight dough method. The dough is kneaded until it is elastic to the touch and does not stick to the board, the object being to incorporate air and to distribute the yeast uniformly. The dough is then covered and allowed to rise until it has doubled its bulk, and does not respond to the touch when tapped sharply, but gradually and stubbornly begins to sink.

At this stage, the dough is "ripe," and ready to be worked down (kneaded). It will require from 2 to 3 1/2 hours to rise, depending on the grade and consistency of the flour used, the temperature of the room in which it is set, and the amount of yeast used. This process is best accomplished at a temperature ranging from 80° to 90°F.

After rising, the bread is again worked down well, turned over in the bowl, and left to rise until about three-quarters its original bulk.

Then it is turned out on a board, kneaded together enough to work out the air, and cut up in loaf-size pieces. It takes 1 pound plus 3 or 4 ounces of the dough to make a one-pound loaf.

Knead the dough until the air has been worked out and leave it on the board a few minutes so it will rise just a little You will find that this improves the texture of the bread.

Then form into loaves and knead just enough to work out the air. Do not knead too much. With a little experience you will become a master at bread making.

Instructions for baking bread are given in the section titled "The Oven," following.

Sponge Bread. Bread is also made by setting a "sponge" at the beginning. That is, by making a batter of the water, the yeast, and part of the flour, and letting it rise until it is light. Then the remaining ingredients are added and the mixture worked into a dough. Bun and cracker dough is usually set with the sponge method, because it produces a very fine and light texture. Ordinary white and whole wheat breads are often made by the same process.

A sponge is light enough when it appears frothy and full of bubbles. The time required will vary with the quantity and quality of yeast used, as well as with the temperature of the room in which it is set to rise.

Yeast. The most convenient yeast is dry yeast, which is always reliable and can be obtained in most grocery stores.

In Bible times families used to keep a little of their dough in an earthen vessel from one baking time to another. This sour dough was used for yeast in bread making. My mother used this kind of yeast.

Sometimes in the early days we would go to a brewery and for two pennies we would get nearly a two-quart pail full of yeast. This yeast was just the same as the Fleischmann's yeast today, only it was in liquid form.

Bread Raising. A proper place for bread to rise when you make your own bread is of great importance in order to have good bread and to have it good every time. I have at different times used an ordinary, clean, wooden dry goods box, put some shelves in it, and made a door through which I could put my big bread pan. Then I made a place below the lower shelf where I could set a lighted lamp with a little dish of water above it to keep the box at an even temperature. You can also put in a large dish of hot water, or heat some soapstones or bricks wrapped in a piece of paper or cloth to heat the box to an even temperature. There must be considerable space between these soapstones and the first shelf upon which your bread is set. In such a compartment the sponge can be raised as well as the bread after it is put in pans.

I have also found a common oats sprouter, made of galvanized iron, very convenient. They are easily obtained and sold everywhere, by Sears, Montgomery Ward, and others. An oats sprouter has a hot water tank over a lamp, which can be regulated to get an even temperature to raise bread. This is a very valuable device to have in any household and will pay for itself in a short time. You can also use this useful device to make malt, as well as to sprout different grains and legumes for table use. Of course, anyone handy with a saw and hammer can make a wooden box, as described in the preceding paragraphs, to serve the same purpose.

Sometimes bread is left standing around on the table subject to drafts and it gets too cold while it is trying to rise. Furthermore, I never advise that bread be set to rise all night, unless the proper yeast cannot be obtained, in which case a slow and long process of rising is made necessary because of the yeast.

Put enough yeast in the bread to cause it to rise in two or three hours. The first time the bread should rise high enough just before it falls so that when it is touched it will go down. Should it happen that it rises so much that it falls, it is necessary that it be kneaded and allowed to rise again before it is put in the pans. After it is in the pans, it should rise half its size before it is put in the oven. If the bread rises too much while in the pan it will be coarse and full of holes. Should it accidentally rise too high, knead it over and let it rise again.

Whole wheat flour bread must not be permitted to rise as light in the pans as white flour bread. Care in this respect will preserve in the bread that sweet, nutty, wheat flavor that is so characteristic of bread made from the entire grain, but which will be lacking if the loaves rise too light in the pans.

Make it a business to have good bread, and do not give up until you do. Be determined, and say as many others have said, "I can make anything that anyone else can."

Some years ago I held a food demonstration in one of the Southern states. A Southern woman who attended one of these demonstrations had never made a loaf of bread in her life. All she had ever learned to make was soda and baking powder biscuits. She learned to make some very fine bread in only a single lesson. I furnished the flour, so I knew it was whole wheat flour. The first batch she made did not turn out very well, for the sole reason that the oven was not hot enough. The second batch was very fine. After one learns how it is very easy to make good bread.

If you will only be determined to have good bread, with a little experimenting you will succeed. I know a twelve-year-old girl who bakes delicious bread.

C. THE OVEN

Daughter's Note: *This section refers to the old wood-burning range in common use at the time this book was written, and not to a modern gas or electric range.*

It is very important that one have a good oven in order to make good bread. I have many times found ovens in which the side of the bread nearest the fire box would burn, or sometimes it would burn on top, or on the bottom. This can be remedied to some extent in most ovens. If the bread does not bake evenly on the top, side, and bottom, there is something wrong with the oven.

If the bread burns too quickly on the side where the fire is, you can take the grate out of the firebox, spread a layer of fire clay next to the oven, or put asbestos paper behind the grate. If the bread burns on the bottom, you can lay a piece of asbestos or a piece of tin on the bottom of the oven. Often if a piece of wire fencing with small mesh is placed on the bottom of the oven, a little bit of air space being left between the bread pan and the bottom of the oven prevents the bread from burning on the bottom. If the bread does not bake enough on the bottom, it is evident that too much soot and ashes are in the oven and the stove needs cleaning out.

For whole wheat bread, the oven should be heated to 450°F., then gradually be reduced to 350° to 300°F. It is well to have an oven thermometer, which you can find for sale in any department store for around $1.50 to $2.50. If you have no thermometer, the oven should be hot enough so the bread will begin to brown in fifteen minutes.

Be sure your oven is hot enough. If it is not, your bread will not be good. After the bread is thoroughly heated, reduce the oven temperature. If the same temperature were kept, it would burn the bread on the outside. Therefore, as mentioned in the preceding paragraph, the temperature should be gradually reduced from 450° to about 350° and then at last to about 300°. Bake your bread thoroughly, allowing an hour to one and one-quarter or one and one-half hours in the oven.

Old-Fashioned Clay Oven. Before the iron stove came into existence, people baked bread in various ways. Sometimes they baked on the hearth of a fireplace, sometimes between two hot stones, and sometimes they baked it in hot ashes, and toasted ears of corn upon the coals. In some countries they made ovens of clay and straw, similar to the way the Egyptians made brick.

My parents had one of these clay ovens. It was made like this: we built a platform about two and a half feet high of 2-inch thick lumber. The platform we had was about 5 feet wide and 6 or 7 feet long. These boards were heavily covered with clay mixed with cut straw, then one layer of brick was laid over them so it left a very smooth and nice surface on top. Then an arch from wooden slats was built over that. The arch was about 2 feet in height in the center. The back was closed except for a short chimney, and this was covered with a small piece of tin to hold the heat after the fire was taken out of the oven. The arch was covered with 2 or 3 layers of clay mixed with cut straw. A door was left in front, through which the oven was fired, and also for putting in and taking out the bread. After the oven was all finished, a slow fire would be started in it, which would dry out the clay. After the clay was partly dried, the fire would be increased, and it would burn this clay into brick in much the same way as bricks are made.

When we wanted to get the oven ready for bread making, we built a fire inside. When the bread was ready to go, all the coals and fire were raked out and the oven cleaned off. Many times the bread was put right on the brick, but we usually put it in pans. In this oven we baked lovely bread with a beautiful crust. We generally arranged the fire so we could leave the bread in the oven from an hour to an hour and a half.

It would be a great blessing if every home had an oven of this kind and people made their own bread today.

The finest bread may be made in this kind of an oven, because it bakes just right. The oven should be hot enough so that in fifteen minutes the bread will begin to brown. Then allow the heat to gradually diminish, as it naturally would in the clay oven, as the fire was all taken out. Such ovens can also be made so there is a little fireplace on the front part that opens into the oven, with a chimney on the opposite side. Then you can fire while you are baking.

Use of Steam in the Oven. It is much easier to get a good crust on bread without burning it if there is steam in the oven. This may be accomplished by placing a small pan of water in the oven. Some of the big bakeries that have chain ovens bake bread in 900° heat in 20 to 25 minutes, using considerable steam in the oven to keep the bread from burning.

D.   ZWIEBACK

No bread is entirely dextrinized, or turned into grape sugar; therefore zwieback or twice-baked bread, in which this process is completed, is very wholesome and very easy to digest. A good way to make zwieback is to slice the bread about one-half inch thick, and let it dry out in the sun, or in a slow oven, until it is entirely dry.

I have kept zwieback an entire year in fine shape in a common barrel lined with heavy brown paper. During this time there was a long period of wet weather, and it seemed as if the zwieback had gathered a little moisture, but there was not a trace of mold; I put it outdoors on paper in the sun and let it dry out thoroughly again, and after it had been heated in the oven, it was just as good as when it was freshly made. I did this for experimental purposes.

Zwieback should be made an important part of our diet, and if rightly handled, will save a great deal of time and expense. I have at times, when I was not in a position to bake my own bread, had some bakery make twenty-five, fifty, and even up to four hundred loaves of good whole wheat bread, using my own recipe, for myself and neighbors to make into zwieback. As mentioned earlier, the bread can be sliced evenly and dried out in an oven or out-of-doors in the sun until it is perfectly dry. Then heat the oven and brown it slightly on both sides. Use for breakfast or lunch time. To make an excellent lunch, serve it with fruits, or fruit juices, soybean milk or malted nut cream. Use it any way you like, but make it a practice to have a large supply of zwieback on hand.

E. COMBINATIONS OF GRAINS AND LEGUMES IN BREADS

In Bible times they used to combine different grains and legumes and make them into bread. "Take thou also unto thee wheat, and barley, and beans, and lentils, and millet and fitches, and put them in one vessel, and make thee bread thereof." (Ezekiel 4:9)

A number of seeds have been used in bread since Abraham's time and are still used by the Germans and others, such as caraway, gimmel, anise, rue, fennel, and dill, All of these have medicinal properties. They are all good for indigestion, and prevent fermentation. For gas and colic, rue was quite frequently used, even by the priests in Christ's time. It has a wonderfully quiet, soothing effect upon tired and weary brains.

People would do well today if they would use more of these things instead of the abundant luxuries that destroy both soul and body.

F. BREAD BAKING IN BIBLE TIMES

In early Bible times when ovens were rare, sometimes a number of women would bake their bread in one oven, as in Leviticus 26:26, where ten women baked bread in one oven. From ancient times until recent years, bread, legumes, and fruit seemed the main diet. In ancient times, bread, raisins, and figs were used a great deal. Abigail brought two hundred loaves of bread, one hundred clusters of raisins, and two hundred cakes of figs with some other things to David. (1 Samuel 25:18)

G.   BREAD RECIPES

Many good bread recipes can be found in almost any cookbook. Leave out the harmful ingredients and use only those that are wholesome.

Where these recipes advise grease or oils of any kind, use a little raw peanut butter, which is very rich in oil; and for the sweetening use malt sugar or Karo syrup, which enriches the bread, gives it a very excellent flavor, and keeps it moist.

The bread is done when it shrinks away from the sides of the pan. Remove at once from the pan and cool on a wire rack, away from drafts.

Whole Wheat Bread
(3 loaves)

1 cake compressed yeast
3 cups warm water
2 tbs. Karo syrup
1 tbs. salt
7 cups whole wheat flour

In a large mixing bowl, crumble the yeast into the warm water. Stir in the Karo syrup, and salt. Add the flour and mix all the ingredients to a medium soft dough. Turn out on a slightly floured board, and knead until elastic to the touch, about 20 to 30 minutes. Then return the dough to the bowl, cover, and let stand in a warm room. The dough should rise until, when tapped sharply, it begins to sink. This takes about two hours. Work the dough down well, turn over in the bowl, and let rise again to half again its size; then shape into loaves and put into pans for baking.

Let rise until half again its original bulk, then bake in a preheated 400° oven at least one hour or longer. These coarse breads must be watched closer during the rising than those made from white flour, as they get light in much less time.

When taking bread from the oven, sponge it off with a cloth that has been dampened in cold water or oil. Soybean or nut milk, however, may be used in place of water to improve the bread. Set the loaf on a wire rack to cool off quickly, and the crust will be brittle and tender.

Rye Bread
(2 loaves)

1 cake compressed yeast
3 cups lukewarm water
1 tbs. caraway seed (optional)
5 cups rye flour
1 cup sifted white flour
1 tbs. salt

The white flour should be flour strong in gluten. It should be the same as that used when making washed gluten for nut foods.

Dissolve the yeast in 1 cup of lukewarm water. Add the caraway seed, if used, and 2 1/2 cups rye flour, or enough to make a sponge. Beat well. Cover and set aside in a warm place, free from drafts, to rise for about two hours.

When the sponge is light, add the white flour, the rest of the rye flour or enough to make a soft dough, and the salt. Turn out on a board and knead for at least ten minutes. Place in bowl, cover, and let rise until it doubles in bulk. This takes about two hours.

Turn out on a board and shape into two long loaves. Place in shallow pans, cover, and let rise again until light — about one hour. Turn on the oven to 375°. With a sharp knife lightly cut three strokes diagonally across the top of each loaf, and place in the oven. Bake at 375°, a slower oven than when making white bread, for 30 to 35 minutes.

Note: By adding 1/2 cup of sour dough, left from a previous baking, an acid flavor is obtained that is considered by many a great improvement for rye bread. This should be added to the sponge. My mother made nearly all her bread from sour dough, saved from previous baking, both rye and whole wheat. As nearly as I can remember now, she would save about a pint of dough from her baking and keep that until the next baking. It would be sour enough to start the yeast germs. Then she would work the bread the same as directed.

Rye bread can be worked much the same as whole wheat bread. Rye flour does not contain as much gluten as wheat, and therefore it does not rise as light as whole wheat flour without the addition of wheat flour strong in gluten. I have made a splendid loaf of rye bread with 3 1/2 cups of rye flour and one-half cup of strong white gluten flour. You may also use 3 cups of whole rye flour and 1 cup of whole wheat flour, strong in gluten, to make a splendid rye loaf.

Whole Wheat Raisin Bread
(2 loaves)

1 cake compressed yeast
1 cup lukewarm water
6 cups whole wheat flour
3/4 cup malt honey, malt sugar, or Karo syrup
1 cup raisins, well-floured
1 tsp. salt
1 cup raw peanut butter
4 tbs. oil

Dissolve the yeast in one cup lukewarm water. Add two cups flour, and the malt honey, and beat until smooth. Cover and set aside to rise in a warm place, free from drafts, until light, which will take about 1 1/2 hours.

When well risen, add the floured raisins, the rest of the flour or enough to make a moderately soft dough, and the remainder of the ingredients. The raw peanut butter should be dissolved in a cup of lukewarm water. If the dough is too soft, add a little more flour, and the next time use less water.

Knead lightly. Place in a well-greased bowl, cover, and let rise again until double in bulk about 1 1/2 hours. Shape into loaves, fill well-greased pans half full, cover, and let rise until light about one hour.

Bake at 400° for 10 minutes and then at 375° for 40 to 50 minutes longer.

Steamed Graham Bread
(2 loaves)

1 cake compressed yeast, dissolved in a little warm water
3 cups nut milk
1 tsp. salt
1 cup malt honey or Karo syrup
2 cups cornmeal
3-1/2 cups of graham flour

Mix the yeast, nut milk, salt, and malt honey together; then mix the cornmeal and flour, and stir into the liquid. Put into two well-greased basins or empty cans and steam under 5 pounds steam pressure for 2 1/2 or 3 hours. Then the bread can be put in a moderate oven and browned a little for 15 minutes, if desired.

Soybean Bread No.1
(2 loaves)

2 lbs. whole wheat flour
1 lb. soybean mash or 1/2 lb. soybean flour
1 cake compressed yeast
1 pint lukewarm water
1/2 cup malt sugar or Karo syrup
salt to taste

Mix 2 pounds fine whole wheat flour and 1 pound soybean mash, after the milk is taken out; or in place of the mash, 1/2 pound soybean flour may be used.

Dissolve one cake of compressed yeast in a little lukewarm water; add 1 pint of water, 1/2 cup of malt sugar or Karo syrup, and salt to taste. Mix this with the flour and mash to make a fairly stiff dough, about the consistency of regular bread dough. If the dough is not stiff enough, a little more flour may be added.

Let it rise to about double its size in a warm place. Then knead the dough down and fold it over toward the inner side. Turn it over and let it rise again to about half again its size. Then knead it and shape into two loaves, put in pans, letting it rise to about double its size. Bake at 400° for 10 minutes, then at 375° for 45 minutes longer. It should begin to brown about 15 minutes after placing in the oven. Bake the bread thoroughly; this gives it a good flavor and makes it easy to digest.

Soybean Bread No.2
(3 loaves)

3 lbs whole wheat flour, finely ground
1 lb. soybean meal (out of which the milk has been washed)
1 cake compressed yeast
1 pint lukewarm water
1 cup malt sugar or Karo syrup
salt

Mix this together following the method given in the recipe for Soybean Bread No.1; work the dough as described above, and bake thoroughly.

About 2 or 3 tablespoonfuls of malt honey added to the water will add very much to the flavor and value of the bread, giving it a deep nutty flavor. Or to make the bread even better, use malt extract, which is high in diastase and aids in the digestion of starch.

When this bread is made into zwieback, thoroughly dried out until it is a light golden brown, diabetics can eat it because the starch has been changed into grape sugar. Zwieback is excellent for everyone.

Health Gems or Crackers

These gems (an old-time name for muffins) are good for those suffering with Bright's disease, diabetes, liver, or kidney troubles and may be made as follows.

Put 2 cups of whole wheat flour in a pan on the stove, over a medium heat. Stir it frequently with a wooden paddle until it is very slightly golden brown or what we call dextrinized. Remove from the heat.

To the whole wheat flour add 1 cup of soybean flour and 1 cup of boiled spinach or 1/2 cup of powdered spinach. Then add some peanut milk, made from raw peanut butter. (To make peanut milk, mix raw peanut butter into a cream with water to the consistency of thin cream or cow's milk.) The batter should be just thick enough so it will drip from a spoon. Salt to taste. Place batter in paper baking cups in a muffin pan or you may grease the pan instead. Bake at 425°F. for 20 minutes or until nicely browned.

If you wish to make a cracker, more flour will need to be added. Roll it out to any thickness you want, and cut it to any size you desire. This makes a most wonderful product, either as a cracker or a gem. Mashed, cooked carrots may be used in place of spinach, and also two or more tablespoonfuls of malt honey or Karo syrup may be added. Bake in the oven at 350° for 15 minutes or until lightly browned.

Soybean Buns

4 cups whole wheat flour
1 cup soybean meal (mash) or 1/2 cup soybean flour
1/2 cup soybean butter
2 packages of dry yeast
1 cup water or soybean milk

To the whole wheat flour and the soybean meal or flour, add the half cup of soybean butter. Dissolve the yeast in the water or soybean milk and add to the flour mixture. After the dough has risen (in 2 or 3 hours) mix it down, turn over, and let rise to half again its size. Now shape into the size of buns that you like and let them rise to about half again their size. Bake from 20 to 30 minutes, according to the size of the buns, at 350°.

H.   UNLEAVENED BREAD

Unfermented or unleavened bread is made light by the introduction of air into the dough or batter. This is done by beating the batter breads and kneading the dough breads.

Unleavened Gems. When making unleavened gems or muffins, have your water, nut milk, and other ingredients as cold as possible and salted to taste. Have your gem pans greased and sizzling hot, and have your batter just stiff enough so that it will drip from the spoon. Place the gems in a preheated oven and bake for 20 minutes at 400°. This will make a very palatable bread.

Cornmeal Gems
1 cup soybean milk
2 tbs. oil
1 tsp. salt
1 cup cornmeal
1 cup whole wheat flour

Place the milk, oil, and salt in a bowl. Now beat the cornmeal and flour into this mixture. The ingredients should be cold as described above, and your gem pans greased and sizzling hot. Bake in a preheated oven at 400° for 20 minutes.

Oatmeal or Soybean Gems
1-1/2 cups milk
3 tbs. oil
1 tsp. salt
1 cup cornmeal
1 cup whole wheat flour
1 cup oatmeal or soybean meal

Follow mixing and baking directions for making cornmeal gems.

Potato or Carrot Gems
1 cup milk
3 tbs. oil
salt to taste
2 cups whole wheat flour
1 cup mashed Irish potatoes, sweet potatoes, or mashed carrots

Follow mixing and baking directions for making cornmeal gems.

In the three foregoing recipes, soybean butter may be used instead of oil. Soybean butter makes a better product, because the oil is emulsified and this renders it more easily digested.

Soybean Gems
1/2 lb. soybean mash (out of which soybean milk has been washed)
1/2 lb. dextrinized cornmeal
1/2 cup soybean milk or water

To dextrinize cornmeal, put the meal in a large baking pan in the oven. Do not have the oven too hot as the meal should not be burned. Stir frequently with a pancake turner or a wooden paddle until it turns a golden brown. This turns the starch into dextrose and makes it palatable and easy to digest.

Mix the mash and the dextrinized cornmeal with the soybean milk. Salt to taste. Pour them in hot, greased cast-iron gem pans and bake for 20 minutes in a hot oven at 400°.

This makes a very wholesome gem, one that diabetics can eat.

This mixture, made thin enough with more milk added, may be spooned out on a greased cookie sheet as drop cookies, and baked in a 375° oven for 10 minutes.

Pones

1/3 lb. cornmeal
1/3 lb. whole wheat flour
1/3 lb. oatmeal flour
1-1/2 cups soybean milk or water
2 tbs. malt honey or Karo syrup

Mix together all the ingredients. Have batter cold and greased gem pans and oven hot (400°). Bake 30 minutes.

Beaten Biscuit

2 cups whole wheat flour
2/3 cup soybean milk
1/2 cup soybean butter
2 tbs. Karo syrup
salt

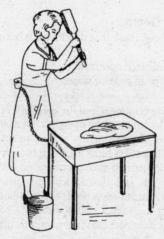

This Woman is Beating the Dough for Beaten Biscuits.

Put your flour into a bowl, add the milk, then the soybean butter, Karo syrup, and salt. Mix into a stiff dough as you would in making ordinary bread. Beat with a rolling pin or any heavy stick. This beating is done to make the biscuit tender and mellow.

Make into sticks or roll about one-half inch thick and cut in sizes to suit your taste. This can be rolled still thinner and made into a cracker if you like. Prick with a fork to keep it from blistering. Bake at 325° for 30 minutes to a light brown.

In the picture, the woman is making beaten biscuits. The table is my own design, made by nailing a board 6 inches thick, 18 inches wide, and 24 inches long to the legs. Then I put a bottom on the table, and filled it with cement, and made the top of the table smooth. Such a table can also be made out of heavy planks.

The club the woman in the picture is using was made from a two by four, about three feet long. She is beating a piece of dough on the table. She keeps folding the dough over and over, and repeating the folding and beating. After it has been well-beaten, about 10 or 15 minutes, make it into little biscuits, or cut it into thin little crackers or sticks, and when it is baked long enough to be thoroughly dextrinized it will be mellow enough to melt in your mouth. It makes one of the finest, most easily digested breads that can be made, without any shortening, baking powder, soda, or yeast. A little shortening may be used, however, such as soybean butter.

When I had a food factory, I made these old-fashioned beaten biscuits, and ran the dough through the dough brake about 20 or 30 times. It was then called a very fine article of food, by those who understood crackers. This would also make very fine pie crust. Always use whole wheat flour to make old-fashioned beaten biscuits. This makes very fine communion bread.

In beating the dough, beat it until it is flattened out, then fold over and beat some more, continuing this way until the process has been repeated at least twenty times or more, depending upon the weight of the beater and the vigor put into beating it.

Whole Wheat Crisps

Mix 5 ounces of raw peanut butter, with 1/2 pint of water, making a milk. Stir 1 pound of whole wheat flour into the raw peanut butter milk, and salt to taste. Make the dough stiff enough so that it can be rolled thin. Cut into squares and bake at 375° for 10 to 15 minutes. This makes a lovely cracker.

It can be improved by adding to the milk about two big tablespoonfuls of malt honey or Karo syrup. This is a complete food and very palatable.

These crisps may also be made from raised dough. Make the dough as for sponge bread. Take a scant 1 1/2 pints of water, 1/2 pound of malt honey or Karo syrup, and about 4 ounces of raw peanut butter. Make the peanut butter into a milk, and set the sponge as for bread, as outlined on the third page of this chapter. Use for this amount about 1 cake of compressed yeast. When it has risen as for bread, knead it and work it into thin rolls. Prick them with a fork so they will not blister, cut into strips and bake in a 350° oven until brown. This makes a very delicious cracker.

These recipes may be divided or multiplied, according to the size of the batch you desire to make.

I.   PIES

Raised Pie Crust
1 yeast cake
warm water, to dilute yeast
1/2 cup cooking or salad oil
malt sugar, small amount
1 cup whole wheat flour
1 cup soybean flour or soybean mash

Dissolve the yeast cake in the warm water and add the oil and malt sugar. Now add the whole wheat flour and soybean flour. Mix in the same way as bread dough and let rise for an hour or more in a warm place. When it has risen, knead down

and let rise again for 10 or 15 minutes before rolling out.
Then roll out thin and put in pie tins, allowing it to rise about
15 minutes. Bake for 10 minutes at 450°.

Soybean Pumpkin Pie
2 cups hot soybean milk
2 tbs. fine zwieback crumbs
1/3 cup malt sugar, malt honey, or regular honey
a few grains of salt
1 cup drained, mashed pumpkin
1/2 tsp., or less, of almond flavoring
prepared pie crust

The crust for this kind of pie should have a built-up edge.
Heat the milk. While the milk is heating, mix the zwieback
crumbs, sugar, and salt and stir them into the mashed pumpkin. Mix thoroughly and add the hot milk. Add seasoning.
Pour into a crust and bake in a moderate oven (350°) until
set, about 35 minutes.
Instead of almond flavoring, 1/2 tsp. each of nutmeg and
cinnamon may be used.

Fig Marmalade Pie
1 cup figs
1 cup pitted dates
1 cup raisins
3 cups soybean milk
prepared pie crust

Mix the figs, dates, and raisins and run together through a
food chopper. The holes in the plate of the mill should be
quite fine so as to puree the fruit, so that it is easier to digest.
Reduce the thickness of the fruit with soybean milk to the
right consistency. Pour this filling into a raised pie crust,
directions for which are given in the foregoing recipes, and
bake for 15 or 20 minutes in a moderate oven (350°). No top
crust is needed for this pie.

To thicken the filling, about 2 teaspoons of agar-agar may be soaked in the cold milk for a short time; then boil this mixture before adding to the fruit.

Vanilla may be added for seasoning, which gives the pie a very different flavor.

If the crust is allowed to rise to the thickness of the filling, it makes a healthful pie, one that would make an excellent school lunch for children. It is something they will like and which will nourish as well as satisfy them.

This pie filling may be prepared without the raisins. It may also be made with pitted dates alone, which makes a very sweet pie.

6

PREPARING WHOLESOME DESSERTS AND BEVERAGES

A. DESSERTS

Fruit pies may be considered healthful when the crust is made of whole wheat flour and well baked. A whole wheat crust has a rich nutty flavor and requires a little less shortening than when made of white flour. But rich starchy pie fillings and custards are among the most objectionable of all desserts.

Unleavened Pie Crust

1 cup whole wheat flour
1 cup soybean flour
1 tsp salt
1/2 cup cooking or salad oil
3 tbs. ice water

Mix flours and salt in a mixing bowl. Add oil and mix well with a large fork. Sprinkle ice water over the mixture and mix well. Press the mixture into a smooth ball with the hands. Divide the ball into halves and flatten both parts slightly. Roll each half between wax paper. Makes one 2-crust pie shell.

Brown Betty

1 1/2 cups seedless raisins
1/2 tsp. salt
1 quart chopped apples
1 tbs. lemon juice
1 scant cup brown sugar
1/2 cup water
1 cup whole wheat zwieback crumbs

Spread half the raisins over the bottom of a greased pudding dish, cover raisins with half the chopped apples, sprinkle over the apples half the sugar and half the crumbs, sprinkle over this the remainder of the raisins and chopped apples. Sprinkle on the rest of the sugar and crumbs, add salt and lemon juice to one-half cup of water and pour this over the top of the pudding. Cover the pudding and set in a pan of water, cover, and bake an hour. Remove from the pan of water and bake without the cover long enough to brown the top slightly. Serve with vanilla sauce.

Vanilla Sauce

To the desired amount of soybean cream you may add malt sugar and vanilla to taste. This makes a delicious sauce, to be used in the place of starchy sauces and whipping cream.

Vegetable Gelatin

To prepare agar-agar for dessert, soak one tablespoon of agar-agar in one pint of warm water thirty minutes, drain and then simmer twenty minutes in another pint of warm water; cook until dissolved. The quantity of liquid will be reduced by boiling. Strain the liquid and add a pint of any desired fresh fruit or fruit juice. Bananas, peaches, or any other fresh fruit may be sliced in the bottom of each mold to give variety. Before serving, decorate with crushed or chopped nuts. For dressing, use either the vanilla sauce or soybean cream.

Orange Jelly
3/4 cup orange juice
1 cup malt sugar
1 tsp. grated orange rind
3/4 cup water
3 tbs. lemon juice
1 tbs. vegetable gelatin (see Vegetable Gelatin)
salt

Mix the orange juice, rind, lemon juice, pinch of salt, and sugar, add the water; when boiled gelatin is ready, add the other ingredients. Mold until firm. Serve with soybean cream.

Strawberry Jelly

1 tbs. agar-agar
1 3/4 cups crushed strawberries
2 tbs. lemon juice
1 cup boiling water for agar-agar
few grains salt
1 cup malt sugar

Prepare as for orange jelly; when cool decorate with strawberry halves, and serve with crushed nuts or soybean cream.

Baked Apples

Wash the apples and remove the cores without cutting completely through the apple. Then fill the cavities with raisins or dates, and bake until done (about 45 minutes) at 350° in a flat baking dish with a little water in the bottom. With the raisins, chopped nuts may also be used, which add to the flavor. Serve with a nut cream.

Stuffed Dates

Remove the pits with a sharp knife, cutting lengthwise, and replace with pecan meats or other nuts if preferred. If you wish to remove the skins, scald them, draining well. As a rule they should always be scalded to remove dirt.

Rice Pudding

1 cup soy cream
1 cup cooked brown rice
pinch of salt
1 cup drained, crushed pineapple

Mix together, chill, and serve. Other fruits may be used in place of pineapple.

Cream Tapioca

1/2 cup tapioca (minute)
2 1/2 cups soybean milk
1/3 cup malt sugar
1 tsp vanilla
pinch of salt
1/2 cup soy cream

Soak the tapioca in soybean milk fifteen minutes. Add the sugar and salt, and bring to a boil, stirring constantly. Place in a double boiler, and cook until tapioca is transparent. Add vanilla, chill, and serve with soy cream.

B. BROTHS AND BEVERAGES

Soybean Coffee

Place the quantity of soybeans you desire in a flat baking pan and heat in a hot oven, stirring frequently to prevent burning.

Watch them closely and thoroughly stir them as they will get much darker inside than on the outside while roasting. The outside hull seems to brown less rapidly than the inner portion, so you will find it necessary to take a few out occasionally, and break them open with a hammer to see just how they are roasting. To get a good-flavored coffee, it is necessary to have an even roast. If some of the beans are not roasted quite enough, and some of them a little too much, it spoils the flavor of the coffee.

After roasting, grind the beans in a mill, to a coarse grind. Brew the coffee in a pot the same as you would regular coffee.

Get some coffee and compare the color so you will know how brown to make it. Half bran and half soybeans may also be used for a good coffee.

Soybean Milk

The recipe for soybean milk is given in Chapter 1 of the section.

Cereal Coffee No.1

Cereal coffee is a product that is used very much nowadays, and can be made very easily at home.

Place the quantity of rye grain you desire in a large flat baking pan and roast in a hot oven. Stir the grain with a wooden paddle until it becomes as brown as coffee. Grind rather coarse in any small hand mill. It is now ready for use.

When roasting the whole grain, take a little out with a spoon when it gets nearly done, lay it on a solid board and break it up with a hammer in order to determine the brownness.

It is helpful to have handy a little regular coffee in a glass container so its degree of brownness can be easily compared with that of the homemade coffee.

Cereal Coffee No.2

Wheat bran is used in this recipe. Mix equal parts water and malt honey. Moisten the bran, a pound or whatever quantity you desire, with the water and malt honey mixture, let it get quite dry, or altogether dry before roasting. You may use Karo syrup in place of malt honey.

It may be placed in the sun or where it is airy to dry, so it does not sour before it gets dry.

When dry place in a flat baking pan, in a hot oven, stirring frequently, until it is as brown as coffee. The flavor of this kind of coffee is very pleasing.

Half bran and half rye may also be used. The rye, however, must be ground before mixing it with the bran. This makes a fine-flavored coffee.

The bran for this coffee may be purchased from a feed

store. It is much cheaper than bran put in packages and sold at the grocery stores. The ordinary bran run in large mills is just as clean as the flour from which the bran is taken, not touched by human hands. It runs out of the spout into a bag, and is perfectly clean and safe to use.

ADDENDUM: There are many good ready-made cereal coffees available on the market today.

Bran Water

To 2 cups of bran add 1 quart of water, and let it stand overnight. In the morning strain through a fine sieve or cheesecloth.

This bran water liquid can be used in any kind of soup stock, stew, or any breads in place of ordinary water.

Bran Broth

Cook 1 1/2 cups of the bran water (see preceding recipe) for about 5 minutes. Add 1/2 cup of soybean milk. More or less of the bran water and soybean milk may be taken, depending, of course, upon the amount required to suit the need, but this is a good proportion to use. Season with vegetable extract or Vegex and parsley.

Oatmeal Water

To 1 quart of water, add 1 cup of oatmeal, and soak it overnight. In the morning, strain through a fine sieve or cheesecloth.

This is to be used in soup stocks, stew, or breads in place of water. It increases the vitamins and makes soups creamy.

Soybean Broth

Place 2 cups of wheat bran in 1 quart of unsweetened soybean milk. In another pan, soak one cup of oatmeal in 1 quart of soybean milk. Place these two containers in the refrigerator overnight. In the morning, stir each one several times and strain.

Pour 1 pint of boiling unsweetened soy milk on 4 heaping tablespoonfuls chickweed; let stand for half an hour and strain.

Mix the wheat bran, oatmeal, and chickweed liquids together, adding 1 quart unsweetened soy milk. Add diced celery and onions for flavoring, to taste. Simmer for thirty minutes, adding 3 tablespoonfuls Kloss's Mayonnaise. A few minutes before it is finished, add 1 cup of very finely cut parsley. This broth contains all the nutrients the body requires.

Oatmeal Broth

Prepare oatmeal water as given in the preceding recipe, and cook 5 minutes. To every 3/4 cup of oatmeal water, add 1/4 cup soybean milk. Season with vegetable extract or Vegex.

A very excellent drink can also be made by mixing one part each of bran water and oatmeal water, heating them, adding soybean milk, and seasoning to taste. A little parsley, onion, or celery lends a pleasing flavor.

Herb Broth
2 cups wheat bran
1 cup oatmeal
4 tbs. chickweed water

Soak 2 cups wheat bran in 1 quart of water, and also one cup oatmeal in 1 quart of water overnight. Stir up each mixture several times; then strain.

Pour 1 pint of boiling water on the chickweed, let steep 1/2 hour; strain.

Mix together the wheat bran, the oatmeal, and 4 tablespoonfuls of the chickweed water, and add one quart soybean milk. Parsley, finely cut, may be added for flavoring, or season with celery or onions as preferred. Let simmer for a few minutes and serve. A little Kloss's Mayonnaise may also be added.

This broth contains all the nutrients the body requires.

Soybean Buttermilk

Buttermilk is an excellent article of diet for everyday use, but is especially beneficial in malnutrition, tuberculosis, toxic conditions, and intestinal infections. Soybean buttermilk has the advantage of producing an alkaline effect in the body and is more nourishing than ordinary buttermilk or yogurt buttermilk used under various names. It is rich in minerals and very palatable.

Use unsweetened soybean milk. Let stand until sour if desired, or until just clabbered and not sour. Beat up with an eggbeater, and add salt to taste.

Potassium Broth

2 cupfuls bran
2 large onions
1 cup oatmeal
2 stalks celery
4 quarts water
1/2 bunch minced parsley
4 potatoes, medium sized
2 vegetable oysters (salsify)
2 large carrots

Mix the first 3 ingredients and soak overnight. Beat up with an eggbeater and strain through a fine sieve.

Wash thoroughly 4 medium-sized potatoes and slice thin, also 2 large carrots, 2 medium-sized onions (optional), 2 large stalks celery with the green leaves cut fine, 1/2 bunch of parsley cut up and 2 good-sized vegetable oysters. Cook these in the bran/oatmeal water. Let simmer in a covered kettle until vegetables are done. Mash up vegetables and strain again through a fine sieve.

C.   HERB DRINKS OR TEAS

Coffee, tea, chocolate, and cocoa are harmful to the system, but all of the teas named in the following list are very fine to drink and take the place of harmful drinks. The herb teas are rich in medicinal and chemical properties. Some are very healing to the stomach and a good tonic. Others prevent fermentation and gas in the stomach and bowels, and also prevent griping. Some are very excellent to overcome nausea and vomiting, and all of them have a splendid beneficial effect on the system. There are some that are nice to take in the evening before retiring to induce sleep. All of them are soothing and quieting to the system.

In order to select the one best suited to your need, look in the index for the description of each of the herbs given. Some are wonderful medicine for children and others are fine for pregnant women, to prevent nausea and vomiting. Others are good for those with diarrhea, or bowel and colon trouble. They are not expensive.

peppermint	fennel
hyssop	spearmint
strawberry leaves	rue
alfalfa	hop blossoms
chickweed	dandelion
sassafras	catnip
green celery leaves	yellow dock
wintergreen	mint
meadowsweet	camomile
sarsaparilla root	juniper berries
birch bark (small twigs)	chicory
red raspberry leaves	sage
calamus root	wild cherry bark
red clover blossoms	(small twigs)

Herb Tea

Use one heaping teaspoon of the herbs granulated, or if powdered use one-half teaspoon, to a cup of boiling water. Place the herbs in a pan, and pour the boiling water over them, allowing it to steep one half hour. Cover. This steeping draws the mineral elements out of the herbs. These elements are very beneficial to the system.

These teas are less expensive than coffee, tea, etc., and they are healthful, beneficial, and not harmful.

Section VII
Effects of Polluted and Adulterated Foods on the Body

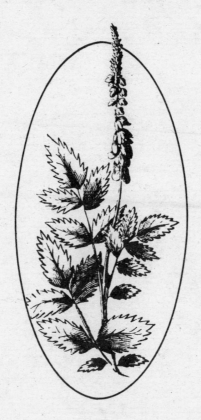

Common Agrimony

1

ADULTERATION OF FOOD

Our health depends on how nearly we live in harmony with Nature's laws. An all-wise God put all the elements in the soil that are necessary for the building of our bodies. Wrong habits of eating and drinking as well as the use of refined and adulterated foods are largely responsible for the intemperance, crime, and sickness that are a curse to the world.

As a result of man's trying to improve on nature, the human race is deteriorating, especially in America where people are accustomed to so-called luxuries. Although food may be ample in quantity, modern methods of refining remove many of the important elements. In many cases, the food is adulterated and preservatives are added to conceal their inferior quality and extend their shelf life.

The food question has not been given its deserved place in the medical world. We are made of what we eat, nothing else; and we should eat to increase our strength and preserve our health and life. All foods do not agree with everyone, but everyone should eat the natural foods that agree best with them. Disease and illness would be rare if our bloodstream was pure and our body was not full of waste matter and toxins. Poisonous waste matter in the system is the result of eating more food than the body can assimilate or eliminate. Foods that are high in protein, such as meats of all kinds, eggs, etc., principally cause this problem. You may eat improperly for a while without any noticeable bad effects, but serious health problems will inevitably follow. Moreover, the use of starchy foods and tea contribute greatly to the occurrence of intestinal ills, constipation, leukorrhea, etc. Acidic-reacting blood is one of the results of excess sugar and starch in the diet. It is not always the amount of food that is eaten that causes trouble; it may be wrong combinations or indigestible food of any kind, especially greasy and fried foods.

ANNOTATION: If you happen to be one of the 10 million or so Americans that suffer from asthma, you have about a 10 percent chance of being specially sensitive to sulfites, a preservative and antioxidant that is commonly added to our food supply. The FDA receives about two complaints each day regarding reactions to sulfites. Through September of 1985 about 850 reactions had been reported, including several deaths. While asthmatics as a group are at the highest risk, nearly one-fourth of all reactions occur in persons with no prior history of asthma.

When a reaction occurs, the first symptom is usually difficulty breathing, followed shortly by nausea, vomiting, diarrhea, abdominal cramps, hives, swelling of the soft tissues, rapid pulse, a drop in blood pressure, and occasionally loss of consciousness and death.

Sulfiting agents are used in food mainly to prevent discoloration and spoilage. See Table 1. Since they help to prevent lettuce from wilting and turning brown so rapidly, they are frequently used in restaurant salad bars. They are found in many packaged potato products as well as in other produce, certain types of seafood, and even in beer and wine. They are also used in over 1,100 drug products, both prescription and nonprescription, to help maintain the potency and stability of the drug. Sulfiting agents are listed on food labels under such chemical names as sulfur dioxide, potassium bisulfite, potassium metabisulfite, sodium bisulfite, sodium metabisulfite or sodium sulfite.

TABLE 1
PREVALENT PRESERVATIVES

Sulfur dioxide and various forms of inorganic sulfites that release sulfur dioxide when used as food ingredients are known collectively as sulfiting agents. On food labels, their presence may be identified as sulfur dioxide, potassium bisulfite, potassium metabisulfite, sodium bisulfite, sodium metabisulfite, or sodium sulfite. Some of the major food catagories in which they are usd include the following:

Avocado dip and guacamole
Beer
Cider
Cod (dried)
Fruit (fresh peeled, dried, or maraschino-type)
Fruit juices, purees and fillings
Gelatin
Potatoes (fresh peeled, frozen, dried or canned)
Salad dressing (dry mix) and relishes
Salads (particularly at salad bars)
Sauces and gravies (canned or dried)
Sauerkraut and coleslaw
Shellfish (fresh, frozen, canned, or dried) including clams,
    crab, lobster, scallops, and shrimp
Soups (canned or dried)
Vegetables (fresh peeled, frozen, canned, or dried),
    including fresh mushrooms
Wine vinegar
Wine and wine coolers

From "FDA Consumer," Dec. 1985 - Jan. 1986, page 20.

Because of the adverse effect of sulfites on vitamin B_1, the FDA has always prohibited their use on foods that are important sources of this vitamin, such as enriched flour and bread. Since they are able to restore a natural red appearance to meat and thus give a false impression of freshness, their use for this purpose is also prohibited.

Foods that are served in restaurants are not usually packaged or labeled, so sulfite-sensitive individuals must be especially careful when eating out. Foods to be particularly wary of are salads, potatoes, seafood, cooked vegetable dishes, wine, beer and bakery products.

The title of an article in *U.S. News and World Report,* July 15, 1985, asks the question, "Is the Food You Eat Dangerous to Your Health?" The answer appears to be a qualified but definite yes; much of the food we eat may certainly be a health hazard. When you add to this the contaminated water we drink and the polluted air we breathe, it's no wonder that the environmentalists, as well as a growing number of doctors, researchers, and concerned citizens, are becoming increasingly worried about the problem.

The opening sentences in this news article are enough to make most people sit up and pay attention. "When an American sits down to a typical breakfast, chances are the menu includes bug spray, weed killer, an embalming agent, and arsenic. It's no joke. Favorite foods such as bananas, cereal, milk, and toast all contain traces of lethal compounds."

Many of these poisons are accumulating in human tissues and it is felt by some doctors that degenerative diseases of the heart and kidneys, as well as many common symptoms, such as indigestion, frequent headaches, dizziness, and insomnia, may be the result of eating chemically contaminated food. While some of the worst of these toxic substances, such as DDT, were banned over a decade ago because of their slow breakdown, small amounts can still be found in the body tissues of the average American.

Some of the pesticides used on farms and in millions of gardens are washed off by the rain and eventually may end up miles away in lakes, rivers, and finally in the ocean. In some areas many species of fish are rapidly becoming, or have already become, unfit for human consumption. Among these are rainbow trout, Chinook and coho salmon, eel, channel catfish, striped bass, Atlantic herring, Pacific salmon, Alaska king crab, California sardines, and English sole. In some locations, entire fish species are being threatened with extinction.

The enormity of this problem may be better comprehended when it is realized that "American farmers use 1 billion pounds of insecticide each year — nearly 4 1/2 pounds of bug killer for every man, woman, and child in the U.S. As a consequence, 52 percent of the average American's food intake contains chemical residues."

On the positive side, there is an increasing concern on the part of government agencies over the widespread environmental pollution; and the allowable levels of many toxic chemicals are being closely examined, while others are being banned entirely. There is also a growing trend to rely more on the insects' natural enemies to keep them under control. Planting crops that insects find unattractive and the development of more natural pesticides that degrade easily are also steps in the right direction to help clean up the mess that man has made of his environment.

A. DEVITALIZED FOODS CAUSE DISEASE

Many people suffer almost continually from ailments, the cause of which they are unable to determine. They know that they feel very miserable and are subject to frequent headaches, indigestion, poor appetite, and many other troubles.

There are causes for all such disturbances. Deficiency of the necessary elements in the body is the cause for many such troubles. The body is composed of more than 30 elements and a shortage of one or more of these impairs the proper functioning of the entire system. There is generally no real organic breakdown in such cases, but the body is not functioning properly. An inadequate supply of any of these important elements is the major cause of a great many ailments. These nutrients are supplied in properly prepared food, but the American diet is very deficient in many of these important elements.

The refined, degerminated, demineralized, and devitalized foods are a curse to humanity. The miller, in making white flour, takes out the vital part of the grain that makes a new plant, the wheat germ, and also removes the bran, the part that contains the minerals and vitamins that supply our bodies with blood-making material. Many other foods that we have eaten daily from childhood have been treated in the same manner.

Furthermore, foods that are improperly prepared lose much of their nutritive value. It is very essential that foods be eaten in their natural state as often as possible. Too much cooking injures food. Certain food elements are destroyed by even a small amount of heat and for that reason such foods as can be eaten raw should be served often. Green leafy vegetables, such as cabbage, spinach, romaine, lettuce, endive, celery, and many others contain those substances that the human body must have to function properly. A lack of such elements in the daily food is a form of starvation. See also Section IV, Chapter 1.

Such vegetables as carrots, tender beets, parsnips, cucumbers, potatoes, young turnips, and others like them should not be peeled. Using a stiff brush is an excellent way to clean such vegetables so that the peels can be eaten. The highest mineral content of such foods lies just under the skin; therefore, vital minerals are lost if these vegetables are peeled.

None of the water left over from cooking vegetables should be thrown away. It contains valuable minerals and vitamins and should be used in soups or other cooking. In cooking leafy vegetables, just enough water should be added to keep them from burning and they should not be cooked any longer than is absolutely necessary. Spinach or beet tops should never be cooked over 4 or 5 minutes. If beets are cooked with tops, it takes much longer to cook the beets than the tops, so the beets should be diced fine and cooked in only enough water to keep them from burning. Use the stems, but cut them in quarter-inch lengths and add them to the beets after they are about half-done (about 8 minutes). Cut the leaves fine and when the beets are about done, add the leaves, for it takes only about 4 minutes to cook them. Sea salt should be added after the stems have come to a boil. A little Kloss Soybean Butter diluted with water to the consistency of cream should be added just as the heat is turned off, or else it can be added when they are served. It takes about 10 to 15 minutes to cook beets in this manner.

Never put soda in your cooking water to make the vegetables tender. Neither should soda be used in cooking dried peas, beans, corn, etc., even if it does shorten the length of time necessary to cook them. The common use of soda

biscuits and cornbread made with baking powder and soda
is a cause of vitamin deficiency disease, because soda destroys much of the vitamin C during cooking. Remember,
disease cannot get a foothold when the body is in the best
condition.

B.   LIST OF REFINED FOODS

The following table lists the consumption of refined foods
in the United States during 1931 and is quoted from a bulletin
published by the Department of Agriculture, reprinted from
Cereal Chemistry, Vol.12, No. 5, September 1935, compiled
by Dr. J. A. LeClerc, senior chemist, and his associates. The
consumption of such large amounts of refined food as long
ago as 1931 is astounding. Everyone should avoid the use of
these commonplace devitaminized foods.

Many staple foods on the market are, according to today's
prevailing standards, legitimate foods and are widely advertised. They are most unhealthful, however, and cannot be
recommended from a health standpoint. Such foods are
candies, white rice, various canned and preserved foods,
sulphured fruits, highly seasoned foods, etc. Most of these
foods are deficient in nutritional value, and substances that
are detrimental to health have been added to preserve or color
them.

YEARLY CONSUMPTION PER CAPITA
IN U.S. (1931)

	1931 TOTAL POUNDS	PER CAPITA POUNDS
Refined sugar	12,017,000,000	98.3
Cornstarch	158,000,000	1.3
Polished rice	719,000,000	5.9
White flour	20,825,000,000	170.7
Corn syrup	707,000,000	5.7
Corn sugar	780,000,000	6.4
Candy	1,439,000,000	11.8
Hominy and grits	341,000,000	2.8
Rye flour	292,000,000	2.4
Cornmeal	2,598,000,000	21.3
Corn breakfast food	378,000,000	3.1
Macaroni and water noodles	451,000,000	3.7
Corn and cottonseed oils	1,403,000,000	11.5
Poultry	2,940,000,000	24.1
Beef, veal	6,893,000,000	56.5
Mutton and lamb	866,000,000	7.1
Lard and lard substitutes	2,720,000,000	22.3

HEALTH-DESTROYING FOODS

Health-destroying foods are such foods as spices, mustard, pepper, vinegar, salt, condiments, salted meats, canned meats, salted fish, Tabasco sauce, Worcestershire sauce, gravies, fried or greasy food, pastries, very hot or ice-cold food, all soft drinks, chewing gum, coffee, tea, cocoa (see Table l), alcohol, white flour and white flour products, cane sugar and cane sugar products. The organs in our body that make blood cannot convert these foods into pure blood. Nerves are nourished by the blood; therefore, the blood must be pure and contain all of the elements necessary for nourishing the nerves as well as every other part of the body.

TABLE I

CAFFEINE CONTENT
OF BEVERAGES AND FOODS

ITEM	Milligrams Average	Caffeine Range
Coffee (5-ounce cup)		
Brewed, drip method	115	60-180
Brewed, percolator	80	40-170
Instant	65	30-120
Decaffeinated, brewed	3	2-5
Decaffeinated, instant	2	1-5
Tea (5-ounce cup)		
Brewed, major U.S. brands	40	20-90
Brewed, imported brands	60	25-110
Instant	30	25-50
Iced (12-ounce glass)	70	67-76

ITEM	Milligrams Average	Caffeine Range
Cocoa beverages (5-ounce cup)	4	2-20
Chocolate milk beverage (8 ounces)	5	1-7
Milk chocolate (1 ounce)	6	1-15
Dark chocolate, semisweet (1 ounce)	20	5-35
Baker's chocolate (1 ounce)	26	26
Chocolate-flavored syrup (1 ounce)	4	4
		(12-ounce serving)
Soft Drinks		
Sugar-Free Mr. PIBB		58.8
Mountain Dew		54.0
Mellow Yello		52.8
TAB		46.8
Coca-Cola		45.6
Diet Coke		45.6
Shasta Cola		44.4
Shasta Cherry Cola		44.4
Shasta Diet Cola		44.4
Mr. PIBB		40.8
Dr. Pepper		39.6
Sugar-Free Dr. Pepper		39.6
Big Red		38.4
Sugar-Free Big Red		38.4
Pepsi-Cola		38.4
Aspen		36.0
Diet Pepsi		36.0
Pepsi Light		36.0
RC Cola		36.0
Diet Rite		36.0
Kick		31.2
Canada Dry Jamaica Cola		30.0
Canada Dry Diet Cola		1.2

Source: FDA, Food Additive Chemistry Evaluation Branch, based on evaluations of existing literature on caffeine levels.

Source: Institute of Food Technologists (IFT), April 1983, based on data from National Soft Drink Association, Washington, D.C. IFT also reports that there are at least 68 flavors and varieties of soft drinks produced by 12 leading bottlers that have no caffeine.

From "FDA Consumer," March 1984, pages 14-15.

A.   BAKING POWDER

Baking powder contains two chemicals, bicarbonate of soda and tartaric acid. These two chemicals do not neutralize each other in any way so as to destroy or render them harmless and there is left in the bread a substance identical to Rochelle salt that is sold at the drug store. As an illustration; two teaspoons of baking powder added to a quart of flour leave in the bread 165 grains of Rochelle salt; that is, 45 grains more than is contained in Seidlitz powder. This has no nutritive value; instead, it retards digestion and gives the organs of elimination extra work to throw off the poison.

In 1908 there was a great national uproar made about the poisonous effects of baking powder. A direct appeal was made to President Theodore Roosevelt and he appointed a committee to investigate the physiological effects of baking powder.

After this investigation, the Department of Agriculture issued bulletin No.103, which contained this final determination by the committee concerning baking powders. "In short, the board concludes that alum baking powder is no more harmful than any other baking powders, but that it is wise to be moderate in the use of foods that are leavened with baking powder." There is nothing in that statement that proves that baking powders are harmless; it simply states that one baking powder is no more harmful than the other, but the physiological action of baking powder was found to be of such a nature "that it is wise to be moderate in the use of foods that are leavened with baking powder."

Our present phosphate beds are exhausted, but phosphate

is still needed for making pancake flour and for manufacturing baking powder. Aluminum compounds are used extensively with phosphates in the manufacture of fully one-half of all the baking powder made in the United States. In the manual of the Parke-Davis Company, one of the largest pharmaceutical houses in America, it states the following concerning aluminum: "Powerful astringent (causes animal tissues to contract), rarely used internally, except in painter's colic." Most baking powders on the market now are real poisons. They eat the lining of the stomach or damage it until inflammation and congestion follow. Soda decreases the pancreatic juices that are needed to digest protein, fats, and carbohydrates.

More than one hundred million pounds of baking powder are used in the United States every year, and less than one million pounds can be said to be free from dangerous poisons.

ONE TEASPOONFUL (5 mg) OF BAKING POWDER

	mg of sodium	mg of potassium
Alum type	500	8
Phosphate type	450	9
Tartrate type	360	250
Low sodium type	2	500

ANNOTATION: The two leading brands of baking powder are Calumet and Clabber Girl. Calumet has sodium aluminum sulfate, cornstarch, calcium sulfate, calcium acid phosphate, and calcium silicate. Clabber Girl has three of the above plus bicarbonate of soda, but it lacks calcium sulfate. Sodium aluminum sulfate has been used in making soap, printing on fabrics, and as a water-softening agent. Calcium sulfate is used in the manufacture of cement, chemical fertilizer, plaster of paris, artificial marble, and as a glaze in paints, enamels, paper, insecticide dusts, and in the manufacture of sulfuric acid. Calcium acid phosphate is used in chemical fertilizer and in enameling. Calcium silicate is used in the manufacture of Portland cement, lime glass, plastics, and in road construction.

B. CONDIMENTS

Condiments are added simply to make food taste better to a perverted appetite. The taste for condiments is decidedly an acquired one. Condiments of all kinds are repulsive to infants and to everyone whose taste has not been perverted. They furnish no nutrition, and are very irritating to the delicate lining of the stomach and digestive tract. They promote a feverish condition in the system that is very injurious to health, causing dyspepsia and nervous irritability.

Mustard and black pepper cause inflammation of the stomach and skin. Habitual use produces intestinal catarrh (a discharge from the mucous membranes) and ruins the digestive juices. Both red and black pepper cause an increase in acid secretion by the stomach. This irritates the delicate lining of the stomach so much that bleeding may occur.

The idea that spices and similar substances aid digestion is erroneous. Condiments hinder rather than aid digestion. The oils found in condiments are all irritating and when they are applied to the skin in a concentrated form they will cause blistering, inflammation, and irritation. If the contact is prolonged, they will destroy the tissue. The effect upon the stomach is similar. When these poisons are absorbed into the blood, they are brought into contact with every cell and fiber of the body. Often the delicate cells of the kidneys undergo degenerative change from the use of condiments, their efficiency is impaired, and as a result we have Bright's disease and other illnesses.

C. PICKLES

Pickles are indigestible and resist the action of the gastric juice as would pebbles. They cause great irritation and chronic diseases. They are hardened by the action of acetic acid, and sometimes by the addition of alcohol. They arrest the action of the saliva and cause gastric catarrh. Acetic acid is an active poison. Stuffed olives, green olives, brandied fruits, etc, are in the same class. Salads in which vinegar is used are far from wholesome and must be excluded from the diet of the sick or invalid. Lemons should be substituted for vinegar, as they are an excellent tonic and cleanser of the system. Many kinds of germs cannot live in lemon juice.

3

DANGERS FROM DISEASE IN ANIMALS

Meat eating is becoming more and more dangerous because of the steady increase in disease among animals. Some time ago I had a nice herd of registered Jerseys and one morning we noticed in the paper that in the adjoining county thousands of cattle had to be killed because of disease. So I decided to sell my stock and keep only three of the best milk cows. One morning about six or eight months later a neighbor said to me: "Did you hear that Anderson had 16 cows die yesterday and could not do anything for them?" So I decided to sell two of my three cows and just keep "old Lizzie," a registered Jersey. Her milk tested 6 percent butterfat. She never had anything but the very best of feed and the very best care possible. A few weeks later she became sick and refused all food. I told my wife not to use the milk for a day or two, hoping there would be a change for the better, but there was none. Old Lizzie walked as if she was afraid to step on her feet and made queer movements with her lower jaw and all at once she fell over and was dead. We decided then that we would never use any more milk.

Some time after this, we noticed in the paper that there were four or five states in which the chickens as well as the cows were so diseased that for a long time the farmers were not permitted to ship any eggs, butter, or livestock. While we had not used any milk for a long time prior to this, we stopped using meat and eggs too, and have not used them since. We found an abundance of good things that take their place. A few years prior to this I was up in the northern states near the clear-water lakes and found millions of fish dead in the water. On being examined they were found to have a live worm along their spine which killed them.

Not long ago while in San Diego, California, I was told by reliable persons that in the ocean nearby dead fish were so thick on the water that the steamers had a hard time running through them.

For many years I have spent much money and time producing articles of food that will perfectly take the place of meat, fish, milk, eggs, and butter. These new foods are very tasty, easily digested, furnish complete nourishment, and are very inexpensive, costing only a fraction of the amount paid for animal proteins. You will find all of them discussed in this book.

ANNOTATION: Following the publication of Upton Sinclair's novel *The Jungle* in 1906, in which he so vividly described the terrible conditions in the nation's meat packing houses, the Federal Meat Inspection Act was signed into law in 1907. The main deficiency of this act was that it did not apply to meat packers who sold their products within the borders of the states where their plants were located (intrastate sales). By the mid–1960s nearly 8 billion pounds of meat was being slaughtered, processed and sold within the states every year, in this way escaping government inspection. This amount of meat is enough to supply the needs of nearly 50 million people. In the early 1960s the U.S. Department of Agriculture conducted a nationwide survey of those packing plants that were selling their meat within state boundaries. The results of this study were not released until 1967 and they described conditions that were as bad as, or worse than, those described in *The Jungle.* "Scenes in which rodents and insects infested meat, in which the meat of dead animals and diseased animals was processed into sausage, in which animal hair, pus, fecal material, and the unwashed hands of workers contaminated meat, were described in the matter-of-fact language of the professional inspectors."From *Citizen Nader,* Charles McCary, Saturday Review Press, New York, 1972.

The results of this study helped to obtain the passage of the Wholesome Meat Act in 1967. The act was signed into law by President Johnson and it required the states to bring their inspection systems up to federal standards within 2 years.

As indicated by several recent newspaper articles, the passage of this law does not mean that the public can become complacent and take for granted that the quality of meat they are buying is good. As a result of a report on TV in September 1983, the Cattle King Packing Company, once one of the largest suppliers of ground beef for the school lunch program, was forced to close. A 21-count indictment charging the owner, several officers and employees, and 2 USDA meat graders with attempting to defraud the government and private firms by selling adulterated or poor quality meat, was handed down by a federal grand jury in April 1984. The manager of the packing company pleaded guilty to charges of concealing damaged or inferior meat from inspectors. People that were interviewed for this NBC TV report said that meat was processed from cattle that were either dead on arrival at the Cattle King Packing Company or that died in the yards before they could be slaughtered. These people also described filthy working conditions at the packing plant.

In an editorial appearing in the *Los Angeles Times* on Sunday, June 16, 1985, Tom Devine reported that Los Angeles meat inspectors recently found some packing plant practices around the Los Angeles area that were quite similar to those described in *The Jungle*, with the exception that there were no reports of packing plant workers falling into lard vats, never to be seen or heard from again. This article also notes that while food contamination and the number of cases of food poisoning from meat are on the increase, the U.S. Department of Agricluture intends to further relax the federal inspection of meat. In fact, all federal inspection of packing plants may soon come to an end, and the packing plants themselves may substitute their own inspection programs. This would not be a pleasant prospect for meat eaters. Even under the present inspection system, much dishonesty and graft have been reported. During the 1970s it was estimated that in some areas of the United States over 90 percent of the meat inspectors were involved in bribery.

The modern, up-to-date, money-making, livestock farm in

the United States can be compared with an assembly line in a modern high-production factory. The cruel and often insensitive way in which the veal calves are treated is enough to make even an average person cringe and join the nearest humane society or ASPCA. From the time that they are able to stand, the calves are made to stand in stalls only about 2 feet wide and just long enough to fit in. They are unable to turn around and sometimes they are even chained into position. In order to give the light-colored and tender-textured meat so prized by meat lovers, the calves are purposely made somewhat anemic by feeding them a diet that is low in iron. They are deprived of roughage and instead are fed on liquids and nonfat milk products. They receive small doses of antibiotics and vitamins to keep them healthy and stimulate rapid growth. Interestingly, the consumption of meat has actually been dropping lately in the United States from about 192 pounds of meat per person each year in 1970 to 181 pounds in 1979.

In 1960 a shipment of rainbow trout from a fish hatchery in Idaho was stopped at the California border for a routine inspection. A large number of the fish were found to have cancer of the liver. This finding led to the inspection of other fish hatcheries in the western United States. The number of trout that were found to have liver cancer varied from 25 to 100 percent in the various hatcheries. These were fish that were being used to stock the streams and lakes in the western states. Trout that have this form of cancer usually appear as normal, healthy, fast-growing fish and live for half to three-fourths of their normal life span. Why liver cancer develops in such large numbers of these trout is not known for sure, but it is thought to be due to some type of chemical that was present in the food pellets that the trout were being fed. The dry food pellets began to replace fresh meat about 10 years prior to this discovery of liver cancer. A variety of additives, vitamins, and growth stimulants was used in the food pellets in an attempt to replace factors that were present in the fresh meat. It would therefore appear that one or more dietary factors or additives were responsible for this disease.

Fish with unexpectedly large amounts of the potentially lethal poison dioxin in their edible parts were recently taken from lakes and streams in southern Michigan. Even though the traces of this poison were extremely small, in some instances the amount was higher than that recommended for human consumption by the FDA. One surprising feature of this finding was that these fish were caught where there was no apparent source for dioxin contamination of the water.

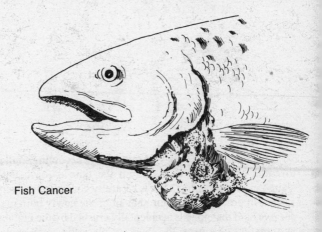

Fish Cancer

In the spring of 1985 the State of California Department of Health Services issued a warning that fish caught in several locations close to the shore near Los Angeles, in Santa Monica and San Pedro bays, could be highly contaminated with DDT or PCB. These two substances may cause cancer or other serious disease and therefore their consumption should be limited. Because of this local problem with contamination, guidelines for fishing in these areas were issued to protect the public. In these guidelines it was made clear that certain kinds of fish could not be eaten at all, and other kinds were limited in the amount that could be eaten each week, specially by pregnant women and young children.

They also recommended that the skin and fat should be removed from the fish while preparing them for eating, and that no liver from any fish should be eaten.

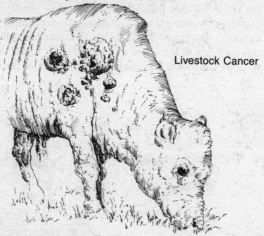

Livestock Cancer

The production of pork is in many ways becoming similar to cattle production, in that from the time of birth until slaughter the young pig's life is carefully controlled in every aspect. In order to make sure that all of the newly born pigs survive, and that none is accidentally crushed by the mother, as sometimes happens, the sows are placed in small enclosures that have openings just large enough so that the small piglets can reach through to nurse. Because the mother's milk is so low in iron content, each newborn pig receives a shot of iron. They also have their teeth clipped in order to keep them from injuring the mother during nursing. As soon as the young pigs are weaned from the mother, which occurs at about 28 days after birth, they are started on low doses of antibiotics in order to prevent the diseases that are frequently fatal to pigs — diarrhea and respiratory failure. It is difficult to believe, but it really happens, that during the marketing and slaughtering process, many pigs actually die from fright before they can be killed. Because the meat turns watery when this happens, and there is an economic loss to the farmers, attempts are now being made to breed the pigs in such a way that this will not happen.

Trichinosis, a disease that is caused by the trichina worm commonly found in hogs, is still a serious health threat, particularly in the southern United States.

In 1953 it was estimated that 350,000 Americans were harboring this worm in their bodies, and while most infected people do not even realize they are carrying this parasite, in 16,000 of these individuals the illness was serious enough to cause symptoms. It was estimated in 1972 that 80,000 pigs containing the trichina parasite were being slaughtered each year. These worms cannot be seen in the carcass of a slaughtered pig before it is stamped "U.S. Inspected Meat." It seems quite evident that since there are still so many cases of trichinosis, some hogs are still being fed raw garbage and housewives or others are serving undercooked pork. When humans eat improperly cooked pork containing the live trichina worms, these parasites are freed from the ingested pork in the victim's intestinal tract and are then carried in the bloodstream to the muscles, heart, and even the brain. Fortunately, the incidence of trichinosis has been decreasing in recent years for two main reasons; first, the nationwide educational effort regarding the necessity of cooking pork thoroughly before it is eaten; uncured pork must be cooked at least one-half hour for each pound of meat. The second reason is the federal prohibition against the feeding of raw garbage to pigs.

More of a mass-produced, assembly line product than even cattle or hog production, the most highly mechanized of all animal production in U.S. agriculture is probably that of the poultry industry. The baby chicks are artificially hatched in gigantic incubators, which hold up to 15,000 eggs. If the chicks are to be raised for cooking purposes, they are kept in huge sheds each holding as many as 50 to 70 thousand birds, with each bird having hardly enough room to move. Because they are packed so close together they frequently rub against each other until they have practically no feathers left. They must also be debeaked by clipping the tip off the beak or by blunting it with a red hot iron in order to prevent pecking and injuring of their neighbors. After they have been fattened for about 2 months, they are taken to an assembly line where as many as 570 chickens a minute are slaughtered. Because of these modern methods of production, it costs only about 20 percent as much today to buy a chicken for broiling as it did in 1940.

The hens that are kept for egg production fare no better. They are placed 4 to a cage that may be as small as 12 by 16 inches in size. Because they are in such close quarters, they also have to have their beaks blunted in order to prevent injury to each other. They are fed a vitamin-enriched diet along with antibiotics and other medicines to prevent disease. They are kept awake under bright lights for 18 to 20 hours a day and produce an egg on the average of every 32 hours, more than double the usual egg production. Because of this very accelerated, strenuous, and extremely debilitating program, the hen is so weak and thin after a year or two that she cannot be used as a broiler but instead ends up in a can of chicken soup.

In 1971 the government accounting office (GAO) examined 68 poultry plants across the country while checking up on the United States Department of Agriculture poultry inspection program. In most of the inspected poultry plants unacceptably dirty conditions were found with unsanitary equipment, floors, and walls and inadequate pest control. In about half of the plants, poultry products were found to be contaminated with fecal material, digestive tract contents, bile, or feathers. The 68 poultry plants that were inspected were responsible for about 20 percent of the total poultry processed yearly in the United States.

Not only have many of the poultry processing plants been found unsanitary, but during the 1960s some very disturbing reports from the poultry industry itself indicated that salmonella infection rates sometimes reached as high as 95 percent.

Not only is this a distressingly high figure, but of additional concern is that many of the processing plants that were found to have contamination rates of 50 percent or more were government inspected plants.

There are two species of bacteria that very frequently cause food poisoning and are often found in meat: salmonella, which is the most common cause of food poisoning, and clostridia, the bacteria that cause the frequently fatal disease called botulism.

The symptoms of salmonella food poisoning range from mild abdominal discomfort to severe pain, cramps, nausea, vomiting, and diarrhea. The latter may lead to dehydration so severe that it may prove fatal to young infants or to elderly persons whose resistance to disease is already low. It has been estimated that about two million Americans suffer from salmonella poisoning every year, usually from eating contaminated food, specially poultry, beef, pork, fish, and eggs. Bacteria and parasites find meat an excellent place in which to grow and multiply; therefore, putrefaction sets in rapidly, specially if the meat is not properly refrigerated. Some of the other serious diseases that may be transmitted by contaminated meat are tuberculosis, tularemia, hepatitis, and brucellosis.

Recently a number of people in the Seattle area came down with a severe illness consisting mainly of diarrhea and bleeding from the colon. Fifteen percent of these people eventually developed serious and permanent kidney damage. The bacteria causing this outbreak were found to be E. coli., a common type of bacteria present in the large intestine of all humans. But the particular type of E. coli. that was responsible for this series of illnesses was a kind that had never been found in the United States before. Further careful investigation traced the origin of these bacteria to some ground hamburger that had been served at a fast-food restaurant. It was not long after this epidemic in Seattle that this same type of bacteria was found scattered throughout the United States.

The long-standing controversy that has been going on since

the 1800s over the advantages and disadvantages of raw (unpasteurized) milk compared with pasteurized milk is still far from settled, and probably never will be to everyone's satisfaction. The proponents of certified raw milk claim that not only does it taste better; that it is more natural; that it contains more vitamins and minerals than pasteurized milk, but it has also been said to contain some special rather nebulous ingredients such as an antistiffness factor, claimed to be good for the treatment of arthritis.

On the other hand, those that advocate the use of pasteurized milk claim that even *certified* raw milk is dangerous because of the possible bacterial contamination, and that it has been definitely proven to harbor certain bacteria that have caused widespread outbreaks of milk-borne disease.

In England, for example, raw milk was found to be the major source for several outbreaks of enteritis (inflammation of the intestines) caused by the bacteria campylobacter jejuni. This same organism has been found to be an important cause of outbreaks of diarrhea in the United States. In 1981 three such outbreaks of enteritis were reported in consumers of raw milk in Oregon, Kansas, and Arizona. The patients all had varying degrees of diarrhea, abdominal pain, fever, headache, nausea, bloody diarrhea, and vomiting. Dogs, cats, poultry, cattle, sheep and pigs can all carry these bacteria. This disease is transmitted by fecal contamination of food or by eating incompletely cooked chicken, hamburgers, clams, or turkey. The raw milk in these cases was probably contaminated by cow feces at the time of milking. Unfortunately, fecal contamination with these bacteria cannot be completely eliminated even with meticulous hygiene in the dairy, and they can survive for weeks in milk kept refrigerated at 4°C. But they are apparently completely eliminated by pasteurization. In the 1800s, before the pasteurization of milk, repeated outbreaks of typhoid fever, scarlet fever, diphtheria, diarrhea, and sore throat were caused by contaminated milk, which was produced and sold under unsanitary conditions.

Raw milk may be sold as either certified or uncertified raw

milk. Certified raw milk is produced in accordance with the standards established by the American Association of Medical Milk Commissions, Inc. and is manufactured by large dairies and sold in some retail stores. Uncertified raw milk, on the other hand, is usually sold by individual dairy farmers on their own farms.

Pasteurization simply refers to heating the milk to a certain temperature and keeping it there for a specified length of time in order to kill the bacteria that are capable of transmitting disease to humans. This process does not sterilize the milk, but does make it quite safe to drink. Both pasteurized and raw milk may be sold with vitamins A and D added and either one may or may not be homogenized (emulsification of the milk fat).

There is no doubt that pasteurization affects the nutritional value of the milk to some degree, as the raw milk advocates claim. Three vitamins are slightly reduced in amount; these are thiamine, vitamin B_{12}, and vitamin C. In each case the loss is less than 10 percent. In addition to the vitamins, approximately 6 percent of the calcium is made insoluble so that it cannot be absorbed by the body and about 1 percent of the protein is coagulated.

The most serious hazard for those who choose to drink raw milk is contamination of the milk with either salmonella or campylobacter bacteria. Both of these organisms have caused serious outbreaks of disease in the United States in recent years. Not only have there been outbreaks of salmonella infection from drinking raw or improperly pasteurized milk, but also from using nonfat dry milk or cheese. Milk is an ideal growth medium for salmonella and some strains of these bacteria can remain alive in such milk products as yogurt for up to two weeks. There are also other bacterial diseases associated with drinking unpasteurized milk; some of these are brucellosis, colibacillosis, listeriosis, tuberculosis, corynebacteriosis, staphylococcosis, streptococcosis, streptobacillosis, and yersiniosis.

A recent widespread outbreak of salmonella food poisoning that involved 5 midwestern states, where thousands were infected and 6 fatalities occurred, was thought to be due to the contamination of pasteurized milk in a modern up-to-date dairy by some raw milk accidentally mixing with it through a faulty connecting pipe. This was reported to be the largest outbreak of salmonella infection in history, with more than 16,000 confirmed cases.

In California a recent epidemic involving about 250 people and resulting in 85 deaths was traced to the bacteria listeria monocytogenes, which had contaminated a certain brand of cheese. The method of contamination was never abolutely determined, but it was believed to be most likely the result of some raw or improperly pasteurized milk causing contamination during the cheese manufacturing process. Many of those who died during this outbreak were pregnant women and young children.

Those who drink raw milk are also at risk in ingesting a virus that has been found to induce leukemia in at least 2 animals – cattle and chimpanzees. This virus is known as the bovine leukemia virus (BLV). It is prevalent in dairy cattle and, once infected, the animal remains a carrier of this virus for life. Nearly one-half of 7,768 dairy cattle in Florida were found to have antibodies to BLV. This indicates either a past or present infection with the virus. In the United States, 20 percent or more of adult dairy cattle are infected with BLV and while the incidence varies considerably among different herds, infection rates of over 80 percent are not uncommon.

While it has not been proven that humans develop leukemia as a result of drinking raw milk, the high incidence of leukemia reported in persons living in areas where BLV is constantly present raises concern. Since at the present time there is no official requirement that milk from cows having lymphosarcoma or BLV be excluded from human consumption, the safest course is to drink pasteurized milk; pasteurization seems to destroy this virus. Most BLV-infected cows release the infectious virus or infected lymphocytes into their milk. (From "Raw Milk In Cancer," Virgil H. Hulse, M.D.,

M.P.H., *The Journal of Health and Healing,* Summer 1983, p. 3.)

Millions of pounds of antibiotics are produced in the United States every year, but less than half of the total amount is used to treat human diseases. The rest, about $270 million worth, is mixed with animal feed and is fed mostly to cattle, poultry, and pigs. The antibiotics were first given over thirty years ago in order to prevent the spread of disease through the closely packed animals while they were being prepared for market; however, a very surprising but beneficial side-effect was soon noticed. For some unexplained reason low doses of antibiotics caused the animals to grow and to put on weight much more rapidly than they would under normal circumstances without the antibiotics. In this way the antibiotics proved to be a double blessing to the cattle growers. At the same time, however, some unfortunate and dangerous results of giving the animals low doses of antibiotics were starting to show up. Antibiotic resistant strains of bacteria rapidly developed in some animals, and it has recently been shown without a doubt that these resistant bacteria can be transmitted to humans who consume the bacteria-contaminated meat, thereby causing disease in humans that is resistant to these same antibiotics. The most common antibiotics fed to the animals are penicillin, tetracycline, and chlortetracycline. Unfortunately, these are the same ones that are most commonly used to treat human disease. At the present time about 80 percent of the pigs and calves, 60 percent of cattle, and 30 percent of the chickens and turkeys eaten in the United States are given feeds that contain small amounts of antibiotics.

The most common group of bacteria that cause food poisoning is salmonella. At one time infection with these bacteria was easily controlled with antibiotics; but now at least 25 percent of salmonella, and some have reported as many as 75 percent, has developed a resistance to the antibiotics that have been fed to the animals. Apparently giving the antibiotics to the animals promotes bacterial resistance by killing off the bacteria that are sensitive to the administered antibiotic but leaves the drug-resistant bacteria to grow and multiply. Although many scientists felt that these resistant bacteria could produce disease in humans, it was not until 1983 that this was proven positively. At that time, an outbreak of gastrointestinal illness that was resistant to the usual antibiotics was traced to hamburger made from a herd of cattle that had been fed chlortetracycline. For the first time the scientists were able to trace how the antibiotic-resistant bacteria made their way from the feed lot to the supermarket, and then to the dinner table.

Just exactly how bacteria build up a resistance to an antibiotic is not known, but that this can occur was recognized years ago in England. Ampicillin, a very common and effective antibiotic, was at one time almost 100 percent effective in treating cases of salmonella infection. Today only one in four patients with a salmonella infection responds to ampicillin treatment. When it was found over ten years ago that resistant new strains of these bacteria were developing in cattle throughout the British Isles, causing thousands of cases of severe diarrhea and several deaths, the British Parliament acted to ban antibiotics that were needed to treat human disease from all animal feeds. Other European and Scandinavian countries have now followed the lead of England.

Up to the present time in the United States powerful lobbies have been successful in preventing Congress from eliminating the use of antibiotics in livestock feed. It was reported in the *American Medical News* of February 8, 1985, however, that the FDA is considering the possibility of urging a government ban on the use of penicillin and tetracycline in livestock feed, not only because of their frequent use in the treatment of human illness but also because of the large number of bacteria resistant to these antibiotics that are appearing in the food of Americans. "The most convincing data in support of a ban have been gathered by the Centers for Disease Control (CDC) in Atlanta, which investigated 52 salmonella outbreaks in the U.S. between 1971 and 1983. 'Salmonella was transmitted from food animals or their products (such as milk) in 69 percent of the outbreaks involving resistant strains and in 46 percent of outbreaks involving antimicrobial susceptible strains,' the CDC's Scott Holmberg, M.D., told a panel of 3 FDA officials."

It is now estimated that from 116 to 264 deaths occur yearly in the United States from the salmonella organisms that are resistant to antibiotics and which originate in food animals that have been given small doses of antibiotics.

Section VIII
Water and Good Health

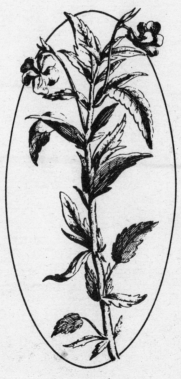

Great Upright Violet

1

HISTORY OF WATER CURE

Water has been used from time immemorial for remedial purposes. The world's oldest medical literature makes numerous references to the beneficial use of the bath in treating various diseases. The learned Greek, Hippocrates, who lived about five hundred years before Christ and is referred to as the "father of modern medicine," was the first to write much on the healing of disease with water. He used water extensively, both internally and externally, in treating illness of all kinds. "When pain seizes the side, either at the commencement or at a later stage, it will not be improper to try to dissolve the pain by hot applications. ... A soft large sponge, squeezed out of hot water and applied, forms a good application. ... A soft fomentation like this soothes pains, even such as shoot to the clavicle." Hippocrates goes on to say: "...for the bath soothes the pain in the side, chest, and back; concocts the sputa, promotes expectoration, improves the respiration, and allays lassitude; for it soothes the joints and the outer skin, and is diuretic, removes heaviness of the head, and moistens the nose. Such are the benefits to be derived from the bath."

Long before Hippocrates recorded his experiences with the healing properties of water, we have learned from the study of ancient history that the Egyptians enjoyed bathing in their sacred river, the Nile. Pictures of ancient Egyptians, found in the tombs, show people preparing for a bath. The baby Moses was found in the rushes when Pharaoh's daughter went down to the river to bathe. Bathing held a prominent place in the instructions that were given by Moses, under divine guidance, for the government of the Hebrew nation. The relation of the bath to the treatment of leprosy would lead us to believe that it was used for its curative effects, and it would seem likely that an agent held in such high regard as a useful remedy would also be highly esteemed as a preventive of disease.

The ancient Persians and Greeks erected stately and magnificent public buildings devoted to bathing. The baths of Darius I (about 558-486 B.C.), one of the earliest Persian kings, are spoken of as being especially remarkable. The Greeks were probably the first nation to use the bath for personal cleanliness as well as for health reasons. Records show that they were using the warm bath more than one thousand years before the birth of Christ. In the ruins of King Nestor's palace in Greece there was found a built-in bathtub and drainage system more than 3000 years old. Rome, however, surpassed all the older nations in the costliness and magnificence of her bathing facilities. The first public bath was erected in Rome in the year 312 B.C. and it used only cold water. It was not long, however, until warm water baths replaced all those using cold water alone. Some of the greatest works of architecture in Rome were the warm public baths, which were supplied with every convenience for increasing the use and luxury of bathing as well as having many rooms for social gatherings. Kings and emperors each endeavored to construct a larger and more ornate public bath than their predecessors. The baths of Diocletian, completed in 302 A.D., were the largest in the world and could accommodate up to 18,000 bathers at the same time. It took 10,000 Christian slaves nearly seven years to complete their construction. When the baths were completed, the slaves had the choice of renouncing their religion or suffering martyrdom. At one time the number of public baths in Rome reached nearly one thousand.

Two noted physicians of the Roman Empire, Celsus and Galen, praised and glorified the bath as being invaluable for the treatment of a number of specific diseases. Galen said that exercise and friction must be used with the bath in order to have a perfect cure. If only the physicians through the following centuries had continued the practice of Galen, as described in his works, what a lot of suffering would have been avoided. Doctors would have refreshed and revived their fever-stricken patients with the use of God-given water, instead of giving them drugs like quinine, mercury, arsenic, etc., and letting them be consumed by fever that parched their lips and disorganized their blood. Many times their suffering was mercifully ended by their deaths. The Emperor Augustus was said to have been cured by water remedies of a disease that had resisted all other methods of treatment.

The Arabians have sometimes been looked upon as a wandering horde of wild men, but about one thousand years ago they had physicians among them that were some of the most learned men of that age. They were very sensible and enthusiastic about the benefits of the bath. Rhazes, one of the most prominent of them, described a method that is scarcely outdone by present-day water treatments. Baths were also used during pestilences.

In Constantinople, Turkish baths were very popular during the fifteenth century.

In the year 1600 A.D., public vapor baths were numerous in Paris, France. They were connected with the barber shops, as many still are in that country at the present time. Dr. Bell, of Paris, stated that, in connection with the city hospitals, nearly 130,000 baths were given in a single year to outside patients. Undoubtedly, patients in the hospitals were steamed and bathed as well. What a marked contrast with present-day hospitals in this country where the use of water treatments is most sadly neglected. Such neglect is inexcusable.

The Germans in olden times were very fond of bathing. According to the records of history, during the Middle Ages when there were many cases of leprosy, it was a religious duty to bathe because of the national faith in bathing. History also tells us that Emperor Charlemagne, who was a giant of a man over seven feet tall with long blond hair, held court while relaxing in a huge warm bath.

During the early part of the eighteenth century, water was used medicinally. Floyer published a history of bathing in which remarkable cures were reported, and he recommended the bath for numerous diseases. A Mr. Hancock, who was a minister, published in 1723 a book called "Common Water, the Best Cure for Fevers." Another book, whose author is unknown, was called "Curiosities of Common Water." It was also published in 1723. In this book water was said to be an "excellent remedy which will perform cures with very little trouble, and without charge, and may be truly styled a universal remedy." French and German writers were also advocating the use of water as a remedy during this same time.

In the early part of the nineteenth century, Vincent Priessnitz popularized the use of cold water as a curative measure. He was a peasant who lived in the Austrian part of Silesia from 1799 to 1851. In the small Austrian town where he grew up, water was used by the people to treat many ailments. When only a young man, Priessnitz suffered a severe injury. Several of his ribs were broken and his chest was caved in on the left side by a loaded wagon. Several of his teeth were also knocked out. The doctors who came to see him did not offer any hope for a cure. But he remembered several years before when he had successfully treated a badly crushed finger by holding it in cold water until the bleeding stopped and the pain was relieved; and he decided to treat his broken ribs in the same way. So by taking deep breaths while leaning over a chair to expand his ribs and using cold water, he was gradually completely cured.

It was not long after this that Priessnitz began to use this cold water treatment on others. His routine course of treatment consisted of cold baths and compresses, along with friction. He used this form of treatment for all manner of disease, since this was what had cured him. He combined the cold water therapy with exercise, deep breathing, and a diet of dark bread, meat, and vegetables that he grew in his own garden. His success greatly encouraged him, but he met with considerable opposition from the doctors when he treated some of their patients and cured them, after the doctors had given them up.

Although Priessnitz had no formal education, he developed various ways of applying cold water to the body to treat different diseases. His fame increased rapidly and in a few years he was known throughout the world. Today he is called the father of modern hydrotherapy. He succeeded in restoring hundreds of people to health who had been pronounced incurable. His friends claimed that he was a great discoverer, but he really didn't discover anything that had not been known for at least a century, if not for thousands of years, before. But since he was an uneducated peasant with no anatomical or medical knowledge, he made many errors, as is shown by some of his cases.

A famous neurologist in Vienna, Dr. Wilhelm Winternitz, went to observe Priessnitz's water cure treatment center in Graefenberg, Austria. He was so impressed with what could be accomplished with such simple means that he spent the rest of his life working to develop new methods of water treatment. The influence of Dr. Winternitz was felt by such well-known American water cure advocates as Dr. Simon Baruch and Dr. John Harvey Kellogg. It was Dr. Baruch who was chiefly responsible for the passage of laws in the state of New York that required the establishment of municipal baths in that state. Dr. Kellogg was the director of the Battle Creek Sanitarium in Michigan, the largest hydrotherapy treatment center in the United States until it was destroyed by fire on February 18, 1902. He developed many new treatments, including the electric light bath, that used natural methods.

The "water cure" spread to America about 1850 and until about 1854 it prospered greatly, but most of the doctors were opposed to this treatment. It seemed almost as though they did not want the people to get hold of any remedy that was practical, inexpensive, and could be used in any home. About 1870 they successfully had a law passed that prevented the water cure practitioners from practicing in New York. Since New York City was the headquarters, as soon as these treatments were stopped there, their use was abandoned nearly everywhere for a while.

Sebastian Kneipp, a Catholic priest in Bavaria who cured Archduke Joseph of Austria of Bright's disease during the late nineteenth century, gained a wide reputation because of his success with the water cure. He also had his patients return to nature, as far as possible. He used herbs with great success because he combined their use with other natural remedies.

The North American Indians used baths for many diseases. They developed original ways of giving both water and vapor baths. The vapor bath was the most commonly used, and it was followed by a plunge into a cold stream. This is similar to the custom so widely practiced at the present time in Finland, of jumping into either the snow or ice-cold water following a hot sauna bath.

The native Mexicans also use a hot-air bath (sauna). They confine themselves in a brick house that is heated by a furnace located on the outside. They seem to have implicit confidence in the efficiency of the sauna bath to destroy disease, using it with much success when ill.

Water is one of the most powerful and yet one of the simplest remedies that can be used by an intelligent mother who understands the effects of hot and cold on the body. If you cleanse and nourish your body properly, and leave nature to itself, it will renovate and heal the body.

Lately, people have been led to believe that there are remarkable virtues in certain spring waters (this refers to water from certain hot mineral springs that is used for external treatments). The claim that these waters are possessed of a miraculous healing power is not true. The healing virtue is in the moist heat that is obtained from the water.

THE WHOLE THING IN A NUTSHELL IS THAT THE USE OF WATER, COMBINED WITH AN ABUNDANCE OF FRESH AIR, SUNSHINE, PROPER DIET, EXERCISE, REST, RECREATION, AND PLEASANT SURROUNDINGS, EFFECTS A CURE.

Unfortunately, in the early days the reputation of water as a remedy was injured because people such as Vincent

Priessnitz used it to extremes. Such practitioners did not understand the human body, the uses of hot and cold water, or the useful and powerful reactions that are produced in the body when it is properly used. People were led to believe that it was a cure-all, and that cold water was the only remedy no matter what the condition or the disease might be. Rest, pure air, nourishing and simple food, sunlight, and exercise are of equal importance to water in all cases. Although water is not a specific, it is one of the most valuable remedies. This is true not only of water, but also of all the other natural remedies. There may be a specific remedy for a particular disease, but there is not one and only one remedy for every disease. Several remedial agents must be combined to suit the condition, and not a single one used to the exclusion of all the others. But even so, water is an important agency in the treatment of nearly every disease when it is correctly applied and used with other forms of treatment.

2

USING WATER TO PRESERVE HEALTH

Water, so valuable for remedial purposes, is fortunately one of the most abundant elements in nature. The human body is composed of about two-thirds water. The fluid secretions and excretions are more than nine-tenths water. Perspiration and saliva are both close to 100 percent water, while blood is 90 percent and muscle is between 80 and 90 percent water.

A. CHARACTERISTICS OF WATER

The composition of water is represented by the chemical formula H_2O, which means that it is composed of two gases, hydrogen and oxygen; proportionately two parts of the former to one of the latter. Both are odorless, colorless, tasteless, and burn readily. Oxygen is the greatest supporter of combustion in life. Hydrogen is one of the lightest gases known.

Water exists in the form of ice when its temperature is below 32°F. When it is at or above 212°F. (the boiling point) it is changed into vapor. Between 32°F. and 212°F. it is a liquid. Water requires a greater amount of heat to elevate its temperature a given number of degrees than any other substance, and it absorbs more heat during temperature elevation than any other substance. When changing from the ice to the liquid state, it absorbs a great amount of heat from the objects it comes in contact with. Water conducts heat much more readily than air does, giving its heat to bodies with which it comes in contact; but it also removes heat when it is at a lower temperature.

Rainwater

Of any water attainable, rainwater comes the nearest to being pure. But even rainwater is often unwholesome because it gathers many impurities as it falls through the atmosphere. Filtered rainwater and distilled water are perhaps the purest forms.

Hard water

When water is hard, it will not produce an abundant lather with soap. The hardness is due to salts of lime, gypsum, chalk, and other minerals, which make it less suitable for use both externally and specially internally.

Hot mineral spring water

This water contains solutions of the salts of magnesium and iron, as well as other chemicals such as iodine, arsenic, and sulphur, which give it a medicinal taste. Such water has been used extensively for cures of chronic ailments in the form of hot baths, etc., but it is absolutely unfit for drinking or cooking purposes. It contains no particular value for cleansing; therefore, one would naturally know that since it is unfit to cleanse the outside of the body it could not be of much benefit internally either.

B. WATER AND THE HUMAN BODY

With the exception of pure air, there is no other element in nature that is so important for sustaining life or that has such an important relation to the human system as pure water. A person can live a week or sometimes even much longer on water alone, but dies quickly if he is deprived of it. A large proportion of our food is composed of from 15 to 90 percent water.

Water undergoes no change in the body, but its presence is absolutely essential for the performance of the vital functions, as it enables various organs to perform their work so that life is sustained. The circulatory system is especially dependent upon water. Water composes a large percentage of the fluid portion of the blood that suspends the blood corpuscles as well as the nutritive and waste elements. With the aid of water, nutrients enter the blood and are conveyed to critical areas of the intricate human mechanism where repair and growth are needed.

There is no other substance that is so well adapted for this exact purpose as water. It circulates through the most delicate capillaries without friction, and even passes through membranes into parts of the body that are not accessible by natural openings. Water is continually passing out of the body through one or more of the organs of elimination — skin, kidneys, lungs, or intestines. If the kidneys become obstructed, we all know there will be serious trouble. The dry air constantly entering the lungs during normal breathing absorbs moisture from the pulmonary membranes. Therefore, it is necessary to supply the body with an abundance of pure water at all times. The average person eliminates about five pints of water in twenty-four hours, and an equal new supply must be provided in order to preserve the fluidity of the blood. People who work hard physically and perspire profusely naturally require more water than others.

It should also be noticed that the diet has a great deal to do with the amount of water demanded by nature. People who eat largely of animal products and use salt, pepper, spices, and condiments freely, require considerably more water to dissolve and cleanse the system of these unhealthful things. On the other hand, people who eat mostly fruit, vegetables and grains, and avoid the use of stimulating foods and drinks, require less water, as a great many vegetables and fruits are composed of more than half water.

Water is the only substance that really quenches the thirst. Other beverages will relieve thirst only in proportion to the amount of water they contain. Most of these drinks are unwholesome because of the injurious substances that are added.

The skin, which is the largest organ in the body, performs several important duties. One of the most important is excretion. This fact could be easily demonstrated if a coat of paint or varnish were applied all over the body, for a person would die almost as quickly as if a dose of poison had been given. The millions of little sweat glands, located just beneath the surface of the skin, are constantly engaged in separating impurities from the blood, which if retained would cause disease and eventually death.

The skin is also an organ of respiration. It absorbs oxygen and eliminates poisonous gases, although by far most of this work is done by the lungs. In some of the lower animals, all the work of respiration is done by the skin. The skin not only absorbs oxygen but it also absorbs liquids to a great extent. Absorption through the skin is increased when it is warm and moist. If a person stays in a warm bath for some time, the weight of the body may be increased. Seamen, when adrift on the ocean and deprived of fresh water, have been known to wet their clothing with seawater, since the skin will absorb some of the water without absorbing the salt.

The skin is a great help in the regulation of body temperature. It is nonconducting and dense, which prevents to a considerable degree the escape of essential body heat. When the body becomes overheated from strenuous vital activity, fever, or external heat, the skin relieves the tissues by favoring the escape of heat. This is exactly what happens in fever when you drink plenty of water or do anything to produce perspiration. The moisture passes from the sweat glands out onto the skin surface where it evaporates, resulting in a powerful cooling action.

The skin is also an organ of touch; in fact, it is the largest organ of sensitivity in the body. Through an extensive network of nerves, the skin is very closely connected with all the great nerve centers in the body. That is why water treatments applied to the body surface are so beneficial and have such a good effect in diseases affecting the nervous system.

The tiny nerve endings that come to the blood vessels in the skin also have a direct connection with the blood vessels deep inside the body. Thus, if either hot or cold is applied to the skin there will be a reaction in the deeper organs also. For example, placing an ice bag over the right lower abdomen in a patient with acute appendicitis will cause a constriction of the blood vessels in the appendix and in this way help to relieve the congestion and inflammation.

Every opening of the body leading to the surface is lined with mucous membrane. Mucous membrane lines the air passages and lungs, the urinary and genital organs, and the whole intestinal tract from the mouth to the rectum. Mucous membrane resembles the skin in that, like the skin, it is made up of several layers. It also secretes and excretes. It excretes foul material (as the exudation in diphtheria) and secretes useful substances when they are in a fluid state.

The importance of the skin as an organ of elimination is made obvious by the offensive odor of perspiration, which will have the distinctive odor of tobacco if the person uses it in any form. This shows that the skin not only eliminates normal body wastes, but may eliminate poisons from the body as well. Urea, sodium chloride, lactic acid, and potassium are some of the substances that are lost in the sweat.

Every movement we make destroys a tiny portion of the living tissues. These dead tissues have a poisonous effect on the body and must be removed. Some of the substances that are normally excreted by the system can be very deadly under certain circumstances, such as some of those contained in the urine, bile, gallbladder, etc. They must be eliminated as quickly as possible and here the marvelous properties of water are again exhibited. Pure water dissolves these poisons whenever it comes in contact with them. Then, after being brought by the circulatory system to the proper organs — liver, skin, kidneys, and lungs — the poisons are expelled.

The skin has millions of pores, from which constantly flows a stream of poisons from the disintegration of body cells. As we perspire, these dead cells or poisons are left on the skin. As time passes, more and more accumulate there. If the skin is normally active, it takes several days for these dead cells to form a layer, which could be compared to a thin coating of varnish. Unless a person bathes properly and often, these dead cells and poisons continue to accumulate and increase until they start to undergo a process of decomposition and subsequent reabsorption into the blood, thus placing an additional load on the organs of excretion.

We all know that a person who does not bathe often has a very unpleasant odor about him, but this offense is not equal to the evil done to oneself. This accumulation obstructs the work of the millions of little pores, and some of the poisons are reabsorbed, thus contaminating the system. Frequent cleansing with water will keep the skin wholly free from poisonous elements. It can easily be understood why so many people have torpid skins, because it is not uncommon to find those who have never taken a real, general cleansing bath in their lives, and most people do not practice it often enough.

A cleansing bath should be taken every day if possible. You wash your face and hands daily, why not your entire body? A cleansing bath taken daily will keep the skin supple and clean. The bath should be as indispensable to a woman as her mirror. Many very refined and fastidious people who spend hours in dressing, including women who use creams, lotions, and makeup to beautify the portions of the skin exposed to view, would be quite shocked to learn the true condition of the unwashed skin. Of course, we do not say that this is true of everyone, but it is true of a great many.

Inactivity of the skin due to improper bathing is one of the main causes of skin disease, especially if coupled with an aggravated condition caused by wrong dietary habits. The relation between the skin and kidneys is very close, and inactivity of the skin is often associated with kidney disorders.

The value of water in preventing disease was recognized by ancient peoples, and baths were used by them to a far greater extent than in modern times. Moses, the great Hebrew lawgiver, required his people to be scrupulously clean, and made bathing a part of their religious duties. His example was followed by Mohammed, who ordered his people to bathe before each of their five daily prayers. Thus, many have believed that cleanliness is next to godliness.

The Greeks regarded the bath as a very essential means of securing physical health. Daily baths were practiced by them, from the youngest to the oldest. The Romans also made a luxury of the bath.

The most renowned physicians from Hippocrates down to Galen, Celsus, Boerhaave, and others such as Sebastian Knieppe and Melville C. Keith, believed that bathing was an invaluable means of preserving health. Nevertheless, as people have become more "enlightened" and "civilized," bathing for health has been more and more disregarded.

During the dark ages in Europe, the bath was unknown. Michelet, a noteworthy historian, tells us that in his opinion, this accounted for the terrible plagues and pestilences of that period.

Mankind then felt the need for something new and started using poisonous drugs. Bathing is a natural instinct, and all nature shows the importance of baths. Rain is the natural shower bath. The influence of it is shown in the fresher, brighter, and more erect appearance of all living plants. Birds and animals do not neglect their baths. If man's instincts had not been perverted by the habits of modern civilization, he would value the bath highly and bathe frequently, as do the more humble creatures whose instincts are still true to nature.

Man's intelligence has made it possible for him to become grossly perverted in almost everything — food, appetite, bathing, etc. Man does not go astray from nature because he lacks intelligence or instinct, but because he wishes to gratify his own desires.

Many are afraid to use one of God's greatest blessings — pure water — because they have never experienced its beneficial effects.

C.   AMOUNT OF WATER NEEDED DAILY

The average person does not drink enough pure water. At least six to eight glasses must be taken daily. More is better, depending upon the kind of food eaten. Cool water is good, but ice water should not be taken. Babies and delicate patients should be given water as carefully as food.

When one drinks an abundance of pure, fresh water the blood and tissues are bathed and purified, thereby being cleansed of all poisons and waste matter. Water is also an essential constituent of the tissue cells and all body fluids, such as the digestive juices, etc.

Water dissolves nutritive material in the course of digestion, so that it can be absorbed into the blood and carried to various parts of the body to repair and build tissues and remove waste.

Water keeps all mucous membranes of the body soft and prevents friction of their surfaces.

Water aids in regulating body temperature and body processes.

Make a special effort to obtain the purest water available.

Recent scientific evidence suggests that elderly people may not feel thirsty even when their bodies are actually in need of water. It was also found that, despite the body's need for more fluid, the kidneys of older people do not tend to conserve fluid as would be expected under these circumstances. These factors may lead to the formation of kidney stones and contribute to constipation, an all-too-common problem in the elderly. Therefore, as you grow older, it is even more important that an adequate supply of fluid be obtained every day.

3

WATER'S EFFECTS AND USE
IN TREATMENT

Water benefits the body in many different ways. When taken by mouth, some of it is absorbed from the intestines and enters the bloodstream to increase its volume. The size of the blood vessels is thus increased (although they are never expanded to their fullest extent), due to an increase in the volume of their contents. The blood becomes more fluid, and as a result the circulation is quickened.

Except for air, water is the most transient substance taken into the body. It is eliminated in four ways: through the lungs, skin, kidneys, and intestines. By its solvent action, the poisons that have been eliminated by the tissue cells are dissolved and then excreted. When the volume of blood is increased, more water comes in contact with the waste matter in every part of the body. Thus, undesirable waste is removed. This is shown by an increase in urinary output and increased activity of the skin (perspiration).

Abundant water drinking increases elimination by the mucous membrane lining of the intestinal tract, an important organ of excretion. The result of this increased activity is that the contents of the intestines become more fluid, thus helping to correct the common problem of constipation. It also removes from the blood some of its poisonous waste material, rendering the blood cleaner for the building up of tissues. In this way both elimination and repair are aided.

The use of water assists in all the vital processes by increasing the renewal of tissues. It is a false idea that bathing renders a person more susceptible to colds. Colds are caused by a disturbance of the circulation. Frequent bathing makes the skin more active, thereby increasing the circulation. A person who takes a daily cold morning bath increases his immunity against colds and is not nearly so susceptible to changes in temperature. Colds contracted after bathing result from not taking proper precautions during and after the bath.

Disease does not exist without some disturbance in the circulation. In health, each part of the body receives its necessary share of blood. Therefore, in any disease, one of the first things to do is to balance the circulation. Prolonged applications of cold water contract the tiny blood vessels and thus the amount of blood in the part is lessened. The same may sometimes be accomplished by applying hot water to some distant part of the body so that the surplus blood will be drawn there and thus relieve the diseased organ.

Applications of heat may be applied to a part where there is not enough blood. At the same time you can apply a cold application to some other part of the body. This will help to send more blood to the deficient area. Very often hot and cold applications can be combined advantageously, because one part of the body cannot contain too much blood without some other part being deprived of its due portion.

Regulation of body temperature is closely associated with circulation, and the two are controlled by the same remedies given in the same way. A part that becomes inflamed and contains too much blood usually causes a fever. A cold application will relieve this.

When you wish to reduce the temperature of any part, the water must not be extremely cold. Use warm or tepid water just a few degrees below body temperature. This can be continued for some time without injury, until the temperature is reduced to normal. Many times one or more organs become torpid or inactive, the skin and liver in particular. When the blood vessels become inactive and distended, congestion results. Alternate hot and cold applications, continued for thirty minutes, will relieve congestion more quickly than any other remedy. Fomentations given as hot as can be tolerated, with cold sponging and drying between each fomentation, is the best method for giving hot and cold treatments.

Pain may be caused by a disturbance of the circulation because the overfilled blood vessels exert pressure upon the nerves. Relief will be obtained from hot applications, which relax the tissues. The nerve fibers will be relieved of pressure, and the circulation will then be stimulated so as to relieve the congestion. In some conditions, such as acute sprains and strains and acute bursitis, a local application of cold may give more relief from pain than applying heat.

A large number of diseases are caused by obstruction of the various organs. Usually the obstruction is due to the accumulation of natural waste products from the tissues or the ingestion of foreign materials, such as one absorbs in hard water or indigestible food. A warm bath opens the pores and removes external obstruction, while water taken by mouth will relieve internal obstruction, because it is the best solvent that we have. Obstruction in the stomach may be removed by emetics. Obstruction in the bowels may be removed by enemas.

With fever, cholera, etc., the blood is usually abnormally thick. This causes slow circulation and the tissues do not obtain proper nourishment. There is nothing as good as water to remedy this condition. If water will not stay in the stomach when taken by mouth, some can be absorbed through the skin by lying in a tub of water of the proper temperature, depending on the difficulty. Hot and cold fomentations applied to the abdomen, with a hot footbath and a cold compress to the head, will often relieve headache. They seem to affect the whole system. Fomentations applied to the abdomen and spine will relieve general nervousness and numerous other ailments. A full, warm bath may be given with equal success.

Water is one of the most powerful means of causing a reaction throughout the entire body in either health or disease. The blood vessels to each organ of the body can be controlled through a reflex arc by the stimulation of a certain area on the skin. For example, the blood vessels overlying the brain can be contracted by taking a hot footbath or dilated by placing a cold pack on the lower part of the spine.

A. EFFECTS OF COLD WATER

The application of cold water to the skin for a short period of time (one to three minutes) will cause the small blood vessels in the area where the cold is applied to contract and the skin will therefore appear pale. The colder the application, the more rapid and complete the contraction will be. Within a few minutes after the cold is removed a reaction will set in and the vessels will dilate, bringing more blood to the area, producing a feeling of warmth and a healthy blush to the skin. Rubbing the skin while the cold is being applied, as in a cold mitten friction rub, will enhance the effects of the cold water. If cold is applied at a more moderate temperature (70° to 80°) for a longer period of time (over five to eight minutes), the vessels in the skin will dilate, while those supplying the internal organs will contract.

When the blood vessels in the skin contract, the blood is forced deep into the internal organs. Just the opposite effect takes place when the surface vessels relax and dilate. The blood is then drawn from the internal organs to the skin. If any of the organs are congested or inflamed, more blood is removed from them than from the healthy organs, in this way relieving the congestion. In any application of cold, the organ nearest the point of application will be affected to the greatest extent.

Prolonged exposure of the body to cold depresses all of the normal physiological reactions in the body, while a short contact of the entire body with cold acts as a general stimulant to all the vital functions, through the action of the central nervous system. Digestive processes, elimination, urine production, respiration, muscle tone, pulse rate, and even some of the endocrine glands such as the thyroid, are all stimulated to greater activity. There is also an increase in the red and white blood corpuscles and in the hemoglobin. It is better to make the application warmer at first and then decrease the temperature gradually so that there will not be a shock or a chilly feeling, and the same results will be obtained. This applies especially to nervous persons, as the sudden application of cold is always a shock. A great many times the body temperature is reduced even though the skin glows and feels warmer. The only accurate way to determine temperature is with a thermometer. It is probably best not to use cold applications at all in persons who are very ill or tired, or in those who dislike or dread cold treatments, or in those who have severe kidney or heart trouble. Before starting any cold treatment, the person should feel warm and not cold or even chilly.

It is important to remember that some people may react poorly to cold, especially if extreme cold is used. In such cases, it is better to stop the treatment or use water at a more moderate temperature.

B. EFFECTS OF HOT WATER

Hot baths or applications should be given above a temperature of 98°F. A short local application of heat causes dilatation of the blood vessels with increased circulation to the part. As with cold water, the effects differ according to the length of the application.

Intense heat acts at first to stimulate the body, but if it is continued a definite depressive reaction occurs. A full hot bath causes an increased pulse rate. A bath given from 106° to 108°F. will increase the pulse from normal to between 100 to 120 beats per minute in a short time. A bath several degrees hotter, up to 112°F., will increase the pulse to more than 150 beats per minute. When the pulse increases to between 80 and 85 beats per minute during the treatment, an ice bag should be placed over the heart. When giving an extremely hot bath, always apply a cold compress to the head, and sponge the entire body with cool water every fifteen or twenty minutes. This will avert faintness. Extremely hot baths are seldom required. It is better, as a rule, to have the water temperature around 102°F. Don't forget to end each hot treatment with some kind of a cool or cold application, in order to close the pores in the skin and reduce the chance of chilling. This will also help to restore the normal alkaline reaction of the blood that applications of heat tend to lower.

There are very few agents that will so rapidly and powerfully excite and stimulate the body metabolism as a short hot bath. The undesirable results of hot baths are due to irrational or incautious use. But these same results are proof of their power.

C. EFFECTS OF WARM WATER

The temperature of a warm bath is between 92° and 98°F. A warm bath never exceeds the temperature of the body. Warm baths decrease the temperature and pulse as do cold baths, but they differ in that there is no shock when taking a warm bath. Therefore, it is not followed by any undesirable reaction. The blood pressure is also decreased.

Warm baths greatly increase the activity of the skin, through perspiration and absorption. When a warm bath is continued for two or three hours, the body weight will be increased as the skin absorbs some of the water. The general effects of a warm bath are mild and soothing, doubtless because of the close approximation to the normal body temperature. It provides favorable conditions for the performance of the natural bodily functions.

Thus, we see that when water is applied at the proper temperature, it is the most natural and powerful means of either depressing or increasing the vital activities of the body. Water applications are wholly of a sympathetic character, and all parts of the body are closely connected by the sympathetic nerves. The skin and mucous membranes are also closely connected, as has been described.

There are many ways of administering water at any temperature, and each different temperature will produce some modification or general effect in the body.

4

WATER'S EFFECTS ON SICKNESS

There are very few substances that possess as many remedial properties as water. Anyone treating the sick should try to accomplish the greatest amount of good with the least expense to the patient's vitality. Following is a list of some of the therapeutic properties of water.

Sedative
Sedative drugs diminish the action of the heart. They affect all the nerve centers controlling the heart, and their action is very often uncertain and detrimental. When water is properly applied, however, it is a very much more efficient sedative, and its use rarely leaves harmful aftereffects. A warm bath will invariably soothe and relax an extremely nervous person and help produce restful sleep.

Antipyretic
There is no drug that will decrease the temperature of the body as quickly, efficiently, and harmlessly as water. The pulse can rapidly be reduced from twenty to forty beats per minute by the use of a cool or cold bath. To decrease body temperature, use water below 98°F.

Anodyne (Analgesic)
Anodynes lessen the nervous sensibilities, thereby relieving pain. Hot water fomentations will always give relief and have often been used when drugs have failed.

Anticonvulsant
Water is unrivaled as a relaxing agent in convulsions and muscle spasm.

Astringent
The use of cold water in arresting hemorrhage is well-known by all physicians.

Laxative
The abundant use of pure water is most effective in helping to overcome constipation, but it never causes violent or unpleasant symptoms such as those that frequently accompany and follow the use of purgatives.

Eliminative
Water is a perfect eliminator. It dissolves poisonous waste materials and foreign elements in the blood, thereby aiding their elimination through the urine, feces, sweat, and lungs.

Diaphoretic (Sudorific)
Water may be used to produce profuse perspiration.

Alterative
For many years mercury was considered the most noteworthy alterative in the materia medica. But it has yielded its place to water. The only thing mercury ever accomplished was to destroy the normal elements of the blood. Water not only preserves and builds up the normal elements, but it also destroys and eliminates the waste elements and increases the circulation.

Tonic
Water used properly will increase the vital activities very quickly and powerfully and restore normal tone to the body. The tonic effect of a cool bath is well-known to everyone.

Stimulant
A stimulant acts to increase the vital functions of the body above what is their usual activity. A short hot bath, lasting five minutes or less, is a very efficient stimulant. It will stimulate the circulation and increase the pulse from 70 to

150 beats within fifteen minutes. Hot baths of a longer duration cause relaxation and even weakness. Short cold baths also act as a very bracing stimulant and tonic.

Derivative

This is a method (in this case, water treatment) for removing blood from a certain part by increasing the blood in another part. This is one of water's most important properties. No application can equal water in efficiency and certainty of action. Water will work wonders. Its use has been terribly neglected, to the great detriment of the human race. Its merits have been well demonstrated and generally acknowledged for years.

Emetic.

Rapidly drinking several glasses of tepid water will often cause vomiting.

Diuretic

The more water that you drink, the greater will be the amount of urine produced.

Expectorant

Heat applied to the chest loosens the secretions so that they can more easily be coughed up.

Anesthetic

The prolonged local use of cold will produce numbness, such as using an ice pack on a sprained ankle.

5

BATHS AND WATER TREATMENTS

Hydrotherapy (water treatment) is not a cure-all. But there is no single drug on the market that can rival water in the great variety of physiological effects it is capable of producing, its wide availability, lack of bad after effects, and relative economy.

Because giving successful treatments with the use of water requires time, effort, and labor, this method of treatment has lost favor in our modern society where "time is money" is more than just a saying; it is frequently also an economic necessity. It is much more convenient to simply take a pill, and disregard the possible ill effects that may be produced in the various systems of the body. The wonderful results that can be obtained from water treatments that are properly given, especially when they are combined with the other true remedies for man's ills — exercise, proper diet, pure air, sunlight, rest, and trust in divine power — cannot be obtained by any other method. Hydrotherapy rarely causes bad side effects or debilitating complications, as many drugs do. Water treatments do, however, take a longer time to produce results, but when the body reacts, it does so in a much more natural way. To give successful water treatments takes time and effort, but this is the price people must sometimes pay to restore and maintain good health. Some of these treatments are so effective, and yet so simple to use, that they should become a part of everyone's daily health program and not be reserved for use only in time of emergency or illness.

A.GENERAL RULES FOR WATER TREATMENTS

In order to obtain the best results, here are some General Rules that *must* be followed when any water treatment is given.

1. The room in which the treatment is given must be warm (70° to 75°F.), clean, and free of drafts.
2. A calm, restful atmosphere without distractions or bright lights should prevail.
3. All articles that are to be used during the treatment must be at hand before starting the treatment.
4. Know ahead of time exactly how the treatment is to be given.
5. Stay with the patient as much of the time as possible and watch for the effects of the treatment. Never go beyond calling distance.
6. Never argue with or irritate the patient by your talking. Be cheerful, express confidence, and converse on pleasant topics. Keep the patient relaxed.
7. Keep the patient covered and warm at all times and avoid chilling.
8. The patient must be warm before the treatment is started. Use a hot footbath beforehand, if necessary.
9. Be sure your hands are warm if it becomes necessary to touch the patient during the treatment.
10. During heat treatments, apply a cold compress on the patient's head when perspiration starts or the temperature reaches 100°F.
11. A cooling procedure should follow any heat treatment.
12. Make sure the patient is thoroughly dry after the treatment.
13. Following the treatment, the patient should be encouraged to relax and take a brief rest.
14. During the course of the treatment, let the patient know what you are doing; especially before using any cold application that may come as a shock.
15. Cold treatments are not tolerated well by infants and young children, aged persons, or those who are extremely weak or exhausted, and such treatments should not be used on these patients.

B. TEMPERATURES

Baths are divided into various classes, according to the water temperature, as follows.

1. Very cold . . . . . 32° to 55°F.
2. Cold . . . . 55° to 65°F.
3. Cool . . . . 65° to 80°F.
4. Tepid . . . . 80° to 92°F.
5. Warm . . . . 92° to 98°F.
6. Hot . . . . 98° to 104°F.
7. Very hot . . . . . 104°F. and above

C. RULES FOR BATHING

1. Never take a full bath within two hours after a meal. Local applications of water such as footbaths, fomentations, compresses, and even sitz baths may be used within a shorter period of time after eating.
2. When preparing baths for the sick, always use a thermometer, when available, to check the water temperature. The method used to test water for babies by placing the elbow in the water will sometimes help when a thermometer is not available.
3. The temperature of the room should be between 70° and 80°F. Patients or invalids may require it somewhat warmer. There should always be good ventilation, but no drafts.
4. Do not use either extremely hot or cold baths for very young, old, feeble, or extremely nervous patients. Although it is permissible to take a cold bath when you are just warm enough to start perspiring, never take a cold bath when you are extremely fatigued or exhausted. It is better to start with a tepid bath and gradually decrease the temperature until the water is cold.

5. Never allow more than three or four days at the most to pass without taking a warm cleansing bath. Take one daily if possible. A cold bath or shower in the morning is an excellent means of stimulating the whole nervous system, as well as preserving bodily cleanliness.

6. Bath attendants should carefully avoid giving a shock to nervous people, or those either afflicted with heart disease or who have had a stroke.

7. The best time for hydrotherapy (water) treatments is about three hours after breakfast.

8. Cold baths should not be taken during menstruation. A shower or warm sponge bath is best.

9. Always use the purest and softest water obtainable.

10. Baths should always be given at an agreeable temperature to sick persons, unless the baths are being used as a treatment to produce some particular effect.

11. If symptoms of faintness appear, apply cold to the head and face, give a drink of cold water, or lower the temperature of the bath by adding cool water.

12. As a precaution against catching a cold, always decrease the temperature of the bath just before finishing, if the person is not strong enough for a shower or cool sponge bath.

13. Cold baths should always be brief, unless given for a specific purpose to a local area of the body.

14. It is extremely important that the patient should be carefully and completely dried. Never leave a patient chilly. Rub him until he is warm.

15. Depending on the patient's condition, it is well to have a little light exercise shortly before bathing.

16 A short rest after bathing will add to its beneficial results. It is best to lie down and keep well covered.

Baths are one of the most powerful means of affecting the human system in either health or disease. Weak patients should have sponge baths, and if necessary these may be given in bed.

If the patient is susceptible to chilliness, sponge one portion of the body at a time, dry and cover that portion, then proceed to the next area.

D. TYPES OF BATHS

Relaxing Bath

This bath is excellent for nervous or agitated persons to help promote sleep and relaxation. It does this by balancing the circulation and relieving congestion in the brain. The temperature of the water should be from 94° to 97°F. It is sometimes best to have the water slightly warmer to begin with and let it cool slowly to the temperature just mentioned, but the patient should never feel chilled.

1. While in the water the patient should attempt to relax. There should be no noise, talking, radio or television.
2. Fill the tub about two-thirds full.
3. Place a folded towel for a headrest on the end of the tub.
4. The lights in the room should not glare in the patient's eyes.
5. A bath towel should be used to cover any part of the patient that is not immersed in the water.
6. Place a cool washcloth over the forehead and eyes.
7. Hot water should be added to maintain the proper temperature.
8. The length of the bath is usually about 30 minutes and never longer than one hour.
9. When finished, the water should be cooled a few degrees by the addition of cold water.
10. Pat the skin dry; do not rub.

Precautions:

Warm the room first to 70° or 75°F. in order to prevent chilling.

A bath thermometer should be used to check the water temperature.

If the patient is not warm, a hot footbath should be given first.

The patient should go to bed in a darkened room immediately afterwards and keep warm.

Tub Baths for Cleanliness

Full tub baths are the most beneficial and pleasant baths that can be taken. The full bath should be taken at least two or three times a week, but preferably every day. Thoroughly scrub the entire body with a coarse washcloth, using a good soap; Ivory is one of the best. This will open the pores and make the skin glands active so that poisons can be eliminated from the system. When this kind of bath is given in disease, good results will be obtained if the patient is rubbed thoroughly while in the water.

A hot tub bath is a specific aid against colds, if taken as soon as they are contracted, making sure that the person does not become exposed or chilled afterwards. For rheumatism, neuralgia, gout, colic, sciatica, or gallstones, the bath must be taken very hot so that the person perspires. Do not make the water hot to start with, but keep increasing the heat. For comfort and good results, when the person becomes too warm, have him stand up and shower off with cool water or rub his body with a towel that has been dipped in cool water. If the person has heart trouble, keep an ice bag over the heart. Keeping a cold compress on the head or around the neck will do much to avoid faintness.

For sick people, it is best to take the bath just before retiring. Baths have a tonic effect. The temperature must be determined by the attendant, and should be suited to the individual patient.

I have taken many cases where persons had been diagnosed by doctors as having heart trouble, and were told that it was dangerous to give them a hot bath. But I have given such persons warm tub baths freely, with beneficial results. Of course, when there is heart trouble, or palpitation of the heart, great care must be taken when beginning the bath not to have it too hot, and not to leave the patient in the tub too long.

Sitz Bath

The sitz bath is also known as the hip or half bath and is one of the most useful. A common washtub may be used, placing under one edge something that will elevate it three or four inches. Protect the skin from contact with the edge of the tub by placing folded towels under the knees and behind the back. A tub made especially for sitz baths has the back raised higher than the front to support the back, the sides slanting down to support the arms. A bathtub is probably the most convenient way for most people to take a sitz bath. The water should reach to the middle of the abdomen. The temperature should be suited both to the condition of the patient and the illness to be treated. The sitz bath acts as an analgesic and derivative. It markedly increases the blood flow.

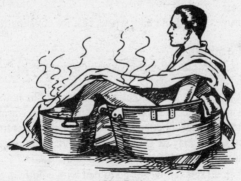

Sitz Bath

The hips and abdomen should be rubbed well by the attendant. The patient must be covered with a sheet or blanket during the bath, and several blankets must be used if sweating is desired. The feet should be placed in a hot footbath at 105° to 110°F. Apply cold compresses to the head when sweating starts and change them every 3 to 5 minutes. The temperature of the water in the footbath should always be higher than the temperature of the sitz bath. An ice bag should be placed over the heart if the pulse is over 80. Begin the bath at a temperature of 90° to 95°F. and increase the temperature to 100° to 110°F. When this temperature is reached, leave the patient in the bath for 5 to 10 minutes more for a tonic effect or 30 to 40 minutes for a regular treatment. Finish by cooling the water to 80° to 90°F. Then pour over the patient some cooler water at about 65° to 70°F. Dry the patient thoroughly, keep him warm and encourage rest for at least 30 minutes. The sitz bath is useful in prostatic diseases, piles, genital and urinary diseases and disorders, urinary retention, cystitis, hemorrhoids and fissures, following hemorrhoidectomy, chronic constipation, diarrhea, congestion in the abdominal or pelvic regions, sinusitis, colds, and headache. It is absolutely indispensable in uterine and many other diseases peculiar to women, such as painful menstruation, pelvic inflammatory disease, etc.

Sometimes a cold sitz bath works best for constipation.

Hot Footbath

This is a simple old-fashioned treatment that has many benefits.

1. It makes the patient feel warm all over. The hotter the water, the more the patient will perspire. A warm patient will react better to any other kind of heat treatment that may be given either with or following the hot footbath.
2. A good relaxer. Never go to bed with cold feet. Sleep comes more readily and you are better able to relax when your feet are warm.

3. Increases the circulation in the feet. Blood is drawn to the feet, relieving other congested organs located inside the body, such as the brain or pelvic organs. It is helpful in the treatment of headaches if used early and with a cold cloth on the forehead.

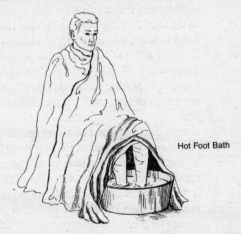

Hot Foot Bath

4. Makes sore feet feel better.
5. Helpful in easing the symptoms of the common cold.
6. Good for the relief of pelvic cramps, abdominal pain, prostatic problems, and menstrual cramps.

How to give a hot footbath:
1. The room should be warm and there should be no drafts. The patient should undress and keep completely covered with a sheet to stay warm.

2. Place both feet in the water. The temperature of the water should be about 100°F. to start with. The container needs to be large enough so that both feet can be placed side by side on the bottom. The water should come up well over the ankles, about halfway to the knees if possible.

3. If the patient is too weak to sit up, this bath can be given in bed.
4. Slowly add hot water as tolerated until the temperature is 115°F., but never hotter.
5. Always add the hot water to one side of the container, making sure that the feet are well protected and out of the way. Stir the water in the container with your hand as additional hot water is added.
6. Keep on with the treatment until the feet are pink. This usually takes from 15 to 30 minutes, but sometimes less. Adding about one tsp. of ground mustard per gallon of water will enhance the effects of the bath.
7. Keep a cold compress on the head and neck.
8. Following the treatment, the feet should be cooled off with cold water and then dried completely, being specially careful to dry well between the toes.
9. If the patient is sweating after the treatment, a cooling procedure such as a neutral shower or alcohol rub should be given.
10. See precautions under hot and cold footbath, following.

Leg Bath

This can be taken by sitting in a bathtub with the water covering the pelvic area. It is useful for chronic ulcers of the leg, swollen knees and ankles, varicose veins, and will also relieve headache and palpitation of the heart.

Alternating Hot and Cold Footbath (Contrast Bath)

This is a very useful remedy for chilblains (mild frostbite of the fingers, toes, or ears) and cold feet. The hot water temperature should range from 100° to 115°F. The cold water should be either cold tap water or ice water. Keep the feet and legs in the hot water for three minutes and in the cold water for not more than one minute. Alternating hot and cold will produce a powerful reaction. The feet should always be rubbed while in the bath. The footbath is most useful in neuralgia, headache, toothache, colds, cold feet, and congestion of the abdominal and pelvic organs (look also under Hot and Cold Contrast Bath, following).

Precautions:

1. The water temperature must be measured accurately with a thermometer.
2. Do not use water hotter than 115°F.
3. Do not leave the patient unattended.
4. Do not use hot water on the feet of diabetics or others with poor circulation, such as in hardening of the arteries, frostbite, etc.
5. Do not end with cold water if the patient is menstruating.

Hot and Cold Contrast Bath

This is one of the easiest and yet most effective water treatments that you can use in your home. The alternating hot and cold dilates and contracts the blood vessels, bringing a supply of fresh new blood to the area being treated. The blood cells that fight infection, the white blood cells, are increased in number and activity and waste products that have collected in the tissues are removed. The healing processes are stimulated and the body is more rapidly restored to a normal condition.

Infections, sprains, strains, bruises, and arthritis are some of the more common conditions that are greatly benefitted by this bath. Contrast baths are used to treat the hands, wrists, feet and ankles and can also be used for the elbows and knees if the container is large enough.

General rules for a contrast bath are as follows.

1. Always use a bath thermometer to check the water temperature.
2. Always treat a larger area than is injured. For example, a sprained ankle should have the water nearly up to the knee.
3. Always start with the hot water and end with the cold, except when treating arthritis, or if the patient is menstruating, or if massage of the part is to follow the treatment. If any of these three situations exist, the hot water should be used last.

How to give a contrast bath:
1. Place the area to be treated in hot water at about 105°F. and leave for 3 minutes.
2. Move the extremity to the ice water for 30 seconds. While it is in the ice water, add hot water to the first tub to increase the temperature to about 110°F.
3. Make eight complete changes, leaving the extremity 3 minutes in the hot water and 30 seconds in the ice water. This will take a total time of about 30 minutes.
4. Keep adding ice and hot water as needed to maintain the proper water temperatures in the two tubs.
5. After the final cold or hot treatment, dry the part thoroughly.
6. This treatment may be given once or twice daily.

Precautions:
1. In acute sprains or strains, it is best to use only cold treatments for the first 24 to 48 hours. After this period, the contrast bath may be used with benefit.
2. Those who have poor circulation due to diabetes or hardening of the arteries should use this bath with care and the water should not be over 105°F.
3. In cases of arthritis the water temperature can be in-

creased to 115° to 120°F. if the patient can tolerate it and the circulation is good.

4. Keep cold compresses on the forehead and neck. These should be changed every 3 or 4 minutes.
5. Check the pulse before starting the treatment and every 5 to 10 minutes thereafter. If the pulse increases or is over 80 beats per minute, place an ice bag over the heart.
6. Cool the patient with an alcohol rub if there is general sweating.
7. Clean and disinfect the containers thoroughly after each treatment, specially if an infection is present.

Emollient and Other Medicated Baths

These baths are very good for treating general skin rashes, specially those that cause itching or burning of the skin, such as poison oak or ivy, allergic reactions, and eczema or local reactions from insect bites. The medications commonly used are oatmeal, cornstarch, and soda, as given in the sections following.

Some general principles for taking a medicated bath are the following.

1. Maintain the temperature of the water in the neutral range of 93° to 98°F. and never warmer than 100°F. or the itching may be increased.
2. Fill the bathtub so that the water will cover as much of the body as possible.
3. Remain in the tub for 10 to 30 minutes.
4. When the bath is completed, pat dry; do not rub. This will tend to leave a thin coating of the agent used on the skin, as well as protecting the sensitive skin from further irritation by rubbing.

Oatmeal Bath

Place three cups of oatmeal in a cheesecloth or coarse

muslin bag. Place it in the tub filled with water. A better way yet is to let very hot water run over the oatmeal bag and into the tub. Then squeeze the bag into the tub. The bag may also be used as a sponge to wash the neck and shoulders. Aveeno, a finely ground oatmeal, is available from some drug stores and makes the bath much easier to do. Place two cups of the Aveeno in a cheesecloth bag and let it soak a short while in hot water; then add it to the bath. This will stop it from getting lumpy, which it may do if it is added directly to the bath water.

Starch Bath

Put one pound of cornstarch in a full tub of water, or you may first mix the starch with enough cold water to make a paste and then add hot water and boil until it is thick.

This mixture may then be added to the bath water. The oatmeal bath is less drying than the starch bath.

Soda Bath

Dissolve one pound (16 ounces) of sodium bicarbonate (soda) in a full tub of water. A mixture of 8 ounces of soda and 8 ounces of starch may be used.

Paraffin Bath

This is an excellent treatment to relieve pain in the hands and wrists. It may also be used for the elbows, feet, or ankles, provided that the container is large enough. The paraffin forms a coating on the skin that prevents the loss of heat; therefore, the temperature of the skin can be increased far more than with the use of just plain water. The penetrating heat produced by the paraffin promotes healing and leaves the skin soft and pliable.

It is specially useful in arthritis and can also be used in bursitis, injury resulting in sprains or strains, and painful joints from other causes such as gout.

To give this treatment you will need a double boiler to melt the paraffin, a bath thermometer, about five pounds of paraffin and one pint of mineral oil.

Place the paraffin and mineral oil in the top of the double boiler and heat until the wax is melted. Then let it cool until a thin film forms on top or it reaches about 125°F. The hands must be clean and dry. Dip the hands and wrists in and withdraw them rapidly, keeping the fingers apart. Do this a few more times until there is a good coating of paraffin on the hands. Then place the hands in the paraffin and leave them there for about 15 to 30 minutes. After the treatment is completed all the paraffin should be peeled from the hands and saved in a closed container. This treatment can be given with benefit every day. It is best to follow with a warm bath or shower and a rest period of about 30 minutes.

Occasionally you may treat a patient whose skin is sensitive to the paraffin, and of course this treatment should not be used for them. Those with skin infections, or conditions resulting in poor blood supply or lack of feeling in the hands or other part to be treated, likewise should not use this treatment.

Eyebath

Water and other solutions may be applied to the eyes in many different ways. A brief treatment can be conveniently given by placing the solution in the cup of the hand, holding it over the eye and blinking, thus bringing the eye directly in contact with the solution. Small glass cups are also made for holding the solution. The solution should be changed frequently.

In any treatment to the eyes, it is essential to learn first the difficulty and the cause, then apply the best thing to remove the cause.

When the membranes that line the eyelid and cover the eyeball become inflamed or there is inflammation of the external structures, cold or cool applications are required. Inflammation of the cornea or iris (the colored membrane behind the cornea) requires hot applications. Compresses made of two or three thicknesses of linen should be used, and changed every five minutes. Cool applications are excellent made in this way. Fomentations are the best method of applying heat. They should be as hot as can be borne. If they give relief, continue for a half hour or more; BUT IF THEY INCREASE THE PAIN, STOP IMMEDIATELY.

Alternate hot and cold applications will give relief in most cases. Leave the hot application on the longest, applying the cool for only a few minutes.

An eyebath using pure cold and hot water is infinitely superior to the patent eyewashes on the market.

An excellent eyewash is made by steeping one teaspoon of golden seal, two heaping teaspoons of boric acid powder, and a half-teaspoon of myrrh in a pint of boiling water. Strain when cool.

Daily eyebaths of tepid water will benefit those who must use their eyes a great deal in working, or who read a great deal. Many people ruin their eyes by neglecting to give them proper care and rest.

Ear Bath

Applications may be made to the ears by using fomentations, compresses, douches, sprays, or poultices. Fomentations and compresses are useful in inflammation of the ear and will restore the hearing in many cases.

Syringing the ear should not be practiced, as it often results in irreparable injury.

The douche is a valuable means of removing foreign substances and insects. Warm water douches at 100°F. are good to remove hardened earwax, and thus restore the hearing. When taking a douche, lean the head over a basin, so that the water can freely run in and out of the ear.

Nose Bath

Close the mouth when drawing any liquid substance into the nose, or when injecting it by means of a fountain syringe. Always apply gently; violent applications often cause great pain and irritation. Never give injections with a piston syringe, as this often forces the substance into the Eustachian tubes and may result in deafness. As a rule, the temperature of nose baths should be tepid or warm.

Turkish Bath

Turkish baths are usually given in a special cabinet and are used to produce fever and profuse perspiration. They are essentially the same thing as our present-day sauna bath. Drink plenty of water before, during, and after the bath to make up for that which is lost by perspiration. The chief agent is hot air. The temperature varies from 105° to 140°F. There are usually unpleasant sensations, but as soon as the patient begins to perspire, these disappear.

After the patient has perspired thoroughly, he is taken to a room at about 90° to 100°F. where the attendant thoroughly rubs and massages the body to remove all of the dead skin, after which the whole body is thoroughly lathered and rubbed, either with the hand or a brush. A shower is given, and then the patient is immersed in a tub of cool water or a spray may be all that is necessary. The patient is then dried, wrapped in a sheet (a blanket sometimes being necessary), and lies down in a room where the temperature is 70° or 80°F.

Besides producing profuse perspiration, the Turkish bath wonderfully stimulates elimination. It is a king of remedies in acute or chronic rheumatism, jaundice, malaria, syphilis, obesity, dropsy, gout, skin disease, eczema, and hydrophobia (rabies). It will break up fevers, typhoid, etc.

The Roman bath is quite similar to the Turkish, with the exception that after the patient has been dried, he is thoroughly rubbed with some sweet oil. This is excellent for persons who are susceptible to colds.

How to give a Turkish bath without a cabinet

Use a common No. 3 washtub. Tilt the tub up by placing a two-by-four or some other kind of strong prop under one edge. Fill the tub with hot water and also fill a large pan with hot water for the feet. Place a folded blanket over the edge of the tub. Place the patient in the tub with his back against the blanket and his feet in the pan of hot water. Cover him well with a sheet, which should be fastened snugly around the neck. As the water cools, take some out and add hot water, being careful not to burn the patient. Keep this up until the patient perspires profusely. Give him plenty of water to drink and wipe the forehead with a cool cloth. This is preferable to a pack if the patient can be moved.

Electric Light Bath

This bath uses simple artificial light. The advantage is that the patient is not subjected to a hot atmosphere, yet it produces profuse perspiration. It is a fine tonic, and is good to use when it is desired to increase the activity of the skin. It is usually used along with some form of hydrotherapy, and since it requires a special electric light cabinet, this treatment is given in a hydrotherapy treatment room by trained personnel.

The patient sits in the light cabinet at a temperature of 125° to 130°F. for 10 to 20 minutes with the head protruding from a hole in the top. This causes profuse sweating, a slight increase in temperature to 101° to 102°, dilatation of the blood vessels, and a decrease in the blood pressure. As soon as sweating begins, a cold cloth should be applied to the face. It is good for the treatment of obesity, some types of kidney disease, neuroses, arthritis, neuritis, hypertension, and symptoms of drug, tobacco, or alcohol withdrawal. It should not be used for those with diabetes, tuberculosis, hyperthyroidism, for severely weakened patients, or persons with heart trouble or hardening of the arteries.

E.   A PERSONAL WATER TREATMENT

One of my favorite personal water treatments is the douche spray. The operator stands ten or fifteen feet away, if we have the room, and the stream of water is turned on with a force strong enough so it will hurt just slightly.

To begin with, the water should be a little warmer than the

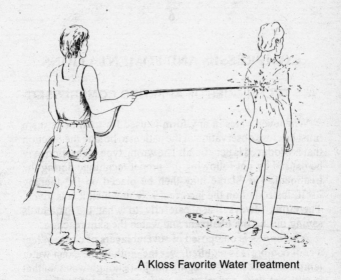

A Kloss Favorite Water Treatment

temperature of the body or as warm as I can comfortably stand it and have the operator start by directing the spray to the back of my head and then spray up and down my spine, clear down to my feet. Then I keep turning and he sprays the side of my neck and face clear around, up and down; and I keep turning around and around and let him spray right in my face.

Then I turn my head down so that the spray will hit on the top and all over the head, and keep turning until I am well warmed up.

Then I have the operator turn the water a little cooler than the body temperature, and start spraying the back of the head again, as well as up and down the spine clear to the feet.

I keep turning around so the water strikes every part of my body. I even hold each foot up so the spray strikes the bottom of the feet and keep turning until the cooler water sprays my entire body.

We keep this up for ten or fifteen minutes. I enjoy this treatment very much.

6

COMPRESSES AND FOMENTATIONS

A. TECHNIQUES OF APPLYING COMPRESSES

Whenever water in any form is used for treatment, there must be close observation of the patient to be sure the reaction that is produced is beneficial. The wrong type of reaction may be caused by not following the proper technique during the treatment. The blame may then be placed on the therapy itself, instead of on the incorrect way in which it was given. Therefore, always listen carefully to what the patient is saying during the treatment and watch the skin reaction.

A compress is composed of several layers of cloth. When a cool compress is required, wet the cloth in the exact water temperature desired, wringing out just enough water so that it will not drip, and place it upon the affected body part. Change the compress every five minutes.

A cold compress is prepared by placing crushed ice between the layers of cloth. This, of course, does not need to be renewed so frequently.

In applying compresses to delicate parts of the body, great care should be taken not to injure the part. A very thin compress should be used in such cases.

The effects of a compress are very similar to those of a poultice.

The wet girdle, leg pack, wet sheet pack, chest pack and wrapper, and half-pack are simply large compresses.

Heating Compress

A heating compress actually feels cold when it is first applied, but after only a short time it starts to heat up as the body reacts against the cold. Such a compress, when applied to the throat, is very good for the treatment of sore throat, tonsillitis, laryngitis, whooping cough, croup, and colds.

1. Use a strip of thin cotton cloth long enough to wrap around the neck four times, or you may use two thicknesses and wrap them around the neck twice. They should be wide enough to cover the entire neck and also should be pulled up well under the ears; usually three or four inches wide is enough.

2. You will also need a strip of flannel or wool cloth to use as a covering and long enough to wrap around the neck twice. It should be about an inch or two wider than the cotton.

3. Cut a piece of plastic, from a disposable trash bag, long enough to go around the neck once and about one-half inch wider than the cotton.

The following steps should be performed to give a heating compress to the throat:

1. Dip the cotton cloth in cold water and wring it out until it no longer drips.

2. Wrap it around the neck, making it fit as close to the skin as possible. It is very important that there are no air pockets or wrinkles. Cover it completely with the piece of plastic.

3. Cover this with the flannel or woolen strip. Be sure that all of the moist cotton cloth is covered. Tighten the cover snugly but not so much that it is uncomfortable for the patient. Pin it securely in place.

4. Leave the compress in place overnight. It should be dry when removed in the morning.

The compress will draw blood to the skin surface that will warm and dry the cotton; and as a result, congestion of the structures deeper in the neck will be relieved.

5. After the compress is removed, rub the neck with a cool cloth and dry thoroughly to prevent chilling.

6. If the patient's circulation is poor, and the cold cotton cloth will not warm up, wring the cloth out of hot water instead and use it in the same way.

The same type of compress may be applied to the abdomen. It is useful in constipation, indigestion, and helps to promote sleep. You will need the same items as for the throat compress, but the cotton strip should be two thicknesses, 8 to 10 inches wide, and long enough to wrap around the abdomen one and a half times, overlapping in the front. The flannel or woolen binder will need to be about 12 inches wide and the same length as the cotton or slightly longer. A strip of plastic 12 inches wide and long enough to wrap around the body once can be used between the cotton and flannel to make the effect of the compress last longer. As noted earlier, a piece of plastic of the proper size cut from a disposable trash bag may be used.

How to give a heating compress to the abdomen:
1. Spread the strip of flannel on the bed so that when the patient lies down on it, it can be folded over the abdomen.
2. If plastic is to be used, it should be spread on the flannel.
3. Wring the cotton out of cold water (or hot, as noted under throat compress) and place it on the flannel (or plastic). Be sure all the wrinkles are smoothed out.
4. Have the patient lie on the compress on his back and fold the layers over the abdomen, the cotton layer first, so that it overlaps on the front of the abdomen. Smooth each layer and remove all air pockets.
5. Cover completely and snugly with the plastic and/or flannel and pin securely in place. Air must not get to the moist cotton or the heating effect will be spoiled.
6. Remove the compress in the morning, rub the skin with a cold cloth, and then dry thoroughly.
7. If the cotton does not heat up as it should, try putting a hot water bottle on the compress for a short time.

Check to make sure that the flannel is snug and that it is completely covering the cotton. If neither of these suggestions seems to help, it may be necessary to apply the cotton compress only over the abdomen and not wrap it completely around the body. If the patient feels chilly during the wet compress treatment, it is usually because air is getting to the moist cotton.

B. FOMENTATIONS

Fomentations are local applications of moist heat and are used to relieve pain and muscle spasm and also to increase the circulation. They may be used with benefit in such conditions as arthritis, colds, influenza, bursitis, sprains, strains, muscle, joint and nerve pain, gout, and infection, to name only a few.

The fomentation cloths can be made of half cotton and half wool or synthetic fabric, or a thick flannel may also be used. Each piece should be about three feet square and folded three times so that the final fomentation pad is three layers thick and about one by three feet in size.

Have all of the following materials ready before starting the treatment:

1. Three fomentation pads, folded and ready to use.
2. Three covers to wrap around the fomentations, made of the same material and about the same size.
3. A pan of ice water and two wash cloths.
4. At least four large Turkish towels.
5. A sheet or blanket to cover the patient.
6. A large pan or other container of boiling water.
7. A large piece of plastic or a rubber sheet to protect the bed.

How to give fomentation treatments:
1. Place a fomentation pad lengthwise on the bed so that

when the patient lies down the pad will be along the spine. Cover it with several layers of towel so it will not burn. The patient should be warm and comfortable, lying on the spinal fomentation and covered with a sheet or blanket. The feet should be in a pan of hot water at 105° to 110°F. Be sure to keep this water in the footbath hot during the treatment.

2. Cover the area to be treated with two of the towels for the first fomentation and with one towel thereafter.

3. Twist one of the folded fomentations slightly and dip it into the boiling water (Fig. 1) until it is thoroughly soaked, leaving four or five inches of each end out of the water. Wring out the fomentation (Fig. 2) as dry as possible by grasping each end and twisting in opposite directions. Pulling on the fomentation by each end and stretching it as much as possible will help get more of the water out. The wetter the fomentation the hotter it will feel to the patient.

4. Untwist it, wrap it quickly in a fomentation cover, (Fig. 3 and Fig. 4) and place it on the towels that you have already positioned on the patient. Cover the fomentation with a towel. (See also Figs. 5 and 6.)

5. Be certain not to burn any protruding bones or sensitive areas. Additional protection may be needed over such areas.

6. If the fomentation starts to burn the patient, raise it briefly and rub the skin with your hand to remove the moisture. As soon as the fomentation starts to cool, usually in three to five minutes, remove it, dry the skin well with a dry towel, and replace the fomentation with a fresh one. Have the new fomentation all ready to use as soon as the cooler one is

HOW TO MAKE A FOMENTATION

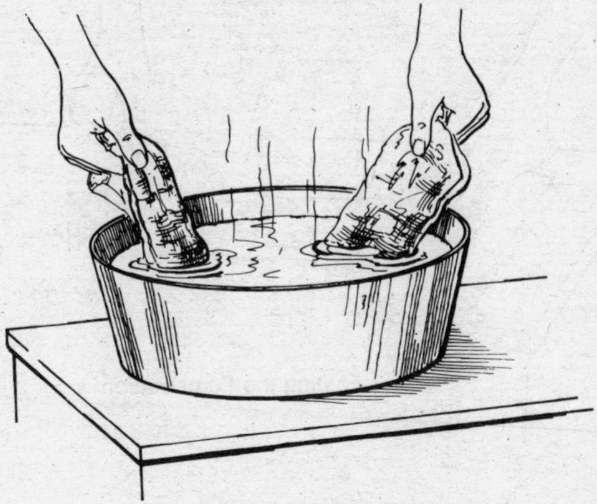

Fig. 1 Heating the Fomentation

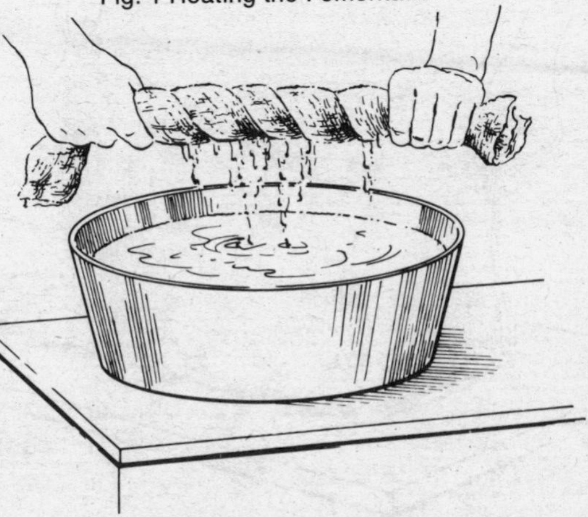

Fig. 2 Wringing the Fomentation.

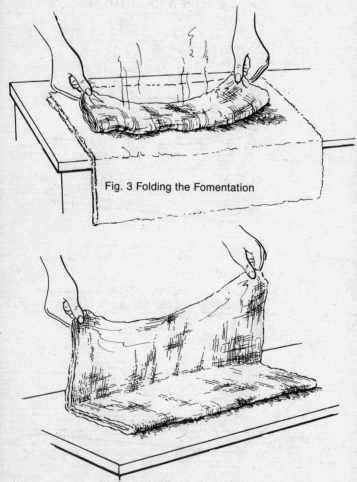

Fig. 3 Folding the Fomentation

Fig. 4 Wrapping the Fomentation

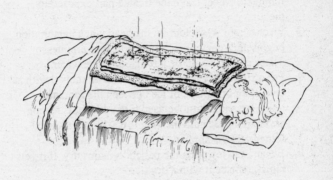

Fig. 5 Fomentation to Spine

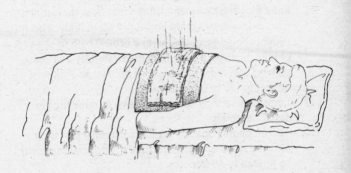

Fig. 6 Fomentation to Upper Abdomen

removed. Never leave the treated part exposed to the air.

7. Place a cold washcloth on the head when perspiration begins and renew it every three to four minutes. These cloths should be wrung out of ice water.

8. For a stronger reaction, the skin can be rubbed with a cold cloth or a piece of ice between the fomentations. Ice should not be used if the patient is having severe pain. Be sure the skin is dry before the next fomentation is applied.

9. Be sure the towel on the patient remains dry. If it gets moist, replace it with a dry one.

10. Usually a total of three fomentations is enough, drying the skin rapidly and thoroughly between each one. After the last fomentation is removed, wipe the skin with a cold cloth and dry thoroughly.

11. Following the treatment, lift the feet from the hot tub, pour cold water over them and dry thoroughly. The patient should be cooled with a neutral bath or shower or with an alcohol rub; then dried carefully and completely; covered with a sheet or blanket and allowed to rest for 30 to 60 minutes.

12. Fomentations may be repeated two or three times a day if necessary.

13. Thermophore pads are available that also provide a moist heat treatment. Their time of application should be limited to 30 minutes.

Fomentations relieve internal congestion by drawing the blood to the skin surface. Very hot applications should be used to relieve pain; hot, short applications (three to five minutes) alternating with cold should be used if a tonic or stimulating effect is desired; five to ten minute treatments with milder heat should be used to produce relaxation.

In addition to those conditions listed earlier in this section, fomentations may also be employed in acute inflammations, local pains, chest congestion, neuralgia, toothache, pleurisy, muscle spasm, to help produce sleep, to increase circulation, and to help eliminate toxins by causing sweating.

The following precautions should be observed when giving fomentations.

Do not use fomentations on unconscious patients, or on the legs and feet of diabetics, or on any part of the body with a lack of feeling or poor blood supply. Use with caution in weak or elderly patients, in children, and in patients who are drowsy or semiconscious. Do not give fomentations to the abdomen on anyone suspected of having acute appendicitis. Fomentations draw blood to the area being treated, so they should not be used if bleeding is present or suspected. Place an ice pack over the heart for patients with a weak heart. Keep the patient well-covered at all times and protected from drafts. Do not leave the patient unattended. Have the patient drink some water at about body temperature during the treatment.

C. HOW TO GIVE A BLANKET PACK

If possible, have two part-wool double blankets and one part-wool single blanket. You will also need a large tub or kettle of boiling water and also a small basin of very cold water (ice water is preferable), to be used in making compresses for the patient's head.

Give a hot footbath while the blanket pack is being prepared. If the patient is able to sit up, have him sit by the bed to have the footbath. If he cannot sit up, have him lie on his back to one side of the bed with his feet in hot water. It is well to give a hot herb tea at this time, such as yarrow, boneset, sage, or catnip, to aid in producing perspiration. Keep the patient covered with a sheet.

Place first a double blanket and then the single blanket on the bed: these are to be wrapped over the wet pack. Take the other double blanket and fold the two longer edges over until they almost meet in the center, then fold one side over the other. This will form a long strip four layers thick, the full length of the blanket. Place the folded blanket in the boiling water and thoroughly saturate it. Do this carefully, so as not to disturb the folds. Leave about ten inches of each end of the blanket out of the water, so that two people can take hold of the ends and twist and pull the blanket in opposite directions, until all the water possible is wrung out. After the blanket has been wrung out, open it and quickly place it on the bed on the single blanket. Remove the footbath. Place the patient on the hot blanket as quickly as possible, as it cools rapidly when opened. Wrap the patient first in the hot wet blanket, then the dry single blanket, and then the dry double blanket. Be sure the feet are well wrapped and warm, and the dry blanket securely wrapped over the wet one. Wrap the blanket so the arms are next to the blanket and not the body.

D. ALCOHOL RUB

An alcohol rub is usually given as a cooling procedure, either after a heating treatment of some kind has been given or to reduce the body temperature in patients with a fever. Sometimes it is used as a tonic.

Rubbing alcohol should be used if it is available, but pure grain alcohol (95 percent) may be used if it is diluted with water, two parts of alcohol to one part of water.

The patient should be kept covered with a sheet, exposing only the part to be rubbed.

Do not pour the alcohol directly onto the patient. Put some in your cupped hand, rub your two hands together and then apply it to the patient's arm, starting with the hand and applying the alcohol up to the shoulder in one stroke. Bring the hands back down the arm, rotating them as you do so that the entire arm is moistened. Stroke rapidly and lightly, using both your hands and be sure that all the alcohol has evaporated and the skin is dry before proceeding to the next part.

After the first arm is finished, cover it with the sheet and proceed to the opposite arm, treating it in the same way. Then rub the chest, legs, abdomen, and back, always using short brisk strokes to hasten the evaporation.

Leave the patient completely dry and comfortable.

Do not apply alcohol on open sores or on irritated skin and do not use on infants or very young children.

E.   ICE PACK

The ice pack is very useful in treating acute sprains, acute bursitis, acute joint inflammation, and bruises. It should be applied as soon after the injury as possible. It contracts the blood vessels, keeps the swelling to a minimum, and relieves pain. The moist cold of an ice pack or compress is of more benefit than the dry cold produced by an ice bag or ice cap, and the ice pack fits more snugly around the joint.

How to use an ice pack:

1. Cover the skin area to be treated with a flannel cloth. Never place ice directly on the skin.
2. Place a layer of crushed ice about one inch thick on a towel or piece of flannel big enough to cover the area completely. Cover this with a second towel and pin in place.
3. Now place the ice pack over the painful area.
4. Pin a piece of plastic or rubber sheet over the compress. Be sure the bed is protected if the treatment is to be given in bed.
5. Leave the pack on for 30 minutes and keep the limb elevated. After the ice pack is removed, dry the skin and keep the area covered with a dry towel or piece of flannel.
6. Repeat this treatment every two hours for a total of 8 to 12 hours or longer if necessary.

7. Make sure that the skin does not freeze.
8. In acute joint sprains, this treatment can be continued for one or two days and then alternate hot and cold may be used, as previously described.
9. If ice is not available, the injured part can be placed in ice water or cold tap water for 30 minutes. This can be repeated every two hours for eight to twelve hours or longer if necessary.

F.   ICE BAG OR ICE CAP

The ice bag is very useful whenever cold treatment is indicated. It should not be left on for longer than 15 or 20 minutes at a time, however. Some of its most common uses are for acute sprains and strains, on the back of the neck for nosebleed and headache, over the heart for palpitation when taking heat treatments, on insect bites and stings, for itching hemorrhoids, and many other conditions.

1. Fill the ice bag about half full with small pieces of ice.
2. Flatten the bag out on a flat surface to remove as much of the air as possible, and then put on the cap.
3. Wrap a thin towel around the bag.
4. Place a piece of plastic or rubber sheeting on the bed for protection.
5. Leave on for 20 or 30 minutes.
6. Remove for the same length of time, keeping the area covered, and then replace the ice bag. This may be continued for 8 to 12 hours as indicated.

G.   COLD MITTEN FRICTION

This is an excellent tonic for the body in the morning and it will greatly improve the general circulation. People who have poor circulation are much more likely to get sick with colds and more serious illnesses than those who have good blood flow to all parts of the body. As people grow older the circulation tends to slow down and the blood vessels become less pliable. This tonic friction bath can be used by nearly anyone. It is simple to learn, requires no expensive equipment, and will certainly improve your health and sense of well-being as well as your general resistance to disease.

Short cold applications or heat treatments followed by cold tend to make the chemical reaction of the blood more alkaline, due to the oxidation of waste products. The blood normally has an alkaline reaction, but during infections, fevers, etc., this alkalinity is reduced and the blood shifts towards an acid reaction, although blood never actually becomes acidic in its reaction. There is also a moderate increase in the number of red blood cells in the circulation as well as an increase in the hemoglobin and a marked rise in the number of white blood cells that fight infection. Not only is there an increase in the number of white corpuscles, but they also become much more active in fighting disease. The effect of a cold treatment lasts about one to three hours and while one treatment cannot be expected to produce a marked or lasting effect, frequent cold treatments, specially with added friction, will produce a permanent and decided improvement in the circulation and an increase in the blood corpuscles and hemoglobin. "Most persons would receive benefit from a cool or tepid bath every day, morning or evening. Instead of the liability to take cold, a bath, properly taken, fortifies against cold, because it improves the circulation; the blood is brought to the surface, and a more easy and regular flow is obtained. The mind and the body are alike invigorated." (*Ministry of Healing,* p.276.)

How to take a cold mitten friction:
1. As always, have the room warm and free of drafts.
2. Fill the washbasin or other container with tepid water at about 85° to 95°F.
3. If you do not have a regular friction mitt and do not wish to purchase one, select a rough washcloth, dip it in the water, and ring it nearly dry.

4. In order to build up a tolerance, you should start gradually. On the first morning rub only one arm from the wrist to the shoulder. Keep rubbing rapidly and vigorously until the skin turns pink and has a tingling sensation.

5. Stop and dry the arm thoroughly with a warm towel.

6. The second morning, rub both arms till pink, first one and then the other, drying each one when completed.

7. On subsequent days add the chest, abdomen, right and left legs, and back. It helps to have someone else rub your back, as rubbing this area vigorously can be quite awkward and tiring.

8. Each day you should make the water a little cooler until you are finally able to use ice water without feeling chilly. The cloth can be a little wetter, but never dripping, if a more vigorous reaction is desired.

9. Eventually you should be able to complete the entire friction bath in under 10 minutes.

10. When giving the treatment to another person, start with one arm until you have produced a good reaction, dry well and do the other arm; then the chest, abdomen, legs, and back. Keep all parts of the body that are not being treated well covered.

Precautions:

1. If at first you get unduly tired from the rubbing, stay on the same part for several days and add other areas of the body at a slower rate. Rest if you need to, but don't give up until you can complete the entire body.

2. Aged or very weak or ill persons may find this treatment too exhausting or they may not be able to obtain a good skin reaction; if that is the case, the cold mitten friction should not be used.

3. Be sure to continue rubbing each area until the skin is pink.

H.   SEDATIVE TREATMENT

This treatment is given to relieve stress and tension:
1. Warm the feet with a hot footbath. If the patient is a diabetic or has poor circulation, wrap the feet in a warm blanket.
2. Use fomentations. (See B. Fomentations, earlier in this chapter for complete directions for making a fomentation.) The fomentations that are used in the sedative treatment should be allowed to cool slightly before being placed on the patient. They should not be used while extremely hot.
3. Have the patient lie on one fomentation that extends the full length of the spine and place a second one across the abdomen.
4. Apply cold compresses to the head and neck, and change them every two or three minutes.
5. As soon as the fomentation begins to cool, remove it, dry the skin, and apply a fresh one. Change the long fomentation on the spine first. Do not rub the skin with ice between fomentations.
6. Change the fomentations three times.
7. Then cool the patient with an alcohol rub or a warm bath or shower.
8. Dry the patient thoroughly, make him comfortable and warm, and encourage rest and sleep.

I.   ARTHRITIS TREATMENT

Alternate hot and cold treatments are many times very helpful in relieving the pain of arthritis. This treatment is mainly for arthritis in the hands, wrists, or feet. The treatment is simple to give and only minimal equipment is needed. You should have two containers large enough to accommodate hands or feet. One of the containers should be filled with hot water at 105° to 110°F. and the other should contain cold water at 60° to 70°F. This is about the temperature of water that comes from the cold water faucet.

1. There should be enough water in the container to reach nearly to the elbows or knees.
2. Use a bath thermometer to determine the water temperature.
3. The extremity should be placed first in the hot water for three minutes and then in the cold water for 30 seconds.
4. Seven complete changes should be made, ending with the hot water.
5. This can be done two or three times a day.
6. If the hot water causes increased swelling, the temperature can be decreased to 105°F. or the time in the hot water can be reduced to two minutes and the time in the cold water increased to one minute.
7. If there is poor circulation, the hot water should never be more than 105°F.
8. For extremely painful joints, an ice pack can be used until the swelling subsides and then the alternate hot and cold treatments may be used.

Many people with arthritis will obtain more relief from the paraffin bath described in Chapter 5, part D, Types of Baths.

J. HEADACHE TREATMENT

Most headaches are caused by stress, muscle tension, dilated blood vessels in the head, or a combination of these. In only one person out of several hundred are headaches likely to be caused by a life-threatening illness such as a brain tumor. The next time you have a headache while at home, try the following program. Better yet, for greater success with this treatment start it as soon as you feel a headache coming on.

1. Warm the bathroom to between 70° and 80°F.
2. Undress and take a hot footbath, as described earlier (in Chapter 5). For this treatment it is best to sit on the edge of the bathtub and fill the tub with hot water over your ankles. Start with water at 105° and increase as tolerated to not more than 115°F.
3. Keep yourself warm by wrapping in a sheet.
4. Have a pan of ice water handy. Dip a washcloth in the ice water, wring it out well and place it over your forehead and eyes. Change the washcloth every two or three minutes.
5. Rub the back of your neck to relax the muscles. Slowly rotate your head in a circle once or twice, relaxing the muscles as much as possible, and then apply a cold cloth to the back of the neck.
6. When your feet have become nice and pink, fill the tub with water at 80° to 95°F. Then get in the tub, place a folded towel behind your head, lean back, and soak for 15 to 20 minutes. Keep the cool cloth over your forehead and eyes.
7. Dry thoroughly. Blot the skin. Do not rub.
8. As soon as you are dry get right into a warm bed. Have the room darkened, with no noises to disturb you. You may even take the phone off the hook if you dare. Close your eyes, relax, and try to remove all irritating, stressful, and unpleasant thoughts from your mind.

K. SALT GLOW

The salt glow is a vigorous peripheral circulatory stimulant and a general tonic. It increases the resistance to disease of all kinds, removes dead skin, and opens and cleans out the pores. Patients obtain a reaction to the salt glow easier than to a cold mitten friction.

Wet two pounds of common coarse salt with water, just enough so that it sticks together. Have the patient stand or sit in the shower or bathtub with the feet ankle deep in a pan of water at 105°F. Keep the patient well covered except for the part that is to be treated. Begin by wetting one arm. Fill your hands with the moist salt, place your hands on each side of the patient's arm and rub up and down the arm vigorously with to-and-fro movements until the skin is aglow. Follow the same procedure with the opposite arm, legs, chest, back, and buttocks. Omit the abdomen if you wish. Use a lighter pressure over bony prominences and sensitive areas. After completion, remove all the salt with a tepid shower or pail pour. Dry thoroughly and have the patient lie down, cover with a sheet or blanket, and encourage rest for a short time.

A salt glow should not be given if skin disease is present.

Section IX
Skills in Caring
for the Sick

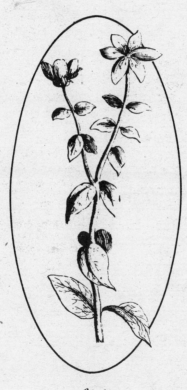

*Stinking
S.ᵗ John's Wort*

1

NURSING

A. CHARACTERISTICS OF A TRUE NURSE

1. Faithful, intelligent, and efficient care of the sick is often responsible in a large measure for recovery.

2. Consideration and kindness characterize a nurse. Irritability, thoughtlessness, and inconsiderate acts are inexcusable. Nurses must be kind in thought, word, and deed.

3. Cheerfulness — a bright and sunny disposition — brings life, hope, and cheer into the sickroom. The sickroom is not a place for a gloomy, morbid nurse.

4. Unselfish, untiring devotion to the interests of the patient is required of a nurse. She or he should be willing to sacrifice herself in behalf of her patient, disregarding personal comfort and convenience.

5. Anyone who is upset by trivial circumstances or who is excitable in trying times should not be a nurse. Good judgment and calmness will tend to inspire confidence in her intelligence.

6. A nurse must always be patient. People who are ordinarily thoughtful and considerate frequently are extremely unreasonable when sick, and demand attention, often unnecessarily. A nurse should always be firm, to secure compliance with her instructions.

7. A nurse should be able to divert the patient's mind from undesirable and depressing thoughts without being obvious about it. She should be discreet and impersonal in her conversations. Reading to the patient is excellent and should be done whenever per-

missible. Avoid any exciting, tiresome, or objectionable topic, either in reading or in conversation. Regulate the matter of visitors without giving offense. Good sound common sense is needed at all times.

8. A nurse should observe changes in the condition of the patient. She must observe anything that is giving discomfort to the patient and change it, if possible; as many times the patient will not say anything for fear of annoying the nurse too often.

9. Physical soundness is most essential in a nurse — good hearing, good vision, and a good sense of smell.

10. A nurse should wear noiseless shoes. Uniforms should not be so stiff as to make a rustling noise with every movement.

11. The nurse should speak distinctly and softly, never in loud tones. Whispering is very objectionable, however, and is always annoying to the patient. The patient's questions should be answered discreetly, and never in a manner that conveys the impression that something he desires to know is being concealed.

12. A nurse's hands should always be warm, clean, and the nails well trimmed. Gentleness and firmness should characterize the touch.

13. Personal neatness and cleanliness should be strictly maintained.

14. All tasks should be accomplished quietly without confusion and noise. But this does not mean to move around on tiptoe, which would invariably be annoying to the patient.

B. NURSING DON'TS

Never sit and tap with the foot or fingers.

Do not make noise when preparing for the night, after the patient is ready for sleep.

Do not disturb the patient when he is settled for a nap by giving food, treatment, drinks, etc.

Do not continually ask patients how they feel and whether they would like something done for them.

Do not let direct rays of light shine in the patient's eyes.

Do not cause unnecessary noise with dishes and papers.

Do not hurry the patient with meals, but encourage him to masticate thoroughly.

Do not jar the bed.

When sitting in a rocking chair, do not rock incessantly. It could be very annoying to the patient.

C.   HOW TO KEEP A CHART

Temperature. At given times during the day the temperature should be taken, usually morning and evening. Use a self-registering thermometer, thoroughly disinfected each time it is used, and be sure that the mercury is below 96° before taking the temperature. If it is not, shake it down, being careful not to hit the thermometer against anything. When taking the temperature, the thermometer is usually held in the mouth beneath the tongue for 3 minutes with the lips tightly closed; or under the armpit for 5 minutes. If taken under the armpit, the arm should be held close to the body to prevent the air from reaching the thermometer. When taking the temperature by mouth, a cold drink should not be given for at least 20 minutes beforehand.

Care must be used when taking a child's temperature so that they do not bite the thermometer. With children it is usually better to take the rectal temperature, which is normally 98.5°, although it may be higher in the early evening. A special thermometer must be used that is made only for taking rectal temperatures.

The temperature rarely rises above 105°F. and if it does, the patient is usually in a perilous condition. In some diseases, such as in inflammatory rheumatism, the temperature may rise above 107° and recovery can still take place. In others diseases, such as inflammation of the bowels, a temperature above 105°F. would indicate great danger.

Pulse. The pulse is usually felt at the wrist over the radial artery, and coincides with the beating of the heart. When it cannot be felt distinctly at the wrist, place the hand over the heart. The average pulse rate in adults is about 72 beats per minute, and in children from 72 to 120 beats per minute. The pulse is usually faster in sickness, though sometimes it may be slower. At times it may reach 140; in that case something must be done at once to lower it. The character of the pulse is as important as its rate, which varies considerably. At times the pulse will be weak, irregular, rapid, slow, or intermittent.

Respiration. Normally the rate of respiration is one-fourth the pulse rate, or about 16 to 20 breaths per minute. It is important to observe not only its frequency, but whether the respiration is noisy, irregular, painful, difficult, or abnormal in any way.

Cough. When a cough is present, it should be noticed at what times it is worse, how frequent, its duration, and character. When there is expectoration, the color, whether profuse or scanty, frothy, bloody, thick, etc., should be noticed.

Discharges. Note bowel discharges and report the size, frequency, color, consistency, and general odor. Note the color, quantity, and odor of the urine, the nature of sediments, the frequency, etc. In saving a specimen for examination, save the first specimen in the morning.

In case of retention in the bladder, so that the bladder becomes distended and the urine flow is not free, a catheter must be used.

Miscellaneous observations. The following information about the patient should also be charted.

The way the patient speaks, whether nervous, restless, rational, irritable.

The strength of the voice.

The hours of sleep.

The locations and character of pain or pains, and whether diminished or aggravated by pressure, whether constant or intermittent, stationary or movable.

The condition of the tongue, whether clean, furred, coated, etc.

The eyes, whether there is swelling of the lids, undue sensitiveness to light, alteration in size of the pupils, color, etc.

The skin, as to warmth of the body, color, moisture, and general appearance.

The expression, whether pinched, anxious, wan, peaceful, or otherwise.

The general attitude and demeanor of the patient.

Record charts can be obtained at most drug stores.

D. GENERAL CARE OF PATIENTS

How to Make a Bed

The mattress should be firm and the sheets large enough to permit them to be well tucked under its edges so they will stay smooth (modern fitted sheets have helped this considerably). It is usually desirable to protect the bed by rubber sheeting placed under the lower sheet.

Place a sheet folded lengthwise across the bed over the lower sheet in the middle of the bed. This is called a draw sheet. Tuck the ends well under the mattress on each side. To change the lower sheet, loosen sheet at both ends and sides. Have patient roll to one side of bed, if possible. Fold soiled sheet up to the patient, follow up by the clean sheet folded and with the outside edge firmly tucked under side and ends of mattress. The patient can then roll back to the other side of the bed onto the clean sheet. Remove the soiled sheet and tuck the clean one in on the other side under the mattress. The draw sheet can be replaced at the same time.

Change the upper sheet by folding crosswise. Tuck the clean sheet in at the foot of the bed and draw into position, the soiled sheet then being drawn to the foot and removed. Strict attention should be paid to having the under sheet perfectly smooth, not only for the patient's comfort, but to prevent bed sores. Also make sure that there are never any crumbs in the bed.

Changing Clothing

In changing a patient's clothes, remove the sleeves first. Lay the clean garment face down on the patient, with the top toward his feet. The sleeves are then put on and as his head is slightly raised the soiled garment can be slipped over his head and the clean one put on at the same time. If the patient is at home and cannot be raised at all, the garment must be cut down the back. Then as one sleeve is taken off the clean one replaces it and the garment can be gradually tucked under the shoulders and body, and the other sleeve changed. Since some patients are very susceptible to changes in temperature as garments are being changed, it is necessary to have a light wrap at hand to throw around the patient's shoulders.

Bathing

Only a small portion of the body should be bathed at a time, and should be dried thoroughly without delay. Use a good soap.

Temperature and Ventilation

The temperature of the room should be kept at about 70°F. In some diseases it may be necessary to keep the room warmer, and in others cooler. The air should always be moist. Air humidifiers may be purchased or rented especially for this purpose. If there is a hot air furnace or stove, keep a dish of water on the radiator or stove. If the nurse sleeps in the patient's room, it should be large and well ventilated.

Disinfection

Lysol or any good disinfectant may be used. The aid of a disinfectant helps materially in keeping the air pure. It should be diluted in water and kept in vessels for receiving discharges.

Disinfection of Clothing

In infectious diseases, all washable clothing, sheets, etc., should be boiled in a covered boiler for at least one-half hour. They should be placed in a disinfectant solution immediately upon removal. Handkerchiefs should not be used. Pieces of soft cloth or disposable tissues should be used and burned.

All sweepings from the room should be burned.

Eating utensils must be boiled, using a good strong laundry soap.

General Instructions

1. When a choice is possible, a bright, sunny, airy room is best in which to nurse the sick. If possible, it should be a room remote from the rest of the house so that noise will not annoy the patient.

2. The room must be kept clean and neat. The sweeping should be done with a dampened broom or dust mop. Dust with a damp cloth to avoid raising dust.

3. In serious illnesses, keep the patient as quiet as possible. It is better to shield him from unpleasant happenings in the household.

4. Prepare and serve food daintily. Feed patient slowly. Give liquids by using a glass drinking tube or drinking straw.

5. Visitors' calls should be brief and not be permitted to weary the patient. It is better to have one caller at a time than to have two present at once.

6. Never jar the bed by knocking against it.

7. When fanning is desired, it should be gentle.

8. The nurse should never dress or undress in the same room with the patient.

9. A nurse should have an opportunity to spend an hour daily in the fresh air and sunshine, and should not for any length of time be on both day and night duty.

10. In fevers, use water freely; give the patient a sip every few minutes, but not too much at one time.

11. For nausea, sips of very hot water or small pieces of chipped ice swallowed whole sometimes give relief.

12. Prepare for a seriously injured patient by having a warm bed with plenty of hot water bottles. In a case of severe shock, keep the head low, stimulate freely, and rub the extremities briskly.

13. In cases of fainting, keep the head low, loosen the clothing about the neck and waist, give plenty of fresh air, bathe the face with cold water, and cautiously let the person inhale smelling salts or ammonia.

14. Heart failure must be treated as shock. Give small doses of red pepper. Either peppermint, skullcap, or lily of the valley tea is very good: take as much as needed. A cold towel rub, given by bathing one part of the body at a time and drying thoroughly, is excellent.

15. Soak sprains immediately in very cold water, apply an ice pack, or use alternate hot and cold water treatments. This will relieve to a great extent the pain and swelling; then apply liniment (see index) freely.

16. Bleeding from the nose can usually be checked by pinching the nose tightly for several minutes while the patient breathes through the mouth. Apply ice packs to the back of the neck and over the nose. Syringing the nostrils with cold salt water is also helpful.

17. Extra covering should always be available during the early morning hours when a patient's vitality is at its lowest.

18. When there is time, bedpans should be warmed before using.

How to Give an Enema in Bed

The bed should be well protected by rubber sheeting. Expel all air from the enema tube by letting some water run through before inserting. The enema tip should be well lubricated with Vaseline or a special lubricating jelly, such as

K-Y jelly. A bed-pan must be available for use when the patient is ready to expel the enema. Have patient lie on the back with knees drawn upward. Insert the tip and let the water run slowly. When there is pain shut off the water and let patient roll from one side to the other. Resume after a few moment's rest. One or two quarts can be injected if care is used, and can be retained from ten to fifteen minutes. After withdrawing the tip, fold a towel and press tightly over the anus for a few minutes to aid in retaining the enema.

Vaginal Douches

Place the patient on her back or sitting in a tub or on a bed-pan at about a 45° angle with the hips well elevated. In cases of infection, it is best to use two to four quarts of water at 105° to 110° two or three times a day for a week, then once a day for three weeks. A douche consisting of two table-spoons of vinegar in one quart of hot water is helpful in cases of ordinary vaginal discharge, but should not be used in thrush (Monilia). In cases of thrush, use one teaspoon of baking soda in one quart of hot water. (See index for herbal douches).

Do not give a douche if the patient is pregnant.

MASSAGE

Massage, when correctly given, is the systematic, well-planned, stroking and manipulation of the tissues; it is *not* simply a haphazard rubbing and pounding of the surface of the body.

This short chapter on massage should be considered only an introduction to this subject; it is not written with the intent of making anyone an expert in this field. Learning massage techniques takes years of special training. It must be emphasized at the outset that improperly given massage can affect patients adversely, making them feel worse instead of better. Therefore, proper care and "intelligent restraint" must be exercised when massage is used, being careful that it is being administered correctly and only in cases where a definite improvement or benefit can be expected.

The structures directly affected by massage are the skin with its underlying fat and connective tissue, muscles, blood vessels (both arteries and veins), lymph channels, nerves, bones, joints, and ligaments. Indirectly affected are the heart, lungs, and large organs within the abdomen.

Massage is one of the most valuable of remedial measures. When used in combination with water treatments, it accomplishes amazing results. It assists in building up the blood by increasing the hemoglobin and the total number of red blood cells, and it rebuilds the tissues in general. Abdominal massage increases the output of urine along with many of its waste products. Some other beneficial effects of massage are: a local and general increase in the flow of blood and lymph fluid through the system; relaxes tense tissues and thereby helps in the treatment of nervous exhaustion and insomnia; prevents stiffness of muscles, maintains their flexibility and nutrition, and helps to eliminate the waste products that have collected in them; breaks down fibrous bands and adhesions in muscles; has a salutary effect on the respiratory and nervous systems; the personal contact exerts a positive psychological effect; can be given in such a way as to promote general sedation and relaxation; restores health and tone to the entire body.

Common sense and consideration for the condition of the patient must be used when giving a massage. For those who are weak or delicate as well as in the very young and old, the length of the treatment should be decreased and the pressure should be light until the muscles become accustomed to the treatment, then more force may be used. The tension should not be so great as to produce pain or injury to the underlying tissues.

A. GENERAL PRINCIPLES AND PRECAUTIONS

There are certain important general principles to remember when giving a massage.

1. The person giving the treatment must have immaculate personal hygiene. He or she must be clean and the hands must be soft and warm, without callouses or sores. The fingernails must be clean and trimmed short.

2. A massage table about 28 inches high with a firm pad or mattress is best, so that the attendant does not have to stoop; however, the floor or the patient's bed may have to be used.

3. The patient should lie flat on the back with all muscles relaxed, a small pillow under the head and a rolled bath towel or small pillow under the knees.

4. After massaging the face, arms, legs, and chest, the patient should lie face down for the back treatment. There should be no pillow under the head, but a small pillow should be placed under the abdomen and a rolled bath towel under the ankles to keep the feet relaxed and comfortable.

5. For a general massage, all clothing should be removed. The patient should be kept warm and covered, except for the part being treated.

6. Some type of lubricant is usually used, such as olive oil, light mineral oil, or one of the products made especially for this purpose. This helps make the skin smooth, prevents the painful pulling of hair, and may help to prevent acne. After massaging a part, any excess lubricant should be removed with a soft towel, rubbing away from the heart.

7. Start and finish the treatment to each area with light stroking.

8. Perform all movements slowly and with a constant rhythm. During stroking, never move faster than about six inches per second, and many times moving even slower will feel better to the patient.

9. Keep your hands in contact with the patient as much as possible. For instance, when you are giving deep stroking from the wrist to the shoulder, return your hands to the wrist by light stroking down the arm.

10. The direction of the massage is important. Contrary to the popular belief during his time, Hippocrates, by careful observation of his patients, found that the effects of massage were much better if the stroking was done toward the heart. His observations have proven to be correct, and all massage should be done in the direction of the flow of blood in the veins; that is, towards the heart. The exception is light stroking, which does not effect the flow of blood or lymph and can be done away from the heart.

11. Massage is usually not given more than once a day.

12. The amount of pressure to use has long been a matter of controversy. In general, it is best not to use enough pressure to injure or bruise the patient. The more

gentle the massage, the more soothing and relaxing will be the results.

13. The number of times any given movement is repeated varies, but is usually between three and six.

Several precautions must be observed when massage is being considered.

1. Massage should not be given if there is a skin disease or rash, or over an open sore, bruise, varicose veins or inflamed joints or muscles.
2. It should not be used if the patient has a fever.
3. Massage of the abdomen should be given with care so as not to injure any of the internal organs.

B.   MASSAGE MOVEMENTS

Over the years many terms have been used to describe the movements used during massage. In some cases different meanings have been applied to the same term by different authors. This has resulted in much confusion.

Following is a simple outline including up-to-date terms for the most frequently used movements, with some of the older terms placed in parenthesis, and followed by a brief description of the various movements.

1. Stroking
    a. superficial or light stroking
    b. deep stroking (friction)
2. Compression
    a. kneading
        (1). superficial kneading or pinching (fulling)
        (2). deep kneading (petrissage)
    b. friction (effleurage)
3. Percussion (tapotement)
    a. clapping or cupping
    b. hacking or chopping
    c. beating

d. tapping
e. spatting
4. Shaking and vibration

Superficial stroking. This movement is performed using very light pressure, even lighter than the weight of the hand. The entire hand should be in contact with the patient, with the fingers together and the thumb in the best position to accommodate to the area being treated. One or both hands may be used. The direction is usually *away* from the heart and a regular rhythm must be maintained. The points at which the hands come in contact with and leave the patient's skin must be barely perceptible to the patient. The hands should be kept flexible so that they conform to the area being treated and produce an equal pressure to all points. The fingers alone may be used for the facial areas.

Deep stroking. The muscles need to be completely relaxed, so it is best to do superficial stroking first. Because one of the main purposes is to hasten the venous and lymphatic circulation, the direction is *toward* the heart. The rhythm, speed of movement, and hand position are the same as for superficial stroking. The amount of pressure need not be great, but thicker areas require more pressure. After the deep stroke is completed, it is sometimes more pleasing to the patient if the hand is returned to its starting position by using a superficial stroke; in this way constant skin contact is maintained.

Superficial kneading. This is done mainly to stimulate the skin. A portion of the skin is grasped between the thumb and first and second fingers, lifted, and then released at the point of greatest strain. In any kneading movement the skin should not slip, but be held securely in the palm or fingers.

Deep kneading. In contrast to stroking, the pressure during kneading is applied intermittently. A muscle is grasped with the entire hand, the palm, or the fingers, and compressed and elevated. Then it is released and the process repeated in an adjacent area. You must be careful not to pinch the tissues. The muscles need to be relaxed and a constant rhythm established. The amount of pressure needed for small muscles is less than for larger ones. The direction of each kneading movement should be toward the heart.

Friction. In some instances the terms friction and deep stroking have been given the same meaning; however, we will use the term friction to mean the movement of the superficial tissues over the deeper ones by keeping the hand or fingers in contact with the skin and making a circular movement over a small area. This helps to break up scars and adhesions and to absorb excess amounts of fluid in the tissues. Use either the palm of the hand or the thumb or fingers. Do not use the fingertips but rather the balls of the fingers. Make several circular motions, then slide the hand or fingers to the adjacent area and repeat, without lifting the hand from the skin surface.

Percussion. This group of movements consists of a series of brisk blows, administered in various ways and with varying degrees of force, using the two hands alternately. Percussion is used most often in healthy persons, although clapping is of benefit to those with respiratory problems when it is used properly. The wrist must be kept loose and flexible in order to give an elastic quality to the blow. Keeping the wrist stiff may produce injury to the patient by bruising the tissues. As a rule the hand should strike the body across the course of the muscles.

Clapping. In this form of percussion, the entire hand is used and the palm is cupped, so that a clapping or explosive sound is produced as the hand comes in contact with the skin.

Hacking. Hold the fingers loosely apart and strike the skin with the little finger surface of the hand only. As contact is made with the skin, the fingers are forced together producing a peculiar vibratory effect. Be sure the wrist is relaxed and flexible.

Beating. The body is struck with the front of the half-closed fist, this includes the heel of the hand and the dorsal (back) surface of the folded fingers. This type of percussion is reserved for the back and thighs.

Tapping. The tips of the fingers alone are used. Be sure the fingernails are short. Either one or all of the fingers of one or both hands can be used. Tapping is usually used on the head and chest.

Spatting. This is done by striking the skin with the fingers, which are held rigid and tightly together. It can be used on nearly any part of the body and is frequently used after water treatments to promote a reaction.

Shaking and vibration. The hands remain in contact with the tissues and a fine vibration or more coarse shaking motion is initiated by the person giving the massage. This technique requires considerable skill as well as the expenditure of much muscular effort and is not used very often.

C.   HOW TO GIVE A GENERAL MASSAGE

By the term "general massage" is meant a massage to the entire body. This should be accomplished in about 45 to 60 minutes. Following the massage, the patient should rest for an hour or so. This is a good sign that the treatment was a success.

During the massage the patient should be asked to turn and move as little as possible. Using the following order of massage will help accomplish this.

Start with the patient on his back and a pillow under the head and knees and then proceed in the following order.

1. Right leg, ankle to hip.
2. Right foot.
3. Left leg, ankle to hip.
4. Left foot.
5. Left arm from hand to shoulder.
6. Right arm from hand to shoulder.
7. Chest and neck.
8. Face. Optional, but good for insomnia and headache.

The patient turns onto the stomach for massage to the back, including the back of the neck and buttocks. The scalp can be included along with the neck and face if desired. The abdomen must be massaged with care, or it may be omitted.

The general principles for giving a massage listed earlier in this chapter should be reviewed and followed. Each movement is usually done on the average of two to four times. Remember to start with light stroking. This will relax the patient and you can apply the lubricant at this time. Then proceed with deep stroking and various types of kneading and end with light stroking. Deep stroking must always be toward the heart.

If desired, one may start by giving the scalp a brisk rub with the fingertips. Massage the face with a rotary motion, beginning with the chin and working upward to the ears. Lubricant is necessary on the face and the tissues should be treated gently. In general, rub across the wrinkles and stroke from the chin to the ears.

Arms. Beginning at the fingertips, stroke the arm upward to the shoulder. Start at the fingertips and rub each finger joint separately with a circular movement. Grasp the arm with your two hands, the thumbs away from each other, and manipulate as if dividing the muscles from the bone. Do this the whole length of the arm.

Next, wring or twist the muscles in the same way that one would wring a wet cloth. This drives the blood from the muscles and stimulates the nerve centers.

Next, knead the muscles by placing one hand on the underside and one on top, grasping firmly, and, using the balls of the thumbs, knead the muscles with a slow rotary motion from left to right.

Now start again at the fingertips and commence a series of squeezes, working on each muscle with a firm, quick grasp. This tends to accelerate the flow of blood to the heart. Strike with the little finger side of the hand, fingers extended and separated.

Now whip the arms with the fingertips, using a light short stroke. This is done by shaking the hands from the wrists.

Legs. Treat in the same manner as the arms, using extra

force on the deeper muscles. The deep leg muscles will stand thumping, hacking, and slapping which the arms cannot stand.

Chest. Lay your hands flat. Give rotary motion from left to right. Grasp the flesh near the lower ribs, working the muscles upward by a rolling motion.

Abdomen. Draw the patient's knees up to relax the abdominal muscles. Place your hands flat on the abdomen near the hips. Using wrist force, roll your hands firmly but gently toward the tips of the fingers, using a rotary motion. Great benefit may be derived from massage in cases of congested liver, constipation, etc.

Back. Commence with the back of the head and neck. Massage the base of the head and down the spinal column very thoroughly. The main movements employed are stroking, pounding, kneading, and percussion.

In giving a massage, there should be a free action from your wrist, the tips of the fingers and balls of the thumbs being used most, except in the pounding and slapping. The movements should always be firm. A halfway-given massage is worse than none at all.

Note: The foregoing is only a very limited description of a general massage as used by my father. If the reader is interested in a more comprehensive treatment of this subject, it would be well to buy a special book such as *Beard's Massage,* published by W. B. Saunders Company, 1981.

Special Colon Massage for Constipation. In performing this special type of massage of the abdomen, remember that the colon begins in the lower abdomen on the right side, passes upward to about the ribs, crosses the abdomen to the left and then passes downward along the left side to the pelvic area where it bends towards the lower mid abdomen.

The lowest part of the colon cannot be reached since it lies too far back in the pelvis, just in front of the sacrum.

The abdominal muscles must be relaxed. Do not use enough force to cause a reflex contraction of these muscles.

Start with lighter stroking and gradually increase the pressure to deep stroking. Move slowly. Lubricate the abdomen and have the patient breathe deeply. Bend the knees up to help relax the abdominal muscles.

Place the fingertips of the right hand over the right lower abdomen with the left hand on top for reinforcement. Press firmly, without hurting the patient, and follow the course of the colon. Repeat from five to ten times.

D. METHOD OF SWEDISH MASSAGE

Arms.
    Lubricate from wrist to shoulder.
    Rub, using friction from hand to shoulder.
    Fulling from shoulder to hand once.
    Apply spiral friction from hand to shoulder, twice to
        each side of the arm, beginning on the inside of the arm.
    Knead from hand to elbow three times, using friction.
    Repeat.
    Rotary kneading to elbow followed by light stroking
        back to the hand. Three times.
    Apply friction from hand to shoulder.
    Percussion from shoulder to hand.
    Hacking, spatting, down and up each side, once.
    Joint movements — bend and then pull the arm, then
        move around in a circle.
    Vibration and stroking.

Chest.
    Lubricate.
    Apply friction.
    Fulling down one side and up the other.
    Apply friction.
    Beginning on neck, palm kneading, twice.
    Apply friction.
    Percussion, tapping, hacking, spatting.
    Stroking.

Abdomen.
>   Lubricate.
>   Deep breathing.
>   Reflex stroking.
>   Deep vibration.
>   Side and circular shaking.
>   Percussion, tapping, hacking, spatting, clapping on colon.
>   Knead colon twice.
>   Use friction.
>   Fulling up and down each side, and up and down the
>   rectus muscles near the middle of the abdomen.
>   Rotary kneading twice to each side, alternating with
>   friction.
>   Stroking.

Leg.
>   Lubricate.
>   Apply friction up.
>   Fulling down.
>   Spiral friction up, twice to each side of the leg, beginning
>   inside.
>   Circular friction up.
>   Rotary kneading to foot, leg, and knee, three times,
>   alternating with friction; repeat.

Back.
>   Lubricate.
>   Apply friction.
>   Fulling down one side and up the other.
>   Apply friction.
>   Knead spine with thumb.
>   Give rotary kneading to both sides twice, alternating
>   with friction.
>   Use heavy friction down spine, twice.
>   Circular heavy kneading down each side of spine, twice.

Knead shoulders with palm. Knead down each side
of spine with palm.
Grasp the muscles up and down the spine.
Heavy wringing up, down, and crosswise.
Percussion, hacking, spatting, clapping.
Stroke entire back. Finish with at least ten light friction
strokes to back.

3

HIGH ENEMAS

There are several different kinds of enemas, such as ordinary enemas taken with only a relatively small amount of fluid in order to cleanse the rectum and lower colon; astringent enemas, taken to relieve inflammation in diarrhea, dysentery, etc.; and nourishing enemas, given in wasting diseases, unconsciousness, and other conditions where it becomes necessary to administer food by rectum. (NOTE: Enemas are no longer used to provide nourishment since more satisfactory and practical methods have been developed.) But high enemas, as recommended in this book, are taken to thoroughly cleanse the entire length of the colon. All the equipment you need to take a high enema is a container that will hold four quarts (one gallon) of fluid, a connecting hose of adequate length, a clamp of some kind to stop the flow of fluid when it becomes necessary, a good lubricant, an ordinary rectal tip, and a bed-pan or readily available toilet.

It is best to administer the enema while lying down. If a suitable treatment table is not available, you may find it most convenient to lie on the floor. Place four quarts of warm water or herbal tea in the container. It is usually not possible to take the entire four quarts at one time, at least not at first. When beginning the enema, inject only enough fluid until you feel full. Hold it as long as you can. Keep adding more fluid until it becomes necessary to expel the entire amount. Repeat this several times until the returns are clear. As soon as the colon is clean, you will be able to retain the full four quarts. You must try again and again until this is possible. When taking the high enema, assume different positions and roll from side to side (as described later in this chapter) so that the water is able to run in, as sometimes there is a kink in the colon, and many times just a change in position allows a great deal more water to flow in.

There are some cases in which there has been a diseased condition of the colon for a long time, or some other difficulty that might make it impossible to ever retain four quarts of water. In those cases, take as much as possible.

If you do not find it possible to retain four quarts of water, even after thoroughly cleansing the colon, don't worry. Getting the entire colon clean is the important thing. The large intestine (colon) varies considerably in size in different people and this has no direct relationship to the size of the individual. A large person may have a relatively short narrow colon that can only hold one or two quarts, while a small person may have a large, long colon capable of holding three or four quarts.

The material used for the enema, whether water, herb tea, etc., should be about body temperature. Otherwise the colon becomes irritated and contracts, causing cramps and making it difficult or impossible to retain the solution.

A flexible, soft, well-lubricated enema tip should be used and inserted several inches into the rectum. Allow the solution in the enema bag or can to fill the tubing before inserting the tip into the rectum.

A great help in filling the entire colon with fluid is to assume the proper positions so that the solution can flow by gravity through the colon by following its natural curves (see Figure 1). Don't forget, there are no two colons exactly alike in position or size, and therefore you may find that you will never be able to hold more than one or two quarts of fluid at a time.

If you follow the directions given here, you will have the best results in completely cleansing the entire colon in the easiest way possible. Staying on a clear liquid diet for 24 hours before taking the enema will not only make it easier to hold the water, but will be a great help in cleansing the colon.

1. Start the solution while lying flat on your back. Allow it to flow slowly and when you start to feel full, turn off the flow.

2. Immediately turn halfway onto your left side and when the pressure eases start the flow again and let as much run in as possible. Again, when you feel quite full turn off the flow and turn all the way onto your left side for several minutes.

3. Start the flow again and slowly turn onto your back and then to your right until you are all the way on your right side. Let as much solution as possible flow in while in this position.

4. When you feel very full, turn off the flow and turn further to your right so you are part way toward your stomach. Stay in this position several minutes, then turn on to your back once more.

5. Leave the enema tip in until just before you are ready to expel the enema.

6. If you have a natural tendency to be constipated, this routine may have to be repeated several times before the entire colon is cleansed.

You may be bothered by cramps while the colon is filling. If this should happen, stop the fluid immediately and take in a slow deep breath through your nose. Hold it for two or three seconds only and then let it out slowly through your mouth. Repeat this several times if necessary until the cramping is relieved. This will usually relax the colon so that the enema may be continued.

In a very small number of patients the colon will prove to be so spastic and irritable that it will contract forcefully and painfully and expel the fluid and perhaps even the enema tip as well. If this should continue to occur after several gentle attempts on different days to introduce the enema solution, or if any blood is noted in the material evacuated from the colon at any time, competent medical advice should be obtained.

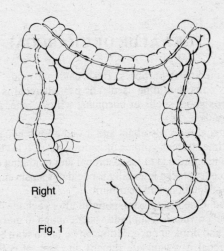

Right

Fig. 1

4

THE VALUE OF CHARCOAL

For medicinal purposes, fresh charcoal made from the finest woods should be used. The best charcoal is obtained from boxwood, shells of coconuts, willow, pine, and other soft woods.

Charcoal is an adsorbent and it will adsorb and condense many times its own volume of various gases. It is very useful as an antiseptic due to its adsorbent and oxidizing qualities. It is excellent taken internally for acid dyspepsia and also for gas, fermentation, and heartburn.

Dose. One heaping teaspoonful after each meal. Put the charcoal powder in a cup, add water enough to make a paste, dilute, and drink at once. More can be taken with benefit.

Charcoal is a valuable remedy in cases of colic due to decomposition of foods in the stomach and bowels, and can be used as either a preventive or curative. Give a tablespoonful in half-a-glass of hot water. As a preventive, take a teaspoonful after each meal in a little hot water.

For inflammation of the bowels or dysentery, give a tablespoonful in half-a-glass of hot water and repeat as often as necessary. Also give charcoal poultices over the bowels and stomach.

Charcoal mixed in a strong smartweed tea makes an excellent poultice for bruises and inflammation.

A charcoal poultice is good for relief of inflammation in the eyes. It is also a most excellent poultice for gangrene, old ulcers, and sores.

I have used charcoal and olive oil mixed to the consistency of paste, or so that it is easy to take. It is very good for some kinds of indigestion. Charcoal also mixes easily with soybean milk, and may be taken in this way for indigestion.

Old charcoal is made more effective if heated before using.

ADDENDUM: Charcoal is truly a universal antidote. Its

use dates back at least to the time of Hippocrates, who lived from 460 to 370 B.C. Activated charcoal is a black, shiny, odorless and tasteless substance made by burning certain types of wood under controlled conditions so that a very large adsorptive surface is produced. All impurities are removed so that it is 100 percent pure vegetable matter. When examined under the microscope, it is seen to be extremely porous, having the appearance of a sponge with rigid walls. Charcoal is adsorptive in its action, rather than being absorptive like a sponge; that is, it acts like a magnet, attracting substances to itself and holding them tightly on its surface, Just how this is accomplished no one knows for sure.

Charcoal can adsorb up to 250 to 350 times its own weight. One quart of charcoal can adsorb nearly 90 quarts of ammonia gas. The surface area of all the particles in a small piece of charcoal only 2/5 of an inch square would cover an area more than 33 yards square. It has a strong affinity for adsorbing impure and toxic gasses which makes it a wonderful remedy for use when fermentation occurs in the intestinal tract with the production of excessive gas, bad breath, heartburn, nausea, sour stomach, and headache. It also adsorbs many poisonous chemicals, drugs, and toxins, such as opium, cocaine, morphine, nicotine, salicylates, strychnine, kerosene, barbiturates, and antidepressant pills, to name but a few. It is of little or no value in lye and caustic alkalis, alcohol, mineral acids, iron, and cyanides; in fact, cyanide actually interferes with the normal adsorptive properties of charcoal.

A dramatic demonstration, conducted in 1813 by the French chemist Bertrand, vividly demonstrated the almost miraculous adsorptive properties of charcoal when he drank five grams of arsenic trioxide mixed with charcoal and survived. A few years later, about 1830, a pharmacist by the name of P. F. Touery, attempting to prove that charcoal was an excellent antidote, took a massive dose of strychnine (ten times the usual lethal dose) with 15 grams (half an ounce) of activated charcoal before the French Academy of Medicine in Paris and suffered no apparent ill effects. But for anyone to try such an experiment today would be considered very foolhardy and dangerous!

During World War I, charcoal was used as an adsorbent in gas masks to protect the soldiers from poisonous gas. Following the war, the use of charcoal in the United States was largely neglected. Two factors that may have contributed to this lack of interest were: (1) the use of burnt toast as a home remedy for poisoning in the place of charcoal gave disappointing results; and (2) the use of the so-called "universal antidote." This consisted of two parts charcoal, one part magnesium oxide, and one part tannic acid. Because of the added substances, it was usually not as effective as using charcoal by itself.

No home should be without charcoal and the knowledge of how to use it effectively. It is a marvelous antidote for many kinds of poisons and is excellent to use for infections. Charcoal is also an excellent air deodorizer when placed in a dish in the refrigerator or anywhere that unpleasant odors are present. It may be used either internally or externally. Charcoal has been found to be harmless when ingested or when used on the skin and may be applied in powdered form directly to skin ulcers or wounds, specially if they are infected.

It can be obtained as a powder, as capsules or as tablets, the powdered form being by far the most effective. Activated charcoal capsules are twice as strong as the tablets, although chewing the tablets before swallowing them increases their effectiveness. The tablets and capsules are used mainly for gas and indigestion. The average adult dose is either 1 tablespoonful of charcoal powder stirred in enough water to make a thick soup-like mixture, or 6 to 8 tablets or 4 capsules twice a day. The charcoal should be kept tightly sealed in a glass or metal container. It is best not to take charcoal when there is food in the stomach if it can possibly be avoided, as the food interferes with its action. In case of poisoning, take five times the weight of charcoal as the estimated weight of the ingested poison. If there is food in the stomach, 8 to 10 times the weight of the poison should be given in the form of finely powdered charcoal. One tablespoonful of charcoal equals about 10 grams. The sooner the charcoal can be taken after the poison is ingested, the more effective it will be. That is why it needs to be readily available in the home, on the camping trip, or wherever it may be needed on a moment's notice. To obtain the maximum effect, it must be ingested before the poison is absorbed from the intestinal tract. As John Holt, M.D., makes clear in the *Journal of Pediatrics:* "It is shown that this agent [charcoal], presently somewhat neglected, has a wide spectrum of activity and when properly used is probably the most valuable single agent we possess … as an emergency antidote for the treatment of ingested poisons… A bottle of charcoal on every medicine shelf would go a long way to combat serious poisonings in the home." A four-ounce jar of activated charcoal powder can be purchased at nearly any drug store for about $3.50. An even more convenient way to have a charcoal mixture ready right when you need it is to purchase a suspension of 30 grams of activated charcoal in four ounces of water already mixed and sealed in a plastic container.

All you have to do when it is needed is to shake the carton a few times, remove the lid and drink the contents. The cost for this premixed, convenient way to have charcoal immediately available is about $5.50. It should be kept in the home emergency medical kit in a conspicuous place.

For a long time there has been some difference of opinion as to whether or not charcoal will adsorb necessary nutrients as well as poisons. Dr. Holt states: "It is now very clear that activated charcoal will adsorb not only poisons but also vitamins, digestive enzymes, amino acids, and other valuable nutrients from the gut. Such losses if continued will seriously affect health, but are of no importance in situations of acute poisoning."

Poultices made of charcoal are excellent for insect bites, stings, poison oak, inflammation around the ears and eyes, to dress and disinfect wounds, cellulitis, boils, carbuncles, and abdominal pain. They also act as a deodorant and anti-septic.

How to make a charcoal poultice:

1. Place equal parts of pulverized charcoal and flaxseed in a pot. Grinding the flaxseed into a fine powder first will make the mixture form a paste faster. This can be done in a blender.
2. Add enough water to form a thick paste and bring it slowly to a boil while stirring.
3. Spread the paste as rapidly as possible on a piece of cotton or muslin of sufficient size to completely cover the area to be treated.
4. The paste should be spread about one-quarter-inch thick and kept about one inch in from the edges of the cloth.
5. Cover this with another cloth of the same size and then place the poultice on the area of the skin to be treated.
6. Cover this with a piece of plastic at least one inch larger on all sides than the poultice.
7. Place a towel over the entire poultice and hold it in place with a roller bandage, strips from an old sheet or towel, an Ace bandage, etc. Pin securely in place with safety pins.
8. Leave on overnight or for 8 to 10 hours during the day.
9. After removing the poultice, rub the skin with a cold cloth.

The amount of material needed for the poultice will depend on the size of the area to be covered. A large area will require about 3 tablespoonsful of charcoal and flaxseed. For small areas, such as a bee sting or spider bite, use only charcoal to make the paste.

Charcoal can be very messy, so be careful as you assemble the poultice.

PRAYER

Unanswered yet? Faith cannot be unanswered.
Her feet were firmly planted on the Rock;
Amid the wildest storms she stands undaunted,
Nor quails before the loudest thunder shock.
She knows Omnipotence has heard her prayer,
And cries, "It shall be done," sometime, somewhere.

Unanswered yet? Nay, do not say ungranted;
Perhaps your part is not yet wholly done.
The work began when your first prayer was uttered,
And God will finish what He has begun.
If you will keep the incense burning there,
His glory you shall see, sometime, somewhere.

                            Robert Browning

Appendix

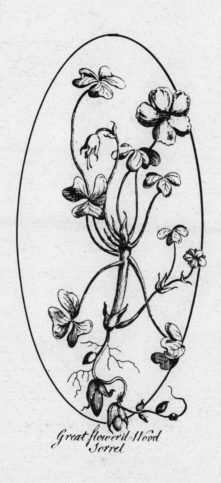

Great flower'd Wood Sorrel

GLOSSARY OF OLD-FASHIONED
MEDICAL TERMS

AGUE: An intermittent fever, sometimes with chills, as in malaria.

APOPLEXY: The result of a stroke (cerebrovascular accident).

BLACK SMALLPOX: The hemorrhagic form of small pox.

CATARRH: An inflammation of the mucous membranes with a free discharge. This has special reference to the air passages of the head and throat. For example, hayfever, rhinitis, influenza, bronchitis, pharyngitis, asthma.

CHOLERA INFANTUM: A common, noncontagious diarrhea seen in young children; occurs most commonly during the summer.

CHOLERA MORBUS: A once popular name for an acute gastroenteritis with diarrhea, cramps, and vomiting, occurring in the summer or autumn. Also called summer cholera or summer complaint.

FARINACEOUS: Of the nature of flour or meal. Starchy or containing starch.

FLUX: Excessive flow or discharge. For example, in dysentery or excessive menstruation.

GLEET: A urethral discharge, either of mucus or pus; commonly seen in the chronic form of gonorrheal urethritis.

HYDROPHOBIA: Rabies.

LEUKORRHEA: A whitish, viscid discharge from the vagina.

LUNG FEVER: A severe lung infection, as pneumonia.

MORTIFICATION: Gangrene.

QUICKSILVER: An old term for mercury.

QUINSY: Peritonsillar abscess or tonsillitis.

SCALD HEAD: Ringworm, or some similar affliction, of the scalp. May also refer to a disease of the hair follicles with formation of small yellow crusts and a very offensive odor; usually affects the scalp.

SCROFULA: Tuberculosis involving the lymph nodes of the neck, usually occurs in early life. Now very rarely seen.

SLEEPING DISEASE: Sleeping sickness; commonly found in Africa. Also viral encephalitis in which lethargy is a prominent feature.

STRANGURY: A slow and painful passage of the urine due to spasm of the urethra and urinary bladder.

SUMMER COMPLAINT: See **CHOLERA MORBUS.**

TETTERS: A once popular name for various eczematous skin diseases. May also refer to a skin disease of animals communicable to man with intense itching.

WHITES: See **LEUKORRHEA.**

ZYMOTIC: Caused by or pertaining to any infectious or contagious disease.

GLOSSARY OF
MEDICAL PROPERTIES OF HERBS

ABORTIFACIENT: Induces the premature expulsion (abortion) of the fetus. Same meaning as **ECBOLIC.** For example: pennyroyal.

ALTERATIVE: Herbs that gradually convert an unhealthy condition of an organ to a healthy one. Gradually facilitates a beneficial change in the body. For example: ginseng.

ANALGESIC: Any substance that relieves pain.

ANAPHRODISIAC: Herbs that decrease or allay sexual feelings or desires.

ANODYNE: Relieves pain and reduces the sensitivity of the nerves.

ANTACID: Neutralizes the acid produced by the stomach.

ANTHELMINTIC: An agent that destroys and expels worms from the intestines. Same as **VERMIFUGE.**

ANTIBILIOUS: An herb that combats biliousness. The term biliousness refers to a group of symptoms consisting of nausea, abdominal discomfort, headache, constipation, and gas that is caused by an excessive secretion of bile.

ANTIBIOTIC: Inhibits the growth of germs, bacteria, and harmful microbes.

ANTIEMETIC: Prevents or alleviates nausea and vomiting.

ANTIEPILEPTIC: An agent that combats the convulsions or seizures of epilepsy.

ANTILITHIC: Aids in preventing the formation of stones in the kidneys and bladder.

ANTIPERIODIC: Prevents the periodic recurrence of attacks of a disease; as in malaria.

ANTIPHLOGISTIC: An agent that counteracts inflammation.

ANTIPYRETIC: Reduces fever. Same as **FEBRIFUGE** or **REFRIGERANT.**

ANTIRHEUMATIC: An agent that relieves or cures rheumatism.

ANTISCORBUTIC: Effective in the prevention or treatment of scurvy.

ANTISEPTIC: Prevents decay or putrefaction. A substance that inhibits the growth and development of microorganisms without necessarily destroying them.

ANTISPASMODIC: An agent that relieves or prevents involuntary muscle spasm or cramps. For example: camomile.

ANTISYPHILITIC: Herbs that improve or cure syphilis. Also called antiluetic.

ANTITUSSIVE: Prevents or improves a cough.

ANTIVENOMOUS: Acts against poisonous matter from animals.

ANTIZYMOTIC: Herbs that can destroy disease-producing organisms.

APERIENT: A mild or gentle laxative. Also called **APERITIVE.**

APHRODISIAC: Restores or increases sexual power and desire.

AROMATIC: An herb with a pleasant, fragrant scent and a pungent taste.

ASTRINGENT: Causes a local contraction of the skin, blood vessels, and other tissues, thereby arresting the discharge of blood, mucus, etc. Usually used locally as a topical application. The word topical pertains to a certain area of the skin or to a substance that affects only the area to which it is applied.

BALSAM: The resin of a tree that is healing and soothing. For example: myrrh.

BALSAMIC: A healing or soothing agent.

BITTER: A solution of bitter, often aromatic, plant products used as a mild tonic.

CARMINATIVE: An herb that helps to prevent gas from forming in the intestines, and also assists in expelling it.

CATHARTIC: Causes evacuation of the bowels. A cathartic may be either mild (laxative) or vigorous (purgative).

CEPHALIC: Referring to diseases affecting the head and upper part of the body.

CHOLAGOGUE: An herb that stimulates the flow of bile from the liver into the intestines.

CONDIMENT: Enhances the flavor of food.

CORDIAL: A stimulating medicine or drink.

DEMULCENT: Soothes, protects, and relieves the irritation of inflamed mucous membranes and other surfaces.

DEOBSTRUENT: Removes obstructions by opening the natural passages or pores of the body.

DEPURATIVE: Tends to purify and cleanse the blood.

DETERGENT: An agent that cleanses boils, ulcers, wounds, etc.

DIAPHORETIC: Promotes perspiration, especially profuse perspiration. Same as **SUDORIFIC.**

DISCUTIENT: An agent that dissolves or causes something, such as a tumor, to disappear. Also called **DISCUSSIVE.**

DIURETIC: Promotes the production and secretion of urine. For example: parsley.

DRASTIC: A violent purgative.

ECBOLIC: See **ABORTIFACIENT.**

EMETIC: Causes vomiting. For example: ipecac, lobelia.

EMMENAGOGUE: An herb that brings on menstruation. For example: camomile.

EMOLLIENT: A substance that is usually used externally to soften and soothe the skin.

ESCULENT: Edible or fit for eating.

EXANTHEMATOUS: Refers to any eruptive disease or fever. An herbal remedy for skin eruptions such as measles, scarlet fever etc.

EXPECTORANT: Promotes the thinning and ejection of mucus or exudate from the lungs, bronchi, and trachea; sometimes the meaning is extended to all remedies that quiet a cough.

FARINACEOUS: Having a mealy texture or surface.

FEBRIFUGE: Reduces body temperature and fever. Same as **ANTIPYRETIC** and **REFRIGERANT.**

HEPATIC: An herb that promotes the well-being of the liver and increases the secretion of bile. For example: golden seal.

HERPATIC: A remedy for skin eruptions, ringworm, etc.

HYPNOTIC: Tends to produce sleep.

LAXATIVE: An herb that acts to promote evacuation of the bowels; a gentle cathartic.

LITHOTRIPTIC: Causing the dissolution or destruction of stones in the bladder or kidneys.

MATURATING: An agent that promotes the maturing or bringing to a head of boils, carbuncles etc.

MUCILAGINOUS: Herbs that have a soothing effect on inflamed mucous membranes.

NARCOTIC: An addicting substance that reduces pain and produces sleep.

NAUSEANT: An herb that causes nausea and vomiting. Somewhat similar to an emetic.

NERVINE: A substance that calms and soothes the nerves and reduces tension and anxiety.

OPTHALMICUM: A remedy for diseases of the eye.

PARTURIENT: A substance that induces and promotes labor.

PECTORAL: Relieves disorders of the chest and lungs, such as an expectorant.

POULTICE: Plant material that is prepared in a special way and applied to the surface of the body as a remedy for certain disorders.

PUNGENT: Irritating or sharply painful. Producing a sharp sensation of taste or smell.

PURGATIVE: A substance that promotes the vigorous evacuation of the bowels. Usually used to relieve severe constipation.

REFRIGERANT: Relieves fever and thirst. A cooling remedy. Lowers body temperature.

RELAXANT: Tends to relax and relieve tension, especially muscular tension.

RESOLVENT: Promotes the resolving and removing of abnormal growths, such as a tumor.

RUBEFACIENT: An agent that reddens the skin by increasing the circulation when rubbed on the surface.

SEDATIVE: Allays excitement, induces relaxation, and is conducive to sleep.

SIALAGOGUE: Promotes the flow of saliva.

SOPORIFIC: Herbs that help to produce sleep.

STIMULANT: An herb that increases the activity or efficiency of a system or organ; acts more rapidly than a tonic.

STOMACHIC: Herbs that give strength and tone to the stomach, stimulate digestion, and improve the appetite.

STYPTIC: Astringent: arrests hemorrhage and bleeding.

SUDORIFIC: Herbs that cause heavy perspiration.

TINCTURE: A solution of the active principal of an herb in alcohol.

TONIC: Herbs that restore and strengthen the entire system. Produces and restores normal tone. A general tonic would be one that braces up the whole system, such as a cold bath.

VERMIFUGE: An agent that expels intestinal worms or parasites. Same as **ANTHELMINTIC.**

VESICANT: An agent that causes blistering, such as poison ivy.

VULNERARY: An herb used in treating fresh cuts and wounds, usually used as a poultice. A healing substance.

GENERAL TABLES

CHILDREN'S DOSE EQUIVALENT TO ADULT DOSE OF 1 TSP. (60 DROPS)

Child's age	Dose
18 or over	1 tsp.
15 to 18 years	3/4 tsp. or 45 drops
9 to 12	1/2 tsp. or 30 drops
4 to 6 years	1/4 tsp. or 15 drops
2 to 3 years	10 drops
1 to 1 1/2 years	7 drops
6 to 9 months	4 drops
0 to 3 months	2 drops

TABLE OF EQUIVALENT FLUID MEASURES

Gallon	Quart	Pint	Glass or cup	Ounce	Table-spoonful	Teaspoonful (dram)	cc (ml)
1	4	8	16	128	256	1024	4000
	1	2	4	32	64	256	1000
	1/2	1	2	16	32	128	500
	1/4	1/2	1	8	16	64	240
				1	2	8	30
				1/2	1	4	15
						1	4

WEIGHTS

Number of grams*		Approximate equivalent
1000 (1 kg.)	. . . .	2.2 lb.
454	. . . .	1.0 lb.
100	. . . .	3.5 oz.
28	. . . .	1.0 oz.
16	. . . .	1.0 tsp.
4	. . . .	1.0 tbs.

*One paper clip weighs about 1 gram.

USEFUL HOUSEHOLD MEASURES (APPROX.)

Measure	Fluid Ounces	Tablespoonful	Fluid Drams	cc (ml)
1 Glassful (cup)	8	16	60	240
1 Teacupful	4	8	30	120
1 Wineglassful	2	4	15	60
1 Tablespoonful (tbs.)	1/2	1	4	15
1 Dessertspoonful	-	-	2	8
1 Teaspoonful (tsp.)	-	-	1	4 (60 drops)

INDEX

INDEX OF COMMON HERB NAMES

<u>NOTE TO READER</u>

Please do not write to us regarding your medical problems for it is unlawful for us to advise you regarding them.